NONSTEROIDAL ANTI-INFLAMMATORY DRUGS

Nonsteroidal Anti-Inflammatory Drugs

Mechanisms and Clinical Uses

Second Edition

Edited by

Alan J. Lewis
Wyeth-Ayerst Research
Princeton, New Jersey

Daniel E. Furst
Virginia Mason Research Center
and University of Washington
Seattle, Washington

Marcel Dekker, Inc. New York • Basel • Hong Kong

Library of Congress Cataloging-in-Publication Data

Nonsteroidal anti-inflammatory drugs: mechanisms and clinical uses / edited by
Alan J. Lewis, Daniel E. Furst. -- 2nd ed.
p. cm.
Includes bibliographical references and index.
ISBN 0-8247-8856-7 (alk. paper)
1. Nonsteroidal anti-inflammatory agents. I. Lewis, Alan. II. Furst, Daniel E.
[DNLM: 1. Anti-inflammatory Agents, Non-steroidal--pharmacology. 2. Anti-Inflammatory Agents, Non-Steroidal--therapeutic use. QV 247 N8143 1994]
RM405.N654 1994
616'.0473--dc20
DNLM/DLC
for Library of Congress 93-34984
CIP

The publisher offers discounts on this book when ordered in bulk quantities. For more information, write to Special Sales/Professional Marketing at the address below.

This book is printed on acid-free paper.

MARCEL DEKKER, INC.
270 Madison Avenue, New York, New York 10016

Current printing (last digit):
10 9 8 7 6 5 4 3 2 1

Printed in the United States of America

Preface

Nonsteroidal anti-inflammatory drugs (NSAIDs) are among the most frequently prescribed drugs that benefit patients with rheumatoid arthritis, osteoarthritis, and related conditions. This volume is an update of our previous book, published in 1987, which reviewed the utility of NSAIDs for the treatment of the arthridites and their potential benefits in unrelated conditions such as dysmenorrhea, ocular inflammatory disease, shock, periodontal disease, and cancer chemotherapy. In this new volume we have chosen to describe important additional clinical applications of NSAIDs, such as migraine, adult respiratory distress syndrome, and stroke, and review the topical and over-the-counter use of these important agents. Although NSAIDs are generally safe and well tolerated, they are associated with a wide spectrum of clinical toxicities. We extensively review the safety and toxicity issues that have been associated with the use of NSAIDs.

Finally, we include a sample of the newer NSAIDs and their current and potential utility. A number of these agents represent potential new classes of anti-inflammatory therapy, and their future role in the treatment of inflammatory diseases remains to be determined.

We hope this book will complement our previous review of this field of research and will provide the reader with a useful reference source for the clinical application of this drug class. We are extremely grateful to all the authors who have contributed to the book and without whom this book would not have been possible. A special thanks also goes to Joe Berkenkopf, who assiduously facilitated the collation of the book.

Alan J. Lewis
Daniel E. Furst

Contents

Preface *iii*
Contributors *ix*

Introduction 1
Alan J. Lewis and Daniel E. Furst

I. Clinical Applications of Nonsteroidal Anti-Inflammatory Drugs

1. Effects of Nonsteroidal Anti-Inflammatory Drugs and Corticosteroids on Cartilage Metabolism in Rheumatoid Arthritis and Osteoarthritis 5
Jean-Pierre Pelletier, Johanne Martel-Pelletier, and Charles J. Malemud

2. Nonsteroidal Anti-Inflammatory Drugs in Migraine 27
Seymour Diamond

3. Nonsteroidal Anti-Inflammatory Agents and the Adult Respiratory Distress Syndrome 43
Hanson B. Cowan and Jean E. Rinaldo

4. Nonsteroidal Anti-Inflammatory Drugs in Stroke 55
Sien T. Chen, Teng-Nan Lin, T. K. Lee, and Chung Y. Hsu

5. Topical Nonsteroidal Anti-Inflammatory Drugs in Skin Diseases and Musculoskeletal Disorders 71
Sydney H. Dromgoole

6. The Over-the-Counter Use of Nonsteroidal Anti-Inflammatory Drugs and Other Antipyretic Analgesics 97
Kay Brune and Keith McCormack

7. Nonsteroidal Anti-Inflammatory Drugs and Their Enantiomers 127
Kenneth M. Williams, Iris Hall, Richard Day, and Franziska Löhrer

II. Toxicity of Nonsteroidal Anti-Inflammatory Drugs

8. Lower Bowel Toxicity of Nonsteroidal Anti-Inflammatory Drugs 145
Ingvar Bjarnason, Andrew Macpherson, Sivagurunathan Somasundaram, and Jeremy Hayllar

9. Prevention and Treatment of Gastric and Duodenal Ulcers Induced by Nonsteroidal Anti-Inflammatory Drugs 159
Esam Z. Dajani and Naurang M. Agrawal

10. Hepatic Injury Associated with Nonsteroidal Anti-Inflammatory Drugs 171
Hyman J. Zimmerman

11. Renal Toxicity of Nonsteroidal Anti-Inflammatory Drugs 195
Andrew Whelton and Cindy W. Hamilton

12. Nonsteroidal Anti-Inflammatory Drugs: Uses in Dermatology and Cutaneous Toxicity 207
Michael Bigby

13. Rare Side Effects of Nonsteroidal Anti-Inflammatory Drugs 217
W. Watson Buchanan and Walter F. Kean

III. New Anti-Inflammatory Drugs and Analgesics

14. Ketorolac 247
John M. Young and James P. Yee

15. Bromfenac 267
Joseph S. Wajdula, Mohamed Osman, Ivan Vavra, Diane Sullivan, and James Ermer

16. Pemedolac 285
Thuy T. Chau, Marie Sanda, and Barry M. Weichman

17. Pravadoline: A Dual-Mechanism Aminoalkylindole Analgesic 297
Susan J. Ward

18. Romazarit 317
David Bradshaw and Peter E. O. Williams

19. Tilomisole 333
Richard P. Carlson, Steven C. Gilman, Francis J. Gregory, W. Craig Daniel, and Richard L. Fenichel

20. Leflunomide: A Novel Immunomodulating Drug 349
Robert R. Bartlett, Thomas Zielinski, H.-Ulrich Schorlemmer, Giles Campion, Predrag Musikic, and Rudolph Schleyerbach

21. Zileuton (A-64077): A 5-Lipoxygenase Inhibitor 367
Judith Cohn

22. Pharmacological Properties of IX 207-887 391
Andrew R. Mackenzie

23. Pharmacological Properties of E5090: An Orally Active Inhibitor of Interleukin-1 Generation 411
Hiroshi Shirota, Ken-ichi Chiba, Masaki Goto, Isao Yamatsu, and Kouichi Katayama

IV. Future Developments

24. Future Therapy for Arthritis 427
Ivan G. Otterness and E. Roy Pettipher

Index *453*

Contributors

Naurang M. Agrawal, M.D. Department of Gastroenterology, Ochsner Clinic, New Orleans, Louisiana

Robert R. Bartlett, Ph.D. Biomedical Research, Hoechst AG Werk Kalle-Albert, Wiesbaden, Germany

Michael Bigby, M.D. Department of Dermatology, Harvard Medical School, Boston, Massachusetts

Ingvar Bjarnason, M.D., M.Sc., M.R.C.Path. Department of Clinical Biochemistry, King's College Hospital, London, England

David Bradshaw, B.Sc., Ph.D. Department of Biology, Roche Products Ltd., Welwyn Garden City, Hertsfordshire, England

Kay Brune, M.D. Department of Experimental and Clinical Pharmacology and Toxicology, The University of Erlangen, Erlangen, Germany

W. Watson Buchanan, M.D. Department of Medicine, McMaster University Faculty of Health Sciences, Hamilton, Ontario, Canada

Giles Campion Biomedical Research, Hoechst AG Werk Kalle-Albert, Wiesbaden, Germany

Richard P. Carlson, Ph.D. Department of Experimental Therapeutics, Wyeth-Ayerst Research, Princeton, New Jersey

Thuy T. Chau, Ph.D. Inflammation Division, Wyeth-Ayerst Research, Princeton, New Jersey

Sien T. Chen, M.D. Department of Neurology, Chang Gung Memorial Hospital, Taipei, Taiwan

Ken-ichi Chiba Eisai Tsukuba Research Laboratories, Eisai Co., Ltd., Tsukuba-shi, Japan

Judith Cohn, M.D., Ph.D. Immunoscience Venture, Pharmaceutical Products Division, Abbott Laboratories, Abbott Park, Illinois

Hanson B. Cowan, M.D. Division of Pulmonary and Critical Care Medicine, Department of Medicine, Vanderbilt University, and Nashville Veterans Administration Medical Center, Nashville, Tennessee

Esam Z. Dajani, Ph.D., F.A.C.G.* G. D. Searle & Co. and Northwestern University School of Medicine, Chicago, Illinois, and University of California at Los Angeles, Los Angeles, California

W. Craig Daniel, Ph.D. Project Management, Inflammation/Immunology, Wyeth-Ayerst Research, Radnor, Pennsylvania

Richard Day, M.B.B.S., M.D., F.R.A.C.P. Department of Clinical Pharmacology and Toxicology, University of New South Wales, and St. Vincents Hospital, Sydney, Australia

Seymour Diamond, M.D. Diamond Headache Clinic, Chicago, and Adjunct Professor, Departments of Pharmacology and Molecular Biology, Chicago Medical School, North Chicago, Illinois

Sydney H. Dromgoole, Ph.D.† Business Development, Allergan Herbert, Irvine, California

James Ermer, M.S. Department of Clinical Pharmacokinetics, Wyeth-Ayerst Research, Philadelphia, Pennsylvania

Richard L. Fenichel, Ph.D. Department of Cardiovascular and Metabolic Disorders, Wyeth-Ayerst Research, Princeton, New Jersey

Daniel E. Furst, M.D. Clinical Research Program, Virginia Mason Research Center, and University of Washington, Seattle, Washington

Steven C. Gilman, Ph.D. Pharmaceutical Research Division, Sterling Winthrop, Inc., Collegeville, Pennsylvania

---

*Present affiliation: International Drug Development Consultants, A Division of Mid Gulf U.S.A., Inc., Long Grove, Illinois.

†Present affiliation: Clinical Operations, Oclassen Pharmaceuticals, San Rafael, California.

Masaki Goto, M.D. Eisai Tsukuba Research Laboratories, Eisai Co., Ltd., Tsukuba-shi, Japan

Francis J. Gregory, Ph.D.* Wyeth-Ayerst Research, Princeton, New Jersey

Iris Hall, Ph.D., B.Sc.(Hons.) Department of Clinical Pharmacology and Toxicology, University of New South Wales, and St. Vincents Hospital, Sydney, Australia

Cindy W. Hamilton, Pharm.D.† Department of Medicine, Johns Hopkins University School of Medicine, Baltimore, Maryland

Jeremy Hayllar, M.R.C.P. Department of Medicine, Mt. Isa Base Hospital, Queensland, Australia

Chung Y. Hsu, M.D., Ph.D. Division of Restorative Neurology and Human Neurobiology, Baylor College of Medicine, Houston, Texas

Kouichi Katayama, Ph.D. Eisai Tsukuba Research Laboratories, Eisai Co., Ltd., Tsukuba-shi, Japan

Walter F. Kean, M.B., Ch.B., M.D.[Glas.], F.R.C.P.[C], F.A.C.P., F.A.C.R. McMaster University Faculty of Health Sciences, Hamilton, Ontario, Canada

T. K. Lee, Ph.D. Department of Medicine, National Taiwan University, Taipei, Taiwan

Alan J. Lewis, Ph.D. Wyeth-Ayerst Research, Princeton, New Jersey

Teng-Nan Lin, Ph.D. Academia Sinica, Institute of Biomedical Sciences, Taipei, Taiwan

Franziska Löhrer, Ph.D. School of Pharmacy, University of Basel, Basel, Switzerland

Andrew R. Mackenzie, B. Tech., Ph.D., D.I.C. Inflammation Biology Division, Bone and Joint Department, Sandoz Research Institute Berne Ltd., Berne, Switzerland

Andrew Macpherson, Ph.D., M.R.C.P. Department of Medicine, King's College Hospital, London, England

Charles J. Malemud, Ph.D. Division of Rheumatic Diseases, Department of Medicine, Case Western Reserve University School of Medicine, Cleveland, Ohio.

Johanne Martel-Pelletier, Ph.D. Rheumatic Disease Unit, Department of Medicine, University of Montreal, and Notre-Dame Hospital, Montreal, Quebec, Canada

---

*Retired.

†Present affiliation: Consultant, Hamilton House®, Virginia Beach, Virginia.

Keith McCormack, M.D. Drug Research Group, McCormack Ltd., Church House, Leighton Buzzard, Bedfordshire, England

Predrag Musikic, M.D. Biomedical Research, Hoechst AG Werk Kalle-Albert, Wiesbaden, Germany

Mohamed Osman, Ph.D. Department of Drug Metabolism, Wyeth-Ayerst Research, Princeton, New Jersey

Ivan G. Otterness, Ph.D. Central Research Division, Department of Immunology and Infectious Diseases, Pfizer Inc., Groton, Connecticut

Jean-Pierre Pelletier, M.D., F.R.C.P.(C.) Arthritis Division, Rheumatic Disease Unit, Department of Medicine, University of Montreal, and Notre-Dame Hospital, Montreal, Quebec, Canada

E. Roy Pettipher, Ph.D. Senior Research Scientist, Department of Immunology and Infectious Diseases, Pfizer Inc., Groton, Connecticut

Jean E. Rinaldo, M.D. Division of Pulmonary and Critical Care Medicine, Department of Medicine, Vanderbilt University, and Nashville Veterans Administration Medical Center, Nashville, Tennessee

Marie Sanda, M.D. Department of Clinical Research and Development, Wyeth-Ayerst Research, Radnor, Pennsylvania

Rudolph Schleyerbach, Ph.D. Biomedical Research, Hoechst AG Werk Kalle-Albert, Wiesbaden, Germany

H.-Ulrich Schorlemmer, Ph.D. Behring Research Laboratories, Marburg, Germany

Hiroshi Shirota, Ph.D. Eisai Tsukuba Research Laboratories, Eisai Co., Ltd., Tsukuba-shi, Japan

Sivagurunathan Somasundaram, Ph.D. Department of Clinical Biochemistry, King's College Hospital, London, England

Diane Sullivan, R.N. Department of Clinical Research and Development, Wyeth-Ayerst Research, Philadelphia, Pennsylvania

Ivan Vavra, M.D., Ph.D. Division of Clinical Research, Department of Clinical Research and Development, Wyeth-Ayerst Research, Philadelphia, Pennsylvania

Joseph S. Wajdula, R.Ph., Ph.D. Department of Clinical Research and Development, Wyeth-Ayerst Research, Philadelphia, Pennsylvania

Susan J. Ward, Ph.D. Departments of Neuroscience and Inflammation, Sterling Winthrop Pharmaceutical Research Division, Rensselaer, New York

Barry M. Weichman, Ph.D. Inflammation Division, Wyeth-Ayerst Research, Princeton, New Jersey

Andrew Whelton, M.D., F.A.C.P., F.C.P. Department of Medicine, Johns Hopkins University School of Medicine, Baltimore, Maryland

Kenneth M. Williams, Ph.D., B.Sc.(Hons.) Department of Clinical Pharmacology and Toxicology, University of New South Wales, and St. Vincents Hospital, Sydney, Australia

Peter E. O. Williams, M.A., Ph.D. Department of Pharmacokinetics and Metabolism, Roche Products Ltd., Welwyn Garden City, Hertsfordshire, England

Isao Yamatsu, M.D. Research and Development Division, Eisai Co., Ltd., Tokyo, Japan

James P. Yee, M.D., Ph.D. Center for Clinical Research Physicians, Syntex Development Research, Palo Alto, California

John M. Young, Ph.D. Institute of Immunology and Biological Sciences, Syntex Discovery Research, Palo Alto, California

Thomas Zielinski Department of Immunology, J. Gutenberg University, Mainz, Germany

Hyman J. Zimmerman, M.D.* Department of Medicine, George Washington University School of Medicine, Washington, D.C.

---

*Professor of Medicine Emeritus and Distinguished Scientist Emeritus.

Introduction

ALAN J. LEWIS
Wyeth–Ayerst Research
Princeton, New Jersey

DANIEL E. FURST
Virginia Mason Research Center
and University of Washington
Seattle, Washington

Nonsteroidal anti-inflammatory drugs (NSAIDs) have become one of the most widely used groups of drugs in the history of medicine. Worldwide, it has been estimated that over 30 million people take NSAIDs daily (1) for relief of symptoms of rheumatoid arthritis, osteoarthritis, and other arthritides; (2) for acute musculoskeletal conditions or miscellaneous injuries; and (3) for dysmenorrhea or postoperative pain. The total worldwide sales for the drugs, estimated to be 17 million dollars in 1960, is expected to reach 1.5 billion dollars per annum by 1995.

The NSAIDs can be classified on the basis of their chemical structure (1). The more traditional NSAIDs, such as aspirin, phenylbutazone, and indomethacin, have excellent anti-inflammatory efficacy, but produce gastric and other side effects. The newer agents may be somewhat better tolerated and may be administered on a once- or twice-daily schedule, which improves patient compliance. Aspirin and ibuprofen are both available without prescription; with extensive safety experience and the loss of patent coverage, other NSAIDs are being considered for over-the-counter use.

All of the commonly used NSAIDs exert their analgesic and anti-inflammatory effects, at least in part, by inhibition of cyclooxygenase, the enzyme that transforms arachidonic acid to prostaglandins, prostacyclin, and thromboxanes. Some recent evidence suggests there are two forms of cyclooxygenase (COX): a constitutive enzyme (COX-1) and a structurally different enzyme (COX-2), which is induced by inflammatory stimuli (2). This important discovery raises the possibility of developing agents that actively suppress COX-2, possibly avoiding the side effects associated with COX-1 inhibition. The NSAIDs also modulate several other cellular processes, including decreases in neutrophil and monocyte migration and phagocytosis, suppression of bradykinin production, and alteration of lymphocyte responses and cartilage metabolism.

Very few "classic" NSAIDs remain in clinical development, a result of saturation of the NSAID marketplace, new scientific information concerning immunoinflammatory processes, and a greater desire to develop drugs that will prevent disease progression.

Over the last few years, several newer agents that have been identified entered clinical trials. These agents affect lipid mediators, such as the leukotrienes and cytokines [e.g., interleukin-1 (IL-1)], which appear to play an important role in inflammatory disease processes. It is too early to know whether these approaches will provide new generations of NSAIDs and whether they will be replacements for currently used NSAIDs or, as is more likely, will be adjunctive to the current therapies.

The purpose of Part I of this book is to focus attention on some of the clinical uses of the NSAIDs in the treatment of the arthritides and to draw attention to the growing potential use of secondary applications of these agents in migraine, adult respiratory distress syndrome, and stroke. The topical uses of NSAIDs and over-the-counter use of these important drugs is also reviewed. Many of the current NSAIDs are racemic mixtures, and the recent regulatory attention placed on development of enantiomers is discussed. Although the currently used NSAIDs are reasonably safe, well tolerated, and effective, their use can be associated with a wide spectrum of clinical toxicities that are probably dose-related. Both common and rare toxicities are discussed in the book.

Finally, future developments in antiarthritic therapy are reviewed. The advent of molecular biology and biotechnology techniques is allowing a better understanding of the etiology and pathogenesis of the arthritides, the genetic basis for rheumatic diseases, the factors regulating cartilage and bone regeneration, and the interaction of inflammatory mediators. As our knowledge base expands, the hope of discovering disease-modifying drugs grows brighter and will usher in important new therapies by the end of the century.

REFERENCES

1. Lombardino JG. Medicinal chemistry of acidic nonsteroidal antiinflammatory drugs. In: Lombardino JG, ed. Nonsteroidal Antiinflammatory Drugs. New York: John Wiley, 1985: 254–431.
2. Xie W, Robertson DL, Simmons DL. Mitogen-inducible prostaglandin G/H synthase: a new target for nonsteroidal antiinflammatory drugs. Drug Develop Res 1992; 25:249–65.

I

Clinical Applications of Nonsteroidal Anti-Inflammatory Drugs

1

Effects of Nonsteroidal Anti-Inflammatory Drugs and Corticosteroids on Cartilage Metabolism in Rheumatoid Arthritis and Osteoarthritis

JEAN-PIERRE PELLETIER and JOHANNE MARTEL-PELLETIER
University of Montreal and Notre-Dame Hospital
Montreal, Quebec, Canada

CHARLES J. MALEMUD
Case Western Reserve University School of Medicine
Cleveland, Ohio

I. INTRODUCTION

Osteoarthritis (OA) and rheumatoid arthritis (RA) are the most common rheumatic diseases. Inasmuch as OA and RA afflict more than 80% of all patients suffering from arthritis, they are a major public health concern (1). Although OA and RA differ fundamentally in several respects, the gradual destruction of joints, primarily the diarthrodial joints, leading to serious morbidity, characterizes them both. Articular cartilage is the major structure responsible for maintaining diarthrodial joint function. Cartilage's viscoelastic properties ensure that normal joint motion is accomplished with minimum friction. Although their etiologies are totally different, OA and RA share some final pathways leading to cartilage degradation, characterized by the gradual and progressive loss of articular cartilage, resulting in erosions to subchondral bone.

Several pharmacological agents with different chemical structures and modes of action are currently available for the treatment of these arthritic diseases. Some, such as corticosteroids and nonsteroidal anti-inflammatory drugs (NSAIDs), are often used to treat both OA and RA. This chapter will examine the different pathways thought to be involved in the synthesis and degradation of articular cartilage extracellular matrix and the effect that these drugs have on these pathways. It will also review studies that have examined their effectiveness in the treatment of OA and RA.

II. CARTILAGE BIOCHEMISTRY AND METABOLISM

Articular cartilage is a tissue consisting of a small number of cells, called chondrocytes, which are embedded in a large volume of extracellular matrix (for review see Ref. 2). The cartilage matrix gives this tissue its physicochemical properties. The chemistry of articular cartilage reflects the composition of the matrix. Cartilage water makes up about

80% of the total wet weight. The remaining weight of the tissue is accounted for mainly by two macromolecules: collagen and proteoglycan.

Proteoglycans comprise linear protein cores to which are linked glycosaminoglycan molecules that consist of polysaccharide chains, primarily chondroitin and keratan sulfates. The chondroitin sulfates are the most abundant glycosaminoglycans. The combination of the glycosaminoglycans and the core protein constitutes the proteoglycan monomer. Only a small fraction of the proteoglycan exists as the free monomer in human articular cartilage. The monomer aggregates by binding to hyaluronic acid, which forms the backbone for the aggregate. The liaison between the hyaluronic acid and the monomers is reinforced by proteins called link proteins. The proteoglycans have several physical and chemical properties considered to be important to the resiliency of articular cartilage. For instance, because of the polyanionic nature of the glycosaminoglycans, the proteoglycans are strongly electronegative and evoke a resistance to compressive force. The water-binding capacity of the proteoglycan macromolecules involves providing water for surface lubrication.

Collagen fibers of articular cartilage have an organization and structure in the form of tension-resisting arcades. The collagen of articular cartilage is considered to be more stable than the proteoglycan. The collagen, which provides the tensile strength, is of several different types. Type II collagen is the main component, but other minor types VI, IX, X, and XI have also been described. The function of these minor collagens is not yet fully understood. However, it seems likely that type IX collagen plays an important role in linking together collagen fibers and proteoglycan macromolecules.

The maintenance of matrix homeostasis is a function of the chondrocytes. Normal tissue function requires that normal architecture of this matrix be maintained (3). This is controlled through the regulation of synthetic and degradative events. In normal tissue, matrix homeostasis is balanced, with the rate of new matrix synthesis being equal to the rate of matrix degradation, so that there is neither net tissue gain nor loss. Both processes are controlled by a variety of extracellular proteins such as growth factors and cytokines. Growth factors, such as insulin-like growth factor-I (IGF-1) and transforming growth factor-β (TFG-β), are most commonly associated with the stimulation of connective tissue formation, whereas cytokines, such as IL-1 and TNF-α, are most commonly associated with the stimulation of matrix degradation.

III. MECHANISMS OF CARTILAGE DEGRADATION

A. Osteoarthritis

Osteoarthritis was thought to occur solely as a consequence of the aging process or by mechanical damage derangement of the joint. However, these concepts have evolved as attention turned to the metabolic activity of articular cartilage (4). In OA, changes occur not only in cartilage, but in other components of the joint (i.e., synovium, periarticular ligaments) (5,6). Synovial inflammation, which is responsible for many clinical symptoms of OA, may also play an important role in the pathological process by interacting with, and thereby accelerating, cartilage catabolism. It is, however, thought that the initial lesions occur at the cartilage level, and that, at a later stage of the disease, the synovium progressively becomes the site of chronic inflammation (7).

The biochemical changes that occur in OA cartilage primarily affect extracellular matrix components: proteoglycan, collagen, and link protein. Proteoglycan is progressively depleted. Chondrocytes appear unable to fully compensate for this depletion, resulting in a net loss in this extracellular component. Proteoglycan structure also changes, with a diminution in the size of proteoglycan aggregates and monomers, and a decrease in the aggregation properties of the monomers and hyaluronate content (4,5,8,9). The latter changes are likely related to degradation of the proteoglycan monomer core protein. The content of type II collagen remains rather stable in OA cartilage. However, the increased cartilage hydration caused by an increase in collagen swelling pressure and the ultrastructural changes of the collagen fibers, as seen by electron microscopy (10), represent important alterations in the collagen fiber network.

It is becoming obvious that enzymatic pathways, in addition to other factors, such as mechanical factors, are involved in OA cartilage extracellular matrix degradation (11). The enzymatic process appears unrelated to a unique system, but rather to a cascade of steps similar to the one seen in the coagulation system. By contrast with RA, in which the synovium is certainly the most important source of degradative enzymes, the chondrocytes in OA seem to be the most important enzymatic source of cartilage extracellular matrix catabolism (3,12). The enzyme families that have now been identified as playing major roles in OA pathophysiology are the metalloproteinases, serine-proteinases, and thiol-proteinases. The two main types of metalloproteinases involved in cartilage degradation are collagenase and stromelysin (13,14). Collagenase appears to be responsible for the breakdown of the collagen network in OA cartilage (13). Stromelysin is the main form of proteoglycanase identified in human articular cartilage (15). These two enzymes showed increased activity in OA cartilage, and their levels correlate with the severity of cartilage lesions (13,16,17). Stromelysin potentially activates procollagenase (18) and, thereby, is likely to play a dual role in OA pathophysiology. Metalloproteinase biological activity is controlled both by physiological inhibitors and activators. In OA cartilage, there is an imbalance between the amount of the specific inhibitor of metalloproteinase, TIMP-1, and metalloproteinases, resulting in a relative deficit of the inhibitor (19); such a deficit is likely responsible for the increase in biologically active enzymes found in this tissue. Enzymes of the serine-proteinase and thiol-dependent proteinase families have been suggested as physiological metalloproteinase activators. Among them, the plasminogen activator (PA)–plasmin system and cathepsin B are the most likely to play such a role (20,21). The possibility that a PA–plasmin system might be involved in the activation of latent metalloproteinases was suggested in a recent ex vivo study, which showed a significant increase in plasmin activity and plasminogen activator (urokinase type) level in OA cartilage (22). Moreover, there was a positive correlation between the level of plasmin and active collagenase. Concomitantly, the level of one of the major physiological inhibitors of plasminogen activators, PAI-1, was decreased. This, in part, may explain the increased level of biologically active PA in OA tissue.

The degradation of the extracellular matrix in OA often occurs in the area surrounding the chondrocytes. Cathepsin B, a lysosomal enzyme with an acid pH optima, is likely to play an important role in that process, as indicated by a recent study showing that the cathepsin B level is increased in cartilage lesions, with a concomitant decrease in cysteine-proteinase inhibitory activity (23). This imbalance between cathepsin B and cysteine-proteinase inhibitor levels may be an important contributing factor in OA cartilage degradation.

Once cartilage degradation begins, the breakdown products, such as fragments of extracellular matrix components, are released into the synovial fluid and phagocytosed by cells from the synovial membrane. These latter cells have a macrophagic function, and this process will result in an inflammatory response. Synovial inflammation stimulates the synthesis of proteolytic enzymes by infiltrating macrophages and activates synovial lining cells and stromal fibroblasts. This phenomenon results in local tissue destruction and cartilage degradation as the enzymes diffuse into the cartilage matrix. Cytokines, synthesized by synovial lining cells, and macrophages, including interleukin-1 (IL-1) and possibly other factors, likely increase synovial and cartilage metalloproteinase synthesis, resulting in further cartilage degradation (see Ref. 3 for review). A vicious circle of compensatory synthesis, chondrocyte activation, and extracellular matrix degradation is in motion.

Although a direct correlation of cytokines and in vivo changes in OA has yet to be established, the presence of IL-1 in arthritic synovial fluid and in OA synovium (24–28) supports a pathophysiological role for this cytokine. Synovium explants, derived from joints of human OA patients, synthesized both isoforms of IL-1 (α and β) (26). Interleukin-1β is the most preponderant form, and its release is greatly enhanced by lipopolysaccharides (LPS). In this study (26), tumor necrosis factor-α (TNF-α) could not be detected in unstimulated synovial membranes. Although a significant level of TNF-α is present in most synovial fluid from RA patients, it is found only occasionally in synovial fluid from OA patients (29). These data indicate that IL-1 is likely to be involved in the increased synthesis of proteinases, such as metalloproteinases and plasminogen activators, in OA synovium, since metalloproteinase level correlates with the severity of synovial inflammation (30), and the latter correlates with the level of IL-1 in the synovial fluid (28).

Interleukin-1 increased the synthesis of prostaglandins (PGE) in several cell types in response to a variety of stimuli, such as endotoxin immune complexes, cytokines, and others. Studies have demonstrated that certain feedback mechanisms exist by which IL-1 synthesis is somewhat regulated by prostaglandin E (PGE). Prostaglandins, under physiological concentration, reduce translation of IL-1 (31), and this suppression is mediated by the induction of cAMP (31,32); however, endogenous PGE_2 formation is involved in IL-1–induced IL-1 synthesis (33).

Cytokines may also be involved in modulating metalloproteinase inhibition and activation in OA. For instance, the imbalance between TIMP-1 and metalloproteinase levels in OA cartilage (19) may be mediated by IL-1, as this cytokine decreases in vitro TIMP-1 synthesis in parallel with an increased metalloproteinase synthesis in articular chondrocytes (34). Plasminogen activator also appears to be similarly modulated by IL-1. In fact, the in vitro effect of IL-1 on articular cartilage showed a dose-dependent PA increase while causing a sharp decrease in the PAI-1 level (34). These in vitro effects of IL-1 on articular cartilage complement the ex vivo findings in OA cartilage and stress the role of this cytokine in OA pathophysiology. Furthermore, the profound effect of IL-1 on PAI-1, together with PA enhancement, are powerful factors in the generation of plasmin and metalloproteinase activation. Along with its role as an enzyme activator, plasmin may also be involved in cartilage matrix degradation by direct proteolysis of the proteoglycan monomer (35). Although now only speculative, recent data suggest that plasmin contributes to the transformation of pro-IL-1 into its biologically active form (36). Finally, IL-1 may be involved in osteophyte formation, by stimulating the proliferation of human osteoblastlike cells, causing increased periarticular bone formation (37).

There is much evidence supporting the involvement of cytokines in OA cartilage degradation. Immunohistochemical studies of normal human cartilage (24,26) showed that IL-1 is synthesized in only a very few chondrocytes and only from those in the superficial layer. However, in OA, a strong positive staining for IL-1α and IL-1β was observed in the upper half of the cartilage in both chondrocytes and the extracellular matrix (24,26,38). These findings support the presence of IL-1 in OA tissue. Together with the studies indicating that IL-1 induces resorption of cartilage both in vitro (39–41) and in vivo (41), the immunolocalization makes IL-1 involvement in the pathophysiology of OA very likely. In addition, evidence also suggests that IL-1 is involved in modulating the chondrocytic synthetic pathway, including synthesis of matrix macromolecules and proteinases. Immunohistochemical studies of OA cartilage showing simultaneous positive staining of chondrocytes for stromelysin, as well as IL-1, strongly suggest that these proteins are secreted by chondrocytes (43).

Although considerable evidence has been accumulated on IL-1's ability to influence chondrocyte metabolism, the exact mechanism(s) by which IL-1 promotes its biological action is not yet completely understood. Interleukin-1 (α and β) is a small globular protein of 17 kilodaltons (kDa) belonging to the polypeptide hormone family (44). Their accepted mode of action on cells is likely mediated through membrane receptors. In articular tissues, interleukin-1 receptor (IL-1R) has been identified on chondrocytes, as well as on synovial fibroblasts (45–48). The sequence of events following IL-1 binding is still largely unknown, but evidence suggests that the IL-1R complex is translocated to the nucleus (49,50). This raises the possibility that this receptor participates directly in the regulation of gene expression. The regulation of IL-1R in chondrocytes is particularly relevant to the development of OA, as these cells can be highly stimulated at picomolar concentrations of IL-1 (45–48). We recently investigated the physical and kinetic properties of IL-1R in human articular normal and OA chondrocytes (51). In the latter, the IL-1 concentration required for half-maximal stimulation of metalloproteinase synthesis was three to four times lower for OA than for normal cells (51). This indicates that OA chondrocytes have a higher sensitivity than normal to the stimulation of metalloproteinase synthesis by IL-1, which could be related to higher levels of IL-1R type 1 in the former. These changes in OA chondrocytes could have important implications for the role of IL-1 and IL-1R in the pathogenesis of OA.

B. Rheumatoid Arthritis

Although OA and RA are two arthritic diseases that differ greatly in several aspects, including their origin and clinical presentation, they do share some common mechanisms leading to cartilage degradation. In RA, synovial inflammation and pannus are, without doubt, major factors in cartilage destruction (52). The synovial membrane histological features in RA and OA patients is characterized by a wide heterogeneity (53–55). At one end of the spectrum, there is marked hyperplasia of the synovial lining layer, with a dense cellular infiltrate composed mainly of lymphocytes and monocytes. At the opposite end, the synovial membrane is thickened by fibrotic tissue, with a very sparse cellular infiltrate. Both RA and OA synovium display a similar spectrum, but there is a somewhat lesser degree of inflammation in OA (54,55).

Considerable information has been gathered on the histology and immunohistology of synovitis in both OA and RA. Studies using cell lineage-specific monoclonal antibodies (MAbs) have helped identify the different mononuclear cell populations present in these tissues. We studied the histological and immunopathological features of the synovial membrane of RA and OA patients who had undergone total knee arthroplasty (7). There were no significant differences in the percentages or the distribution pattern of the infiltrating T-cell subsets (CD4, CD8), HLA-DR, or interleukin-2 receptor-bearing cells. However, inflammatory indexes, which included the thickness of the lining cell layer and the density of the mononuclear cell infiltrate, were significantly higher in the RA patients. Few studies have addressed the issue of the inflammatory infiltrate's cell subsets and their distribution in the synovial membrane of patients with OA. It is interesting that, despite a tendency for a lower cell density, the percentage, distribution, and organization of the different cell populations were similar to those in the RA synovium. Moreover, some OA synovial membranes are so heavily infiltrated by inflammatory cells that they are indistinguishable from RA synovium (7,55,56). Thus, the histological picture in a subset of OA may mimic that of RA, despite a clear clinical, immunological, and radiological exclusion of RA.

One of the major characteristics of joint destruction in RA is the presence of bone erosion. Interleukin-1 and TNF are among the most potent polypeptide hormones that regulate bone resorption (see ref. 57 for review). The effect of IL-1 is mediated not only through PGE synthesis, which is a potent stimulator of bone resorption, but also through prostaglandin-independent resorption (57). The action of TNF-α and β is mediated by the osteoclasts and is blocked by inhibitors of PGE synthesis.

The mechanisms thought to mediate cartilage degradation involve the release of humoral factors by the inflamed synovium. These mechanisms are somewhat similar to those described in the OA section (58). Hyperplasia of the synovial lining cells (involving both type A and type B) results from an as yet unknown antigenic stimulus. Proliferation of the synovial cells proceeds in intimate association with subintimal inflammatory cell migration in which activated macrophages, T and B lymphocytes, neutrophils, and mast cells are involved. These cell populations participate in complex immunological reactions contributing to the pathophysiology. A scenario for the reactions occurring in the synovial joint in RA, for which cytokines are believed to play a central role, proceeds according to this current view. Activated macrophages within the pannus, predominantly the synovial lining cells, synthesize and release proteolytic enzymes, such as collagenase and stromelysin (59). Stimulated macrophages also synthesize cytokines, such as IL-1 and TNF-α (58). These cytokines not only locally stimulate synovial cells in the pannus, such as synovial fibroblasts, to synthesize metalloproteinases, but also contribute to further cartilage degradation by stimulating at a distance, through diffusion into the synovial fluid, the synthesis of proteolytic enzymes by chondrocytes. Among other things, IL-1 may inhibit chondrocyte synthesis of proteoglycans, further compromising cartilage structure. In the synovial fluid, polymorphonuclear leukocytes attracted into the joint space by chemotactic factors, such as leukotriene-B_4 (LTB_4) and C5a, degranulate, thereby releasing proteolytic enzymes such as elastase, collagenase, cathepsin G, and other lysosomal hydrolases that saturate the capacity of the endogenous proteinase inhibitors (α_2-macroglobulin and α_1-antiproteinase) in synovial fluid (60).

The elaboration of free-oxygen radicals by polymorphonuclear neutrophils (PMN) is also believed to play a role in tissue destruction by causing depolymerization of hyaluronic acid, inactivation of proteinase inhibitors, and producing chemotactic factors (61). Alterations in cartilage extracellular matrix proteins may arise nonenzymatically through the generation of oxygen-dependent free radicals (62,63). The principal extracellular matrix protein components of cartilage can be degraded in several ways; hyaluronic acid can be depolymerized by hydroxyl radicals (64) or by the generation of singlet oxygen species in vitro (65). Whether or not cartilage hyaluronate and synovial fluid hyaluronate are altered in structure by the same pathway is unknown. It has been suggested that some anti inflammatory drugs, including NSAIDs, act pharmacologically in part because they are scavengers of free radicals (66–68).

Cartilage hyaluronate changes, seen as a reduction in average molecular size in an experimental lapine model of osteoarthritis, may have resulted from hyaluronate degradation (69), and this could potentially play an important role in the reduction of large proteoglycan aggregates in this experimental model (70).

Several studies suggest that "chondroprotective" measures that would spare the proteoglycan aggregate from degradation would be of benefit to cartilage. Nonenzymatic cleavage of link protein has been demonstrated in vitro with hydrogen peroxide (71,72), but recent studies indicate that cleavage products of human link protein made in this manner and those occurring in situ are different (73). Thus, even though chondrocytes synthesize hydrogen peroxide in cell culture (74), it is not known if it plays any role in altering the tertiary complex of link protein, hyaluronate, and proteoglycan monomer in the cartilage.

The effects of oxygen-derived free radicals on collagen structure must also be considered. Here is remains to be seen whether the oxygen radical effects on collagen are direct or indirect. The role of oxygen-derived free radicals may be to provide an augmentative environment that enhances the biological activity of enzyme systems that can degrade type II collagen. For example, the activation of neutrophil collagenase may occur through the action of hypochlorous acid on the latent procollagenase (75). As reviewed by Greenwald (63), no specific studies on the direct susceptibility of type II to oxygen-derived free radicals has been performed. Oxygen-derived free radicals could also alter structures of accessory matrix proteins before gaining access to other potential targets in the proteoglycan aggregate complex.

IV. EFFECTS OF NONSTEROIDAL ANTI-INFLAMMATORY DRUGS AND CORTICOSTEROIDS ON CARTILAGE METABOLISM

This section will address the effects of NSAIDs and corticosteroids both in vitro and in vivo on the main pathophysiological mechanisms leading to cartilage repair and degradation in OA and RA. We will also examine studies that have investigated the therapeutic effectiveness of these drugs both in experimental models and in humans.

A. Effects of Nonsteroidal Anti-Inflammatory Drugs on Cartilage Anabolism

The potential of NSAIDs to alter the synthesis of proteoglycan and collagen has been explored by using cartilage and chondrocyte cell cultures (76–78). Because of the increasing interest in the effect of cytokines on mediating cartilage changes, NSAIDs' reversal of cytokine-induced suppression of proteoglycan and collagen would be of considerable importance in designing future strategies for treating the arthritic joint.

Interleukin-1 has been reported to reduce proteoglycan and collagen synthesis in vitro (79,80). Some studies suggest that analyses on chondrocytes derived from young individuals cannot be directly extrapolated to cartilage derived from older individuals (81); but evidence to the contrary has been presented when murine responses to IL-1 have been compared as a function of the animal's age (82). In preliminary studies, recombinant forms of IL-1α and IL-1β did not suppress proteoglycan synthesis using high-density cultures of chondrocytes derived from osteofemoral heads (our unpublished data). Evidence has been presented that animal and human cartilages are sensitive to specific NSAIDs in their ability to diminish compensatory matrix responses in the presence of IL-1 (24,83). In porcine articular cartilage organ cultures, inhibition of proteoglycan synthesis with salicylic acid ($IC_{50} \approx 100$ μg/ml), ibuprofen ($IC_{50} \approx 4$ μg/ml), and indomethacin ($IC_{50} \approx 2$ μg/ml) could be partially reversed by the prostaglandin E_1 analogue, misoprostol (83). Misoprostol also appeared to be effective in aiding recovery from the suppressive effects of IL-1 on proteoglycan synthesis (83). The NSAIDs have variable effects on proteoglycan synthesis. This has been borne out by extensive studies using both cartilage explants and chondrocytes in culture. Usually, total proteoglycan synthesis is affected. In cell culture, altered compartmentation of proteoglycan has been reported (84).

Some NSAIDs appear to have favorable effects on cartilage. Four NSAIDs, namely, sulindac sulfate, benoxaprofen, tiaprofenic acid, and naproxen have been distinguished from other NSAIDs for their effects on proteoglycan synthesis. Benoxaprofen ($IC_{50} \approx 10$ μg/ml) actually augmented proteoglycan synthesis in vitro when normal cartilage was used (85). Sulindac sulfate, at concentrations ranging from 1.5 to 30 μg/ml, caused a slight increase (average 13%) in proteoglycan synthesis; however, this was not concentration-dependent (86). Tiaprofenic acid did not increase or decrease proteoglycan synthesis in human or rabbit chondrocyte cultures (78,87,88). Naproxen did not suppress proteoglycan synthesis in canine cartilage when administered orally (89), but at high concentration (100 μg/ml), it suppressed "matrix" proteoglycan (read out as keratan sulfate concentration) in first-passage rabbit chondrocytes (84). Thus, the concentration of NSAID, mode of administration, and test system, all have the potential to alter the given results with any NSAID. Even given this caveat, many NSAIDs have proteoglycan and/or collagen synthesis-suppressing activity. Among those NSAIDs acting in this way are indomethacin (89–92), tolmetin (93), phenylbutazone (94), the salicylates (91,95,96), and diclofenac (92). The indomethacin and salicylate effect on proteoglycans is correlated with the physical state of cartilage. Fibrillated tissue is more susceptible to the effects of the drugs (96). Interestingly, ketoprofen, which augments proteoglycan synthesis (84), and fenoprofen, which suppresses proteoglycan synthesis (91), belong to the proprionic class of NSAIDs. Thus, NSAIDs' structural similarities cannot predict their effects on cartilage proteoglycan synthesis. In addition, the test system (i.e., cell culture, organ culture, in vivo testing, and dose range) will affect the interpretation of the results.

The mechanisms responsible for the augmentative or suppressive effects of NSAIDs on proteoglycan synthesis probably do not proceed through a single common pathway. Among the NSAIDs tested, only sodium salicylate failed as a cyclooxygenase inhibitor in first-passage monolayer cultures of rabbit chondrocytes (97). Several other NSAIDs in this study, including indomethacin and sodium meclofenamate, inhibited eicosanoid synthesis, which was coupled to a decrease in the synthesis of cAMP (97). Coupled with recent evidence that agonist-stimulated increases in cAMP resulted in elevated proteoglycan production, a mechanism involving activation of cAMP-dependent protein kinase (A kinase) or phosphorylation of selected target intracellular substrates activated by A kinase must be considered.

Studies showed that simple increases in, or accumulation of, cAMP (i.e., by forskolin and isoproterenol) did not always result in stimulated proteoglycan synthesis (98). Forskolin stimulated proteoglycan synthesis (99), and isoproterenol did not (98). Preferential binding of cAMP to either of the regulatory subunits (R_I or R_{II}) of the A kinase could not be demonstrated (100). Recent findings (100) suggested that NSAIDs augment intracellular protein phosphorylation by activation of A-kinase in monolayer cultures of rabbit and in human nonarthritic and osteoarthritic chondrocytes (personal observations). In measurements of A-kinase–driven phosphorylation, sodium salicylate, sodium meclofenamate, indomethacin, and tiaprofenic acid, all augmented phosphorylation of selected substrates. This result makes it highly unlikely that augmented substrate phosphorylation by NSAIDs is related to the cyclooxygenase inhibitory capacity of the NSAID.

In assessing in vitro effects of NSAIDs on proteoglycan and collagen synthesis in cell culture, it is instructive to keep in mind whether therapeutic doses of the drug were used. Recent studies (92,101) have assessed NSAIDs effects on rabbit chondrocytes. Concentrations of diclofenac, indomethacin, ketoprofen, piroxicam, and tiaprofenic acid ranged from 0.1 to 100 μg/ml. The highest concentration of NSAID inhibited proteoglycan synthesis and secretion in both explant and cell culture, which was reversible in the cell cultures, but not in the explants when the cultures were washed free of the drug. This emphasizes the need to consider that NSAIDs can avidly bind to components with extracellular matrices. Thus, NSAIDs can retain their activity in cartilage long after they are administered. The reported adverse effect of indomethacin and other NSAIDs on the progression of osteoarthritis is an example of this phenomenon (102).

B. Effect of Nonsteroidal Anti-Inflammatory Drugs on Cartilage Catabolism

Despite skepticism over the therapeutic effectiveness in altering the progression of arthritides, NSAIDs are among the most commonly prescribed drugs for these medical conditions. At present, no evidence has been obtained to support contention that these drugs, which relieve symptoms, may also induce remission of RA or OA. Although NSAIDs have been available for years, most studies, until recently, have addressed only their anti-inflammatory properties. Work in spontaneous and experimental animal models (103–108) indicates that some NSAIDs, such as diclofenac and pirprofen, may reduce the progression of OA lesions. These and other studies exploring the effect of drugs on the metabolism of normal and OA cartilage have sparked renewed interest in therapeutic intervention.

There have been several in vivo and in vitro studies on the effects of NSAIDs on normal and OA cartilage metabolism of different animal species. To date, studies on normal animal cartilage have shown that NSAID, such as sodium salicylic, indomethacin and piroxicam, have no significant effect on cartilage catabolism (109). This could partly be due to the very slow catabolic rate of normal cartilage, which makes the effect of drugs difficult to determine. In vivo studies using experimental animal models have shown that not all NSAIDs affect OA cartilage lesions the same way (103–108). For instance, in C57 black mice, a spontaneous OA model, diclofenac and pirprofen reduced the incidence and severity of OA lesions, whereas sodium salicylate and several other NSAIDs (acetylsalicylic acid, phenylbutazone, indomethacin, ibuprofen, naproxen) increased the incidence and severity (108). In the rabbit meniscectomy model, pirprofen, among several other NSAIDs tested, effectively reduced OA lesions (106,107).

Only a few studies with human cartilage have been performed [e.g., McKenzie et al. (110]), showing that, with aged cartilage from femoral heads, indomethacin and sodium salicylates suppressed proteoglycan synthesis. This observation is also supported by recent studies that indicate a similar effect of salicylate on human OA knee cartilage (87). This effect on OA chondrocytes may be due to a general cytotoxicity, as indicated by morphological studies.

Recent in vitro studies indicate that some NSAIDs may reduce the degradation of human OA cartilage by actually inhibiting cartilage metalloproteinase activity (87). These studies show that therapeutic serum (26 μg/ml) and synovial fluid (2.6 μg/ml) concentrations of tiaprofenic acid significantly reduced cartilage proteoglycan catabolism by decreasing metalloproteinase synthesis. The effect of tiaprofenic acid was also noted when metalloproteinase synthesis was stimulated by IL-1. This could be reversed by pharmacological doses of PGE_2 (24). These results strongly support a connection between the effect of tiaprofenic acid on cartilage catabolism and its inhibition of cyclooxygenase. In vivo studies by Vignon et al. in OA patients demonstrated that tiaprofenic acid taken orally significantly reduced the stromelysin activity in articular cartilage harvested at the time of hip replacement surgery (111). A recent study showed that tiaprofenic acid reduced the incidence and severity of cartilage lesions in an experimental OA canine model (112). Similar results were also reported by Mahmud et al. for naproxen (113). Preliminary in vitro data on human cartilage explants also suggest that piroxicam (114) may have some inhibitory effect on cartilage catabolism.

Indomethacin suppresses metalloproteinase synthesis in human OA synovium and in synovial cells in culture (115). The synthesis of metalloproteinases and plasminogen activators (a likely candidate in the physiological activation of proenzymes) was inhibited by NSAIDs by an inhibitory action on cyclooxygenase (116). In vivo, tiaprofenic acid also decreased the plasminogen activator level in the synovial fluid of patients with OA (117).

Many in vitro and in vivo experiments have clearly demonstrated the capacity for cytokines, such as IL-1 and TNF-α, to induce cartilage degradation. Moreover, the presence of these cytokines in situ in arthritic diseases has been clearly established (3,58). Over the last few years, there have been numerous experiments examining the effect of drugs, such as NSAIDs and corticosteroids, on the synthetic release and effect of cytokines on target tissues or cells. Several in vitro experiments using cell culture (mainly macrophages) have indicated that drugs that inhibit cyclooxygenase, such as NSAIDs, do not suppress IL-1 synthesis and may even induce a slight stimulation of IL-1 production (118,119). However, with dermal fibroblasts, Mauviel et al. showed that indomethacin can prevent the increased transcription of the IL-1β gene in response to stimulation by IL-1 (120). The effects of molecules that can inhibit both the cyclooxygenase and lipoxygenase pathways seem to hold more promise. Several compounds that suppress both pathways of arachidonate metabolism have been observed to downregulate IL-1. Tenidap (CP-66,248), at an unbound concentration as low as 1 μg/ml, specifically inhibited the synthesis of IL-1 in mouse peritoneal macrophages and human peripheral blood monocytes (121,122). In recent experiments on peripheral blood mononuclear cells, tenidap not only inhibited IL-1 production but also IL-6 and TNF-α (123). This drug inhibited the response of murine T-cell line induced by recombinant IL-1 (121) and reduced the synovial fluid IL-1 level in RA patients (124). The compound SK&F 86002, which inhibits both cyclooxygenase and lipoxygenase pathways, also reduced the synthesis and secretion of IL-1 from human peripheral blood monocytes (125). In addition, this compound, in ex vivo experiments, suppressed the increased production of IL-1 by splenocytes obtained from adjuvant arthritic rats (126).

Interleukin-1 is present in increased amounts in OA cartilage and synovium (24–26) and is likely responsible for increased metalloproteinase synthesis and cartilage degradation. Herman et al. demonstrated that the synthesis of cartilage catabolic factor(s) by OA synovial membranes in vitro was consistently reduced, by therapeutic concentrations of piroxicam (27). A similar effect was also reported by Rainsford on porcine synovial tissue, using diclofenac, indomethacin, piroxicam, and sulindac sulfide (127). Tiaprofenic acid, in vivo, also reduced the level of IL-1β in human OA synovial fluid (128). A recent study indicated that tenidap reduces the stimulatory effect of IL-1 on chondrocyte metalloproteinase synthesis by down-regulating the IL-1 receptor level (129).

No data are available concerning NSAIDs' effects on the natural course of RA. However, several in vitro studies and in vivo analyses in experimental RA animal models have been reported. From these, some data have emerged on how NSAIDs may affect important pathophysiological pathways that lead to cartilage degradation. Several NSAIDs were found, in vitro, to reduce the activity, production, or both, of IL-1 by human monocytes at pharmacological concentrations, but not at therapeutic concentrations (130). Although indomethacin reduces the in vitro synthesis of metalloproteinases by RA synovium explants when introduced in vitro (115), this effect was not observed when synovial proteinases were studied after oral administration of indomethacin. Whether or not these contradictory results reflect the decay of the drugs action has not been determined (131). Piroxicam reduced the production of cartilage catabolic factors by RA synovium explants in culture (27). The results of recent in vivo studies in murine antigen-induced arthritis showed that several NSAIDs had no effect in protecting joint damage in this model of inflammatory arthritic disease (132, 133). However, tenidap (IC_{50} 6.1 μg/ml, free form), in contrast with several NSAIDs, such as naproxen, ibuprofen, piroxicam, and indomethacin, inhibited the in vitro the release of activated neutrophil collagenase (134).

In summary, several in vitro and in vivo studies in experimental models support the hypothesis that certain NSAIDs, may have chondroprotective effects in OA by modulating several pathophysiological mechanisms leading to cartilage degradation. In contrast, the results of studies in RA seem to support the general impression that the conventional NSAIDs, although helpful in relieving some of the symptoms of the disease, are ineffective in preventing its progression. However, the introduction of new antirheumatic drugs may very well challenge this concept.

V. EFFECT OF CORTICOSTEROIDS ON CARTILAGE METABOLISM

Among the treatments used for rheumatic disorders, corticosteroids are used most often, principally because they provide prompt, and effective relief of clinical symptoms. The administration of these agents is either orally or intra-articular, with the latter preferred for cases of osteoarthritis. Despite their current heavy use in clinical practice, a review of the literature indicates that few data are available on the therapeutic efficacy and effectiveness of oral corticosteroids. Animal models, however, have provided some useful data on the chondroprotective effects of steroids in controlling pathophysiological changes in inflammatory arthritides (132,133).

In human investigations, several studies suggest that oral steroids alter disease progression (135,136). Evidence for a reduction in the progression of cartilage erosions by use of oral steroid (135), as measured by radiographic analysis, has corroborated earlier studies suggesting that oral corticosteroids reduce cartilage breakdown, as measured by serum keratan sulfate levels (136). Coupled with a lack of strong support that steroids affect the underlying process in RA (137) and the significant side effects associated with oral administration of corticosteroids, the use of these agents remains open to further scrutiny.

The reluctance to use steroids must be balanced by the clinical responses following intra-articular steroid injection. Acute flares respond significantly when single or a few joints fail to respond to other treatment regimens. It is generally agreed that the same joint not be injected more than two or three times per year.

The potential damaging effects of corticosteroids on joint cartilage must also be considered. In in vitro studies, corticosteroids have decreased cartilage proteoglycan synthesis (138,139). Some studies have even suggested that oral or intra-articular corticosteroids worsen cartilage defects or cause lesions to form in normal cartilage (138–142). Several of these conclusions are based on studies in which the experimental conditions used nonphysiological doses of steroid or required repeated injections. This makes these conclusions unlikely to be relevant to the clinical situation.

When steroids are used in a narrow range of therapeutic doses, substantial palliative effects have been reported. This has been especially true in therapy of osteoarthritis. In experimentally induced models of osteoarthritis, such as the partial medial meniscectomy model in the rabbit, low-dose intra-articular steroid injection reduced the severity of cartilage ulcers and osteophyte formation (106,143). In a guinea pig model, a similar finding was reported (104). In the anterior cruciate ligament transection model of canine osteoarthritis, low-dose oral corticosteroids (prednisone, 0.20–0.25 mg/kg) or intra-articular steroids (triamcinolone hexacetonide, 5 mg/month) significantly reduced the incidence and severity of cartilage lesions and osteophytic spurs (144). These results were well correlated with those from human investigations (145) in which it was shown that repeated steroid injections in knees of individuals with chronic arthritis showed no evidence of exacerbated cartilage destruction or progressive deterioration of the joint.

In the inflammatory arthritides, recent animal model results indicated that oral or intra-articular steroids "normalized" proteoglycan synthesis and reduced the severity of cartilage lesions in the mouse in which inflammation was induced by antigen (132,133). Once more, a correlative human investigation provides evidence for the efficacy of steroids in inflammatory arthritis. Glucocorticoid injections reduced the proteoglycan content in synovial fluid from patients with RA or inflammatory arthritis (146), suggesting a protective effect on reducing cartilage breakdown.

The effects of steroids in limiting cartilage destruction may relate to their potent effects on altering cartilage catabolism. Both in vivo and in vitro, metalloproteinase synthesis in inflamed synovium (30,115,147) and osteoarthritic cartilage (16,87) is suppressed by steroids. Steroids also suppress putative physiological activators of latent metalloproteinases, such as plasminogen activator (148), and inducers of metalloproteinase gene expression, such as cytokines (i.e., IL-1) (127,149). Glucocorticoids have reduced the release of IL-1 from lipopolysaccharide-stimulated macrophages in a dose-related fashion (150). The mechanisms through which the corticosteroids exert their action include the suppression of the transcription of the IL-1 gene and a decrease in IL-1 mRNA stability (150).

The effectiveness of glucocorticoids in the treatment of OA is not surprising, as corticosteroids may act on different catabolic mechanisms involved in the development of this disease, including the enzymatic degradation of cartilage, in which metalloproteinases are of importance (3,12). Endogenous glucocorticoids, through their binding to the cognate intracellular receptor (GR), may be important homeostatic bioregulators that could provide a control mechanism against the overproduction of metalloproteinases and, secondarily, cartilage matrix degradation. Our laboratory demonstrated the presence of glucocorticoid receptors (GR) on human chondrocytes and established that the chondrocytic action of glucocorticoids on metalloproteinases requires GR occupancy (151). Moreover, the recent finding of a down-regulation of GR expression and level in OA cartilage chondrocytes may be responsible in vivo for chondrocytes being underresponsive to endogenous glucocorticoids, contributing to the overproduction of metalloproteinases. In addition, we also showed (152,153) that the synthesis of collagenase is significantly less responsive to glucocorticoid suppression in human OA chondrocytes than in normal ones, and that this finding is probably because the GR level is significantly reduced in OA cells (153). Because, in every glucocorticoid responsive cell the effectiveness of the response is dependent of the cellular levels of GR (154), factors that modulate the GR level within a target cell are of primary importance. The decreased biological response of OA chondrocytes to corticosteroids may be responsible for a suboptimal therapeutic response to the drug. The administration of an agent that could reverse the down-regulation of GR expression may have therapeutic application in the treatment of OA.

The effect of prostaglandins and cAMP on normal and osteoarthritic chondrocytes was analyzed. Studies were done looking at the effect of dibutyryl cAMP, PGE_2, and the PGE_1 analogue, misoprostol, on the GR-binding level of normal articular chondrocytes. The PGE_2 and dibutyryl cAMP induce a statistically significant elevation of the GR-binding level by 1.6- and 1.7-fold, respectively. The PGE_1 analogue provoked a twofold increase in the steroid-binding level. The OA chondrocytes in primary culture expressed fewer GR than normal chondrocytes; sensitivity of OA cells to the action of PGE_2 and cAMP was similar to that of normal cells (155).

Agent(s) capable of increasing the GR level may be efficacious in slowing the progression of OA and allowing endogenous corticosteroids to exert their full biological effect. Injectable glucocorticoids are an important pharmacological therapy in the management of OA. Their efficacy may be dependent on adequate GR expression in chondrocytes or synoviocytes. Thus, a knowledge of those factors that influence the expression of GR, and with it the ability to manipulate such levels, may be important in the successful treatment of OA.

Of considerable interest is the recognition that, although steroids potently suppress synovial joint catabolism, they do not appear to augment anabolic responses required for repair. This viewpoint has significance in the treatment of arthritis. Maintenance of steroid concentrations in tissues is apparently important to maximize therapeutic benefit and minimize potential deleterious effects on chondrocytes. Thus, there is substantial evidence from experimental and clinical studies to support the contention that steroid injections, used as appropriate therapeutic doses, are unlikely to cause damage to articular cartilage. The recent data support an optimistic view of steroid use in the treatment of OA.

ACKNOWLEDGMENT

Supported by grants from the Canadian Arthritis Society, the Medical Research Council of Canada, and a grant from the National Institute on Aging, AG-02205 (USPHS).

REFERENCES

1. Masi AT, Medsger TA. Epidemiology of the rheumatic diseases. In: McCarty DJ, ed. Arthritis and allied conditions. Philadelphia: Lea & Febiger, 1989:16–54.
2. Mankin HJ, Brandt KD. Biochemistry and metabolism of cartilage in osteoarthritis. In: Moskowitz R, Howell DS, Goldberg VM, Mankin HJ, eds. Osteoarthritis diagnosis and management. Philadelphia: WB Saunders, 1984:43–80.

3. Pelletier JP, Roughley PJ, DiBattista JA, McCollum R, Martel-Pelletier J. Are cytokines involved in osteoarthritis pathophysiology? Semin Arthritis Rheum 1991; 20(suppl 2):12–25.
4. Mankin HJ. The reaction of articular cartilage to injury and osteoarthritis. N Engl J Med 1974; 291:1285–92.
5. Mankin HJ, Treadwell BV. Osteoarthritis: an 1987 update. Bull Rheum Dis 1986; 36:1–10.
6. Sokoloff L. Osteoarthritis as a remodeling process. J Rheumatol 1987; 14:7–10.
7. Haraoui B, Pelletier JP, Cloutier JM, Faure MP, Martel-Pelletier J. Synovial membrane histology and immunopathology in rheumatoid arthritis and osteoarthritis. In vivo effects of antirheumatic drugs. Arthritis Rheum 1991; 4:153–63.
8. Tyler JA. Chondrocyte-mediated depletion of articular cartilage proteoglycans in vitro. Biochem J 1985; 225:493–507.
9. Martel-Pelletier J, Pelletier JP, Malemud CJ. Activation of neutral metalloprotease in human osteoarthritic knee cartilage: evidence for degradation in the core protein of sulphated proteoglycan. Ann Rheum Dis 1988; 47:801–8.
10. Pelletier JP, Martel-Pelletier J, Altman RD, Ghandur-Mnaymneh L, Howell DS, Woesnner JF Jr. Collagenolytic activity and collagen matrix breakdown of the articular cartilage in the Pond–Nuki dog model of osteoarthritis. Arthritis Rheum 1983; 26:866–74.
11. Proceedings of the international symposium on osteoarthritis. Proteases: their involvement in osteoarthritis. J Rheumatol 1987; 14:1–133.
12. Dean DD. Proteinase-mediated cartilage degradation in osteoarthritis. Semin Arthritis Rheum 1991; 20(suppl 2):2–11.
13. Pelletier JP, Martel-Pelletier J, Howell DS, Ghandur-Mnaymneh L, Enis J, Woessner JF Jr. Collagenase and collagenolytic activity in human osteoarthritic cartilage. Arthritis Rheum 1983; 26:63–8.
14. Sapolsky AI, Malemud CJ, Norby DP, Moskowitz RW, Matsuta K, Howell DS. Neutral proteinases from articular chondrocytes in culture. 2. Metal-dependent latent neutral proteoglycanase, and inhibitory activity. Biochim Biophys Acta 1981; 658:138–47.
15. Sapolsky AI, Keiser H, Howell DS, Woessner JF Jr. Metalloproteases of human articular cartilage that digest cartilage proteoglycan at neutral and acid pH. J Clin Invest 1976; 58:1030–41.
16. Pelletier JP, Martel-Pelletier J, Cloutier JM, Woesnner JF Jr. Proteoglycan-degrading acid metalloprotease activity in human osteoarthritic cartilage, and the effect of intra-articular steroid injections. Arthritis Rheum 1987; 30:541–8.
17. Martel-Pelletier J, Pelletier JP, Cloutier JM, Howell DS, Ghandur-Mnaymneh L, Woessner JF Jr. Neutral proteases capable of proteoglycan digesting activity in osteoarthritic and normal human articular cartilage. Arthritis Rheum 1984; 27:305–12.
18. Murphy G, Cockett MI, Stephens PE, Smith BJ, Docherty AJ. Stromelysin is an activator of procollagenase. A study with natural and recombinant enzymes. Biochem J 1987; 248:265–8.
19. Dean DD, Martel-Pelletier J, Pelletier JP, Howell DS, Woessner JF Jr. Evidence for metalloproteinase and metalloproteinase inhibitor (TIMP) imbalance in human osteoarthritic cartilage. J Clin Invest 1989; 84:678–85.
20. He CS, Wilhelm SM, Pentland AP, Marmer BL, Grant GA, Eisen AZ, Goldberg GI. Tissue cooperation in a proteolytic cascade activating human interstitial collagenase. Proc Natl Acad Sci USA 1989; 86:2632–6.
21. Werb Z, Mainardi CL, Vater CA, Harris ED Jr. Endogenous activation of latent collagenase by rheumatoid synovial cells. Evidence for a role of plasminogen activator. N Engl J Med 1977; 296:1017–23.
22. Martel-Pelletier J, Faure MP, McCollum R, Mineau F, Cloutier JM, Pelletier JP. Plasmin, plasminogen activators and inhibitor in human osteoarthritic cartilage. J Rheumatol 1991; 18:1863–71.
23. Martel-Pelletier J, Cloutier JM, Pelletier JP. Cathepsin B and cysteine protease inhibitors in human osteoarthritis. J Orthop Res 1990; 8:336–44.

24. Pelletier JP, Martel-Pelletier J. Evidence for the involvement of interleukin 1 in human osteoarthritic cartilage degradation: protective effect of NSAID. J Rheumatol 1989; 18(suppl 27):19–27.
25. Wood DD, Ihrie EJ, Hamerman D. Release of interleukin-1 from human synovial tissue in vitro. Arthritis Rheum 1985; 28:853–62.
26. Martel-Pelletier J, Cloutier JM, Pelletier JP. Cytokines, interleukin-1 and the tumor necrosis factor in human osteoarthritic tissues [abstract]. Trans Orthop Res Soc 1990; 15:111.
27. Herman JH, Appel AM, Hess EV. Modulation of cartilage destruction by select nonsteroidal anti-inflammatory drugs. In vitro effect on the synthesis and activity of catabolism-inducing cytokines produced by osteoarthritic and rheumatoid synovial tissue. Arthritis Rheum 1987; 30:257–65.
28. Wood DD, Ihrie EJ, Dinarello CA, Cohen PL. Isolation of interleukin-1 like factor from human joint effusions. Arthritis Rheum 1983; 26:975–83.
29. Hopkins SJ, Meager A. Cytokines in synovial fluid. II. The presence of tumor necrosis factor and interferon. Clin Exp Immunol 1988; 73:88–92.
30. Martel-Pelletier J, Cloutier JM, Pelletier JP. Neutral proteases in human osteoarthritic synovium. Arthritis Rheum 1986; 29:1112–21.
31. Knudsen PJ, Dinarello CA, Strom TB. Prostaglandins post-transcriptionally inhibit monocyte expression of interleukin 1 activity by increasing intracellular cyclic adenosine monophosphate. J Immunol 1986; 137:3189–94.
32. Hurme M. Modulation of interleukin-1β production by cyclic AMP in human monocytes. FEBS Lett 1990; 263:35–7.
33. Sirko S, Dinarello CA. A role for arachidonic acid metabolites of cyclooxygenase in IL-1 induced synthesis of IL-1 in vitro. Lymphokine Res 1990; 9:608.
34. Martel-Pelletier J, Zafarullah M, Kodama S, Pelletier JP. In vitro effects of IL-1 on the synthesis of metalloproteases, TIMP, plasminogen activators and inhibitors in human articular cartilage. J. Rheumatol 1991; 18(suppl 27):80–4.
35. Mochan E, Keler T. Plasmin degradation of cartilage proteoglycan. Biochim Biophys Acta 1984; 800:312–5.
36. Matsushima K, Taguchi M, Kovacs EJ, Young HA, Oppenheim JJ. Intracellular localization of human monocyte associated interleukin 1 (IL-1) activity and release of biologically active IL-1 from monocytes by trypsin and plasmin. J Immunol 1986; 136:2883–91.
37. Bunning RA, Richardson HJ, Crawford A, Skjodt H, Hughes D, Evans DB, Gowen M, Dobson PR, Brown BL, Russell RG. The effect of interleukin-1 on connective tissue metabolism and its relevance to arthritis. Agent Actions 1986; 18(suppl):131–52.
38. Shinmei M, Masuda K, Kikuchi T, Shimomura Y. The role of cytokines in chondrocyte mediated cartilage degradation. J Rheumatol 1989; 18(suppl):32–4.
39. Campbell IK, Piccoli DS, Butler DM, Singleton DK, Hamilton JA. Recombinant human interleukin-1 stimulates human articular cartilage to undergo resorption and human chondrocytes to produce both tissue- and urokinase-type plasminogen activator. Biochim Biophys Acta 1988; 967:183–94.
40. Saklatvala J. Tumor necrosis factor alpha stimulates resorption and inhibits synthesis of proteoglycan in cartilage. Nature 1986; 322:547–9.
41. Campbell IK, Piccoli DS, Roberts MJ, Murdin KD, Hamilton JA. Effects of tumor necrosis factor α and β on resorption of human articular cartilage and production of plasminogen activator by human articular chondrocytes. Arthritis Rheum 1990; 33:542–52.
42. Henderson B, Pettipher ER. Arthritogenic actions of recombinant IL-1 and tumour necrosis factor alpha in the rabbit: evidence for synergistic interactions between cytokines in vivo. Clin Exp Immunol 1989; 75:306–10.
43. Pelletier JP, Faure MP, DiBattista JA, Wilhelm S, Visco D, Martel-Pelletier J. Coordinate synthesis of stromelysin, interleukin-1, and oncogene proteins in experimental osteoarthritis. An immunohistochemical study. Am J Pathol 1993; 142:95–105.
44. Dinarello CA. Biology of interleukin-1. FASEB J 1988; 2:108–115.

45. Chin JE, Horuk R. Interleukin-1 receptors on rabbit articular chondrocytes: relationship between biological activity and receptor binding kinetics. FASEB J 1990; 4:1481–7.
46. Chin JE, Rupp E, Cameron PM, MacNaul KL, Lotke PA, Tocci MJ, Schmidt JA, Bayne EK. Identification of a high-affinity receptor for interleukin-1α and interleukin-1β on cultured human rheumatoid synovial cells. J Clin Invest 1988; 82:420–6.
47. Bird TA, Saklatvala J. Identification of a common class of high affinity receptors for both types of porcine interleukin-1 on connective tissue cells. Nature 1986; 324:263–6.
48. Chandrasekhar S, Harvey AK. Induction of interleukin-1 receptors on chondrocytes by fibroblast growth factor: a possible mechanism for modulation of interleukin-1 activity. J Cell Physiol 1989; 138:236–46.
49. Curtis BM, Widmer MB, deRoos P, Qwarnstrom EE. IL-1 and its receptor are translocated to the nucleus. J Immunol 1990; 144:1295–303.
50. Qwarnstrom EE, Page RC, Gillis S, Dower SK. Binding, internalization, and intracellular localization of interleukin-1β in human diploid fibroblasts. J Biol Chem 1988; 263:8261–9.
51. Martel-Pelletier J, McCollum R, DiBattista J, Faure MP, Chin JA, Fournier S, Sarfati M, Pelletier JP. The interleukin-1 receptor in normal and osteoarthritic human articular chondrocytes. Identification as the Type 1 receptor and analysis of binding kinetics and biologic function. Arthritis Rheum 1992; 35:530–40.
52. Harris ED. Pathogenesis of rheumatoid arthritis. In: Kelly WN, Harris ED Jr, Ruddy S, Sledge CB, eds. Textbook of rheumatology. Vol. 1. 3rd ed. Philadelphia: WB Saunders, 1989:905–42.
53. Martel-Pelletier J, Cloutier JM, Pelletier JP. In vivo effects of antirheumatic drugs on neutral collagenolytic proteases in human rheumatoid arthritis cartilage and synovium. J Rheumatol 1988; 15:1198–204.
54. Lindblad S, Hedfors E. Arthroscopic and immunohistologic characterization of knee joint synovitis in osteoarthritis. Arthritis Rheum 1987; 30:1081–8.
55. Revell PA, Mayston V, Lalor P, Mapp P. The synovial membrane in osteoarthritis: a histological study including the characterization of the cellular infiltrate present in inflammatory osteoarthritis using monoclonal antibodies. Ann Rheum Dis 1988; 47:300–7.
56. Goldenberg, DL, Egan MS, Cohen AS. Inflammatory synovitis in degenerative joint disease. J Rheumatol 1982; 9:204–9.
57. Lorenzo JA. Cytokines and bone metabolism: resorption and formation. In: Kimball ES, ed. Cytokines and inflammation. Boca Raton: CRC Press, 1991:145–68.
58. Arend WP, Dayer JM. Cytokines and cytokine inhibitors or antagonists in rheumatoid arthritis. Arthritis Rheum 1990; 33:305–15.
59. Gravallese EM, Darling JM, Ladd AL, Katz JN, Glimcher LH. In situ hybridization studies of stromelysin and collagenase messenger RNA expression in rheumatoid synovium. Arthritis Rheum 1991; 34:1076–84.
60. Harris ED Jr, Faulkner CS II, Brown FE. Collagenolytic systems in rheumatoid arthritis. Clin Orthop 1975; 110:303–16.
61. Fridovich I. The biology of oxygen radicals. Science 1978; 201:875–80.
62. McCord JM. Free radicals and inflammation: protection of synovial fluid by superoxide dismutase. Science 1974; 185:529–31.
63. Greenwald RA. Oxygen radicals, inflammation, and arthritis: pathophysiological considerations and implications for treatment. Semin Arthritis Rheum 1991; 20(suppl 2):219–40.
64. Myint P, Deeble DJ, Beaumont PC, Blake SM, Phillips GO. The reactivity of various free radicals with hyaluronic acid: steady state and pulse radiolysis studies. Biochim Biophys Acta 1987; 925:194–202.
65. Andley UP, Chakrabarti B. Role of singlet oxygen in the degradation of hyaluronic acid. Biochem Biophys Res Commun 1983; 115:894–901.
66. Puig-Parellada P, Planas JM. Synovial fluid degradation induced by free radicals. In vitro action of several free radical scavengers and anti-inflammatory drugs. Biochem Pharmacol 1978; 27:535–7.

67. Betts WH, Cleland LG. Effect of metal chelators and anti-inflammatory drugs on the degradation of hyaluronic acid. Arthritis Rheum 1982; 25:1469–76.
68. Carlin G, Djursater R, Smedegard G, Gerdin B. Effect of anti-inflammatory drugs on xanthine oxidase and xanthine oxidase-induced depolymerization of hyaluronic acid. Agents Actions 1985; 16:377–84.
69. Manicourt DH, Howell DS, Moskowitz RW, Goldberg VM, Malemud C, Pita JC. Application of new techniques to separation of proteoglycan aggregates from normal and destabilized rabbit articular cartilages. Acta Biol Hung 1984; 35:137–42.
70. Manicourt DH, Howell DS, Pita JC, Moskowitz RW, Goldberg V, Malemud C. Studies of cartilage proteoglycans in an osteoarthritic rabbit model. In: Peyron JG, ed. Osteoarthritis—current clinical and fundamental problems. Paris: CIBA-Geigy Press, 1985:192–202.
71. Roberts CR, Mort JS, Roughley PJ. Treatment of cartilage proteoglycan aggregate with hydrogen peroxide. Relationship between observed degradation products and those that occur naturally during aging. Biochem J 1987; 247:349–57.
72. Roberts CR, Roughley PJ, Mort JS. Degradation of human proteoglycan aggregate induced by hydrogen peroxide. Protein fragmentation, amino acid modification and hyaluronic acid cleavage. Biochem J 1989; 259:805–11.
73. Nguyen Q, Liu J, Roughley PJ, Mort JS. Link protein as a monitor in situ of endogenous proteolysis in adult human articular cartilage. Biochem J 1991; 278:143–7.
74. Tiku ML, Liesch JB, Robertson FM. Production of hydrogen peroxide by rabbit articular chondrocytes. Enhancement by cytokines. J Immunol 1990; 145:690–6.
75. Weiss SJ, Peppin G, Ortiz X, Ragsdale C, Test ST. Oxidative autoactivation of latent collagenase by human neutrophils. Science 1985; 227:747–9.
76. Hess EV, Herman JH. Cartilage metabolism and anti-inflammatory drugs in osteoarthritis. Am J Med 1986; 81(suppl):36–43.
77. Bjelle A. NSAID and cartilage metabolism. Scand J Rheumatol 1988; 77(suppl):43–52.
78. Fujii K, Tajiri S, Kajiwara T, Tanaka T, Murota K. Effects of NSAID on collagen and proteoglycan synthesis by cultured chondrocytes. J Rheumatol 1989; 16(suppl 18):28–31.
79. Benton H, Tyler JA. Inhibition of cartilage proteoglycan synthesis by interleukin 1. Biochem Biophys Res Commun 1988; 154:421–8.
80. Tyler JA, Benton HP. Synthesis of type II collagen is decreased in cartilage cultured with interleukin 1 while the rate of intracellular degradation remains unchanged. Coll Relat Res 1988; 8:393–405.
81. Bayliss MT, Vilim V, Hardingham TE, Muir H. Age-related changes in the biosynthetic response of human articular cartilage to IL-1 [abstract]. Trans Orthop Res Soc 1989; 14: 329.
82. van Beuningen HM, Arntz OJ, van den Berg WB. In vivo effects of interleukin-1 on articular cartilage: age-related differences [abstract]. Trans Orthop Res Soc 1990; 15:327.
83. Dingle JT. Cartilage maintenance in osteoarthritis: interaction of cytokines, NSAID and prostaglandins in articular cartilage damage and repair. J Rheumatol 1991; 18(suppl 28):30–7.
84. Bjelle A, Eronen I. The in vitro effect of six NSAIDs on the glycosaminoglycan metabolism of rabbit chondrocytes. Clin Exp Rheumatol 1991; 9:369–74.
85. Palmoski MJ, Brandt KD. Benoxaprofen stimulates proteoglycan synthesis in normal canine knee cartilage in vitro. Arthritis Rheum 1983; 26:771–4.
86. Palmoski MJ, Brandt KD. Effects of some nonsteroidal anti-inflammatory drugs on proteoglycan metabolism and organization in canine articular cartilage. Arthritis Rheum 1989; 23:1010–20.
87. Pelletier JP, Cloutier JM, Martel-Pelletier J. In vitro effects of tiaprofenic acid, sodium salicylate and hydrocortisone on the proteoglycan metabolism of human osteoarthritic cartilage. J Rheumatol 1989; 16:646–55.
88. Muir H, Carney SL, Hall LG: Effects of tiaprofenic acid and other NSAIDs on proteoglycan metabolism in articular cartilage explants. Drugs 1988; 35(suppl 1):15–23.
89. Ratcliffe A, Azzo W, Saed-Nejad F, Lane N, Rosenwasser MP, Mow VC. In vivo effects

of naproxen on composition, proteoglycan metabolism, and matrix metalloproteinase activities in canine articular cartilage. J Orthop Res 1993; 11:163–171.

90. McKenzie LS, Horsburgh BA, Ghosh P, Taylor TKF. Effect of anti-inflammatory drugs on sulphated glycosaminoglycan synthesis in aged human articular cartilage. Ann Rheum Dis 1976; 35:487–97.
91. Palmoski MJ, Brandt KD. Relationship between matrix proteoglycan content and the effects of salicylate and indomethacin on articular cartilage. Arthritis Rheum 1983; 26:528–31.
92. Collier S, Ghosh P. Comparison of the effects of non-steroidal anti-inflammatory drugs (NSAIDs) on proteoglycan synthesis by articular cartilage explant and chondrocyte monolayer cultures. Biochem Pharmacol 1991; 41:1375–84.
93. Brandt KD, Palmoski MJ. Effect of salicylates and other non-steroidal anti-inflammatory drugs on articular cartilage. Am J Med 1984; 77(suppl 1A):65–9.
94. Bostrom H, Bernsten K, Whitehouse MW. Biochemical properties of anti-inflammatory drugs. II. Some effects on sulphate-^{35}S metabolism in vivo. Biochem Pharmacol 1964; 13:413–20.
95. Lowther DA, Handley CJ, Gundalach A. Effect of salicylic acid on articular cartilage in organ culture. Pharmacology 1978; 17:50–5.
96. Palmoski MJ, Brandt KD. Effect of salicylate on proteoglycan metabolism in normal canine articular cartilage in vitro. Arthritis Rheum 1979; 22:746–54.
97. Malemud CJ, Moskowitz RW, Papay RS. Correlation of the biosynthesis of prostaglandin and cyclic AMP in monolayer cultures of rabbit articular chondrocytes. Biochim Biophys Acta 1982; 715:70–9.
98. Malemud CJ, Papay RS. Stimulation of cyclic AMP in chondrocyte cultures: effects on sulfated proteoglycan synthesis. FEBS Lett 1984; 167:343–51.
99. Malemud CJ, Mills TM, Shuckett R, Papay RS. Stimulation of sulfated proteoglycan synthesis by forskolin in monolayer cultures of rabbit articular chondrocytes. J Cell Physiol 1986; 129:51–9.
100. Malemud CJ, Papay RS, Hasler P, Kammer GM. cAMP-dependent protein kinase in chondrocyte cultures: holoenzyme activation, phosphorylation of cellular proteins, effects of NSAIDs and possible role in proteoglycan synthesis. Semin Arthritis Rheum 1990; 19(suppl 1):10–5.
101. Collier S, Ghosh P. Evaluation of the effects of anti-arthritic drugs on the secretion of proteoglycans by lapine chondrocytes using a novel assay procedure. Ann Rheum Dis 1989; 48:372–81.
102. Rashad S, Revell P, Hemingway A, Low F, Rainsford K, Walker F. Effect of nonsteroidal anti-inflammatory drugs on the course of osteoarthritis. Lancet 1989; 2:519–22.
103. Kalben DA. Chemical model of osteoarthritis: a pharmacological evaluation. J Rheumatol 1987; 14(suppl):130–1.
104. Williams JM, Brandt KD. Triamcinolone hexacetonide protects against fibrillation and osteophyte formation following chemically induced articular cartilage damage. Arthritis Rheum 1985; 28:1267–74.
105. Williams JM, Brandt KD. Benoxaprofen reduces osteophyte formation and fibrillation after articular cartilage injury. J Rheumatol 1985; 12:27–32.
106. Butler M, Colombo C, Hickman L, O'Byrne E, Steele R, Steinetz B, Quintavalla J, Yokoyama N. A new model of osteoarthritis in rabbits: III. Evaluation of antiosteoarthritic effects of selected drugs administered intra-articularly. Arthritis Rheum 1983; 26:1380–6.
107. Colombo C, Butler M, Hickman L, Selwyn M, Chart J, Steinetz B. A new model of osteoarthritis in rabbits: II. Evaluation of anti-osteoarthritic effects of selected antirheumatic drugs administered systematically. Arthritis Rheum 1983; 26:1132–9.
108. Maier R, Wilhelmi G. Preclinical investigations of drug effects in models of osteoarthrosis. In: Munthe E, Bjelle A, eds. Effects of drugs on osteoarthrosis. Proceedings of the 10th European congress of rheumatology, Moscow, 1983. Berne: Hans Huber 1984:90–6.
109. Herman JH, Appel AM, Khosla RC, Hess EV. The in vitro effect of select classes of

nonsteroidal antiinflammatory drugs on normal cartilage metabolism. J Rheumatol 1986; 13:1014–8.

110. McKenzie LS, Horsburgh BA, Ghosh P, Taylor TKF. Effect of anti-inflammatory drugs on sulphated glycosaminoglycan synthesis in aged human articular cartilage. Ann Rheum Dis 1976; 35:487–97.
111. Vignon E, Mathieu P, Broquet P, Louisot P, Richard M. Cartilage degradative enzymes in human osteoarthritis: effect of a nonsteroidal antiinflammatory drug administered orally. Semin Arthritis Rheum 1990; 19(suppl 1):26–9.
112. Pelletier JP, Martel-Pelletier J. In vivo protective effects of prophylactic treatment with tiaprofenic acid or intra-articular corticosteroids on osteoarthritic lesions in the experimental dog model. J Rheumatol 1991; 18(suppl 27):127–30.
113. Mahmud F, Rosenwasser MP, Nesad-Saed F, Lane N, Mow VC, Rateliffe A. The in vivo effect of naproxen on canine OA articular cartilage. Arthritis Rheum 1991; 34:S=86.
114. Verbruggen G, Veys EM, Malfait AM, Cockez P, Schatteman L, Wieme N, Heynen G, Broddelez C. Proteoglycan metabolism in tissue-cultured human articular cartilage: influence of piroxicam. J Rheumatol 1989; 16:355–62.
115. McGuire MB, Murphy G, Reynolds JJ, Russell RGG. Production of collagenase and inhibitor (TIMP) by normal, rheumatoid and osteoarthritic synovium in vitro: effects of hydrocortisone and indomethacin. Clin Sci 1981; 61:703–10.
116. Mochan E, Uhl J, Newton R. Evidence that interleukin-1 induction of synovial cell plasminogen activator is mediated via prostaglandin E_2 and cAMP. Arthritis Rheum 1986; 29:1078–84.
117. Fibbi G, Serni U, Pucci M, Caldini R, Magnelli L, Del Rosso M. Plasminogen activators and tiaprofenic acid in inflammation. A preliminary study. Drugs 1988; 35(suppl 1):9–14.
118. Persico FJ. Low molecular weight inhibitors of interleukin-1. In: Kimball ES, ed. Cytokines and inflammation. Boca Raton FL: CRC Press, 1991:59–87.
119. Kovacs EJ. Control of IL-1 and TNF-α production at the level of second messenger pathways. In: Kimball ES, ed. Cytokines and inflammation. Boca Raton FL: CRC Press, 1991:89–107.
120. Mauviel A, Temime N, Charron D, Loyau G, Pujol JP. Interleukin-1α and β induce interleukin-1β gene expression in human dermal fibroblasts. Biochem Biophys Res Commun 1988; 156:1209–14.
121. Otterness IG, Bliven ML, Downs JT, Hanson DC. Effects of CP-66,248 on IL-1 synthesis by murine peritoneal macrophages. Arthritis Rheum (abstract) 1988; 31:S90.
122. McDonald B, Loose L, Rosenwasser LJ. The influence of a novel arachidonate inhibitor, CP66,248 on the production and activity of human monocyte IL-1. Arthritis Rheum (abstract) 1988; 31:S17.
123. Sipe JD, Bartle LM, Loose LD. Modification of proinflammatory cytokine production by the antirheumatic agents tenidap and naproxen. A possible correlation with clinical acute phase response. J Immunol 1992; 148:480–4.
124. McDonald B, Loose L, Rosenwasser LJ. Synovial fluid IL-1 in RA patients receiving a novel arachidonate inhibitor CP66,248. Arthritis Rheum (abstract) 1988; 31:A88.
125. Lee JC, Griswold DE, Votta B, Hanna N. Inhibition of monocyte IL-1 production by the anti-inflammatory compound, SK&F 86002. Int J Immunopharmacol 1988; 7:835–43.
126. DiMartino MJ, Griswold DE, Berkowitz BA, Poste G, Hanna N. Pharmacologic characterization of the anti-inflammatory profiles of a new dual inhibitor of lipoxygenase and cyclooxygenase. Agents Actions 1987; 20:113–23.
127. Rainsford KD. Effects of antiinflammatory drugs on the release from porcine synovial tissue in vitro of interleukin 1 like cartilage degrading activity. Agents Actions 1987; 21:337–40.
128. Vignon E, Mathieu P, Couprie N, Cloppet H, Herbage D, Louisot P, Richard M. Effects of tiaprofenic acid on interleukin-1, phospholipase A_2 activity, prostaglandins, neutral protease and collagenase activity in rheumatoid synovial fluid. Semin Arthritis Rheum 1989; 18(suppl 1):11–5.

129. Pelletier JP, McCollum R, DiBattista J, Loose LD, Cloutier JM, Martel-Pelletier J: Regulation of human normal and osteoarthritic chondrocyte interleukin-1 receptor by antirheumatic drugs. Arthritis Rheum, 1993 (In Press).
130. Chang DM, Baptiste P, Schur PH. The effect of antirheumatic drugs on interleukin 1 (IL-1) activity and IL-1 and IL-1 inhibitor production by human monocytes. J Rheumatol 1990; 17:1148–57.
131. Haataja M, Fräki JE, Vainio E. Effect of antirheumatic drugs on proteinases in synovia of patients with rheumatoid arthritis. Int J Clin Pharmacol Biopharm 1978; 16:417–9.
132. De Vries BJ, van den Berg WB. Impact of NSAIDs on murine antigen induced arthritis. II. A light microscopic investigation of antiinflammatory and bone protective effects. J Rheumatol 1990; 17:295–303.
133. De Vries BJ, van den Berg WB. Impact of NSAIDs on murine antigen induced arthritis. I. An investigation of antiinflammatory and chondroprotective effects. J Rheumatol 1989; 18(suppl):10–8.
134. Blackburn WD Jr., Loose LD, Heck LW, Chatham WW. Tenidap in contrast to several available nonsteroidal anti-inflammatory drugs, potentially inhibits the release of activated neutrophil collagenase. Arthritis Rheum 1991; 34:211–6.
135. Harris ED Jr, Emkey RD, Nichols JE, Newberg A. Low dose prednisone therapy in rheumatoid arthritis: a double blind study. J Rheumatol 1983; 10:713–21.
136. Campion G, Schnitzer T, Zcitz H, Lenz ME, Lindeman M, Thonar E. The effect of oral administration of prednisone and the non-steroidal anti-inflammatory drugs piroxicam and naproxen on serum levels of keratan sulfate (KS) [abstract]. Trans Orthop Res Soc (abstract) 1990; 15:334.
137. Glass D, Russel AS, Snaith ML, Daly JR. Possible unnecessary prolongation of corticosteroid therapy in rheumatoid arthritis. Lancet 1971; 2:334–7.
138. Behrens F, Shepard N, Mitchell N. Metabolic recovery of articular cartilage after intra-articular injections of glucocorticoid. J Bone Joint Surg 1976; 58A:1157–60.
139. Mankin HJ, Conger KA. The acute effects of intra-articular hydrocortisone on articular cartilage in rabbits. J Bone Joint Surg 1966; 48A:1383–8.
140. Moskowitz RW, Davis W, Sammarco J, Mast W, Chase SW. Experimentally induced corticosteroid arthropathy. Arthritis Rheum 1970; 13:236–43.
141. Salter RB, Gross A, Hall JH. Hydrocortisone arthropathy: an experimental investigation. Can Med J 1976; 97:374–7.
142. Silberberg M, Silberberg R, Hasler M. Fine structure of articular cartilage in mice receiving cortisone acetate. Arch Pathol 1966; 82:569–82.
143. Moskowitz RW, Goldberg VM, Schwab W, Berman L. Effects of intra-articular corticosteroids and exercise in experimental models of inflammatory and degenerative arthritis [abstract]. Arthritis Rheum 1975; 18:417.
144. Pelletier JP, Martel-Pelletier J. Protective effects of corticosteroids on cartilage lesions and osteophyte formation in the Pond–Nuki dog model of osteoarthritis. Arthritis Rheum 1989; 32:181–93.
145. Keagy RD, Keim HA. Intra-articular steroid therapy: repeated use in patients with chronic arthritis. Am J Med Sci 1967; 253:45–51.
146. Saxne T, Heingegård D, Wollheim FA. Therapeutic effects on cartilage metabolism in arthritis as measured by release of proteoglycan structures into the synovial fluid. Ann Rheum Dis 1986; 45:491–7.
147. Firestein GS, Paine MM, Littman BH. Gene expression (collagenase, tissue inhibitor of metalloproteinases, complement, and HLA-DR) in rheumatoid arthritis and osteoarthritis synovium. Quantitative analysis and effects of intra-articular corticosteroids. Arthritis Rheum 1991; 34:1094–105.
148. Hamilton JA, Bootes A, Phillips PE, Slywka J. Human synovial fibroblast plasminogen activator: modulation of enzyme activity by antiinflammatory steroids. Arthritis Rheum 1981; 24:1296–303.

149. Snyder DS, Unanue ER. Corticosteroids inhibit murine macrophage Ia expression and interleukin 1 production. J Immunol 1982; 129:1803–5.
150. Lee SW, Tsou AP, Chan H, Thomas J, Petrie K, Eugui EM, Allison AC. Glucocorticosteroids selectively inhibit the transcription of the interleukin 1β gene and decrease the stability of interleukin-1β mRNA. Proc Natl Acad Sci USA 1988; 85:1204–8.
151. DiBattista JA, Martel-Pelletier J, Wosu LO. Sandor T, Antakly T, Pelletier JP. Glucocorticoid receptor mediated inhibition of interleukin-1 stimulated neutral metalloprotease synthesis in normal human chondrocytes. J Clin Endocrinol Metab 1991; 72:316–326.
152. DiBattista JA, Martel-Pelletier J, Antakly T, Tardif G, Cloutier JM, Pelletier JP. Reduced expression of glucocorticoid receptor levels in human osteoarthritic chondrocytes. Role in the suppression of metalloprotease synthesis. J Clin Endocrinol, 1993 (in press).
153. DiBattista JA, Martel-Pelletier J, Faure MP, Antakly T, Pelletier JP. Reduced expression of glucocorticoid receptors in osteoarthritis (OA) chondrocytes [abstract]. Arthritis Rheum 1990; 33:S30.
154. Bloom E, Matulick DT, Lan NC, Higgins SJ, Simons SS, Baxter JD. Nuclear binding of glucocorticoid receptor: relations between cytosol binding, activation and the biological response. J Steroid Biochem 1980; 12:175–84.
155. DiBattista JA, Martel-Pelletier J, Cloutier JM, Pelletier JP. Modulation of glucocorticoid receptor expression in human articular chondrocytes by cAMP and prostaglandins. J Rheumatol 1991; 18(suppl 27):102–5.

2

Nonsteroidal Anti-Inflammatory Drugs in Migraine

SEYMOUR DIAMOND
Diamond Headache Clinic
Chicago, Illinois
and Chicago Medical School
North Chicago, Illinois

I. INTRODUCTION

The nonsteroidal anti-inflammatory agents (NSAIDs) play a vital role in treatment of migraine headaches. By becoming familiar with the indications for their use, the clinician can facilitate successful therapy for many refractory types of migraine. The various pharmacological actions of these drugs provide evidence for utilizing these agents in the treatment of migraine headache.

II. MIGRAINE HEADACHES

The debate over the etiology of migraine has continued to flare for many centuries. Headache researchers have assumed sides on whether migraine is a vascular or neurogenic disorder. The role of the vasoactive substances in migraine has also been contested.

Researchers have identified the role of the prostaglandins in triggering an acute migraine attack (1). As prostaglandin inhibitors, the NSAIDs vary widely in chemical structure; however, they do affect a uniform decrease in prostaglandin synthesis by the inhibition of cyclooxygenase. The potency of the NSAIDs may be attributed to this action (2).

In migraine, the release of vasoactive substances has been observed with abnormal platelet aggregation (3). Most NSAIDs are known to have platelet antiaggregant action (4). Migraine researchers have continually implicated serotonin in the etiology of migraine. Serotonin is almost entirely transported in the blood by the platelets. During the initial stage of a migraine attack, plasma serotonin increases, and the level decreases as the attack continues to peak (5). Indoleacetic acid (5HIAA) is the primary breakdown product of serotonin and is excessively excreted in the urine of some patients during an acute migraine episode (6).

The use of NSAIDs in the treatment of migraine is not a recent innovation. The analgesic action of aspirin has long sanctioned its use in the abortive treatment of headaches, including migraine. Its use as a platelet antagonist has long been recognized. In 1964, Sicuteri's group reported on the antimigraine properties of indomethacin (7). Anthony and Lance, in 1968, also investigated the use of indomethacin in migraine (8). Studies concerning these agents in the abortive and prophylactic treatment of migraine have increased as the number of available NSAIDs have multiplied.

A. Abortive Therapy

In their classic treatment review of the NSAIDs in migraine, Pradalier's group noted that a drug must have certain characteristics to be effective in treating an acute migraine attack (4), including a high level of bioavailability, with an early and high serum peak and an absence of serious side effects. Various researchers have conducted investigations into the use of NSAIDs in the treatment of acute migraine attacks. In most studies, the NSAID agent has been superior to placebo and equivalent reference drugs. The following will summarize reports on specific agents.

1. Aspirin

The availability of aspirin has afforded its easy access to migraine patients in their quest for relief of an acute attack. During an initial interview, many patients will relate that aspirin is not effective for their severe attacks, and the associated nausea and vomiting precluded the use of this agent. In Volans' study (9), the salicylate levels were lower during acute migraine attacks in patients using aspirin for migraine abortive therapy. The plasma salicylate levels increased when the aspirin was given in combination with intramuscular (IM) metoclopramide (an antinauseant that increases normal gastric motility). The author suggested that aspirin absorption was delayed, and possibly diminished, during migraine attacks because of altered gastric motility.

Ross-Lee's group (10) felt that Volans study was limited, and examined both plasma salicylate and plasma aspirin levels during a migraine attack treated with aspirin, 900 mg; aspirin, 900 mg, and oral metoclopramide, 10 mg; or aspirin, 900 mg, and IM metoclopramide, 10 mg. For those patients receiving aspirin and metoclopramide, increases were observed in both plasma aspirin and plasma salicylate levels. Aspirin appeared earlier in the plasma of patients receiving aspirin and oral metoclopramide, than in those receiving aspirin alone or aspirin with intramuscular metoclopramide. The group receiving aspirin and oral metoclopramide also reported more rapid relief than the other groups; however, 1 h after receiving therapy, the patients receiving aspirin and IM metoclopramide reported a higher level of pain relief.

In a later study, Ross-Lee's group conducted a retrospective study of 61 patients, examining the use of soluble aspirin in the treatment of acute migraine (11). Complete or almost complete relief of the attacks was achieved by 44% of the patients. Sixteen percent of the patients reported adverse effects, such as nausea and vomiting, which may have been due to the migraine, rather than the drug. Patients experiencing an aura preceding the attack demonstrated a better response to aspirin, possibly owing to the absorption of the drug early in the attack. The authors did note that in contrast with a double-blind study, a retrospective study is limited in its scope. The study was further limited, as the patients were all migraine patients referred to a consultant neurological practice, and thus it did not offer the broad base of a multicenter study.

The studies by Ross-Lee's group (10,11) prompted Japanese researchers to report on the efficacy of intravenous (IV) aspirin in acute migraine attacks (12). In three patients receiving IV aspirin during a migraine attack, the pain disappeared within 15 min. The authors suggested that the rapid effect could be attributed to prompt inhibition of prostaglandins, as the headache was established by the time the aspirin was administered. In considering these studies on the use of aspirin and acute migraine attacks, the necessity for further studies is apparent. These results also imply that simple analgesics, including aspirin and other NSAIDs, may be substituted, in some patients, for the habituating analgesics and ergotamine preparations.

2. *Ibuprofen*

The popularity of ibuprofen as an analgesic has boomed since its introduction to the over-the-counter market. In 1984 alone, about 1 billion prescription tablets were used, and 1.5 billion over-the-counter preparations of ibuprofen were sold in the United States (13). Studies have reviewed the benefits of this agent in tension-type headaches, and the need for investigations with acute migraine did emerge.

In an 1983 study, ibuprofen was evaluated in a randomized double-blind, controlled trial in comparison with paracetamol (acetaminophen) in the abortive treatment of migraine (14). At the onset of an acute migraine attack, each of the 30 patients was instructed to use two capsules of either ibuprofen 200 mg or paracetamol 450 mg. The patients were to maintain a monthly diary to report up to ten migraine attacks during the month of treatment. In the final analysis of 27 patients, only 22 completed the crossover, 23 completed treatment with ibuprofen, and 26 with paracetamol. Although both drugs reduced the severity of the headache, ibuprofen also decreased the duration of the attack. No statistically significant differences were demonstrated between the two agents for side effect profile. These investigators believed that ibuprofen was a welcome addition to the armamentarium of migraine abortive agents.

A more recent study examined the efficacy of a prescription dose (800 mg) of ibuprofen for the abortive treatment of migraine (15). Forty patients, diagnosed with either migraine with aura (classic) or migraine without aura (common), participated in a double-blind, crossover, randomized clinical trial. At the onset of the attack, the patient would take either ibuprofen, 800 mg, or placebo and, if needed, could take an additional 400-mg dose 30–60 min after the initial dose. If the headache persisted 3 h after the first dose, the patient could use rescue medications, which were the same agents they used before entry to the study. Each treatment protocol was used for five migraine attacks. A total of ten migraine attacks were studied for 27 patients, and 12 were studied for five to nine attacks. The mean duration of migraine attacks treated with ibuprofen was 4.9 ± 2.9 h, compared with 11.2 ± 8.6 for placebo. In grading the severity of the attacks, ibuprofen showed a significant improvement rate over placebo. Of those treated with ibuprofen, 33% graded the headache as mild, 53% as moderate, and 14% as severe. The placebo group noted mild headache in 7%, moderate in 67%, and severe in 26%. The need for rescue medication was noted by 22% of the ibuprofen group and 81% of the placebo group. The differences between the groups for side effects, such as nausea and vomiting, was insignificant.

3. *Naproxen and Naproxen Sodium*

Several investigators have examined the efficacy of naproxen and naproxen sodium in the treatment of acute migraine. Naproxen is considered a potent NSAID that strongly inhibits prostaglandin synthesis, platelet aggregation, and serotonin release. Because earlier studies had demonstrated its effectiveness in the prophylactic therapy of migraine

(16), Johnson's group undertook a randomized, double-blind parallel group study comparing the efficacy of naproxen sodium and placebo in migraine attacks (17). Seventy patients with migraine, with or without aura, participated in the study. Each patient was treated for ten attacks with either 3 tablets of naproxen sodium, 275 mg, or placebo, to be used at the first signs of an acute migraine. If the headache had improved or remained the same, the patient could use an additional 2 tablets of naproxen sodium, 275 mg, or placebo. However, if the patient's symptoms had increased, the patient was offered a rescue combination analgesic of paracetamol, 1000 mg, and metoclopramide, 10 mg. The patients were assessed on a monthly basis. Significant improvement was demonstrated in both severity and duration of headaches in patients using naproxen sodium. The need for rescue analgesics had also decreased in the active drug group. Side effects, including gastrointestinal symptoms, were reported by 10% of the patients, and could also be attributed to the rescue medications.

In a Scandinavian study, naproxen was compared with placebo in the treatment of acute migraine attacks (18). The protocol involved a double-blind, crossover, randomized trial using naproxen, 750 mg, or placebo at the onset of an acute migraine attack. Of the 40 patients enrolled in the study, 32 completed the two treatment periods of either six migraine attacks or 3 months, whichever occurred first, and were then switched to the alternate treatment. At the initial symptom of an attack, the patient was to use 3 tablets of either naproxen, 250 mg, or placebo. The patients were permitted to use an additional tablet, up to 5 tablets in any 24-h period. Rescue medication, which had been used before entry to the study, could be used within 2 h after onset of the attack. In reviewing the results, the investigators noted that naproxen was superior, in comparison with placebo, in reducing the severity and duration of the headaches. Side effects, including nausea, vomiting, lightheadedness, and photophobia, were also reduced in patients using naproxen. The need for rescue medication was also diminished, and both patients and physicians preferred naproxen.

These results were confirmed in a later study by Andersson's group (19), with a similar double-blind, crossover trial. The headache severity was significantly decreased with naproxen ($p = 0.047$) in the first 2 h of the migraine attack.

The efficacy of naproxen sodium in migraine attacks versus placebo prompted Pradalier's group to compare this agent with an ergotamine tartrate compound (20), the most widely used therapy for migraine abortive therapy. A randomized, parallel trial involving 114 patients was undertaken with treatment periods of 3 months or six attacks, whichever occurred first. At the first signs of a migraine attack, patients consumed either 3 tablets of naproxen sodium, 275 mg, or 1 tablet of a combination agent containing ergotamine tartrate, 2 mg; caffeine, 91.5 mg; and cyclizine chlorhydrate, 50 mg. The duration and severity of the attacks were substantially decreased by both agents. If the study medications were consumed within 2 h of the onset of the attack, naproxen sodium demonstrated significant improvement over the ergotamine agent in reducing headache severity, nausea, and lightheadedness. An increase in vomiting, the need for rescue medications, and side effects was associated with ergotamine consumption. The tolerance for naproxen sodium was judged superior to ergotamine by investigators and patients. They concluded that naproxen sodium was a safe and effective agent for migraine abortive therapy.

A similar study was conducted in a multicenter United States study that employed a double-blind, parallel protocol investigating six headaches over a 3-month period (21). At the enrollment of the 161 subjects, each patient was randomly assigned to one of three treatment protocols: naproxen sodium, 825 mg; ergotamine tartrate, 2 mg, with caffeine; or placebo. The study medication was to be used at the first sign of a headache. A second dose could be repeated 30 min later, if needed, and rescue medication could be employed 30 min after the second dose. Final analysis of the data was conducted on 122 patients, with 39 patients in the naproxen sodium group, 41 treated with ergotamine, and 42 in the placebo group. At 1 h following the first dose, naproxen sodium showed superior efficacy over placebo ($p = 0.032$). The difference was not statistically significant for ergotamine versus placebo ($p = 0.084$), nor for naproxen sodium versus ergotamine ($p = 0.65$). Increased nausea was noted in the ergotamine group from 30 to 120 min after the first dose. However, a decrease in nausea was noted in the same time period for the naproxen sodium group. Better relief of nausea, photophobia, lightheadedness, and motor symptoms was noted for the naproxen sodium group at 1 h after the first dose, in contrast with the results demonstrated by the ergotamine group. Vomiting was also decreased in the naproxen sodium group, compared with the other two groups. The authors concluded that naproxen sodium is superior in efficacy to placebo, is as effective as ergotamine, and is better tolerated than ergotamine. The decreased frequency and severity of nausea and decreased vomiting was significant in the naproxen sodium group.

4. *Mefenamic Acid*

The efficacy of naproxen in migraine abortive therapy prompted investigators to study other NSAIDs. The derivatives of fenamic acid have been demonstrated to reduce the synthesis of prostaglandins, but also the actions of exogenous prostaglandins in vitro (22). Mefenamic acid was the first of this group to be developed. In an open trial in 1968, it was found to be effective as an analgesic in migraine therapy (23). A double-blind, controlled study of this agent in migraine abortive therapy was not undertaken until 1983 (24). Forty migraine patients were enrolled in the study, which would consist of six consecutive migraine attacks. The patients were randomly selected for two groups, and for each migraine attack, they were provided metoclopramide, 10 mg; mefenamic acid, 500 mg, or a matching placebo; and paracetamol, 500 mg, or matching placebo. In the first three attacks, they would take either of the active drugs and would switch in the last three attacks. The medications were to be taken as early as possible in the attack. Aspirin, 600 mg, was used as a rescue medication, to be taken 3 h after the trial medication, if the symptoms had not resolved. The aspirin could be repeated every 4 h, if necessary.

Twenty-two patients completed the study; 12 patients used mefenamic acid for the first three attacks and 10 used paracetamol for the first three attacks. Headache intensity was reduced by 36 ± 11% with mefenamic acid, and 27 ± 10% with paracetamol. Although this difference is not statistically significant, the authors noted a 28% probability exists that mefenamic acid is twice as potent as paracetamol as an analgesic. They concluded that the minimal difference between the two analgesics could suggest that peripheral prostaglandin-mediated pain pathways, in which paracetamol is inactive, may be less significant than central pathways, which are inhibited by both drugs.

5. *Diclofenac Sodium*

Investigations of the NSAID, diclofenac sodium, in the treatment of acute migraine, were initiated owing to its action of inhibiting prostaglandin biosynthesis (25), thereby increasing the release of plasma β-endorphins (26). In the United States, this drug is available only in an oral preparation. However, an Italian study examined its effectiveness in a parenteral form (27). In a double-blind, crossover trial, diclofenac sodium was compared with placebo (physiological solution) in 40 migraine patients who were experiencing at least one migraine attack per week. For the treatment of three consecutive migraine attacks, the patients were randomly given diclofenac sodium, 75 mg IM, or matched placebo, IM. The alternative preparation was administered for the next three consecutive attacks. If the headache was still present 6 h after administration, the patient was given diclofenac sodium, 100 mg, by rectal suppository. No other rescue drugs were to be taken during the study period. Patients treated with diclofenac sodium were significantly improved ($p < 0.001$) over those patients given placebo. A decrease in associated symptoms, such as photophobia, nausea, and vomiting, was also superior in patients treated with diclofenac sodium ($p < 0.01$), compared with those given placebo. The patients also expressed a preference for diclofenac sodium ($p < 0.001$). Because of this preference for the active drug, the authors suggested that the tolerance to the drug was similar to placebo.

In a recent study, the oral form of diclofenac sodium was evaluated in the treatment of acute attacks of migraine without aura (28). A double-blind, placebo-controlled, crossover protocol was used in a multicenter trial. The 107 patients enrolled in the study had been experiencing two to eight migraine attacks on a monthly basis for at least 2 years. Each patient was treated for four consecutive migraine attacks; two attacks with diclofenac, 50 mg tablets, and two with matching placebo. The patients were instructed to use the medication within 30 min of the onset of the headache. At 1 h after the first dose, the patient was permitted to use another tablet if the symptoms warranted a repeat dose. Rescue medications, excluding aspirin and other NSAIDs, were permitted 2 h after the initial dose. Ninety patients were included in the final analysis. The need for a second tablet was demonstrated in 87% of the patients treated with placebo, whereas 78% of the patients treated with diclofenac sodium required a second dose. At 2 h after the initial dose, the treatment was considered a success if the pain had decreased significantly or the duration of the attack was less than 2 h. The therapy was considered a failure if the patient's symptoms had decreased within 2 h after the initial dose, but relapsed within 24 h. Of the 186 attacks treated with diclofenac, 51 (27%) aborted within 2h, whereas only 35 (19%) of the attacks resolved on placebo. In 54% of the patients treated with diclofenac, escape medications were needed. However, 66% of those treated with placebo required rescue medications 2 h after the initial dose. Evaluation of the drug efficacy by both the physician and the patient was superior for the diclofenac ($p < 0.005$). Many patients complained of gastrointestinal distress following treatments; however, owing to the nature of migraine, it was difficult to attribute the gastrointestinal symptoms to the drug or to the actual migraine attack.

During this investigation, the proposed guidelines of the International Headache Society (IHS) on controlled studies in migraine were formulated. According to the recommendations of the IHS, the main parameter of efficacy is the number of attacks aborted within 2 h of drug intake. This parameter was selected because it is clinically relevant, simple, and is not affected by rescue medications (29). According to this criterion, diclofenac was significantly more effective than placebo in aborting migraine attacks. Diclofenac also demonstrated better results than placebo in reducing the intensity of the headache attack after 2 h, as well as duration of the attack, and need for rescue medications. The authors concluded that oral diclofenac is a viable agent for migraine abortive therapy. Unfortunately, oral preparations may not be the preferred route owing to the gastrointestinal symptoms, and the development of diclofenac suppositories may be indicated.

6. *Miscellaneous*

Other NSAIDs have been investigated for efficacy in migraine abortive therapy; however, these agents are not available in the United States. The NSAIDs include tiaprofenic acid (30), pirprofen (31), and tolfenamic acid (32). Each agent was beneficial in the treatment of the acute migraine attack.

Ketorolac is the first parenteral NSAID available in the United States. Although no definitive studies have been conducted on its use in migraine abortive therapy, the popularity of this drug is increasing in acute headache management. In an open-label trial conducted at an emergency department, ketorolac was administered to 12 consecutive patients presenting with the chief complaint of headache (33). After undergoing a complete history and physical examination, and ascertaining that the patient did not have a sensitivity to ketorolac or any other NSAID, the patient received ketorolac, 60 mg IM. The response to this drug was evaluated at 1 h after its administration. None of the patients required rescue medications, and they were sufficiently improved to leave the emergency department. The authors noted that ketorolac offers the advantage of being nonnarcotic, nonhabituating, and it has a low side effect profile. Double-blind investigations are necessary to determine the efficacy of ketorolac in the abortive treatment of migraine.

B. Prophylactic Therapy

Migraine prophylactic therapy is indicated for patients experiencing two or more attacks per month. This type of therapy should also be considered for patients with less frequent headaches, but whose attacks last 2 days or more, or the acute attacks completely disrupt their daily lives. The goals of prophylactic therapy include preventing the onset of the acute attacks and reducing the frequency and severity of these episodes. The drugs of choice in the prophylaxis of migraine are the β-blockers and, in particular, propranolol. Alternative or adjunct therapeutic agents include the NSAIDs.

1. *Indomethacin*

The first NSAID investigated for migraine prophylaxis was indomethacin (8). The authors recognized its effectiveness as an antipyretic and as an anti-inflammatory in rheumatic diseases. In an earlier study, Sicuteri's group identified headache as a side effect of indomethacin therapy (7). They considered the vasoactive properties of indomethacin and demonstrated that indomethacin, 20 mg injected IV, triggered a decrease in cerebrospinal fluid pressure for several minutes, an episode that could be related to intracranial vasoconstriction. Similar changes were produced by the oral administration of indomethacin, 200 mg.

In the study by Anthony and Lance (8), 38 patients participated in a randomized, double-blind, parallel study comparing indomethacin and placebo in the prophylaxis of migraine. The patients were given either indomethacin, 25 mg, or identical placebo capsules three times daily. At the end of 1 month of treatment, the patients were assessed, and the trial continued with all patients taking indomethacin. During the controlled trial, patients in both groups demonstrated similar results. Fourteen patients demonstrated improvement after 1 month of open trial. After 9 months of active treatment, only three patients remained headache-free. Of the remaining patients, five were lost to follow-up; nine were considered improved, although the acute attacks continued to be very severe; and the remaining patients demonstrated no benefit from indomethacin. Fifteen patients reported side effects, such as indigestion, lightheadedness, insomnia, and feelings of fullness in the head. The authors concluded that indomethacin, 75 mg/day, was not superior to placebo in the management of frequent and severe migraine attacks.

2. Aspirin

In recognition of aspirin's action as a potent inhibitor of prostaglandin synthesis and platelet aggregation, its use in migraine prophylaxis has been investigated. In 1978, a double-blind, crossover study was undertaken comparing aspirin, 650 mg, versus matched placebo, given twice daily (34). Twelve migraine patients participated in the trial, in which each agent was given for 3 consecutive months. Patients were permitted to use abortive therapy for acute migraine attacks. For this study, the investigators defined a positive clinical response as a greater than 50% decrease in migraine frequency over 3 months. Nine patients (75%) demonstrated a positive response to aspirin therapy. The remaining three patients were judged nonresponders. Side effects were limited to three patients who experienced mild gastritis, of which two of the patients were helped with antacid therapy. The authors noted that aspirin inhibits platelet aggregation and secretion of platelet factors, such as serotonin, by preventing synthesis of prostaglandin and thromboxane A_2. No evidence has been documented that human platelets become refractory to the inhibitory effects of aspirin after long-term treatment. If an abnormal platelet function was inherent in migraine patients, then aspirin and similar agents would always be effective. However, previous studies have demonstrated that indomethacin is not always an effective treatment in migraine (33). If the efficacy of aspirin in migraine was related to its analgesic effect alone, acetaminophen could also be a candidate for migraine prophylactic therapy, and this agent has not demonstrated efficacy in migraine prevention. The authors suggest the need for further investigation into aspirin in migraine prophylaxis as it relates to hyperaggregable platelets. They concluded that aspirin is a viable therapeutic agent for migraine prophylaxis. The patient receiving this therapy should be monitored for persistent gastrointestinal complaints and any signs of bleeding in the gastrointestinal tract.

In a recent study, aspirin was compared with metoprolol, a β-blocker, in migraine prophylaxis (35). Twenty-eight migraine patients participated in a double-blind, crossover study. The trial consisted of a run-in period of 8 weeks, with two active treatment periods, each lasting 3 months, one with aspirin and one with metoprolol. During the run-in period, the patients received no prophylactic therapy. For treatment of acute attacks, the patients could use a combination agent of metoclopramide, 10 mg, with acetaminophen, 500 mg. Aspirin was not permitted for abortive therapy. During active treatment, patients were given either 3 capsules of aspirin, 500 mg/day, or 1 capsule of metoprolol, 200 mg, with 2 matched placebo capsules per day. Final analysis was done on the 21 patients who completed the study. In comparison with the run-in period, the frequency of attacks was decreased with aspirin an average of 26 ± 22%, and with metoprolol at 50 ± 18%. The decrease with metoprolol was significantly greater than aspirin ($p < 0.01$). The authors noted that aspirin does demonstrate efficacy in migraine prophylaxis. However, metoprolol was superior in reducing the frequency of acute attacks. They concluded that aspirin should be considered for migraine prophylaxis only in those patients with contraindications to β-blockers or other standard therapeutic agents.

Another study presented during 1990 (36) investigated the effect of low-dose aspirin (325 mg every other day) among 22,071 male physicians in the United States. Follow-up questionnaires were sent annually after the subjects had participated in a randomized, double-blind, placebo-controlled study. The questionnaire requested information on the occurrence of numerous medical conditions, including migraine. Participants in the aspirin group were followed, on average, for 60 months. At the end of this period, 86% of the initial group had received aspirin, and 14% were using placebo. Six percent (661) of those in the aspirin group, reported episodes of migraine during the trial. In the placebo group, 7.4% (818) complained of migraine attacks. With this survey, information could not be gleaned on frequency and severity of migraine attacks. The authors believe that this data suggest low-dose aspirin is indicated for migraine prophylactic therapy.

An editorial in the same issue of *Journal of the American Medical Association* identified some weaknesses in the low-dose aspirin study (37). Primarily, all study subjects were male, and a female preponderance in this condition is universally recognized. Also, the absence of data on aspirin's effects on migraine severity, frequency, and duration, renders some of the findings dubious. Finally, the diagnosis of migraine was based on a self-report questionnaire, and not according to unbiased procedures according to standard criteria. The physicians may have been experiencing chronic tension-type headaches, but classified their attacks as migraine.

3. Naproxen and Naproxen Sodium

In conducting investigations of therapies for variants of cluster headache, including chronic paroxysmal hemicrania, a Norwegian group noted the wide range of clinical effects of the various NSAIDs (38). The efficacy of naproxen in migraine abortive therapy prompted these investigators to examine its efficacy in migraine prophylaxis. The authors acknowledged that naproxen is a potent inhibitor of PGE and $PGE_{2\alpha}$, and would possibly be an excellent choice in the prevention of migraine attacks. Twenty-eight patients participated in a double-blind placebo-controlled crossover trial, including a 2-month drug-free interval. The patients were randomly assigned to two treatment groups; the groups were given naproxen, 250 mg bid, or matching placebo for 6 weeks, and were then switched to the alternate treatment for 6 weeks. All patients received placebo for 1 week between the treatment periods to minimize any carryover effect from the active drug. Dextropropoxiphen, 65 mg, was provided for therapy of acute migraine attacks. In reviewing the data, the investigators found that naproxen did decrease the number of migraine attacks. However, the reduction in attacks was statistically significant only in those patients who initially received placebo. No decrease in migraine attacks was demonstrated in those patients who remained on the placebo regimen during the entire study. There was no statistically significant difference between naproxen and placebo in their effect on the duration of the attacks or the side effect profile. The authors concluded that naproxen may slightly modify the longitudinal pattern of migraine. Naproxen, in the dosage used in this trial, is not a potent prophylactic agent, but is well tolerated. They believed that investigation into the NSAIDs in migraine prophylaxis should continue. Currently, however, these drugs would not replace more conventional therapies in the migraine treatment hierarchy.

Naproxen sodium has been the subject of various reports in migraine prophylaxis. Again, its success in migraine abortive therapy encouraged researchers to investigate its possible role in migraine prevention. Ziegler and Ellis reported the results of a double-blind, placebo-controlled crossover study in 34 patients (39). The study continued for 20 weeks, starting with a 1- to 2-week period in which all of the patients received placebo in a single-blind design. During the next 7 weeks, the patients received either 2 tablets of naproxen sodium, 275 mg, or matching placebo twice daily. The therapy was switched during the last 7 weeks. Each patient underwent a 2-week washout period between treatment phases, in which they received placebo to resolve any residual pharmacological effects of the active drug. Therapeutic effectiveness was rated by both patients and investigators by an approximate 3:1 ratio. Naproxen sodium was superior to placebo ($p = 0.02$ and 0.01, respectively). Again, no statistically significant difference was observed in the side effect profile of either therapy. These investigators suggested that naproxen sodium demonstrated a moderate effect in migraine prophylaxis, in particular in reducing the frequency and duration of the migraine attacks. They could not conclude if the efficacy of naproxen sodium derived from its antiplatelet effect, antiprostaglandin activity, or both. The need for further studies was recognized, as they felt that there was no substantial evidence that any of the NSAIDs, including naproxen sodium, would be preferred to the more standard therapies for migraine prophylaxis.

In a United States multicenter trial, naproxen sodium was compared with the primary agent used in migraine prophylaxis, propranolol (40). In a double-blind, randomized, parallel trial, 161 migraine patients entered a study in which they received either naproxen sodium, 550 mg bid, propranolol HCl, 40 mg tid, or placebo. The trial consisted of a 2-week washout period, in which all patients received placebo. During the next 2 weeks, the patients were randomized to either the naproxen, propranolol, or placebo groups, and the naproxen sodium group received the full dosage. In the next phase, lasting 12 weeks, patients received the full dosage of either active drug, or continued on placebo. The fourth phase lasted one week, in which propranolol patients were tapered to 40 mg bid, and the remaining patients continued their previous dosage regimen. Final analysis was completed on 129 patients; 42 patients received naproxen sodium, 44 were in the propranolol group, and 43 continued in the placebo group. The clinical effectiveness of both active drugs were viewed by patients and investigators alike as superior to placebo in the following four headache categories: frequency, severity, associated nausea, and visual disturbances. In overall evaluations for tolerance, propranolol hydrochloride was preferred over naproxen sodium by patients ($p = 0.053$) and investigators ($p = 0.032$). The naproxen sodium group reported more gastrointestinal complaints, but these symptoms were mild and transient. In reviewing the data, the investigators noted a significant response in the naproxen sodium group relative to menstrual migraine. Again, the need for further studies, particularly in menstrual migraine, was identified.

During the same year, Welch's group sought to establish the efficacy of naproxen sodium in migraine prophylaxis (41). They investigated the actions of this agent as a potent inhibitor of prostaglandin biosynthesis and platelet aggregation. The trial employed a randomized, double-blind, placebo-controlled, crossover protocol with a 2-week run-in phase in which all patients received placebo. The two active phases consisted of 8-week treatment periods, in which one-half of the patients were randomly assigned to the naproxen sodium group, and the remaining to placebo. A 2-week washout period divided the two treatment phases, and the patient groups were switched during the second treatment period. The patients were treated with naproxen sodium, 550 mg bid, or matching placebo. Of the 40 patients who originally entered the first washout period, 35 completed the trial. In global assessment, both patients and investigators judged naproxen sodium superior over placebo ($p < 0.03$). Naproxen sodium was effective in reducing the number of days with severe headache. These investigators also analyzed platelet function tests during the trial. Naproxen demonstrated efficacy in inhibiting platelet aggregation response in most patients. However, the authors found no correlation between the degree of inhibition and clinical efficacy. Also, naproxen sodium demonstrated no effect on platelet adhesiveness or microemboli formation. They concluded that naproxen sodium could be selected as a first-line agent in migraine prophylaxis.

Other studies have compared naproxen sodium and the serotonin and histamine antagonist, pizotifen (42). In a more recent study, naproxen sodium was compared to pizotyline (a synonym for pizotifen) and placebo (43). Pizotifen is not available in the United States, but has been used extensively in Europe and Canada for the prophylactic treatment of migraine. In each study, the active drugs were judged superior over placebo in prevention of migraine. Behan and Connelly did not demonstrate any statistically significant difference between the two drugs (43); however, Bellavance and Meloche observed that naproxen sodium was slightly more effective than pizotyline during the first month of therapy (44).

4. *Mefenamic Acid*

The fenamate compounds are known to inhibit both the biosynthesis and biological action of the prostaglandins. These agents have demonstrated efficacy in the abortive therapy of migraine (23), but few investigations have analyzed their usefulness in migraine prophylaxis. Johnson's group compared the efficacy of mefenamic acid and propranolol with placebo in migraine prevention (44). The study employed a double-blind, crossover protocol, which enrolled 29 migraine patients who experienced at least one migraine attack per month, with an average headache history of 20 years. Each of the three treatment phases lasted 3 months, and the following medication sequences were provided: (a) mefenamic acid, 250 mg, or matching propranolol placebo, 2 tablets tid; (b) propranolol, 40 mg, or matching mefenamic acid placebo, 2 tablets tid; and (c) mefenamic acid placebo or propranolol placebo, 2 tablets tid. The patients were randomly selected for the treatment sequences. Seventeen patients completed the three phases of the trial. Mefenamic acid ($p < 0.05$) and propranolol ($p < 0.01$) significantly reduced the total frequency and duration of the acute migraine attacks, compared with placebo. However, there was no significant effect on the average duration of the attacks. No significant difference was demonstrated between the drugs in their effects on migraine frequency or duration. These investigators noted that mefenamic acid was equally as effective as propranolol in reducing migraine frequency. They did observe that a few patients reported gastrointestinal complaints while taking mefenamic acid. These symptoms were severe, and indicate that mefenamic acid should be discontinued for severe gastrointestinal complaints.

5. *Fenoprofen Calcium*

The propionic acid derivative, fenoprofen calcium, was also investigated as a migraine prophylactic agent because of the previously demonstrated NSAID efficacy in this therapy. At our clinic, 110 patients participated in a double-blind, randomized, placebo-controlled trial comparing the efficacy of fenoprofen calcium, 200 mg tid; fenoprofen calcium, 600 mg tid; or matching placebo (45). Following a 4-week baseline phase, in which all patients received placebo, the patients participated in a 12-week parallel treatment phase. They were randomly selected for the treatment groups. In the fenoprofen 200-mg group (n = 32), 22% had more than a 50% improvement in reducing migraine frequency, whereas the fenoprofen 600-mg group (n = 36), 36% had more than a 50% improvement. Twenty percent of the placebo group (n = 34) demonstrated more than a 50% improvement in decreasing migraine frequency. The 600-mg dose significantly decreased the severity and duration of the headaches, and the need for relief medications. Gastrointestinal complaints were the most frequently cited side effect. We consider fenoprofen calcium a viable agent in migraine prophylaxis, and well tolerated.

6. Ketoprofen

Ketoprofen is a rapidly absorbed NSAID, with a relatively short plasma half-life antiprostaglandin actions, and antibradykinin activity. In 1974, a Norwegian study was conducted with this drug to evaluate a possible role in migraine prophylaxis (46). A double-blind, crossover protocol was employed in 26 consecutive migraine patients. The treatment phases consisted of two 6-week periods in which patients received either ketoprofen, 50 mg tid, or matching placebo, divided by 1 drug-free week. The sequence of treatment was randomized. Final analysis was conducted on 24 patients, 16 of whom reported improvement in headache frequency and severity. Ketoprofen demonstrated efficacy over placebo ($p < 0.05$), although the improvement with the active drug was moderate. A more than 50% decrease in headache parameters was noted in only 5 patients (21%). The authors noted that ketoprofen was well tolerated and suggested its possible consideration in migraine prophylaxis.

A retrospective study on ketoprofen in migraine prophylaxis was recently reported (47). Eighty-nine patients, with a migraine diagnosis, were reviewed. 40 patients experienced pure migraine, and 49 had the mixed-headache syndrome, that is migraine and tension-type headaches. These 49 patients were selected because they could differentiate between the two types of attacks. The average daily dose of ketoprofen for the migraine group was 198.2 mg in divided doses, and the average length of treatment was 8.2 months. In the mixed-headache syndrome group, patients consumed an average daily dose of 215.7 mg in divided doses for an average of 7.3 months. Physicians were asked to complete global evaluations and improvement was based on decreases in the frequency of acute migraine attacks. In the pure migraine group, 46.7% of the patients reported a decrease in frequency from 4.67 to 2.49 attacks per month. A decrease in frequency of migraine attacks was noted by 65.7% of the patients in the mixed-headache group. Adverse effects were reported by 24 patients from both groups, and 18 patients discontinued ketoprofen therapy because of these symptoms. The authors concluded that ketoprofen was an effective agent in migraine prophylaxis.

C. Menstrual Migraine

Most headache experts concur that a female preponderance exists in migraine, with estimates that 60% of migraineurs are women. These experts also report that 70% of female migraineurs indicate a menstrual relation with their migraine attacks. In addition to the awareness of the role of prostaglandins in headache, researchers have also focused on the relationship of dysmenorrhea and prostaglandin inhibitors (48). Aspirin and other over-the-counter analgesics have demonstrated efficacy in relieving dysmenorrhea (49). Research into the NSAIDs and menstrual migraine naturally evolved.

In reviewing the results of an investigation into naproxen sodium in migraine prophylaxis, the authors noted improvement in menstrual migraine during therapy with this NSAID (41). In the final analysis, 36 patients included menstrual dates during the 17-week trial. In both active treatment groups, headaches occurring during the premenstrual week were less frequent and less severe than during the week after onset of menses. The placebo group demonstrated more headaches during the week before menses than after the onset of menses. Headache severity did demonstrate a greater decrease in the naproxen sodium group than the placebo groups ($p = 0.01$). The patients in the naproxen sodium group also experienced less severe premenstrual headaches than the propranolol group, although the difference was not statistically significant. The authors noted that a long-term study was needed to evaluate NSAID treatment of menstrual migraine.

Pendergrass' group examined the effect of small doses of aspirin and acetaminophen on total menstrual loss as well as dysmenorrhea and headache (50). During the 4-month investigation, 90 women recorded data on their menstrual periods. No pain relievers were used during the first two periods. The patients were permitted during the last two periods to use 2 tablets of aspirin, 325 mg; acetaminophen, 325 mg; or matching placebo, every 4 h, for a total of 8 tablets during the first 24 h after spotting. Neither drug altered the degree of menstrual loss. However, both analgesics were more effective than placebo ($p = 0.0072$) in decreasing the pain of the menstrual cramps, which is specifically attributed to an overabundance of $PGF_{2\alpha}$ (50). Neither active drug was effective in relieving the menstrually associated headaches. The authors indicated that this response reflects the difference in the physiological mechanisms involved in the two pain disorders. The pain of headache is considered to be due to a spillover of prostaglandins into the general circulation during menstruation and may be potentiated by other substances, such as histamine (49). The authors noted that their study was limited, as patients were not questioned about when the headaches occurred, and if they were related to the onset of the menses or the cramps. The headaches may have occurred before or after taking the analgesic and could not be linked to the effects of the medications.

A double-blind, placebo-controlled study was undertaken on the use of naproxen sodium in menstrual migraine prophylaxis (51). These investigators acknowledged that menstrual migraine often is refractory to standard prophylactic therapies. Forty women participated in this study, who had a diagnosis of migraine without aura. The headaches occurred at each menstrual period and lasted from 1 to 4 days. During the other weeks of the cycle, these patients were headache-free. The treatment period was preceded by a 2-month run-in phase. During the second phase, the patients were given naproxen sodium, 550 mg, or matching placebo, bid, starting 7 days premenses and continuing through the sixth day of menstrual flow, for three menstrual cycles. In the next three menstrual cycles, all patients were given active drug in an open trial.

Final analysis was conducted on 35 women: 18 receiving naproxen sodium for six menstrual cycles, and 17 receiving placebo for three periods and the active drug for the last three menstrual cycles. In both groups, an improvement of over 50% was reached after only 3 months of active treatment. Analgesic consumption significantly decreased during the first 3 months of active drug therapy. Although 25% of the patients taking naproxen sodium experienced mild or moderate adverse effects, such as nausea and epigastric distress, the medication was not discontinued. Overall, naproxen sodium demonstrated superiority over placebo in relieving menstrual migraine. Its rapid absorption and attainment of therapeutically effective serum concentrations enhance the efficacy of naproxen sodium in short-term therapy, such as that required for menstrually related headaches. Naproxen sodium is also well tolerated and is a viable agent in the prevention of menstrual migraine.

Clinically, the use of mefenamic acid has also demonstrated efficacy in the prophylactic treatment of menstrual migraine. The dose is 250 mg tid, starting 3 days premenses and continued through the flow.

III. CONCLUSION

The results of these various trials indicate that the NSAIDs are effective and well-tolerated therapies in the treatment of migraine. The NSAIDs may not replace standard therapies in migraine prophylaxis, such as the β-blockers or the calcium channel blockers. For those patients who are refractory or cannot tolerate these other therapeutic agents, the NSAIDs provide an excellent alternative. The NSAIDs may also serve as effective adjuncts to other types of therapy. At the present time, I believe that the NSAIDs are the treatment of choice for menstrual migraine, starting 2–3 days premenses and continuing through the flow. Long-term investigations are needed to analyze any continuing effects from NSAID therapy.

REFERENCES

1. Amano T, Meyer JS. Prostaglandin inhibition and cardiovascular control in patients with headache. Headache 1982; 22:52–9.
2. Boghen D, Desaulniers N. Background vascular headache: relief with indomethacin. Can J Neurol Sci 1983; 10:271–1.
3. Deshmukh SV, Meyer JS. Cyclic changes in platelet dynamics and the pathogenesis and prophylaxis of migraine. Headache 1977; 17:101–8.
4. Pradalier A, Clapin A, Dry J. Treatment review: non-steroid anti-inflammatory drugs in the treatment and long-term prevention of migraine attacks. Headache 1988; 28:550–7.
5. Anthony M, Hinterberger H, Lance JW. The possible relationship of serotonin to the migraine syndrome. Res Clin Stud Headache 1968; 2:29.
6. Sicuteri F, Testi A, Anselmi B. Biochemical investigations in headache; increase in hydroxyindoleacetic acid excretion during migraine attacks. Int Arch Allergy Appl Immunol 1961; 19:55.
7. Sicuteri F, Michelacci S, Anselmi B. Characterisation of the vasoactive and antimigraine properties of indomethacin, a new anti-inflammatory agent derived from indole. Settim Med [Italy] 1964; 52:335.
8. Anthony M, Lance JW. Indomethacin in migraine. Med J Aust 1968; 1:56–7.
9. Volans GN. The effect of metoclopramide on the absorption of effervescent aspirin in migraine. Br Clin Pharmacol 1975; 2:57–63.
10. Ross-Lee L, Heazlewood V, Tyrer JH, Eadie MJ. Aspirin treatment of migraine attacks: plasma drug level data. Cephalalgia 1982; 2:9–14.
11. Ross-Lee L, Eadie MJ, Tyrer JH. Aspirin treatment of migraine attacks; clinical observations. Cephalalgia 1982; 2:71–6.
12. Noda S, Itoh H, Umezaki H, Fukuda Y. Successful treatment of migraine attacks with intravenous injection of aspirin. J Neurol Neurosurg Psychiatry 1985; 48:1187.
13. Peterson DI. Headache: Part IX. Nonsteroidal antiinflammatory drugs for the treatment of headache. IM 1986; 7:69–77.
14. Pearce I, Frank GJ, Pearce JMS. Ibuprofen compared with paracetamol in migraine. Practitioner 1983; 227:465–7.
15. Havanka-Kannianinen H. Treatment of acute migraine attack: ibuprofen and placebo compared. Headache 1989; 29:507–9.
16. Lindegaard KF, Ovreli W, Sjaastad O. Naproxen in the prevention of migraine attacks. A double blind placebo-controlled cross-over study. Headache 1980; 20:96–8.
17. Johnson ES, Ratcliffe DM, Wilkinson M. Naproxen sodium in the treatment of migraine. Cephalalgia 1985; 5:5–10.
18. Nestvold K, Kloster R, Partinen M, Sulkava R. Treatment of acute migraine attack: naproxen and placebo compared. Cephalalgia 1985; 5:115–9.
19. Andersson PG, Hinge HH, Johansen O, Andersen CU, Lademann A, Gøtzsche PC.

Double-blind study of naproxen vs placebo in the treatment of acute migraine attacks. Cephalalgia 1988; 9:29–32.
20. Pradalier A, Rancurel G, Dordain G, Verdure L, Rascol A, Dry J. Acute migraine attack therapy: comparison of naproxen sodium and an ergotamine tartrate compound. Cephalalgia 1985; 5:107–13.
21. Sargent JD, Baumel B, Peters K, Diamond S, Saper JR, Eisner LS, Solbach P. Aborting a migraine attack: naproxen sodium v ergotamine plus caffeine. Headache 1988; 28:263–6.
22. Grimmer AJ, Leathard HL, Peatfield RC, Rose FC. The effects of mefenamic acid on tone and evoked responses in human isolated cerebral arteries. Br J Pharmacol 1982; 75:67.
23. Hall DW. Migraine—mefenamic acid in the treatment of attacks. J R Coll Gen Pract 1968; 15:321–4.
24. Peatfield RC, Petty RG, Rose FC. Double blind comparison of mefenamic acid and acetaminophen (paracetamol) in migraine. Cephalalgia 1983; 3:129–34.
25. Fowler PD. Diclofenac sodium. In: Huskisson EC, ed. Anti-rheumatic drugs. New York: Praeger, 1983:117–56.
26. Martini A, Bondiolotti GP, Sacerdote P, et al. Diclofenac increases beta-endorphin plasma concentrations. J Int Med Res 1984; 12:92–5.
27. Del Bene E, Poggioni M, Garagiola U, Maresca V. Intramuscular treatment of migraine attacks using diclofenac sodium: a crossover clinical trial. J Int Med Res 1987; 15:44–8.
28. Massiou H, Serrurier D, Lasserre O, Bousser M-G. Effectiveness of oral diclofenac in the acute treatment of common migraine attacks: a double-blind study versus placebo. Cephalalgia 1991; 11:59–63.
29. Bousser MG, Baron JC. The clinician's view on end points. Neuroepidemiology 1987; 6:228–33.
30. Pini L-A, Bertolotti M, Bergonzini G, Casalgrandi L, Giroldi L, Sternieri E. Pharmacokinetics of tiaprofenic acid after oral administration in fasting patients during and between migraine attacks. Headache 1990; 672–5.
31. Guidotti M, Zanasi S, Garagiola U. Pirprofen in the treatment of migraine and episodic headache attacks: a placebo-controlled crossover clinical trial. J Int Med Res 1989; 17:48–54.
32. Tokola RA, Neuvonen P. Effects of migraine attack and metoclopramide on the absorption of tolfenamic acid. Br J Clin Pharmacol 1984; 17:67–75.
33. Harden RN, Carter TD, Gilman CS, Gross AJ, Peters JR. Ketorolac in acute headache management. Headache 1991; 31:463–4.
34. O'Neill BP, Mann JD. Aspirin prophylaxis in migraine. Lancet 1978; 2:1179–81.
35. Grotemeyer K-H, Scharafinski H-W, Schlake H-P, Husstedt IW. Acetylsalicylic acid vs. metoprolol in migraine prophylaxis—a double-blind cross-over study. Headache 1990; 30:639–41.
36. Buring JE, Peto R, Hennekens CH. Low-dose aspirin for migraine prophylaxis. JAMA 1990; 264:1711–13.
37. Dalessio DJ. Aspirin prophylaxis for migraine [editorial]. JAMA 1990; 264:1721.
38. Lindegaard K-F, Övrelid L, Sjaastad O. Naproxen in the prevention of migraine attacks. A double-blind placebo-controlled cross-over study. Headache 1980; 20:96–8.
39. Ziegler DK, Ellis DJ. Naproxen in prophylaxis of migraine. Arch Neurol 1985; 42:582–4.
40. Sargent J, Solbach P, Damasio H, et al. A comparison of naproxen sodium to propranolol hydrochloride and a placebo control for the prophylaxis of migraine headache. Headache 1985; 25:320–4.
41. Welch KMA, Ellis DJ, Keenan PA. Successful migraine prophylaxis with naproxen sodium. Neurology 1985; 35:1304–10.
42. Behan PO, Connelly K. Prophylaxis of migraine: a comparison between naproxen sodium and pizotifen. Headache 1986; 26:237–9.
43. Bellavance AJ, Meloche JP. A comparative study of naproxen sodium, pizotyline, and placebo in migraine prophylaxis. Headache 1990; 30:710–5.

44. Johnson RH, Hornabrook RW, Lambie DG. Comparison of mefenamic acid and propranolol with placebo in migraine prophylaxis. Acta Neurol Scand 1986; 73:490–2.
45. Diamond S, Solomon GD, Freitag FG, Mehta ND. Fenoprofen in the prophylaxis of migraine: a double-blind, placebo controlled study. Headache 1987; 27:246–9.
46. Stensrud P, Sjaastad O. Clinical trial of a new antibradykinin, anti-inflammatory drug, ketoprofen, in migraine prophylaxis. Headache 1974; 14:96–100.
47. Diamond S, Freitag FG, Gallagher RM, Feinberg DT. Ketoprofen in the prophylaxis of migraine. Headache Q 1990; 1:75–7.
48. Halbert D, Demers L, Jones D. Dysmenorrhea and prostaglandins. Obstet Gynecol Surv 1976; 31:77–81.
49. Chan W. Prostaglandins and nonsteroidal antiinflammatory drugs in dysmenorrhea. Annu Rev Pharmacol Toxicol 1983; 23:131–49.
50. Pendergrass PB, Scott JN, Ream LJ, Agna MA. Effect of small doses of aspirin and acetaminophen on total menstrual loss and pain of cramps and headache. Gynecol Obstet Invest 1985; 19:32–7.
51. Sances G, Martignoni E, Fioroni L, Blandini F, Facchinetti F, Nappi G. Naproxen sodium in menstrual migraine prophylaxis: a double-blind placebo controlled study. Headache 1990; 30:705–9.

3

Nonsteroidal Anti-Inflammatory Agents and the Adult Respiratory Distress Syndrome

HANSON B. COWAN and JEAN E. RINALDO
Vanderbilt University
and Nashville Veterans Administration Medical Center
Nashville, Tennessee

I. INTRODUCTION

Despite major advances in the technology of intensive care and an increased understanding of the pathophysiology of acute respiratory failure, mortality associated with the adult respiratory distress syndrome (ARDS) remains unacceptably high (1–3). The cause of ARDS appears to be multifactorial and is associated with the sepsis syndrome, aspiration of gastric contents, trauma, pancreatitis, and a variety of other conditions (2,3). Although its exact pathogenesis remains uncertain, ARDS appears to be an inflammatory disorder of the lung parenchyma associated with increased endothelial and epithelial permeability, with exudation of plasma protein-rich fluid into the interstitial and alveolar spaces of the lungs (4,5). This increased permeability and fluid accumulation in the lungs results in the associated clinical findings of severe dyspnea, and hypoxia, diffuse roentgenographic chest infiltrates, and decreased lung compliance, without evidence of elevated left atrial pressure (4). Treatment of ARDS remains supportive, consisting of oxygen therapy, mechanical ventilation, and the use of positive end-expiratory pressure (PEEP). No specific pharmacologic treatment of the syndrome has been shown to be efficacious.

Because ARDS has long been thought to result from lung inflammation, there has been considerable interest in the use of anti-inflammatory agents as potential therapy (5–7). Corticosteroids were formerly employed empirically by many physicians, but two large randomized prospective trials did not show that they were helpful (6,7). Further interest in nonsteroidal anti-inflammatory agents (NSAIAs) followed.

The purpose of this chapter is to review the laboratory and clinical experience with NSAIAs that have been tried in the treatment of the sepsis syndrome and ARDS. First, we will present an overview of the current status of research on the mechanisms of acute lung injury, with special reference to the chemical mediators that produce the endothelial injury and associated changes, emphasizing mechanisms that might be amenable to modification by NSAIAs. Second, we will discuss the experimental animal models frequently used to examine lung injury, with a special reference to those studies that have used one of three specific NSAIAs. Finally, we will present the most current data available concerning the use of NSAIAs in human clinical trials for ARDS.

II. MEDIATORS OF ACUTE LUNG INJURY

Several potent mediators likely contribute to the initiation and progression of the injury and inflammation that lead to acute respiratory failure and that may culminate in multiorgan failure and death of the patient (5,8). Conclusions on the likely role of the various putative mediators of experimental acute lung injury are inferred mainly from (a) the effects of blocking mediator synthesis or action; (b) temporal or quantitative correlations between defined parameters of lung injury and the levels of these mediators in the blood, lymph, or lavage fluid from the experimental animals; and (c) similarities between the actions of mediators ex vivo and certain features of acute lung injury in animals. The exact role of each of the various mediators in lung injury is often difficult to ascertain. One is never sure of the relative importance of each individual mediator in an inflammatory setting in which multiple mediators are involved, nor is one sure to what extent a given compound that is released during the acute injury is a mediator of injury, as opposed to being a marker of injury. These limitations have made the choice of potentially useful pharmacological agents and the interpretation of the experimental studies very difficult.

A. Cellular Mediators of Injury

Sequestration of *neutrophils* in the pulmonary microvessels and their subsequent migration into the interstitial and alveolar spaces are typical histological findings in ARDS (5). Bronchoalveolar lavage fluid from patients with ARDS contains numerous neutrophils and high concentrations of neutrophil products, especially neutrophil elastase (8). Upon being activated, neutrophils as well as macrophages contribute to the acute lung injury by releasing lipid and enzyme mediators and generating reactive oxygen species (8). The critical role of the neutrophil was clearly demonstrated in studies with depletion of neutrophils or inhibition of their function. This depletion or inhibition protected against several forms of experimental acute pulmonary edema (9). Furthermore, neutrophils with impaired function are incapable of inducing pulmonary edema under conditions for which normal, activated neutrophils do so (10). However, severe neutropenia is not a guarantee against the development of ARDS (11). Two products of neutrophils—reactive oxygen species and neutrophil elastase—have received the most recent attention as potential contributors to acute lung injury.

Reactive oxygen species (superoxide anion, hydrogen peroxide, hydroxyl ion, and singlet oxygen) are among the principal mediators of acute lung injury and are frequently produced in quantities sufficient to overwhelm normal host antioxidant defenses. These toxic oxygen species are produced mainly by activated neutrophils and alveolar macrophages (8,12).

Several lines of evidence suggest a link between reactive oxygen species and the pathogenesis of acute lung injury (10,12–15): (a) experimental generation of free radicals leads to acute pulmonary edema in vitro (12); (b) increased oxidant activity is present in bronchoalveolar lavage fluid from patients with ARDS (15); (c) neutrophils from a patient with chronic granulomatous disease could not induce acute pulmonary edema (14); and

(d) pretreatment with free-radical scavengers protects against acute pulmonary edema in experimental preparations (12–15).

Similar to reactive oxygen species, proteolytic enzymes are released mainly by neutrophils and macrophages. Proteinases, particularly neutrophil elastase, are major factors in the production of experimental lung injury (8,12,16,17). The pathogenetic potential of elastase and other proteinases is normally counteracted by proteinase inhibitors. This normal balance may be tipped in favor of proteolytic enzymes if proteinase inhibitors are inactivated, as by cigarette smoke or other oxidants. Some recent studies have shown the ability of activated neutrophils to solubilize human alveolar extracellular matrix (18). The proteolytic enzyme thrombin, which catalyzes the formation of fibrin from fibrinogen, is a potent agonist for platelet aggregation through release of adenosine diphosphate (ADP), serotonin, and thromboxane A_2 (TXA_2). Infusion of thrombin in vivo induces experimental lung injury by causing pulmonary microembolism with fibrin clots (19).

Activated *lymphocytes*, *monocytes*, and *macrophages*, by releasing a variety of cytokines, can accentuate or modulate acute lung inflammation. As briefly discussed later, these cytokines, especially tumor necrosis factor (TNF), interleukin-1 (IL-1), and IL-6, are released mainly by macrophages and are currently the subject of intense investigation as mediators of acute lung injury and inflammation (20–22).

The role of *platelets* in the production of increased permeability pulmonary edema has recently been reexamined. Although platelet aggregation is often associated with events that lead to lung injury, normal platelets may be important in maintaining vascular integrity, and pharmacological manipulation of platelets may not be beneficial in maintaining this vascular integrity (17).

B. Soluble Mediators: Peptides and Lipid Mediators

Proteins that may contribute directly in mediating pulmonary injury include cytokines, chemotactic proteins, proteolytic peptides, and activated complement (5). Additional peptides present in the airways and parenchyma of the lung, such as the kinins and substance P, which constrict the airways and pulmonary vessels, may contribute to these effects in acute lung injury. Other peptides, such as the opioid peptides, may play a major role in the mediation of the systemic hypotension and shock caused by endotoxemia, hemorrhage, spinal trauma, aspiration, and anesthesia. As such, these opioid peptides may predispose the lung to acute injury (16,17,19).

1. Cytokines

Cytokines have become a major focus of current research aimed at determining the cause and propagation of inflammation. The term *cytokine* refers to a variety of cell-derived peptide molecules that are released by effector cells and cause an alteration in the functional activities of the target cells. These soluble cytokines bind to target cells through specific cell surface receptors and generate one or more internal receptor-coupled second messages. These second-message systems generate the functional responses of the target cells.

Of the known cytokines, tumor necrosis factor (TNFα), also known as cachectin and released by monocytes and macrophages on stimulation by bacteria or endotoxin, is now thought to be the principal and, possibly, the essential mediator of septic shock and its consequences, including acute lung injury (20–22). Injections of recombinant human

TNFα (rhTHFα) into rats produces systemic shock hypovolemia, hemoconcentration, metabolic acidosis, pulmonary edema, intestinal ischemia, renal tubular necrosis, and death (23). Also, serum or plasma levels of TNFα are markedly increased in experimental models of lethal endotoxemia and in normal human volunteers injected with *Escherichia coli* endotoxin (22,24).

Another cytokine capable of inducing many of same pathophysiological effects noted with TNFα, including the marked high-permeability pulmonary edema, is the monokine interleukin-1β (IL-1β). Like TNFα, IL-1β is secreted mainly by activated macrophages. Infusions of recombinant IL-1β into unanesthetized rabbits causes granulocytopenia, wet-to-dry weight gain, pulmonary extravasation of radiolabeled albumin, and electron microscopic evidence of pulmonary endothelial injury (21,22,25).

Levels of IL-6, another cytokine in the host immune response to infection and inflammation, are elevated in patients with sepsis and are correlated with the severity of the illness and mortality rate (26). The TNFα and IL-6 levels are significantly higher in nonsurvivors than in survivors of sepsis and were independent of the severity of illness at presentation. In addition, levels of TNFα and IL-6 were sustained for longer than 24–48 h in nonsurvivors (22,26). These cytokines have been reviewed elsewhere and will not be discussed further here (21,22,27,28).

2. *Lipid Mediators*

Among the principal mediators of injury and inflammation in the lung and other organs are two groups of potent lipids: platelet-activating factors (PAF) and arachidonic acid metabolites (5,8,27). The biosynthesis of both of these groups of compounds may be triggered by one reaction: the activation of membrane phospholipase A_2. Recent evidence indicates that, in human neutrophils, both arachidonic acid and PAF are probably derived from a common precursor, arachidonate-containing phosphoglycerides, especially phosphatidylcholine (29,30).

a. Platelet-Activating Factor. Chemically, PAF is 1-*O*-hexadecyl/octadecyl-2- acetyl-*sn*-glycero-3-phosphocholine, sometimes abbreviated AGEPC. Synthesized and released by blood cells (neutrophils, monocytes, eosinophils, basophils, and platelets), vascular endothelium, alveolar macrophages, and mast cells, PAF activates not only platelets, but neutrophils and other inflammatory cells (29–31). Its biological actions on these cells include increased intracellular calcium concentrations and stimulation of prostaglandin, thromboxane, and leukotriene synthesis; formation of superoxide anion; chemotaxis; adherence; and lysosomal enzyme release. Furthermore, in minute physiological concentrations (10^{-11}–10^{-10} M), PAF primes neutrophils to respond to subsequent stimulation by other agonists and, thereby, become more effective as endothelial cytotoxins (32). The role of PAF in acute lung injury has been extensively reviewed and will not be reviewed further here (31,33,34). Among the systemic effects of PAF in vivo are increased vascular permeability, hemoconcentration, decreased cardiac output, systemic shock, and ischemic bowel necrosis. Pulmonary effects include airway constriction, decreased pulmonary compliance, airway hyperreactivity, pulmonary hypertension and edema (31,33).

b. Arachidonate Metabolites. Generated by leukocytes, macrophages, and mast cells, as well as pulmonary endothelial and epithelial cells, arachidonic acid is metabolized to several compounds (eicosanoids) with various and potent actions (28). Metabolites, the formation of which is catalyzed by the enzyme cyclooxygenase, include thromboxane A_2 (TXA_2), prostacyclin (PGI_2), and prostaglandins (PG) D_2, E_2, and $F_{2\alpha}$. Arachidonic acid products catalyzed by the lipoxygenase enzymes include hydroperoxyeicosatetraenoic acid (HPETE), the leukotrienes (LK), and the lipoxins. Different cells and tissues are associated with different patterns of arachidonic acid metabolites (30). More recently, the cytochrome P-450 products from arachidonic acid metabolism have been reviewed, with particular focus on their functional effects (35–37).

The most extensively studied, and probably most important in producing the pulmonary responses to injury, are TXA_2 and the leukotrienes (30,38). As a bronchoconstrictor, pulmonary vasoconstrictor, and platelet-aggregating compound, TXA_2 is believed to contribute to pulmonary hypertension, decreased pulmonary compliance, and complement activation during *E. coli* endotoxemia (30,38). Pulmonary thromboxane synthesis is markedly stimulated during experimental acute lung injury, and inhibition of this synthesis partially protects against some of the features of the injury, including bronchoconstriction and pulmonary hypertension, although usually not against the increased endothelial permeability (39).

Of the leukotrienes, the cysteinyl leukotrienes (formerly the slow-reacting substance of anaphylaxis), LTC_4, LTD_4, and LTE_4 induce airway and pulmonary vasoconstriction, increase systemic and pulmonary microvascular permeability, and decrease cardiac contractility (40,41). Leukotriene-B_4 stimulates leukocyte migration, aggregation, and adherence to endothelium (40). Increased concentrations of cysteinyl leukotrienes have been found in the bronchoalveolar fluid from mice with hyperoxia lung injury (42) from patients with ARDS, and from patients who appeared to be developing ARDS (43).

The lipoxins are products synthesized by human leukocytes through the action of 5- and 15-lipoxygenases on arachidonic acid (40). These compounds stimulate neutrophil chemotaxis and superoxide anion generation, contract guinea pig lung strips (small airways), and dilate systemic microvessels (40).

III. ANIMAL STUDIES

A wide variety of insults to the alveolocapillary membrane by direct (e.g., aspiration) and indirect (e.g., sepsis, endotoxin, drug overdose) methods have been used in various animal species, from rodents to primates, to model the clinical syndrome of ARDS. Common to most of these models has been the description of a diffuse and intense inflammatory reaction in the microvasculature of the lung (5). The recognition that neutrophils, macrophages, and other components of the inflammatory cascade contribute and participate in the progression of the acute lung injury, resulted in the use of anti-inflammatory agents, including NSAIA, as pharmacological probes to further define the pathophysiology of the acute inflammation. The data from these animal studies with NSAIA have generated interest in clinical trials of the anti-inflammatory therapy for ARDS (44). We will discuss three specific agents.

A. Ibuprofen

Ibuprofen is a cyclooxygenase inhibitor that is alleged to have additional direct effects on leukocyte function (45,46). These specific properties, including the ability of high concentrations of ibuprofen to chelate iron, diminish platelet and neutrophil aggregation, and attenuate leukocyte lysosomal and oxygen radical release, suggest that ibuprofen may be of potential therapeutic benefit for leukocyte (neutrophil)-mediated acute lung injury in animals, such as occurs with sepsis induced by gram-negative organisms.

Multiple studies of nonbacteriologically infusion-induced pulmonary injury with pretreatment protocols are reported in the literature (47,48). Pretreatment of animals with ibuprofen inhibited the formation of both TXA_2 and PGI_2 (49). Generally, the systemic and pulmonary circulatory responses to injury were attenuated by ibuprofen, as anticipated increases in both mean pulmonary artery pressure (PPA) and the calculated pulmonary vascular resistance (PVR) were consistently blunted or blocked.

Pretreatment with ibuprofen has also modified direct effects of acute lung injury in the pulmonary microcirculation, as well as sequelae of the insult on arterial oxygenation. Thus, the deterioration the PaO_2 that followed the induction of acute lung injury has been substantially prevented by pretreatment with ibuprofen (48). Following ibuprofen pretreatment in large animals, changes in indexes of altered microvascular fluid flux, as measured by pulmonary lymph flow (QL) and lymph/plasma total protein ratio ([L/P]TP), have been interpreted as demonstrating the ability of this anti-inflammatory drug to significantly prevent the development of increased pulmonary microvascular permeability (50). Finally, pretreatment with ibuprofen reduced neutrophil adherence to both skin and pulmonary endothelium, following the administration of chemotactic agents such as LTB_4, zymosan-activated plasma, or thrombin (49). A concentration-dependent reduction in neutrophil superoxide anion generation was also demonstrated following ibuprofen administration (49).

These studies suggest that ibuprofen alters neutrophil adherence to endothelial surfaces. This alteration of adherence may be a direct effect of ibuprofen on neutrophils, but as yet, we have no such evidence. Neutrophil adherence appears to be highly regulated by glycoprotein receptor expression, and there is now no evidence that ibuprofen affects expression of cell surface adhesion molecules and receptors.

Since pretreatment therapy is not clinically useful for ARDS, the previous studies might be of only limited clinical use. A few studies have investigated infusion-induced lung injury and the use of ibuprofen posttreatment (51–53). A study using vascular-sclerosing agents with ibuprofen (51) demonstrated the same general patterns of protection and amelioration of lung injury that was reported in the aforementioned pretreatment studies. Specifically, ibuprofen prevented anticipated increases in mean PPA, QL, and lung wet/dry ratios, which otherwise followed the infusion of the sclerosing agents (51). A second study employed monocrotalin to induce acute lung injury in rats. This induced injury is characterized by an increase in pulmonary microvascular permeability, pulmonary hypertension, and the development of right ventricular hypertrophy, but is different from the infusion models of acute lung injury in that the pulmonary pathophysiology develops 5 days after administration of the monocrotalin (52). When compared with untreated control animals, 14 days of therapy with ibuprofen did not result in a significant decrease in either lung wet/dry ratios or right ventricular hypertrophy (52). Since ARDS is a protracted process in most patients, this would suggest that ibuprofen would have little effect on the later progress of the disease, despite its transient physiological effects in the early phases.

Most acute lung injury models that have investigated the effects of ibuprofen have employed a bacteriologically induced insult. Most of these studies have used live *E. coli*, *E. coli* endotoxin, or live *Pseudomonas aeruginosa* in a large animal model (ovine or porcine). These models are reported to manifest two "phases" of response to the bacteriological insult (54). During the phase 1 response (at 30 min), an increase in pulmonary QL is thought to be primarily the result of an abrupt increase in the microvascular hydrostatic pressure (p_{mv}) complicating acute pulmonary hypertension.

During the phase 2 response (at about 4 h), the mean PPA falls, yet both QL and (L/P)TP ratios remain elevated or increase further. This phase 2 response describes a time in the progression of acute lung injury that is considered to represent an increase in pulmonary microvascular permeability (37).

Overall, the effects of ibuprofen pretreatment in bacteriologically induced acute lung injury are most impressive during the acute or phase 1 response (5,53,54). During this stage, an increase in vasoconstrictor prostanoids (e.g., TXA_2) is thought to contribute to both the immediate pulmonary hypertensive response and the accompanying ventilation–perfusion mismatch that underlies arterial hypoxemia in animal models of acute lung injury. As noted earlier in the infusion–injury models, pretreatment of the animals with ibuprofen in these studies of bacteriologically induced acute lung injury attenuated both the injury-related arterial hypoxemia and the acute pulmonary hypertension. Thus, the phase 1-induced decrease in Pa_{O_2} and increase in mean PPA have been entirely prevented or attenuated by ibuprofen pretreatment in large-animal models of acute lung injury.

In studies wherein pulmonary microvascular fluid flux was assessed by measuring changes in lung QL, ibuprofen pretreatment also significantly modified the expression of the pathophysiology. Extension of benefit into phase 2 response, or the period of altered permeability in acute lung injury, was demonstrated when treatments with ibuprofen and diphenhydramine were combined (53). Both in vitro neutrophil adherence and the degree of neutrophil accumulation in bronchoalveolar lavage fluid were significantly reduced with ibuprofen pretreatment (53). As with infusion-induced lung injury models, a dose-dependent effect on neutrophil function was probable, as low doses of ibuprofen enhanced neutrophil function, whereas higher doses had an inhibitory effect (53).

When compared with pretreatment protocols, studies that have used ibuprofen treatment postinsult have not resulted in the same magnitude of protection from the sequelae of acute lung injury, in spite of the demonstrated inhibition of cyclooxygenase activity. Some attenuation in the anticipated increase in mean PPA accompanied postinsult treatments when ibuprofen was combined with either PGE_1 or methylprednisolone. Other than the improvement in the stroke volume index, the combination of PGE_1 and ibuprofen did not provide additive benefit.

B. Indomethacin

In infusion injury models of acute lung injury, the effects of pretreatment with indomethacin were generally similar to those discussed with ibuprofen. Increases in pulmonary QL during the early phase 1 response to thrombin-induced lung injury were blunted by indomethacin, although this effect did not extend into the phase 2 response of the injury process (50). In the single canine model reported (55), indomethacin was effective at preventing anticipated arterial hypoxemia and minimized the abrupt increase in mean PPA, seen with the infusion of zymosan-activated plasma.

In bacteriologically induced infusion models of acute lung injury, indomethacin pretreatment prevented the accumulation in plasma of PGE and PGF_2, whereas injury-induced pulmonary hypertension and acute arterial hypoxemia were simultaneously prevented (56). Indomethacin enhanced the accumulation of leukotrienes in a rat model of neutrophil activation (57). Pretreatment with indomethacin also blunted the expected increase in free-oxygen radical production that accompanied cellular stimulation with phorbol myristate acetate (57).

C. Meclofenamate

Studies that employed meclofenamate in infusion-induced models of ARDS were all pretreatment protocols. Meclofenamate was effective in inhibiting the production of TXB_2 and 6-keto-$PGF_{1\alpha}$ (50). The effects of meclofenamate on the pathophysiology of acute lung injury was, in general, less effective in both phase 1 and phase 2 responses than has been reported with either ibuprofen or indomethacin (58).

In the two studies reported that employed *E. coli* endotoxin infusion in sheep (59,60), pretreatment with meclofenamate prevented the phase 1 response increase in mean PPA and QL. The combination of methylprednisolone and meclofenamate in one of these studies attenuated most of the phase 1 as well as the phase 2 response to *E. coli* infusion (59).

Taken as a group, these animal studies using ibuprofen and meclofenamate would suggest that the most dramatic and reproducible effects of these agents are on the immediate acute bronchospastic or vasoactive responses to sepsis, which result in pulmonary hypertension and ventilation–perfusion mismatching. These are short-lived and probably result from cyclooxygenase inhibition. There is no convincing effect on lung injury per se. Ibuprofen is more problematic because of its many other poorly defined effects (other than cyclooxygenase inhibition). However, even for ibuprofen, evidence for inhibition of endothelium injury is sparse. Combinations of agents may work better, but are even more difficult to evaluate (53,61). Little is known about the effects of ibuprofen on lung injury from nonsepsis-induced models, and further research in these areas is needed.

IV. CLINICAL TRIALS: IBUPROFEN AND INDOMETHACIN

Clinical trials with the NSAIAs in acute lung injury and ARDS are lacking. Two clinical reports of experience with oral ibuprofen may be relevant to understanding the potential of this drug in ARDS (62,63). Normal volunteers, rendered hypoxic through breathing a mixture of 12.5% oxygen in nitrogen, experienced a rise in PVR when PaO_2 fell below 55 mmHg. Pretreatment with ibuprofen resulted in an 85% reduction in serum TXB_2, without any short-term effect on arterial hypoxemia (62). The second clinical report was a single case study of a patient with ARDS (63). Treatment with an oral dose of ibuprofen was followed by an infusion of ibuprofen for 24 h. Within 4 h after initiating treatment, the patient experienced an increase in PaO_2 and a concomitant decrease in mean PPA. Termination of treatment resulted in a dramatic increase in mean PPA (63).

A small clinical pilot using ibuprofen in patients with established sepsis syndrome showed that ibuprofen, administered as a rectal solution, decreased body temperature, heart rate, and minute ventilation, and increased blood pressure (44). Each of these effects might have been related to ibuprofen's pronounced antipyretic effect. In addition there was a trend toward a decrease in peak airway pressure. A large prospective multicenter trial of ibuprofen in sepsis is currently underway and will undoubtedly shed more light on the effects of ibuprofen on sepsis-induced ARDS.

Indomethacin treatment in patients with ARDS has been investigated and reported in a single study (64). Ten patients with established ARDS were randomized to receive either indomethacin as a single dose or placebo. In comparing 1-h postinfusion levels with baseline observations in the indomethacin-treated group, patients experienced an increase in PaO_2, and a decrease in Qs/Qt. These alterations returned to baseline over the ensuing 8 h following treatment. No changes were noted in the placebo group (64).

No clinical studies have employed meclofenamate.

V. CONCLUSIONS

Anti-inflammatory therapies and pulmonary hypertension: Cyclooxygenase inhibition has been demonstrated with each of the anti-inflammatory drugs reviewed. Blocking the increase in plasma levels of the potent vasoconstrictor TXA_2 was associated with blunting of the anticipated rise in mean PPA, regardless of the pretreatment or posttreatment protocol.

Anti-inflammatory therapies and arterial hypoxemia: In both pretreatment and post-treatment protocols using anti-inflammatory agents, the magnitude of hypox- emia accompanying an acute lung injury insult was not as severe as in control groups not receiving this treatment.

Anti-inflammatory therapies and the neutrophil in ARDS: In animal studies, treatment with ibuprofen or indomethacin attenuated the depressed neutrophil counts observed in control animals receiving *E. coli* infusions. Meclofenamate did not exhibit this effect. Accumulation of neutrophils in the lung's microcirculation may be an important precipitating event in the development of increased pulmonary microvascular permeability in these animal models of ARDS as well as in the clinical condition.

VI. SUMMARY

The pathogenesis of ARDS is complex and poorly understood. There is, as yet, little reason to expect that NSAIAs will dramatically alter the progression of the process, although they may affect certain vasoactive components mediated by cyclooxygenase products. Much research has been completed on the effects of NSAIAs in sepsis and ARDS, but the results have been inconclusive to date. We hope that the large clinical trial currently underway will shed definitive light on the usefulness of ibuprofen in sepsis and ARDS.

ACKNOWLEDGMENT

Supported by the Department of Veterans Affairs.

REFERENCES

1. Ashbaugh DG, Bigelow DB, Petty TL, et al. Acute respiratory distress in adults. Lancet 1967; 2:319–23.
2. Fowler AA, Hamman RF, Good JT, et al. Adult respiratory distress syndrome: risk with common predisposition. Ann Intern Med 1983; 98:593–7.
3. Pepe PE, Potkin RT, Hotlman-Reus D, et al. Clinical predictors of the adult respiratory distress syndrome. Am J Surg 1982; 144:124–30.
4. Fowler AA, Hamman RF, Serbe GO, et al. Adult respiratory distress syndrome. Am Rev Respir Dis 1985; 132:472–8.
5. Brigham KL, Meyrick B. Endotoxin and lung injury. Am Rev Respir Dis 1986; 133:913–27.

6. Bernard GR, Luce JM, Sprung CL, et al. High dose corticosteroids in patients with the adult respiratory distress syndrome. N Engl J Med 1987; 317:1565–70.
7. Bone RC, Fisher CJ, Clemmer TP, et al. A controlled clinical trial of high-dose methylprednisolone in the treatment of severe sepsis and septic shock. N Engl J Med 1987; 317:653–8.
8. Repine JE. Neutrophils, oxygen radicals and the adult respiratory distress syndrome. In: Said SI, ed. The pulmonary circulation and acute lung injury. Mt Kisco, NY: Futura Publishing, 1985:249–81.
9. Heflin AC, Brigham KL. Prevention by granulocyte depletion of increased vascular permeability of sheep lung following endotoxemia. J Clin Invest 1981; 68:1253–60.
10. Shasby DM, Vanbenthuysen KM, Tate RM, et al. Granulocytes mediate acute edematous lung injury in rabbits and in isolated rabbit lung perfused with phorbol myristate acetate: role of oxygen radicals. Am Rev Respir Dis 1982; 125:443–7.
11. Ognibene FP, Martin SE, Parker MM, et al. Adult respiratory distress syndrome in patients with severe neutropenia. N. Engl J Med 1986; 315:547–51.
12. Schraufstatter IU, Revak SD, Cochrane CG. Proteases and oxidants in experimental pulmonary inflammatory injury. J Clin Invest 1984; 73:1175–83.
13. Ward PA, Till GO, Kunkel SR, et al. Evidence for role of hydroxyl radical in complement and neutrophil-dependent tissue injury. J Clin Invest 1983; 72:789–801.
14. Taylor AE, Matalon S, Ward PA, eds. Physiology of oxygen radicals. Bethesda: American Physiological Society, 1986.
15. Cochrane GC, Spragg RG, Revak SD. Studies on the pathogenesis of the adult respiratory syndrome: evidence of oxidant activity in bronchoalveolar lavage fluid. J Clin Invest 1983; 71:754–61.
16. Said SI. Influence of neuropeptides on airway smooth muscle. Am Rev Respir Dis 1987; 136:S52–8.
17. Lo SK, Burhop KE, Kaplan JE, et al. Role of platelets in maintenance of pulmonary vascular permeability to protein. Am J Physiol 1988; 254:H763–71.
18. Palmgren MS, deShazo RD, Carter RM, et al. Mechanisms of neutrophil damage to human alveolar extracellular matrix: the role of serine and metalloproteases. J Allergy Clin Immunol 1992; 89:905–15.
19. Malik AB. Mediators of pulmonary vascular injury and edema after thrombin. In: Said SI, ed. The pulmonary circulation and acute lung injury. Mt Kisco, NY: Futura Publishing, 1985:429–54.
20. Stephens KE, Ishizaka A, Larrick JW, et al. Tumor necrosis factor causes increased pulmonary permeability and edema. Am Rev Respir Dis 1988; 137:1364–70.
21. Wendel A. Reactive oxygen species, antiproteases, and cytokines in sepsis. Klin Wochenschr 1991; 69:969–74.
22. Billiau A, Vanderkerckhove F. Cytokines and their interactions with other inflammatory mediators in the pathogenesis of sepsis and septic shock. Eur J Clin Invest 1991; 21:559–73.
23. Tracey KJ, Beutler B, Lowry SF, et al. Shock and tissue injury induced by recombinant human cachectin. Science 1986; 234:470–4.
24. Michie HR, Manogue KR, Spriggs DR, et al. Detection of circulating tumor necrosis factor after endotoxin administration. N Engl J Med 1988; 318:1481–6.
25. Goldblum SE, Jay M, Yoneda K, et al. Monokine-induced acute lung injury in rabbits. J Appl Physiol 1987; 63:2093–100.
26. Sullivan JS, Kilpatrick L, Costarino AT, et al. Correlation of plasma cytokine elevations with mortality rate in children with sepsis. J Pediatr 1992; 120:510–5.
27. Martin MA, Silverman HJ. Gram-negative sepsis and the adult respiratory distress syndrome. Clin Infect Dis 1992; 14:1213–28.
28. Zentella A, Manogue K, Cerami A. The role of cachectin/TNF and other cytokines in sepsis. Prog Clin Biol Rev 1991; 367:9–24.
29. Chilton FH, Murphy RC. Remodeling of arachidonate-containing phosphoglycerides within the human neutrophil. J. Biol Chem 1986; 261:7771–7.

30. Henderson WR. Eicosanoids and lung inflammation. Am Rev Respir Dis 1987; 135:1176–85.
31. Braquet P, Paubert-Braquet M, Bourgain RH, et al. PAF/cytokine auto-generated feedback networks in microvascular immune injury: consequences in shock, ischemia and graft rejection. J Lipid Mediat 1989; 1:75–112.
32. Vercellotti GM, Yin HQ, Gustafson KS, et al. Platelet activating factor primes neutrophil responses to agonists: role in promoting neutrophil-mediated endothelial damage. Blood 1988; 71:1100–7.
33. Koltai M, Hosford D, Guinot P, et al. Platelet activating factor (PAF). A review of its effects, antagonists and possible future clinical implications (part I). Drugs 1991; 42:9–29.
34. Vanhoutte PM, Rubanyi GM, Miller VM, Houston DS. Modulation of vascular smooth muscle contraction by the endothelium. Annu Rev Physiol 1986; 48:307–20.
35. Capdevila JH, Falck JR, Estabrook RW. Cytochrome P450 and the arachidonate cascade. FASEB J 1992; 6:731–6.
36. McGiff JC, Carroll MA. Cytochrome P450-dependent arachidonate metabolites: biological activities. Adv Prostaglandin Thromboxane Leukotriene Res 1989; 19:34–41.
37. Fitzpatrick FA, Murphy RC. Cytochrome P-450 metabolism of arachidonic acid: formation and biological actions of "epoxygenase"-derived eicosanoids. Pharmacol Rev 1988; 40:229–41.
38. Ogeltree ML. Overview of physiological and pathophysiological effects of thromboxane A_2. Fed Proc 1987; 46:133–8.
39. Gee MH, Perkowski SZ, Tahamont MV, et al. Arachidonate cyclo-oxygenase metabolites as mediators of complement-initiated lung injury. Fed Proc 1985; 44:46–52.
40. Samuelsson B, Dahlen SE, Lindgren JA, et al. Leukotrienes and lipoxins; structures, biosynthesis and biological effects. Science 1987; 237:1171–6.
41. Voelkel NF, Stenmark KR, Reeves JT, et al. Actions of lipoxygenase metabolism in isolated rat lungs. J Appl Physiol 1984; 57:860–7.
42. Smith LJ, Shamsuddin M, Anderson J, et al. Hyperoxic lung damage in mice: appearance and bioconversion of peptide leukotrienes. J Appl Physiol 1988; 64:944–51.
43. Stephenson AH, Lonigro AJ, Hyers TM, et al. Increased concentrations of leukotrienes in bronchoalveolar lavage fluid of patients with ARDS or at risk for ARDS. Am Rev Respir Dis 1988; 138:714–9.
44. Bernard GR, Reines HD, Metz CA, et al. Effects of a short course of ibuprofen in patients with severe sepsis [abstract]. Am Rev Respir Dis 1988; 137:A138.
45. Romson JL, Bush LR, Haack DW, Luechesi BR. The beneficial effects of oral ibuprofen on coronary artery thrombosis and myocardial ischemia in conscious dogs. J Pharmacol Exp Ther 1980; 215:271–8.
46. Brown KA, Collins AJ. Action of nonsteroidal anti-inflammatory drugs on human and rat peripheral leukocyte migration in vivo. Ann Rheum Dis 1977; 36:239–43.
47. Snapper JR, Hutchinson AA, Ogeltree ML. Effects of cyclooxygenase inhibitors on the alterations in lung mechanics caused by endotoxemia in the unanesthetized sheep. J Clin Invest 1983; 72:63–76.
48. Fuhrman TM, Holloy MF, Reines HD, et al. Beneficial effects of ibuprofen on oleic acid induced injury. J Surg Res 1987; 42:284–9.
49. Perlman MB, Johnson A, Malik AB. Ibuprofen prevents thrombin-induced lung vascular injury: mechanism of effect. Am J Physiol 1987; 242:H605–15.
50. Johnson A, Malik AB. Pulmonary transvascular fluid and protein exchange after thrombin-induced microembolism. Am Rev Respir Dis 1985; 132:70–6.
51. Hammond B, Fairman RP, Monroe P. The pulmonary hypertension of sclerosing agents is prevented by cyclo-oxygenase inhibitors. Am J Med Sci 1985; 290:98–101.
52. Ganey PE, Roth RA. Ibuprofen does not alter the cardiopulmonary effects of monocrotaline pyrole. Am J Physiol 1987; 252:H743–8.
53. Traber DL, Adams T, Henriksen N, et al. Ibuprofen and diphenhydramine reduce the lung lesion of endotoxemia in sheep. J Trauma 1984; 24:835–40.

54. Brigham KL, Owens P. Increased sheep lung vascular permeability caused by histamine. Circ Res 1975; 37:647–57.
55. Borg T, Gerdin B, Hallgren R, et al. The role of polymorphonuclear leukocytes in the pulmonary dysfunction induced by complement activation. Acta Anesthesiol Scand 1985; 29:231–40.
56. Cafalo RC, Lewis PE, O'Brien WF, et al. The role of prostaglandins in endotoxemia: comparisons in response in the nonpregnant, maternal, and fetal models. Am J Obstet Gynecol 1980; 137:53–7.
57. Ward P, Sulavik MC, Johnson KJ. Rat neutrophil activation and effects of lipoxygenase and cyclooxygenase inhibitors. Am J Pathol 1984; 116:223–33.
58. Konstam MA, Hill NS, Bonin JD, et al. Prostaglandin mediation of hemodynamic responses to pulmonary microembolism in rabbits: effects of ibuprofen and meclofenamate. Exp Lung Res 1987; 12:331–45.
59. Begley CJ, Ogletree ML, Meyrick B, et al. Modification of pulmonary responses to endotoxemia in awake sheep by steroidal and nonsteroidal anti-inflammatory agents. Am Rev Respir Dis 1984; 130:1140–6.
60. Snapper JR, Bernard GR, Hinson JM, et al. Endotoxemia-induced leukopenia in sheep. Am Rev Respir Dis 1983; 127:306–9.
61. Sielaff TD, Sugerman HJ, Tatum JL, et al. Successful treatment of adult respiratory distress syndrome by histamine and prostaglandin blockade in a porcine *Pseudomonas* model. Surgery 1987; 102:350–7.
62. Hallemans R, Naelje R, Melot C, et al. Do cyclooxygenase products mediate hypoxic pulmonary vasoconstriction in man? [abstract]. Am Rev Respir Dis 1984; 129:A341.
63. Hasselstrom LJ, Ellasen K, Mogensen T, et al. Lowering pulmonary artery pressure in a patient with severe acute respiratory failure. Intensive Care Med 1985; 11:48–50.
64. Steinberg SM, Rodriguez JL, Bitzer LG, et al. Indomethacin treatment of human adult respiratory distress syndrome. Circ Shock 1990; 30:375–84.

4

Nonsteroidal Anti-Inflammatory Drugs in Stroke

SIEN T. CHEN
Chang Gung Memorial Hospital
Taipei, Taiwan

TENG-NAN LIN
Institute of Biomedical Sciences
Taipei, Taiwan

T. K. LEE
National Taiwan University
Taipei, Taiwan

CHUNG Y. HSU
Baylor College of Medicine
Houston, Texas

I. INTRODUCTION

Preceding the era of nonsteroidal anti-inflammatory drugs (NSAIDs), aspirin was found anecdotally to be effective in prevention of cerebral thrombosis (1). Inhibition of cyclooxygenase has now been identified as a prime mechanism of action of NSAIDs, including aspirin (2). Following the discoveries of thromboxane (TX) A_2, and prostacyclin (PGI_2) in the 1970s (3,4), our understanding of the physiology of platelets and vessel walls has been greatly enhanced. The potent opposing biological actions of TXA_2 and PGI_2 on platelets and vessel walls have prompted a hypothesis that explains many facets of cerebrovascular diseases on the basis of disturbances in the balance of these two cyclooxygenase metabolites (5–8). The observations that NSAIDs may block TXA_2 and PGI_2 synthesis with differential potencies raises the possibility of pharmacological modification of platelet–vessel wall interactions by these drugs in cerebrovascular diseases (8). In fact, many experimental and human studies have been conducted using various kinds of NSAIDs to treat or prevent postischemic hypoperfusion, vasospasm, ischemic neuronal damage, and even neonatal intraventricular hemorrhage (IVH). However, the most promising results, so far, have been restricted to the use of aspirin in the prevention of transient ischemic attacks (TIAs) and ischemic stroke (9,10).

This chapter will begin with a brief description of arachidonic acid (AA) metabolites, particularly those derived from the cyclooxygenase pathway, and their relevance to platelet–vessel wall interactions that are important in the pathophysiology of cerebrovasreviewed to provide the foundation for current concepts concerning the pharmacological intervention of cerebrovascular disease using NSAIDs. Finally, trials of NSAIDs in different types of strokes will be reviewed, focusing on aspirin, which has been the only dominant NSAID in clinical stroke trials so far.

II. BIOLOGICAL ACTIONS OF ARACHIDONIC ACID METABOLITES ON PLATELETS AND VESSEL WALLS

A. Effects on Platelet Aggregation

Thromboxane A_2 (TXA_2), a major AA metabolite in platelets, was named for its platelet-aggregating action (11). Thrombin, collagen, and epinephrine stimulate platelet production of TXA_2, whereas TXA_2 is blocked by cyclooxygenase inhibitors, notably NSAIDs. Platelet aggregation is a complex process, and TXA_2 is only one of several factors, so that inhibition of its synthesis alone may not prevent aggregation (12). Prostacyclin (PGI_2) is the most potent endogenous inhibitor of platelet aggregation (13) and is also the main AA product in vessel walls. When PGI_2 is released from the endothelial surface, it limits the growth of platelet thrombi and, at high concentration, prevents adhesion (14). The antiplatelet effect of NSAIDs is through inhibition of cyclooxygenase (15,16), which catalyzes the conversion of AA to the labile endoperoxides PGG_2 and PGH_2, which is the precursor of PGI_2 and TXA_2. Other AA metabolites derived from the cyclooxygenase pathway, including PGE_2 and $PGF_{2\alpha}$, may also affect platelet aggregability, but are much less potent than TXA_2 and PGI_2.

B. Effects on Cerebral Vessels

Thromboxane A_2 is the most potent naturally occurring cerebral vasoconstrictor (17), and PGI_2 is a potent opposing dilator (18). In isolated cerebral arteries, TXA_2, at 0.03–0.15 nM, causes vasoconstriction, whereas PGI_2, at 0.2–0.8 nM, produces dilation (18).

C. Platelet–Vessel Wall Interaction and Thromboxane A_2–Prostacyclin Balance

An active vascular endothelium is necessary for maintaining vascular integrity and potency (19–21). There is a delicate and complex interaction of vessel walls and platelets. Protacyclin inhibits platelet aggregation and removes preformed aggregates. A balance of TXA_2 and PGI_2 production occurs during the contact of platelets with vessel walls and serves to prevent adhesion and aggregation of platelets and other blood cells (Fig. 1). Damage to endothelium and exposure of the collagenous subendothelial surface promote platelet aggregation and trigger the coagulation cascade. Thrombosis may develop if the TXA_2–PGI_2 balance favors TXA_2 (7,8). Although TXA_2–PGI_2 imbalance is an oversimplified and only partial explanation for the thromboembolic proclivity (22), it provides a useful framework for exploration of the relevant pharmacology of NSAIDs in cerebrovascular diseases.

III. ARACHIDONIC ACID METABOLITES AND CEREBROVASCULAR DISEASES

A. Contribution to Acute Ischemic Injury

In cerebral ischemia, AA metabolites may contribute to postischemic hypoperfusion, brain edema, and irreversible neuronal damage (23,24). Ischemia triggers (Fig. 2) an initial rise

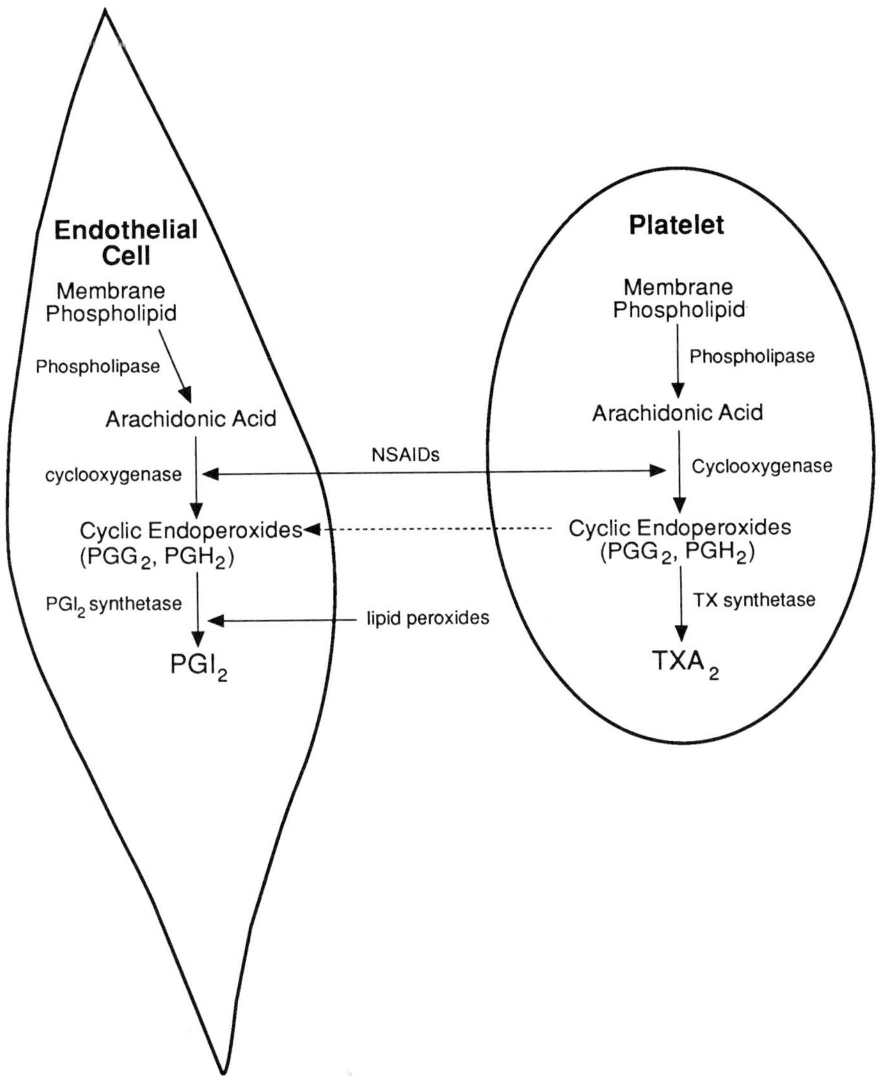

Figure 1 Major metabolic pathways of arachidonic acid metabolism in endothelial cells and platelets. Horizontal arrows indicate sites of enzyme inhibition. Dashed line with arrow denotes shunting of cyclic endoperoxides from platelets to endothelial cells for PGI_2 production.

in intracellular calcium ions (25), leading to activation of phospholipases. Phospholipid breakdown results in increase in free fatty acids, including AA (26), which is rapidly converted to eicosanoids (PGs, TXA_2, and leukotrienes). Oxygen free radicals are generated early in both the cyclooxygenase and lipoxygenase pathways (27), and some of the AA byproducts (e.g., lipid peroxides) are also free radicals. Excessive free-radical production may inhibit PGI_2 synthesis (28), fostering TXA_2–PGI_2 imbalance. Cerebral TXB_2 formation increases after ischemia in gerbils (29) and rats (30); increased urinary levels of TXB_2 also occur with human stroke (31). This sequence could contribute to formation of platelet microthrombi (32) as well as impairment of microcirculation (33–35),

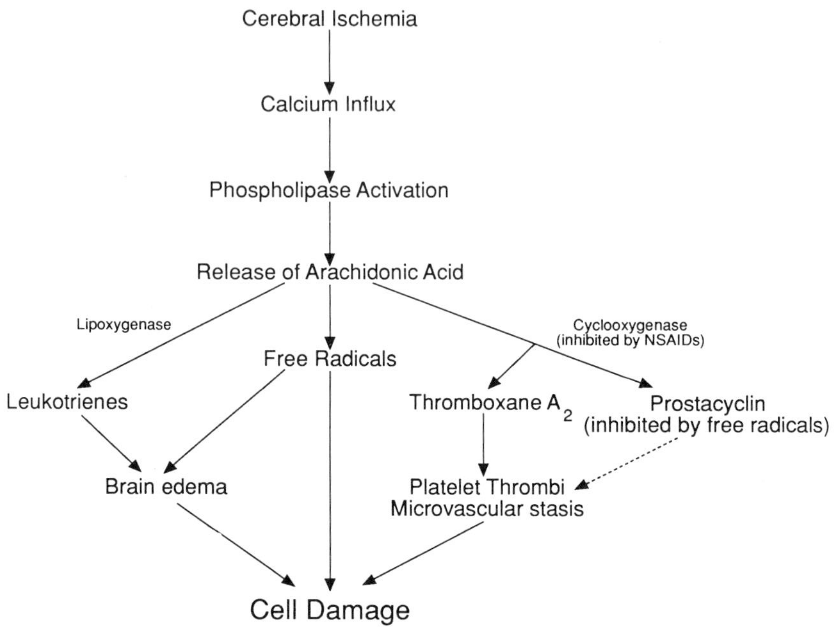

Figure 2 Possible mechanism of ischemic neuronal damage involving arachidonic acid cascade. Dashed line with arrow denotes inhibition.

leading to prolonged severe depression of cerebral blood flow and irreversible neuronal damage. These detrimental effects may be amplified by leukotriene-induced brain edema (36,37) and free–radical-mediated brain injury (38–40).

B. Contribution to Cerebral Vasospasm

Because TXA_2 and PGI_2 have potent effect on vascular tone, a TXA_2–PGI_2 imbalance may also cause vasospasm. The role of vasospasm in cerebral ischemia has not been established. Although focal spasm is the most usual explanation for cerebral infarction in migraine (41), it is thought to be a rare cause of TIA and transient monocular blindness (42,43). In stroke patients without a cardiac source of emboli or angiographic evidence of arterial occlusion, vasospasm is among the possible mechanisms of cerebral ischemia (10).

Delayed vasospasm after subarachnoid hemorrhage (SAH) is a well-known phenomenon, and is one of the major causes of morbidity and mortality following SAH caused by rupture of an intracerebral aneurysm (44,45). Despite vigorous investigation for years, the cause of vasospasm remains obscure. A possible mechanism involving AA metabolism has been proposed. During experimental SAH, there is a significant decrease of PGI_2 and increase of TXA_2, PGE_2, D_2, and $F_{2\alpha}$ production in cerebrospinal fluid (CSF), correlating with endothelial damage and lysis of subarachnoid blood clot (46–48). This TXA_2–PGI_2 imbalance has also been demonstrated during the clinical course of SAH in humans (48–50). Thus, an alteration of TXA_2–PGI_2 balance may be one of the mechanisms leading to prolonged cerebral vasospasm following SAH.

C. Contribution to Neonatal Intraventricular Hemorrhage

Intraventricular hemorrhage (IVH), caused by rupture of the fragile germinal layer capillaries, is a catastrophic perinatal event among preterm neonates and has been reported to occur in 40–50% of infants of less than 34-weeks gestational age (51–53). The pathophysiology is not well understood. However, its linkage with perinatal asphyxia has led to the hypothesis that increases in cerebral arterial blood volume following hypoxia and hypercapnia may be responsible for the hemorrhage (54–56). Since cerebral blood flow is controlled in part by PGs synthesized from cerebral microvasculature, a role for PGI_2, a potent vasodilator, involvement in this pathological condition has been postulated. This concept is supported by the findings that premature infants with respiratory distress syndrome and IVH have high circulating levels of PGI_2 (57,58).

D. Contribution to Thromboembolic Events

The role that AA metabolites may play in thromboembolism is mainly through their effects on platelet function. Platelets are involved in the development of atherosclerosis (59,60). Atherosclerotic lesions develop at sites of arterial orifices or bifurcations (61,62), at which disturbed flow favors platelet accumulation (63,64). Mural thrombi composed of platelets and fibrin on the atherosclerotic lesions are incorporated into the vessel walls (65). Platelets release serotonin and TXA_2 (66). Both cause vasoconstriction and may lead to endothelial cell contraction with exposure of the thrombogenic subendothelium (60). Atherosclerotic arteries produce less PGI_2 than normal (67,68), perhaps as a result of accumulation of lipid peroxides in the vessel wall (69). Lipid peroxides may shift the balance of TXA_2 and PGI_2 to favor thrombus formation by inhibiting vascular PGI_2 synthetase (69). It is also noteworthy that high-density lipoproteins that protect against ischemic heart disease stimulate PGI_2 (70,71); the low-density lipoproteins, an atherogenic factor, reduce PGI_2 output (70).

Artery-to-artery embolism has merged as a major mechanism of TIAs and strokes (42). Atherosclerotic disease in the large cervical and intracranial arteries is a major source of emboli. Platelet emboli have been observed in retinal vessels during attacks of transient monocular blindness (72). Platelet thrombi have been found in atherosclerotic plaques removed by carotid endarterectomy (73,74). Emboli of cardiac origin may contain largely platelets and fibrin (75). The induction of platelet–fibrin thrombi by experimental injury of vessels is inhibited by aspirin and other NSAIDs; this suggests that platelet aggregation mediated by TXA_2 plays a major role in thrombus generation (76).

IV. USES OF NONSTEROIDAL ANTI-INFLAMMATORY DRUGS IN STROKE

A. In Acute Cerebral Ischemia

Pharmacological interventions to salvage ischemic neurons from dying during acute stage of cerebral ischemia have, as yet, met with limited successes. Although the ischemic cascade involving AA metabolism is an intriguing biochemical process contributing to acute ischemic neuronal damage, inhibition of cyclooxygenase by NSAIDs in animal models of acute ischemia did not yield consistent results. In dogs, indomethacin alone or with PGI_2 treatment improved postischemic reperfusion after global cerebal ischemia (78,79); indomethacin with PGI_2 and heparin promoted neuronal recovery (80). In rats, pretreatment with PGI_2 and indomethacin prevented cerebral ischemia after extracranial vascular injury (81). In contrast, indomethacin pretreatment in baboons reduced basal cerebral blood flow and increased brain edema (82). Prostacyclin and indomethacin also had no beneficial effect in acute focal cerebral ischemia in dogs (83). There has been no clinical trial of NSAIDs in the treatment of acute ischemic stroke. Several reasons may account for the lack of efficacy of NSAIDs in treating acute cerebral ischemia. First, NSAIDs block the cyclooxygenase in different tissues so that synthesis of PGI_2 in the endothelium is also inhibited. Second, NSAIDs do not inhibit the lipoxygenase pathway. Production of leukotrienes is not affected or may even be increased by NSAIDs because of shunting of AA from the cyclooxygenase to the lipoxygenase pathway. Leukotrienes derived from the lipoxygenase pathway alter vascular permeability, constrict cerebral arterioles, and are potent chemoattractants (84–86). All these may contribute to ischemic brain edema, postischemic hypoperfusion, and leukocyte-mediated cellular damage (37). Finally, other mechanisms for ischemic neuronal injury may exist and include the neurotoxic effect of excitatory neurotransmitters (87), calcium-mediated proteolysis (88), and free–radical-induced injury (38–40). These detrimental effects, except for free-radical scavenging, are not deterred by NSAIDs.

B. In Cerebral Vasospasm

Cerebral vasospasm may play a role in causing thromboembolic stroke, but it is a problem of great clinical importance following SAH. The basic functional abnormality is unclear, and pharmacological attempts to prevent or to treat vasospasm have been disappointing (89). Although the theory of an imbalance between TXA_2–PGI_2 production is attractive, the effects of NSAIDs in experimental cerebral vasospasm are inconsistent. The NSAIDs that have been tested included aspirin (90–93), indomethacin (90,92,95–97), meclofenamate (90–92,94), ibuprofen (94,98), naproxen (90), sudoxicam (90), and piroxicam (94). Conflicting results have been noted even for the same NSAID. For example, indomethacin markedly inhibits AA-induced sustained contractions of isolated dog basilar arteries in one report (92), but was unable to diminish such contractions induced by bloody CSF in another (94). The pathogenesis of delayed cerebral vasospasm after SAH remains to be determined and is likely to involve multiple vasoactive factors. More than two-dozen substances in the circulating blood have been implicated in the pathogenesis of vasospasm following SAH (46). A PG-mediated effect is only one of numerous factors contributing to this complex phenomenon. Thus, it is not surprising that vasospasm may not be prevented or reversed by NSAIDs alone. Further investigation in this field is clearly needed.

C. In Neonatal Intraventricular Hemorrhage

Indomethacin is effective in closure of the patent ductus arteriosus (PDA) in premature infants (99,100). Infants with PDA are also at increased risk for developing IVH (54). Given the finding that newborn infants receiving indomethacin for treatment of a PDA also had a lower incidence of IVH (99,101,102), several prospective clinical trials have been carried out to examine the efficacy of indomethacin in preventing neonatal IVH (102–108); however, the results were conflicting. Some investigators found that low-dose indomethacin decreased the incidence of IVH, without significant reductions in urinary output or other major side effects (106,107). Hanigan et al. reported that indomethacin decreased the incidence of IVH in infants weighing 1000–1500 g at birth, but not in infants of lower weights (105). Some investigators, on the contrary, showed no significant effect of indomethacin on IVH (102,104), and side effects, such as prolonged bleeding time (control: 2.7; indomethacin: 5.5 min, $p < 0.001$), elevation of serum creatinine level (control: 96; indomethacin: 121 mmol/L, $p = 0.01$), and gastrointestinal bleeding (control: 0; indomethacin: 29%) were more frequent in the indomethacin-treated infants (104). A recent study demonstrated that indomethacin prophylaxis reduced the relative risk of severe IVH, but other perinatal variables, such as lower birth weight, lower 5-min Apgar score, higher fraction of inspired oxygen, and so on, also contributed to the overall risk of IVH (108). Interpretation of these trial reports are confounded by differences in entry criteria, indomethacin doses, and care practices. There is a need for a multicenter study using a standardized protocol to clarify the issue on the exact effect of indomethacin on IVH. Until more data are available, the generalized use of indomethacin in preventing neonatal IVH cannot be recommended.

D. In Prevention of Ischemic Stroke

The use of NSAIDs in stroke, so far, has been limited to the successful application of aspirin in preventing TIAs and ischemic stroke. Aspirin (acetylsalicylic acid) is one of the world's oldest and most widely used drugs. It prolongs bleeding time and inhibits platelet aggregation. Aspirin inhibits PG synthesis by irreversibly acetylating cyclooxygenase (109) and prevents the conversion of platelet AA to TXA_2. Since platelets cannot synthesize protein, the inactivation of cyclooxygenase by aspirin affects platelets permanently. Inhibition by other NSAIDs, however, is reversible (110). As a result, inhibition of platelet cyclooxygenase by aspirin is cumulative on repeated dosing. This may account for the advantage of using aspirin over other NSAIDs in stroke prevention.

Numerous large-scale randomized trials of antiplatelet treatment for patients with a history of TIA, occlusive stroke, unstable angina, or myocardial infarction have been reported (see Ref. 9 for overview). These trials are characterized by diversity in study population for ages, cardiovascular and cerebrovascular status, and concurrent medical management to control stroke risk factors, and by substantial difference in trial protocols. It is difficult to compare the results from one study with another to draw a conclusion on the effect of antiplatelet therapy in the secondary prevention of stroke. A trialists' overview attempting to solve this problem has been published (9). It included 25 completed trials with a total of 29,000 patients. Most of the trials used aspirin as the antiplatelet agent. The meta-analysis revealed that antiplatelet treatment reduced vascular mortality by 15% and nonfatal vascular events (stroke or myocardial infarction) by 30%, but had no apparent effect on nonvascular mortality. No significant difference was observed between the effects of 300–325 mg aspirin daily versus higher aspirin doses, with or without sulfinpyrazone, or aspirin in combination with dipyridamole. Thus, a moderate effect of aspirin in secondary prevention of occlusive vascular disease has been firmly established. However, many questions remain concerning the use of aspirin for stroke prophylaxis. A few important clinical issues will be discussed here.

1. *Is Aspirin Effective in Primary Prevention of Stroke?*

The issue of primary prevention of stroke by aspirin has been evaluated in two randomized trials of healthy male physicians, one in the United States (111) and another in the United Kingdom (112). The American trial of 325-mg aspirin every other day reported a trend in the increase in risk of stroke among those receiving aspirin; hemorrhagic stroke was observed more frequently in this group than placebo, but the difference was not significant. The British study of 500-mg aspirin daily showed a significant reduction in TIA, compared with placebo but, disturbingly, also indicated a nonsignificant increase in stroke rate. Taken together, these two primary prevention studies demonstrate no reduction in the overall risk of stroke; to the contrary, there is a trend in the increase in disabling strokes

(113). Thus, despite the seemingly universal effectiveness of aspirin in the secondary prevention of stroke, aspirin is not beneficial in primary stroke prevention among healthy individuals.

2. How Much Aspirin is Adequate?

Aspirin inhibits formation of PGI_2 in blood vessels as well as TXA_2 in platelets, constituting what can be termed the "aspirin dilemma" (114). One widely held solution to this is based on the following: Platelet cyclooxygenase is more sensitive to aspirin inhibition than its vascular counterpart (115), and the inhibition of the platelet enzyme is permanent (109), whereas, that of the endothelial enzyme is reversible (116,117). Accordingly, smaller and less frequent doses of aspirin have been advocated in an effort to spare the beneficial endothelial PGI_2 production (118). However, complete sparing of vascular PGI_2 inhibition by adjusting the aspirin dose has not been achieved. Aspirin inhibits PGI_2 production in a single dose as low as 20 mg (119). Most of the trials in the secondary prevention of stroke used relatively large doses of aspirin (900–1300 mg/day). The preliminary report of the UK-TIA trial indicated that 300 mg of aspirin is just as effective as 1200 mg in preventing myocardial infarction and stroke in patients with cerebrovascular diseases (120). Gastrointestinal side effects, however, are fewer with the lower dose. Although 75 mg of aspirin in a single dose significantly inhibits platelet hyperfunction and suppresses the mean plasma TXB_2 levels without significantly altering plasma 6-keto-$PGF_{1\alpha}$ levels (121), doses lower than 300 mg have not had a therapeutic effect in secondary stroke prevention studies. Only one trial using a very low dose (40–75 mg) of aspirin has been completed, and it was a negative study (122). The optimal dose of aspirin has thus not been established. One can only tentatively conclude that a dose of 300 mg daily may be optimal for secondary stroke prevention, but for patients with a history of peptic ulcer, lower doses (75–100 mg) have been recommended (123,124). Information on the dosing and schedule described in the foregoing is applicable to male patients. Effects of aspirin in stroke prevention in female patients are less certain (Sect. IV.D.4)

3. What Dosing Schedule is Optimal?

Because aspirin inactivates cyclooxygenase for the life span of the platelets (half-life: 6–7 days), the benefits of a dosing schedule less frequent than once-a-day have been entertained (125). However, about 10–15% of the platelets are replaced in the circulation every day, and only 2–10% of nonacetylated platelets are needed to restore platelet-mediated thrombotic process (126,127). The benefits of less frequent dosing is probably questionable.

4. Is Aspirin Effective in Women?

Two trials of aspirin in TIA (128,129) showed a lack of effect in women. Animal experiments also showed a reduced effect of aspirin in the female (130). The sex difference in aspirin protection is difficult to explain on the basis of known effect of aspirin on AA metabolism and has not been found in other clinical trials (131,132). Our recent study also showed that 300 mg of aspirin, in a single dose, significantly depressed plasma TXB_2 levels, without any differential effect between sexes (133). The validity of the claim in the two trials showing lack of aspirin effect in women has been questioned because of the small number of female patients enrolled and the relative benign natural course of atherosclerosis in women (134). The UK-TIA trial demonstrated no significant gender differences in response to aspirin (120). We continue to prescribe aspirin as indicated, regardless of sex. Alternative antiplatelet regimen (ticlopidine) has been shown to be effective in secondary stroke prevention and may be desirable in selected female patients (see next section).

5. Is It Advantageous to Add Other Antiplatelet Agents?

In the Canadian Cooperative Study of TIA, the combination of sulfinpyrazone with aspirin offered no significant advantage over aspirin alone (128). Sulfinpyrazone inhibits cyclooxygenase reversibly and is less potent than aspirin. Failure of this combination is not surprising, since pharmacologically there is no advantage in using two drugs acting on the same enzyme (135).

Dipyridamole inhibits phosphodiesterase and blocks the uptake of adenosine into red blood cells (136). Both actions result in an increase of cAMP, which is inhibitory to platelet aggregation. Although there is a theoretical advantage of adding dipyridamole to potentiate the antiplatelet effect of aspirin, such combination has not shown any superiority over aspirin alone in stroke prophylaxis (132,137). Moreover, the high cost, side effects, and the need of frequent dosing, all are unfavorable for prescribing dipyridamole as an adjunct treatment in stroke prevention.

Two multicenter randomized trials of ticlopidine in secondary prevention of ischemic stroke have been completed (138,139). Both showed a significant effect of ticlopidine in stroke prevention; ticlopidine was as effective in women as men. In one of the two studies (140), ticlopidine was superior to aspirin. The mechanism of action of ticlopidine is still unknown. It inhibits adenosine diphosphate (ADP)-induced platelet aggregation, but does not inhibit AA-mediated platelet aggregation. Combination of aspirin and ticlopidine is potentially a better antiplatelet regimen that markedly inhibits platelet aggregation induced by ADP, AA, and platelet-activating factor (139). The role of ticlopidine, alone or in combination with aspirin, in stroke prevention seems promising.

V. SUMMARY

Our understanding of the roles of AA metabolites in the pathophysiology of cerebrovascular disorders has led to the exploration of inhibitors of AA metabolism, notably NSAIDs, in the prevention and treatment of strokes. With the exception of aspirin in stroke prevention, therapeutic efficacy of NSAIDs in different types of strokes remains to be fully proved. Ischemic and hemorrhagic strokes invoke a multitude of pathophysiological and biochemical changes leading to brain injury. Future studies of the roles of NSAIDs in stroke should consider NSAIDs in conjunction with agents affecting other biochemical cascades (e.g., lipoxygenase pathway or excitotoxins) that are also known to cause brain injury. Investigation of the delayed inflammatory reaction following ischemic or hemorrhagic brain injury has just begun (37). The potential therapeutic roles of NSAIDs in strokes may not be fully appreciated until we have better understanding of the contribution of inflammation in the ultimate brain injury.

REFERENCES

1. Craven LL. Prevention of coronary and cerebral thrombosis. Miss Valley Med J 1956; 78:213–5.
2. Paulus HE, Furst DE. Aspirin and other nonsteroidal antiinflammatory drugs. In: McCarty DJ, ed. Arthritis and allied conditions. 11th ed. Philadelphia: Lea & Febiger, 1989:507–41.

3. Hamberg M, Samuelsson B. Prostaglandin endoperoxides: novel transformation of arachidonic acid in human platelets. Proc Natl Acad Sci USA 1976; 71:3400–4.
4. Moncada S, Gryglewski R, Bunting S, Vane JR. An enzyme isolated from arteries transforms prostaglandin endoperoxides to an unstable substance that inhibits platelet aggregation. Nature 1976; 263:663–5.
5. Moncada S, Vane JR. Arachidonic acid metabolites and interactions between platelets and blood-vessel walls. N Engl J Med 1979; 300:1142–7.
6. Mitchel JRA. Clinical aspects of the arachidonic acid–thromboxane pathway. Br Med Bull 1983; 39:289–95.
7. Halushka PV, Dollery CT, MacDermot J. Thromboxane and prostacyclin in disease: a review. Q J Med 1983; 208:461–70.
8. Chen ST, Hsu CY, Hogan EL, Halushka PV, Linet OI, Yatsu FM. Thromboxane, prostacyclin, and leukotrienes in cerebral ischemia. Neurology 1986; 36:466–70.
9. Antiplatelet Trialists' Collaboration. Secondary prevention of vascular disease by prolonged antiplatelet treatment. Br Med J 1988; 296:320–31.
10. Hsu CY, Hogan EL. Antiplatelet agents in acute cerebral ischemia. In: Fisher M, ed. Medical therapy of acute stroke. New York: Marcel Dekker, 1989:73–95.
11. Moskowitz MA, Coughlin SR. Basic properties of the prostaglandins. Stroke 1981; 12:696–701.
12. Bertele V, Falanga A, Tomasiak M, Chiabrando C, Cerletti C, Gaetano G. Pharmacologic inhibition of thromboxane synthetase and platelet aggregation: modulatory role of cyclooxygenase products. Blood 1984; 63:1460–6.
13. Moncada S. Biologic importance of prostacyclin. Br J Pharmacol 1982; 76:3–31.
14. Higgs EA, Moncada S, Vane JR. Effect of PGI_2 on platelet adhesion to rabbit arterial subendothelium. Prostaglandins 1978; 16:17–22.
15. Vane JR. Inhibition of prostaglandin synthesis as a mechanism of action for aspirin-like drugs. Nature 1971; 231:232–5.
16. Smith JB, Willis AL. Aspirin selectively inhibits prostaglandin production in human platelets. Nature 1971; 231:235–7.
17. Ellis EF, Nies AS, Oates JA. Cerebral arterial smooth muscle contraction by thromboxane A_2. Stroke 1977; 8:480–3.
18. Von Holst H, Granstrom E, Hammarstrom S, Samuelsson B, Steiner L. Effect of leukotrienes C_4, D_4, prostacyclin, and thromboxane A_2 on isolated human cerebral arteries. Acta Neurochir 1982; 62:177–85.
19. de Gaetano G, Cerletti C, Dejana E, Vermylen J. Current issues in thrombosis prevention with antiplatelet drugs. Drugs 1986; 31:517.
20. Silver MJ. Mechanisms of hemostasis and therapy of thrombosis: new concept based on metabolism of arachidonic acid by platelets and endothelial cells. Adv Pharmacol Chemother 1981; 18:2.
21. Wu KK. Microvascular thrombosis: pathophysiology and new strategies. Hosp Pract 1985; May 15:47.
22. FitzGerald GA, Smith B, Pedersen AK, Brash AR. Increased prostacyclin biosynthesis in patients with severe artherosclerosis and platelet activation. N Engl J Med 1984; 310:1065–8.
23. Raichle ME. The pathophysiology of brain ischemia. Ann Neurol 1983; 13:2–10.
24. Hsu CY, Liu TH, Xu J, Hogan EL, Chao J, Sun G, Tai HH, Beckman JS, Freeman BA. Arachidonic acid and its metabolites in cerebral ischemia. Ann NY Acad Sci 1989;
25. Chen ST, Hsu CY, Hogan EL. Calcium and calcium antagonists in cerebral ischemia. Chang Gung Med J 1985; 88:43–9.
26. Aveldano MI, Baazan NG. Rapid production of diacylglycerols enriched in arachidonate and stearate during early brain ischemia. J Neurochem 1975; 25:919–20.
27. Wolfe LS. Eicosanoids: prostaglandins, thromboxanes, leukotrienes, and other derivatives of carbon-20 unsaturated fatty acids. J Neurochem 1982; 38:1–14.

28. Warso MA, Lando WEM. Lipid peroxidation in relation to prostacyclin and thromboxane physiology and pathophysiology. Br Med Bull 1983; 39:277–80.
29. Gaudet RJ, Alam I, Levine L. Accumulation of cyclooxygenase products of arachidonic acid metabolism in gerbil brain during reperfusion after bilateral common carotid artery occlusion. J Neurochem 1980; 35:653–8.
30. Shohami E, Rosenthal J, Lavy S. The effect of incomplete cerebral ischemia on prostaglandin levels in rat brain. Stroke 1982; 13:494–9.
31. Fisher M, Zipser R. Increased excretion of immunoreactive thromboxane B_2 in cerebral ischemia. Stroke 1985; 16:10–4.
32. Petito C. Platelet thrombi in experimental cerebral infarction. Stroke 1979; 10:192–6.
33. Levy DE, Uitert RL, Pike CL. Delayed postischemic hypoperfusion: a potentially damaging consequence of stroke. Neurology 1979; 29:1245–52.
34. Crowell RM, Olsson Y. Impaired microvascular filling after focal cerebral ischemia in monkeys. J Neurosurg 1972; 36:303–9.
35. Ames A, Wright RL, Kowada M, Thurston JM, Majino G. Cerebral ischemia: II. The no-reflow phenomenon. Am J Pathol 1968; 52:437–53.
36. Black KL, Hoff JT. Leukotrienes increase blood–brain barrier permeability following intraparenchyma injections in rats. Ann Neurol 1985; 18:349–51.
37. Hsu CY, Liu TH, Xu J, Hogan EL, Chao J. Lipid inflammatory mediators in ischemic brain edema and injury. In: Bazan NG, ed. Lipid mediators in ischemic brain damage and experimental epilepsy. vol 4. Basel: S Karger, 1990:85–112.
38. Liu TH, Beckman JS, Freeman BS, Hogan EL, Hsu CY. Polyethylene glycol-conjugated superoxide dismutase and catalase reduce ischemic brain injury. Am J Physiol 1989; H589-93.
39. Imaizumi S, Woolworth V, Fishman RA, Chan PH. Liposome-entrapped superoxide dismutase reduces cerebral infarction in cerebral ischemia in rats. Stroke 1990; 21:1312–1317.
40. Kinouchi H, Epstein CJ, Mizui T, Carlson E, Chen SF, Chan PH. Attenuation of focal cerebral ischemic injury in transgenic mice overexpressing CuZn superoxide dismutase. Proc Natl Acad Sci USA 1991; 88:11158–62.
41. Hachinski V, Norris JW. The acute stroke. Philadelphia: FA Davis, 1985:149.
42. Barnett HJM. Progress towards stroke prevention: Robert Wartenberg lecture. Neurology 1980; 30:1212–25.
43. Burger SK, Saul RF, Sehorst JB, Thurston SE. Transient monocular blindness caused by vasospasm. N Engl J Med 1991; 325:870–3
44. Heros RC, Zervas NT, Varsos V. Cerebral vasospasm after subarachnoid hemorrhage: an update. Ann Neurol 1983; 14:599–608.
45. Kiwak KJ, Heros RC. Cerebral vasospasm after subarachnoid hemorrhage. Trends Neurosci 1987; 10:89–92.
46. Maeda Y, Tani E, Miyamoto T. Prostaglandin metabolism in experimental cerebral vasospasm. J Neurosurg 1981; 55:779–85.
47. Gaetani P, Marzatico F, Baena RR, Pacchiarini L, Vigano T, Grignani G, Crivellari MT, Benzi G. Arachidonic acid metabolism and pathophysiologic aspects of subarachnoid hemorrhage in rats. Stroke 1990; 21:328–32.
48. Walker V, Pickard JD, Smythe P, Eastwood S, Perry S. Effects of subarachnoid hemorrhage on intracranial prostaglandins. J Neurol Neurosurg Psychiatry 1983; 46:119–25.
49. Seifert V, Stolke D, Kaever V, Dietz H. Arachidonic acid metabolism following aneurysm rupture: evaluation of cerebrospinal fluid and serum concentration of 6-keto-prostaglandin F_1 and thromboxane B_2 in patients with subarachnoid hemorrhage. Surg Neurol 1987; 27:243–52.
50. Baena RR, Baetani P, Folco G, Branzoli U, Paoletti P. Cisternal and lumbar CSF concentration of arachidonate metabolites in vasospasm following subarachnoid hemorrhage from ruptured aneurysm: biochemical and clinical considerations. Surg Neurol 1985; 24:428–32.
51. Ahamann PA, Lazzara A, Dykes FD, et al. Intraventricular hemorrhage in the big-risk preterm infant: incidence and outcome. Ann Neurol 1980; 7:118–24.

52. Papile LS, Burstein J, Burstein R, et al. Incidence and evolution of the subependymal intraventricular hemorrhage: a study of infants with weights less than 1500 grams. J Pediatr 1978; 92:529–34.
53. Dykes FD, Lazzara A, Ahmann P, et al. Intraventricular hemorrhage: a prospective evaluation of etiopathogenesis. Pediatrics 1980; 66:42–9.
54. Hambleton G, Wigglesworth JS. Origin of intraventricular hemorrhage in the preterm infant. Arch Dis Child 1976; 51:651–9.
55. Lou HC, Lassen NA, Friis-Hansen B. Impaired autoregulation of cerebral blood flow in the distressed newborn infant. J Pediatr 1979; 94:118–21.
56. Kenny JD, Garcia-Prats JA, Hilliard JL, et al. Hypercardia at birth: a possible role in the pathogenesis of intraventricular hemorrhage. Pediatrics 1978; 62:465–7.
57. Rennie JM, Doyle J, Cooke RWI. Elevated levels of immunoactive prostacyclin metabolite in babies who develop intraventricular hemorrhage. Acta Pediatr Scand 1987; 76:19–23.
58. Hutchison AA, Ogletree ML, Palmo CJH, et al. Plasma 6-keto prostaglandin F_1 and thromboxane B_2 concentrations in preterm neonates during the first three postnatal days: association with intracranial hemorrhage, the idiopathic respiratory distress syndrome and patent ductus arteriosus. Prostaglandins Leukotrienes Med 1985; 18:163–81.
59. Packham MA, Mustard JF. The role of platelets in the development and complications of atherosclerosis. Semin Hematol 1986; 23:8.
60. Liu MC, Chen YC, Lee TK, Lien IN. Studies of platelet hyperactivity in patients with ischemic cerebrovascular disease. III. Platelet hyperactivation in the chronic phase of cerebral thromboembolism. J Formosan Med Assoc 1985; 84:468–73.
61. Grady P. Pathophysiology of extracranial cerebral arterial stenosis—a critical review. Stroke 1984; 15:224–36.
62. Fry DC. Acute vascular endothelial changes associated with increased blood velocity gradients. Circ Res 1968; 22:165–97.
63. Mustard JF, Murphy EA, Rowsell HC. Factors influencing thrombus formation in vivo. Am J Med 1962; 33:621.
64. Lewis JK, Kohke BA. Endothelial damage and thrombocyte adhesion in pigeon atherosclerosis. Science 1977; 196:1007–9.
65. Barnett HJM. Platelet and coagulation function in relation to thromboembolic stroke. In: Thompson RA, Green JR, eds. Advances in neurology. vol 16. New York: Raven Press, 1977:45–70.
66. Packham MA, Mustard JF. Clinical pharmacology of platelets. Blood 1977; 50:555–73.
67. D'Angelo V, Villa S, Myslixies M, Donati MB, deGaetano G. Defective fibrinolytic and prostacyclin-like activity in human atheromatous plaques. Thromb Haemost 1978; 39:535.
68. Sinzinger H, Silberbaner K, Feigl W, Wagner O, Winter M, Auerswalk W. Prostacyclin activity is diminished in different types of morphologically controlled human atherosclerotic lesions. Thromb Haemost 1979; 42:803.
69. Moncada S, Vane JR. Pharmacology and endogenous roles of prostaglandin endoperoxides, thromboxane A_2 and prostacyclin. Pharmacol Rev 1979; 30:293.
70. Beigz J, Foster W. Influence of human low density and high density lipoprotein cholesterol on the in vitro prostaglandin I synthetase. Acta Biochem Biophys 1980; 620:352.
71. Fleischer LN, Tall AR, Whitte LD, Miller RW, Cannon PJ. Stimulation of arterial endothelial cell prostacyclin synthesis by high density lipoproteins. J Biol Chem 1982; 257:6653–5.
72. Fisher CM. Observations of the fundus oculi in transient monocular blindness. Neurology 1959; 9:333–47.
73. Harrison MJG, Marshall J. The finding of thrombus at carotid endarterectomy and its relationship to the timing of surgery. Br J Surg 1977; 64:511–2.
74. Gunning AJ, Pickering GW, Robb-Smith AHT, et al. Mural thrombosis of the internal carotid artery and subsequent embolism. Q J Med 1964; 33:155.
75. Chesler E, King RA, Edwards JE. The myxomatous mitral valve and sudden death. Circulation 1983; 67:632–9.

76. Folts JD, Crowell EB, Rowe GG. Platelet aggregation in partially obstructed vessels and its elimination with aspirin. Circulation 1976; 54:365–70
77. Folts JD, Gallagher K, Rowe GG. Blood flow in stenosed canine coronary arteries: vasospasm or platelet aggregation? Circulation 1982; 65:248–55.
78. Furlow TW Jr, Hallenbeck JM. Indomethacin prevents impaired perfusion of the dog's brain after global ischemia. Stroke 1978; 9:591–4.
79. Hallenbeck JM, Furlow TW Jr. Prostaglandin I_2 and indomethacin prevent impairment of postischemic brain reperfusion in the dog. Stroke 1979; 10:629–37.
80. Hallenbeck JM, Leitch DR, Dutka AJ, Greenbaum LJ Jr, McKee AE. Prostacyclin, indomethacin and heparin promote postischemic neuronal recovery in dogs. Ann Neurol 1982; 12:145–56.
81. Dougherty JH Jr, Levy DE, Rawlinson DG, Ruff R, Weksler BB, Plus F. Experimental cerebral ischemia produced by extracranial vascular injury: protection with indomethacin and prostacyclin. Neurology 1982; 32:970–4.
82. Harris R, Bayran M, Branston NM, Watson A, Symon L. Modulation of the pathophysiology of primate focal cerebral ischemia by indomethacin. Stroke 1982; 13:17–24.
83. Awad I, Little JR, Lucas F, Skrinska V, Slugg R, Lesser RP. Modification of focal cerebral ischemia by prostacyclin and indomethacin. J Neurosurg 1983; 58:714–9.
84. Peck MJ, Piper PJ, Williams TJ. The effect of leukotrienes C_4 and D_4 on the microvasculature of guinea-pig skin. Prostaglandins 1981; 21:315–21.
85. Rosenblum WI. Constricting effect of leukotrienes on cerebral arterioles of mice. Stroke 1985; 16:262–3.
86. Ford-Hutchinson AW, Bray MA, Doig MV, Shipley ME, Smith MJH. Leukotriene B, a potent chemokinetic and aggregating substance released from polymorphonuclear leukocytes. Nature 1980; 286:264–5.
87. Choi DW, Rothman SM. The role of glutamate neurotoxicity in hypoxic–ischemic neuronal death. Annu Rev Neurosci 1990; 13:171–182.
88. Chen ST, Hsu CY, Hogan EL, Banik NL, Balentine JD. Brain calcium content in ischemic infarction. Neurology 1987; 37:1227–9.
89. Wilkins RH. Attempts at prevention or treatment of intracranial arterial spasm: an update. Neurosurgery 1987; 37:1227–9.
90. Chapleau CE, White RP, Robertson JT. Effects of prostaglandin synthetase inhibitors (PSI) on contraction induced by arachidonate, prostaglandin F_2 and serotonin in basilar arteries [abstract]. Fed Proc 1979; 38:559.
91. Chapleau CE, White RP, Robertson JT. Cerebral vasodilation and prostacyclin: effect of aspirin and meclofenamate in vitro. J Neurosurg 1980; 63:188–92.
92. Chapleau CE, White RP, Robertson JT. Cerebral vasospasm: effects of prostaglandin synthetase inhibitors in vitro. Neurosurgery 1980; 6:155–9.
93. Okamoto S, Handa H, Toda N. Role of intrinsic arachidonate metabolites in the vascular action of erythrocyte breakdown products. Stroke 1984; 15:60–4.
94. White RP, Robertson JT. Comparison of piroxicam, meclofenamate, ibuprofen, aspirin, and prostacyclin efficacy in a chronic model of cerebral vasospasm. Neurosurgery 1983; 12:40–6.
95. Fujita Y, Shingu T, Gi H, Araki O, Matsunaga M, Handa H. Mechanism of cerebral vasospasm induced by oxyhemoglobin. In: Brock M, ed. Modern neurosurgery I. Berlin: Springer-Verlag, 1982:539–74.
96. Fukomri T, Tani E, Maeda Y, Sukenaga A. Effects of prostacyclin and indomethacin on experimental delayed cerebral vasospasm. J Neurosurg 1983; 59:829–34.
97. Okwausaba FK, Weir BKA, Cook DA, Krueger CA. Effects of various intracranial fluids on smooth muscle. Neurosurgery 1981; 9:402–6.
98. Chyatte D, Rusch N, Sundt TM Jr. Prevention of chronic experimental cerebral vasospasm with ibuprofen and high-dose methylprednisolone. J Neurosurg 1983; 59:925–32.
99. Gersony WM, Peckham GJ, Ellison RC, Miettinen OS, Nadas AS. Effects of indomethacin

in premature infants with patent ductus arteriosus: results of a national collaborative study. J Pediatr 1983; 102:895–906.

100. Harris JP, Merrit TA, Alexson CG, Longfield L, Manning JA. Parenteral indomethacin for closure of the patent ductus arteriosus. Am J Dis Child 1982; 136:1005–8.
101. Setzer ES, Morse BM, Goldberg RN, Smith M, Bancalari E. Prophylactic indomethacin and intraventricular hemorrhage in the premature. Pediatr Res 1984; 18:345A.
102. Mahony L, Caldwell RL, Girod DA, Hurwitz RA, Janse RD, Lemous JA, Schreiner RL. Indomethacin therapy on the first day of life in infants with very low birth weight. J Pediatr 1985; 106:801.
103. Ment LR, Duncan CC, Ehreukranz RA, Kleinman CS, Pitt BR, Taylor KJW, Scott DT, Stewart WB, Gettner P. Randomized indomethacin trial for prevention of intraventricular hemorrhage in very low birth weight infants. J Pediatr 1985; 107:937–43.
104. Rennie JM, Doyle J, Cooke RWI. Early administration of indomethacin to preterm infants. Arch J Dis Child 1986; 61:233–8.
105. Hanigan WC, Kennedy G, Roemisch F, Anderson R, Cusach T, Powers W. Administration of indomethacin for the prevention of periventricular–intraventricular hemorrhage in high-risk neonates. J Pediatr 1988; 112:941–7.
106. Ment LR, Duncan CC, Ehrenkranz RA, Kleinman CS, Taylor KJW, Scott DT, Gettner P, Sherwonit E, Williams J. Randomized low-dose indomethacin trial for prevention of intraventricular hemorrhage in very low birth weight neonates. J Pediatr 1988; 112:948–55.
107. Bandstra ES, Montalvo BM, Goldberg RN, Facheco I, Ferrer PL, Flynn J, Gregorios JB, Bancalari E. Prophylactic indomethacin for prevention of intraventricular hemorrhage in premature infants. Pediatrics 1988; 82:533–42.
108. Bada HS, Green RS, Pourcyrous M, Leffler CW, Korones SB, Magill HL, Arheart K, Fitch CW, Anderson GD, Somes G, Tullis K, Campbell J. Indomethacin reduces the risks of severe intraventricular hemorrhage. J Pediatr 1989; 115:631–7.
109. Roth CJ, Majerus PW. The mechanism of the effect of aspirin on human platelets. 1. Acetylation of a particular fraction protein. J Clin Invest 1975; 56:624–32.
110. Patrono C, Ciabattoni G, Patrignani P, et al. Clinical pharmacology of platelet cyclooxygenase inhibition. Circulation 1985; 72:1177–84.
111. Steering Committee of the Physicians' Health Study Research Group. Final report on the aspirin component of the ongoing physicians' health study. N Engl J Med 1989; 321:129–35.
112. Peto R, Gray R, Colins R, Wheatley K, Hennekens C, Jamrozik K, Marlow C, Hafner B, Thompson E, Norton S, Gilliland J, Doll R. Randomized trial of prophylactic daily aspirin in British male doctors. Br Med J 1988; 296:313–6.
113. Hennekens CH, Peto R, Hutchison GB, Doll R. An overview of the British and American aspirin study. N Engl J Med 1988; 318:923–4.
114. Marcus AJ. Aspirin and thromboembolism: a possible dilemma. N Engl J Med 1977; 297:1284–5.
115. Weksler BB, Pett SB, Alonso D, Richter RC, Stelzer P, Subramanian V, Tack-Goldman K, Gay WA Jr. Differential inhibition by aspirin of vascular and platelet prostaglandin synthesis in atherosclerotic patients. N Engl J Med 1983; 308:800–5.
116. Jaffe EA, Weksler BB. Recovery of endothelial cell prostacyclin production after inhibition by low dose aspirin. J Clin Invest 1979; 63:532–5.
117. Burch JW, Baenziger NL, Stanford N, Maajerus PW. Selective cumulative inhibition of platelet thromboxane production by low-dose aspirin in healthy subjects. Proc Natl Acad Sci USA 1978; 75:5181–4.
118. Hirsh J. Progress review: the relationship between dose of aspirin, side-effects and antithrombotic effectiveness. Stroke 1985; 16:1–4.
119. Davi G, Custro N, Novo S, Mattina H, Strano A. The effect of two low doses of aspirin on whole blood thromboxane and prostacyclin generation in healthy subjects. Thromb Haemost 1982; 50:669–70.

120. UK-TIA Study Group. United Kingdom transient ischemic attack (UK-TIA) aspirin trial: interim results. Br Med J 1988; 296:316–20.
121. Lee TK, Chen YC, Lien IN, Liu MC, Huang ZS. Inhibitory effect of acetylsalicylic acid on platelet function in patients with completed stroke or reversible ischemic neurologic deficit. Stroke 1988; 19:566–70.
122. Boysen G, Sorense PS, Juhler M, Anderson AR, Boas J, Olsen JS, Joensen P. Danish very low-dose aspirin after carotid endarterectomy trial. Stroke 1988; 19:1211–5.
123. Sandercock P. Aspirin for strokes and transient ischemic attacks. Br Med J 1988; 297:995–6.
124. Lee TK, Lien IN, Ryu SJ, Lee KY, Hu HW, Tchen PH, Chen CJ, Wu SC, Chen YC. Secondary prevention of ischemic stroke with low dose acetylsalicylic acid. J Formosan Med Assoc 1990; 89:634–44.
125. Viinikka L. Acetylsalicylic acid and the balance between prostacyclin and thromboxane A_2. Scand J Clin Lab Invest [Suppl] 1990; 50:103–8.
126. Cerskus AL, Ali M, Davies BJ, McDonald JWB. Possible significance of small numbers of functional platelets in a population of aspirin-treated platelets in vitro. Thromb Res 1980; 18:389–97.
127. Di Minno G, Silver MJ, Murphy S. Monitoring the entry of new platelets into the circulation after ingestion of aspirin. Blood 1983; 61:1081–5.
128. The Canadian Cooperative Study Group. A randomized trial of aspirin and sulfinpyrazone in threatened stroke. N Engl J Med 1978; 299:53–9.
129. Candelise L, Landi G, Perrone P, Bracchi M, Brambilla G. A randomized trial of aspirin and sulfinpyrazone in patients with TIA. Stroke 1982; 13:175–9.
130. Kelton JG, Hirsh J, Carter J, Buchanan MR. Sex difference in the antithrombotic effects of aspirin. Blood 1978; 52:1072.
131. Fields WS, Lemak NA, Frankowski RF, Hardy RJ. Controlled trial of aspirin in cerebral ischemia. Stroke 1977; 8:301–16.
132. Bousser MG, Eschwege E, Haguenau M, Lefauconnier JM, Thibult N, Toubout PJ. "AICLA" controlled trial of aspirin and dipyridamole in the secondary prevention of atherothrombotic cerebral ischemia. Stroke 1983; 14:5–14.
133. Lee TK, Chen YC, Kuo TL. Comparison of the effect of acetylsalicylic acid on platelet function in male and female patients with ischemic stroke. Thromb Res 1987; 47:295–304.
134. Eichner ER. Platelets, carotids and coronaries: critique on antithrombotic role of antiplatelet agents, exercise and certain diets. Am J Med 1984; 77:513–23.
135. de Gaetano G, Cerletti C, Bertele V. Pharmacology of antiplatelet drugs and clinical trials of thrombosis prevention or difficult link. Lancet 1982; 2:974–7.
136. FitzGerald GA. Dipyridamole. N Engl J Med 1987; 316:1247–57.
137. The American-Canadian Cooperative Study Group. Persantin–aspirin trial in cerebral ischemia. Part II. Endpoint results. Stroke 1985; 16:406–15.
138. Hass WK, Easton JD, Adams HP, Pryse-Phillips W, Molony BA, Anderson S, Kamm B. A randomized trial comparing ticlopidine hydrochloride with aspirin for the prevention of stroke in high-risk patients. N Engl J Med 1989; 321:501–7.
139. Gent M, Easton JD, Hachinski VC, Panak E, Sicurella J, Blakely JA, Ellis DJ, Harbison JW, Robert RS, Turpie AGG. The Canadian American Ticlopidine Study (CATS) in thromboembolic stroke. Lancet 1989; 1:1215–20.
140. Uchiyama S, Sone R, Nagayama T, Shibagaki Y, Kobayashi I, Maruyama S, Kusakabe K. Combination therapy with low-dose aspirin and ticlopidine in cerebral ischemia. Stroke 1989; 20:1643–7.

5

Topical Nonsteroidal Anti-Inflammatory Drugs in Skin Diseases and Musculoskeletal Disorders

SYDNEY H. DROMGOOLE*
Allergan Herbert
Irvine, California

I. INTRODUCTION

Topical nonsteroidal anti-inflammatory drugs (NSAIDs) have been used clinically to treat many skin conditions, including psoriasis, eczema, atopic dermatitis, and other inflammatory dermatoses, as well as soft-tissue injuries and rheumatic pain.

Numerous NSAIDs have been formulated for topical application (Table 1), and the clinical studies associated with these topical NSAIDs are summarized in Tables 2 through 5. Several topical NSAID formulations are currently available in Europe for use in the treatment of selected dermatoses, soft-tissue injuries, and rheumatic conditions (see Table 6). In the United States, none of the topical formulations have been approved for the treatment of dermatological disorders, although there are several over-the-counter (OTC) products that are used for the treatment of soft-tissue injuries and rheumatic pain (see Table 7). Although these products are labeled according to the appropriate monograph guidelines, the Food and Drug Administration (FDA) has recently suggested that clinical trials with topical OTC NSAIDs should be conducted to prove the effectiveness of these drugs (1). Three clinical models were suggested: patients with acute painful injuries (parallel design); chronic painful conditions—headache or dysmenorrhea; and a surrogate group in whom muscle pain was induced by overexertion (crossover-design).

II. PHARMACOKINETICS OF TOPICAL NONSTEROIDAL ANTI-INFLAMMATORY DRUGS

The pharmacokinetics of several topical and oral NSAIDs (benzydamine, piroxicam, felbinac, and ibuprofen) have been recently reviewed by White (2) and demonstrate differences between the pharmacokinetics of the NSAIDs administered by these two routes. In general, topical administration results in (a) slower drug absorption into the systemic circulation, (b) lower plasma concentrations, (c) lower bioavailability—about

*Present affiliation: Oclassen Pharmaceuticals, San Rafael, California.

Table 1 Topical NSAIDs

Name	Concentration (%)	Form	Trade name(s)
Ketoprofen	2.5	Gel	Fastum
Piroxicam	0.5	Gel	Feldene
Benzydiamine	3	Cream	Difflam
Etofenamate	10	Cream	Flexium Bayrogel
Diclofenac	1	Gel	Emulgel, Voltarol
Indomethacin	2.5	Gel	Indocid
Flurbiprofen	5	Solution	
Bufexamac	5	Cream	Parfenac
Salicylic acid	6	Gel	
Ketorolac	2	Gel	
Flunoxaprofen	5	Gel	Priaxim
Fentizac	5	Cream	
Bendazac	3	Cream, Ointment	
Naproxen	10	Gel	Naprosyn
Niflumic acid	3	Gel	Flunir
Ibuprofen	5	Cream	Dolgit, Proflex, Ibuleve
Phenybutazone	5	Ointment	Midy
Felbinac	3	Gel	Traxam

5% of that following oral administration, (d) prolonged plasma elimination half-lives, and (e) measurable drug levels in the tissues and synovial fluids.

III. MODELS OF SKIN INFLAMMATION

The efficacy of various topical NSAIDs have been studied in several models of skin inflammation. Specific models include erythema induced by ultraviolet (UV) light (3–10), scald burns (11–13), and inflammatory responses induced by chemicals, such as methyl nicotinate (14–16), cinnamic aldehyde (14), benzoic acid (14), and anthralin (17).

Topical NSAIDs, including indomethacin, piroxicam, flurbiprofen, and etofenamate, were all effective in reducing erythema when applied after UV irradiation (Table 2).

Table 2 NSAIDs in Models of Inflammation

Model	NSAID	Results	Ref.
UV-induced erythema	2.% INDO solution 0.05% FA cream VEH	INDO > FA = VEH INDO blanched erythema more than either FA or VEH at 4 and 24 h postirradiation.	5
UV-induced erythema	2.5% INDO	INDO decreased dermal damage (erythema, skin temperature and hyperalgesia) but epidermal damage (changes in DNA synthesis, sunburn cell formation) was unchanged.	6

Table 2 NSAIDs in Models of Inflammation

Model	NSAID	Results	Ref.
UV-induced erythema	2.5% DFMD solution 2.5% INDO solution VEH	NSAIDs inhibited erythemal response.	7
UV-induced erythema	1% INDO gel	INDO produced a dose-dependent suppression of UVB and UVC induced erythema. The degree of inhibition was dependent on the time of observation after UV irradiation.	8
UV-induced erythema	5% FLUB solution	Concentration-dependent suppression of erythema.	9
UV-induced erythema	0.5% PIR cream 1% PIR cream 1% PIR gel 1.5% PIR cream 5% BEN 5% ETOF gel 5% INDO cream	Decrease in erythema. PIR creams = INDO cream = ETOF gel. BEN and PIR gels were ineffective.	10
UV-induced erythema	1% INDO gel	INDO produce dose-response reduction in erythema.	17
Methyl nicotinate-induced inflammation	1.5% INDO gel 3% NIF cream 10% CPA cream	All NSAIDs reduced inflammation.	15
Methyl nicotinate-induced inflammation	5% BUF cream 1% DICLO gel 5% IBU cream 2.5% INDO cream 5% PBZ ointment 3% NIF cream 0.05% CLOB cream 1% HC cream 0.1% HCB cream	NSAIDs were more effective than steroids in inhibiting increases in blood flow. DICLO and INDO showed prolonged effects up to 48 h.	16
Chemical-induced inflammation	1% DICLO gel 10% NAP gel 5% SA gel	NSAIDs inhibited erythema induced by benzoic acid, cinnamic aldehyde, dimethyl sulfoxide, and methyl nicotinate, and edema induced by methyl nicotinate.	14
Anthralin-induced inflammation	1% INDO gel 0.05% CLOB cream	CLOB completely inhibited edema, but had little or no effect on erythema. INDO had no effect on edema, but produced significant reduction in erythema.	17

Abbrev: BEN, benzydamine; BUF, bufexamac; CLOB, clobetasol propionate; CPA, collagenic palmitoyl acid; DFMD, diflumidone; DICOL, diclofenac; ETOF, etofenamate; FA, fluocinolone acetonide; FLUB, flurbiprofen; HC, hydrocortisone; HCB, hydrocortisone butyrate; IBU, ibuprofen; INDO, indomethacin; NAP, naproxen; NIF, niflumic acid; PBZ, phenylbutazone; PIR piroxicam; SA, salicylic acid; VEH, vehicle.

When 1% indomethacin gel was applied immediately after irradiation, dose-dependent suppression was observed up to 36 h postirradiation, with maximal effectiveness being observed between 4 and 12 h. Suppression of erythema was also observed when indomethacin was topically applied 24 h postirradiation (8). Several studies have indicated that the topical NSAIDs, indomethacin and flurbiprofen, were more effective than midpotency steroids in reducing the erythematous response (9,18–20). The inhibitory effects of the topical NSAIDs were also similar to those reported following oral administration of NSAIDs (3).

Torrent et al. reported that, although piroxicam cream, etofenamate gel, and indomethacin cream were effective in reducing UV-induced erythema, piroxicam gel and benzydamine cream were ineffective (10). The ineffectiveness of the piroxicam gel demonstrates the effect of vehicle ingredients on the pharmacokinetics or pharmacodynamics of topically applied drugs and underscores the importance of the vehicle in formulating topical drugs.

The mechanism of action of the NSAIDs in reducing UV-induced erythema is probably related to the suppression of a UV-induced increase in prostaglandins (PG), as reported by Black et al. (21). This mechanism would explain the time-dependent suppression of erythema reported by Farr and Diffey (8), but does not fully account for the erythematous response.

In methyl nicotinate-induced inflammation, Duteil reported that NSAIDs (diclofenac, indomethacin, nuflumic acid, and ibuprofen) proved more effective than the corticosteroids—0.05% clobetasol propionate, 1% hydrocortisone butyrate, and 1% hydrocortisone creams—in inhibiting the increases in skin blood flow, with diclofenac and indomethacin showing prolonged inhibitory effects up to 48 h postirradiation (16). As in UV-induced erythema, prostaglandins and free arachidonic acid are involved in nicotinate-induced skin inflammation, and suppression of these inflammatory mediators could account for the observed effects.

Inflammation induced by anthralin produced differential responses with indomethacin and clobetasol dipropionate (17). Clobetasol completely inhibited edema, but had little effect on the erythema, whereas indomethacin produced the opposite effect—inhibited erythema, but had no effect on edema. The authors state that the results suggest either that anthralin inflammation is not due to prostaglandin production, or, if it is, it occurs by a pathway other than the cyclooxygenase one.

IV. CLINICAL EFFICACY OF TOPICAL NONSTEROIDAL ANTI-INFLAMMATORY DRUGS

A. Psoriasis

Several years ago it was hypothesized that the arachidonic acid cascade may play an important role in the pathogenesis of psoriasis and other dermatoses (22–24). Evidence to support this hypothesis included reports of elevated levels of proinflammatory eicosanoids [e.g., arachidonic acid (AA), prostaglandins (PGE_2, $PGF_{2\alpha}$), leukotrienes (LTB_4, LTC_4, LTD_4, and hydroxyperoxyacids (5- and 12-HETE)] in involved psoriatic epidermis (25–32).

Consequently, one might expect that NSAIDs would be useful in the treatment of psoriasis. However, clinical experience with NSAIDs in this disorder is variable. Both topical and oral NSAIDs have been administered. Table 3 summarizes the topical studies

Table 3 Topical NSAIDs in Psoriasis

NSAID(s) (+ controls)	Study Design (No. subjects)	Results	Ref.
1% INDO gel VEH	Open study bid × 2 wk (n = 11)	INDO = VEH	33
1% INDO gel VEH	Double-blind, paired comparison bid × 2 wk (n = 8)	INDO = VEH	33
1% INDO ointment DITH ointment	Double-blind, paired comparison qd × 5 wk (n = 10)	INDO < DITH INDO-treated lesions remained unchanged	34
5% BUF cream VEH	Double-blind, paired comparison qd × 10 d (n = 20)	BUF > VEH Treatments applied under occlusion 14 BUF- and 4 VEH-treated areas had good or excellent responses Adverse reactions: allergic dermatitis (1); local irritation (4)	35
0.5% INDO in 50% ethanol	Open study (n = 5)	INDO exacerbated the condition in all patients.	40
1% INDO cream VEH	Double-blind, paired comparison bid × 4 wk (n = 20)	INDO < VEH INDO caused exacerbation in 14/20 subjects.	50
1% MECLO cream VEH	Double-blind, paired comparison bid for 4 wk (n = 10)	MECLO < VEH MECLO caused exacerbation in 7/10 subjects	50
1% LONAP gel 0.025% FA gel	Double-blind, paired comparison tid × 4 wk (n = 30)	LONAP = FA After 4 wk 90% of the patients in both groups had good, excellent, or complete clearing of the disease. No adverse reactions were seen.	59
2% LONAP gel VEH	Double-blind, paired comparison bid × 4 wk (n = 10)	LONAP > VEH Adverse reactions: burning, tenderness, swelling, lesional erosion, and perilesional erythema and pruritus	61
2% R68151 cream VEH	Double-blind qd × 4 wk (n = 73)	R68151 > VEH After 4 wk, significant reduction in scaling and erythema.	62
2% R70795 cream 0.05% CLOB cream VEH	Double-blind qd × 4 wk	R70795 = CLOB Lasser-Doppler measured temperature changes were similar in both groups.	62

Abbrev: See Table 2; bid, twice daily; DITH, dithanol; LONAP, lonapalene; MECLO, meclofenamate; tid, three times daily; qd, once daily.

of NSAIDs in this disease. Several studies have reported the exacerbation of the disease after application of topical NSAIDs, whereas others have reported no beneficial effects (33,34), and one study with topical bufexamac reported good to excellent results in 60% of the patients (35).

The NSAIDs that have been reported to exacerbate psoriasis after oral administration include meclofenamate (36,37), phenylbutazone (38), salicylates (39), and indomethacin (40,41). Oral NSAIDs that have been reported to be beneficial include meclofenamate (42) and benoxaprofen (43), whereas the addition of oral indomethacin to anthralin (dithranol) treatment offered no significant benefit (44,45).

The role of lipoxygenase products of arachidonic acid in psoriasis, atopic dermatitis, and experimental arthritis has been recently reviewed (46), and an attempt was made to assign a role for lipoxygenase products as mediators of inflammation using criteria proposed by Dale (47) and later modified by Vane (48). Fogh concluded that LTB_4 appeared to fulfil the criteria for putative inflammatory mediators, whereas the role of 12-hydroxyeicosatetraenoic acid (12-HETE) is, as yet, unknown. On the other hand, 15-HETE appeared to inhibit the formation of LTB_4 and 12-HETE, suggesting an anti-inflammatory role for this metabolite (49). It has been hypothesized that the exacerbation of psoriasis by NSAIDs may be the result of inhibition of cyclooxygenase, leading to decreased PG synthesis, but an increase or accumulation of other inflammatory arachidonic acid metabolites, such as leukotrienes or hydroxyperoxyacids (50). Worsening of psoriasis by NSAIDs would support the role of lipoxygenase products in the disease process, but as Green and Shuster have pointed out (33), the absence of worsening does not exclude the hypothesis.

Although evidence is now limited, one class of NSAIDs that may be an effective topical treatment in psoriasis is the 5-lipoxygenase inhibitors (51,52). Repeated intralesional injections of the biologically active AA metabolite, 15-HETE found in psoriatic skin (53–55), can improve psoriasis (46), and benoxaprofen, an NSAID that inhibited the formation of LTB_4 in vitro (56,57), was effective in psoriasis after oral administration (43). Unfortunately, benoxaprofen was withdrawn from the market, for toxicity reasons, shortly after its introduction as a antirheumatic agent. More recently, several 5-lipoxygenase (5-LO) inhibitors, including lonapalene, currently under development, have been reported to be effective in psoriasis after topical application (58–62). The pharmacological changes induced by lonapalene included reduction in LTB_4, which would support the role of the this leukotriene in the pathogenesis of the disease. DeJong et al. have recently reported (63) that short-term (10 days) oral administration of MK-886—a leukotriene biosynthesis inhibitor (by binding to the 5-LO-activating protein -FLAP)—to 16 psoriatic patients produced no clinical changes or reduction in lesional LTB_4 levels. However, at the end of 10-day treatment, a significant reduction (>70%) in urinary LTE_4 excretion was noted, signaling reduction in systemic leukotriene biosynthesis. Similar investigations with a topical formulation of MK-866 would help determine if the insignificant clinical changes were due to nonpharmacological doses of the drug in the psoriatic lesions.

In summary, earlier studies with topical NSAIDs that inhibit cyclooxygenase reported exacerbation of psoriasis, whereas later studies reported a lack of effect or no change, rather than exacerbation. However, it is possible that NSAIDs that inhibit the lipoxygenase pathway (either 5-lipoxygenase inhibitors or lipoxygenase–cyclooxygenase inhibitors) may provide useful topical treatments for psoriasis, and several such pharmacological agents are currently under development.

B. Dermatitis

In a double blind study of 5% bufexamac cream and 0.025% fluocinolone acetonide, Achten et al. reported that 48 patients with contact dermatitis and atopic dermatitis responded equally to both treatments (Table 4) (64). Bufexamac is currently marketed in 11 countries (Australia, Austria, Belgium, Canada, Carribean, France, Germany, Italy, Netherlands, South Africa, and the United Kingdom) (65) and is indicated for the treatment of contact dermatitis, eczema, atopic dermatitis, and radiodermatitis.

C. Eczema

Bendazac provided good or excellent responses in 52% of patients with eczematous dermatoses who had applied the topical formulation twice daily for up to 12 days (66). The therapeutic effect of the drug was evident in the reduction of erythema, edema, itching, and scaling. Tolerance to the 3% topical preparation was generally good, with only three patients noting increases in erythema, vesiculation, itching, and burning (see Table 4).

D. Epidermolysis Bullosa Simplex

Preliminary data (67) in several patients with epidermolysis bullosa simplex (EBS) suggested that topical bufexamac caused a lower incidence of skin blisters and reduced pain intensity. However, a recent double-blind, placebo-controlled crossover study in ten subjects with EBS demonstrated that 5% bufexamac cream was ineffective (68) (see Table 4).

E. Acne

Topical products that can reduce inflammation associated with acne include antibiotics [erythromycin (69) and clindamycin (70)] and some retinoids [13-*cis*-retinoic acid (71) and CD-271 (72,73)]. There are also many topical antiacne products that contain salicylic acid (e.g., Salac and Stridex Pads). Although these products are marketed as acne cleansers, it is possible that the well-documented inhibitory effect of salicylic acid on prostaglandin synthesis may contribute to the products beneficial effect in acne.

F. Fungal Infections

The primary mode of action of topical antifungal agents is related to their ability to inhibit the biosynthesis of ergosterol, resulting in sterol deficiency and fungistatic or fungicidal activity. However, recent research has indicated that some of these antifungal agents can inhibit the cellular release of various arachidonic acid metabolites (PGE_2, 5-HETE, and LTB_4) in vitro (74), whereas other studies have reported inhibition of chemotaxis in vitro (75). These in vitro data suggest that these anti-inflammatory effects may contribute to the clinical efficacy of these drugs.

G. Sunburn

Sunburn is the delayed inflammatory response that occurs after irradiation with UV light. The wavelengths of light that are most effective lie in the UVB region (290–320 nm). Evidence suggests that prostaglandins play a role in this inflammatory response, and this indicates that NSAIDs (both topical and systemic) may be useful treatments for sunburn. Several studies have indicated that NSAIDs (given topically, orally, and intradermally) are effective in reducing UVB-induced erythema (3,5,6,20,76–78). However, it has been

Table 4 Topical NSAIDs in Inflammatory Skin Disorders

Skin disorder	NSAID(s) (+ controls)	Study design (No. subjects)	Results	Ref.
Atopic dermatitis	5% BUF cream 0.025% FA cream	Double-blind qd × 4 wk (n = 24)	BUF = FA	64
Contact dermatitis	5% BUF cream 0.025% FA cream	Double-blind qd × 4 wk (n = 24)	BUF + FA	64
Eczema	3% BEN cream	Open study bid up to 12 d (n = 44)	Excellent or good response in 52% patients; fair response in 34%	66
Eczema	3% BEN cream 3% BEN + 3% HC cream	Double-blind, paired comparison bid × 2 wk (n = 24)	BEN = BEN + HC	66
Eczema	3% BEN cream VEH	Double-blind, paired comparison bid × 2 wk (n = 19)	BEN > VEH Tolerance was good	66
Epidermolysis bullosa simplex (EBS)	5% BUF cream VEH	Double-blind qid × 2 wk (n = 10)	BUF + VEH Ineffective	68
Various dermatoses	5% BUF cream	Open tid × 7 d (n = 71)	Treatment of pruritus ani and vulvae, urticaria, otitis externa, and napkin rash were successful. Contact dermatitis: largely successful Eczema: limited success	82
Various dermatoses	5% BUF cream 0.025% FA cream	Double-blind (n = 50)	BUF = FA	83

Various dermatoses	5% BUF cream 0.1% TAC cream	Double-blind bid–qid × 7 d (n = 23)	BUF = TAC	84
Various dermatoses	5% BUF cream 0.1% BMV ointment	Double-blind tid × 20 d (n = 50)	BUF = BMV	85
Various dermatoses	5% BUF ointment	Open bid–qid up to 4 wk (n = 59)	Treatment resulted in significant reduction in pain and resolution of lesions in 10–14 d, no side effects	
Various dermatoses	5% BUF cream 0.025% FA	Double-blind, parallel bid for at least 2 wk (n = 44)	BUF = FA Adverse reaction in 5 patients (2 FA- and 3 BUF-treated) included increase in erythema and vesiculation.	87
Various dermatoses	5% BUF cream 0.025% FA	Double-blind bid up to 4 wk (n = 35)	BUF = FA	88
Various dermatoses	5% BUF cream TAC cream HC cream VEH	Double-blind (n = 193)	TAC > VEH HC > VEH BUF = VEH	89
Various dermatoses	0.6 mg/ml superoxide dismutase (SOD) cream	Open label tid–qid up to 2 wk (n = 20)	Lesions associated with progressive systemic sclerosis, systemic lupus erythematosus, herpes simplex, and burns responded to treatment with SOD cream.	91
Ichthyosis and various parakeratotic disorders	2% R68151 cream VEH	Double-blind qd × 4 wk (n = 4)	Good rapid response to R68151.	62

Abbrev: See Table 2 and 3; BMV, betamethasone valerate; qid, four times daily; TAC, triamcinolone valerate.

noted (78) that many of these studies have limited clinical relevance because responses were confined to small areas of skin or there were inadequate controls. In a double-blind crossover study in 19 psoriatics, Stern and Dobson concluded that the observed anti-inflammatory effect following oral ibuprofen was of limited usefulness in treating sunburn (77). However, in light of the reported exacerbation of psoriasis by NSAIDs, the clinical model used by these authors may be flawed.

Preliminary data in animals and humans with topical iron chelators has indicated that these compounds may be useful in preventing UV-induced erythema and UVB-induced increases in skin iron levels (79,80). These chelators are thought to bind iron in tissues and inhibit iron-catalyzed production of free radicals. These compounds may represent a new class of topical anti-inflammatory agents.

H. Other Cutaneous Disorders

Although there are several topical formulations of NSAIDs marketed outside the United States, there are only limited clinical data to demonstrate the safety and efficacy in the treatment of various inflammatory dermatoses (81–89) (see Table 4). The treatment period ranged from 1 to 4 weeks and daily application from two to four times. Several studies have indicated that bufexamac was as effective as several corticosteroid formulations [betamethasone valerate (BMV), triamcinolone acetonide (TAC), and fluocinolone acetonide (FA). There are as yet no topical NSAIDs marketed in the United States that are indicated for treatment of inflammatory dermatoses. Other NSAIDs approved outside of this country for treatment of skin disorders include enoxolone, gualenic acid, oxaceprol, and ufenamate (65) (Table 5).

Preliminary data with a new topical 5-lipoxygenase inhibitor (R68151), in four patients with ichthyosis, suggested that this class of NSAIDs may be useful in the management of this disorder (62), but further data are needed to confirm this finding.

Superoxide dismutase (SOD) has been used both topically and systematically for the treatment of inflammatory skin disorders (90,91). Mizushima et al. (90) reported that a topical cream formulation, containing 0.6 mg/ml bovine superoxide dismutase, reduced inflammation associated with progressive systemic sclerosis, systemic lupus erythematosus, Behcet's disease, herpes simplex, and burns, but the cream appeared to have no effect on psoriasis or dermatomyositis (see Table 4). The SOD cream was applied three to four times per day to selected lesions in 20 subjects for up to 14 days. Although this study was not well-controlled, it should be mentioned that many of the treated lesions, in which SOD was effective, were refractory to conventional therapy. This preliminary data with topical SOD is very interesting and merits further evaluation in adequate well-defined populations under double-blind conditions.

Finally, there are several topical OTC formulations containing high concentrations of salicylic acid for the removal of common and plantar warts, whereas lower concentrations of salicylic acid are incorporated in many medicated shampoos, gels, and acne cleansing products. The primary effect of salicylic acid in these products is related to its keratolytic action, which causes the cornified epithelium to swell, soften, and macerate, leading to desquamation.

I. Inflammatory Musculoskeletal Disorders

Numerous clinical studies have been conducted with topical NSAIDs in the treatment of soft-tissue injuries, including sprains, bursitis, tendonitis, contusions, and epicondylitis

Table 5 Topical NSAIDs in Soft-Tissue Injuries and Rheumatic Conditions

Type of Injury	NSAIDs	Design	Results	Ref.
Acute traumatic injuries	0.5% PIR gel VEH	Double-blind, parallel tid–qid × 7 d (n = 139)	PIR > VEH	92
Soft-tissue injuries	0.5% PIR gel VEH	Double-blind, parallel qid × 7–21 d (n = 200)	PIR > VEH	93
Osteoarthritis	0.5% PIR gel VEH	Randomized, parallel study	PIR = IBU	94
	oral IBU (400 mg × tid)	tid up to 4 wk (n = 235)	Both groups—oral and topical—showed 30% reduction in pain intensity	
	PLAC		Overall efficacy judged to be good or excellent in 64% PIR-treated subjects and in 60% of IBU-treated subjects	
Sprains, tendonitis of the ankle, shoulder, and elbow	0.5% PIR gel	Open, parallel study qid up to 14 d (n = 173)	PIR = DICLO	95
	1% DICLO gel		Pain, tenderness, and restriction of joint pain was markedly improved with both drugs after 3 d of treatment. Side effects: mainly mild/moderate local reactions	

(continued)

Table 5 Continued

Type of Injury	NSAIDs	Design	Results	Ref.
Muscular pain	0.5% PIR gel VEH	Double-blind, parallel tid–qid for up to 2 wk (n = 191)	PIR > VEH Marked improvement in 31% PIR and 15% VEH-treated patients	96
Osteoarthritis of the knee	0.5% PIR gel VEH	Double-blind, parallel tid–qid for up to 2 wk (n = 212)	PIR > VEH	97
Rheumatic pain and traumatic pain	1% DICLO Emulgel 1% DICLO regular gel	Double-blind, parallel study in conjunction with ultrasonic therapy tid × 4 wk (n = 120)	DICLO (Emulgel) = DICLO (regular gel) in relief of pain Tolerability was good in both groups, local irritation reported in 3 patients	98
Epicondylitis of the elbow	1% DICLO gel VEH	Double-blind, parallel qid × 14 d (n = 32)	DICLO > VEH Pain level was lower in DICLO-treated group at the end of treatment. Tolerability of DICLO was good. Local adverse reactions included erythema, irritation, sensation of heat, burning or pruritus, allergy, or desquamation	99
Ankle sprain	2% KROL gel VEH 5% ETOF gel	Double-blind parallel tid × 14 d (n = 37)	KROL > VEH KROL = ETO Early relief of pain and reduction in ankle swelling	100

Tendonitis, bursitis	2.5% KETO gel 5% ETO gel	Double-blind, parallel bid × 1 w (n = 36)	KETO = ETO No side-effects reported	101
Ankle sprains	3% BEN cream	Open (n = 86)	No benefit	102
Acute soft-tissue injuries	3% BEN cream VEH	Double-blind, parallel qid × 6 d (n = 43)	BEN > VEH Significant improvement in symptoms (pain, tenderness, swelling, and function) after day 2	103
Soft-tissue injuries	3% BEN cream VEH	Double-blind, parallel bid × 6 d (n = 50)	Benefit observed after 2 days treatment	104
Soft-tissue injuries and fractures	3% BEN cream VEH	Double-blind, parallel tid × 6 d (n = 50)	Signs and symptoms were less severe after day 4 Overall therapeutic benefit: 72% BEN vs 32% VEH	105
Soft-tissue injuries (sprains, ankle injuries)	3% FEL gel	Open label tid × 7 d (n = 30)	Treatment rated as good or very good by 83% of the patients	106
Soft-tissue injuries (sprains, contusions)	3% FEL gel VEH	Double-blind, parallel tid × 7 d (n = 231)	FEL > VEH Significantly greater improvement noted after 4 days. Mild local skin irritation noted in 3 FEN- and 2 VEH-treated patients	107

(continued)

Table 5 Continued

Type of Injury	NSAIDs	Design	Results	Ref.
Enthesiopathy, bursitis, tendonitis, fibromyalgia syndrome	3% FEL gel VEH	Double-blind, parallel tid × 2 w (n = 281)	FEL > VEH Pain severity score change was greater in FEL-treated group Global efficacy: Good/very good 50% FEL-treated subjects) vs 29% (VEH-treated subjects)	108
Acute soft-tissue injuries	3% FEL gel VEH	Double-blind, parallel tid × 7 d (n = 82)	FEL > VEH Good/very good response in 81% FEL- and 28% VEH-treatment groups	109
Localized extra-articular rheumatism	3% FEL gel VEH	Double-blind, parallel tid × 14 d (n = 279)	FEL > VEH	110
Acute tendonitis	3% NIF gel VEH	Double-blind, parallel tid × 7 d (n = 56)	NIF > VEH Tolerability good: itching, erythema, skin prickling in 2 NIF-treated patients	111

Tendonitis	4% INDO spray VEH	Double-blind, parallel (n = 30)	INDO > VEH	112
Sprains, contusions, tendonitis epicondylitis	5% FEN cream VEH	Double-blind, parallel bid–tid × 10 d (n = 20)	FEN > VEH FEN significantly changed the course of the injury, leading to early attenuation and resolution of signs and symptoms	113
Accident and sports-related injuries	5% IBU cream VEH	Double-blind, parallel tid–qid × 10 d (n = 80)	IBU = VEH	114
Soft-tissue injuries (strains/sprains)	10% ETOF cream oral NAP	Randomized study tid × 2 wk or 275 mg NAP tid × 2 wk (n = 60)	ETOF = NAP Overall pain score (none to mild pain 65% ETO vs 86% NAP) Incidence of side effects ETOF (3%) vs NAP (20%)	115
Soft-tissue injuries	10% NAP gel VEH	Double-blind qd × 7 d (n = 120)	NAP > VEH Response produced by NAP was more rapid and all symptoms were improved by day 3.	116

Abbre: See Tables 2-4; DICOL, diclotenac; FEL, felbenac; FEN, fentazac; KETO, ketoprofen; KROL, ketorolac tromethamine

(92–116). Most of these studies (Table 6) showed that NSAID topical formulations are well tolerated and can produce significant symptomatic relief in these conditions. In the United Kingdom, there are five topical NSAIDs that are currently marketed—benzydamine cream, piroxicam gel, felbinac gel, diclofenac gel, and ibuprofen cream. In the United States, there are numerous OTC preparations that are indicated for the relief of minor musculoskeletal discomfort (Table 7), but there are no prescription NSAIDs, such as bufexamac, that are indicated for the treatment of soft-tissue injuries. However, there are at least two topical formulations that are currently in development—benzydamine (InterAmerica Pharm) and etofenamate (Rorer) (65).

The recent review by White (2) provides extensive information on the pharmacology, pharmacokinetics, and clinical usefulness of topical benzydamine, felbinac, piroxicam, and ibuprofen formulations in the treatment of inflammatory musculoskeletal diseases. Pharmacokinetics following the topical administration of these NSAIDs demonstrate that these drugs can penetrate the skin and reach the underlying tissues, including the synovial fluid. Data suggest that the levels of NSAIDs in the subcutaneous tissue can reach pharmacologically active concentrations and thus account for their therapeutic effects in soft-tissue injuries. Concentrations of some NSAIDs reported in the synovial fluid are lower than those that exert pharmacological activity in vitro, but two clinical studies with topical NSAIDs in osteoarthritis (94,115) suggest that adequate anti-inflammatory activity

Table 6 Marketed Topical NSAIDs

NSAID (and synonyms)	Formation	Indications
Bendazac (AF-983, Bindazac)	3% cream, ointment 0.5% collyrium	Skin disease, cataracts
Benzydamine (AF-864)	3 and 5% cream	Musculoskeletal pain, contusions
Bufexamac	5% ointment cream	Contact dermatitis, atopic dermatitis, radiodermatitis, eczema
Clobenoside	2.5% gel	Edema
Enoxolone (glycyrrhetinic acid)	2% ointment	Sunburn, diaper rash, vulvar pruritus, seborrheic dermatitis, atopic dermatitis
Etofenamate (B577, TV 485)	0.5% gel, 1% gel, 0.5% solution	Rheumatic pain, muscle pain
Felbinac (BPAA)	3% gel	Sprains, strains, soft-tissue injuries
Flunoxaprofen	20% gel	Rheumatic disorders, vulvovaginitis
Gualenic acid	0.02%	Skin inflammation
Ibuprofen	5% cream	Rheumatic pain, soft-tissue injuries
Ibuproxam	5% ointment	Tendonitis, tenosynovitis, bursitis
Morniflumate	3% ointment, gel	Rheumatic disorders, gingivitis
Nifenazone	5% ointment	Arthritic disorders
Niflumic acid	3% ointment	Inflammation
Oxaceprol	10% cream	Wheals, burns, sores
Piketoprofen	1.8% cream	Rheumatic disorders, muscle pain, rheumatic pain
Piroxicam	0.5% gel	Rheumatic pain, soft-tissue injuries
Pranosal	5% ointment	Muscle pain
Purazinobutazone		Rheumatic disorders
Ufenamate		Eczema, seborrhea, atopic dermatitis

Table 7 Topical OTC Analgesic and Anti-Inflammatory Products

Brand name	Formulation	Active ingredients	Uses
Aurum the Gold	Lotion	Methyl salicylate, menthol, camphor	Topical analgesic
Therapeutic Gold	Lotion	Methyl salicylate, menthol, camphor	Topical analgesic
TheraGold	Lotion	Methyl salicylate, menthol, camphor	Topical analgesic
BenGay	Ointment, balm, gel	Methyl salicylate, menthol	External analgesic
Icy Hot	Balm, cream, stick	Methyl salicylate, menthol	Topical analgesic
Flex-All 454	Gel	Menthol	Topical analgesic
Medicone Derma	Ointment	Menthol	Antipruritic, analgesic
Noxema Medicated Skin Cream	Cream	Camphor, phenol, clove oil, eucaliptus oil, method	Antipruritic, antiseptic, and counterirritant
Rhuligel	Gel	Benzyl alcohol, menthol, camphor	External analgesic

is achieved in the arthritic joints. Percutaneous absorption studies of piroxicam gel in normal volunteers demonstrated adequate drug levels after topical application (117).

There are only two studies that compare the efficacy of topical and oral NSAIDs (94,115). Unfortunately, neither study investigated the efficacy of the same NSAID given topically and orally.

Dickson compared the efficacy of oral ibuprofen (400 mg tid) to that of topical 0.5% piroxicam gel in patients with mild osteoarthritis of the knee (94). After 4 weeks of therapy, both treatments produced a marked reduction in pain intensity and notable improvement in functional capacity. There were no statistically significant differences in response to treatment (as measured by both physician and patient), and overall efficacy was judged to be good or excellent by 64% of the patients receiving piroxicam gel and 60% receiving ibuprofen. Most adverse reactions were gastrointestinal, with a few local effects attributable to treatment. This double-blind, parallel group study suggests that topical treatment is a useful alternative to oral NSAIDs in the treatment of osteoarthritis.

Vanderstraeten et al. compared the effect of etofenamate 10% cream and oral naproxen (275 mg tid) in 60 subjects with strains and sprains from sports injuries (115). Etofenamate gel was as effective as oral naproxen in the overall clinical evaluation and in reducing the overall pain score, and had a better side effect profile than naproxen (3 vs 20% incidence).

The benefit of topical NSAIDs in the treatment of sports injuries has been recently questioned (118,119). For example, although the double-blind study comparing piroxicam gel with oral ibuprofen in patients with osteoarthritis (94) showed comparable safety and efficacy, the topical formulation was about five times more expensive.

V. ADVERSE REACTIONS TO TOPICAL NONSTEROIDAL ANTI-INFLAMMATORY DRUGS

The most common adverse reactions associated with oral administration of NSAIDs are gastrointestinal bleeding and perforations, and acute deterioration of renal function (120).

Table 8 Adverse Reactions Associated with Topical NSAIDs

Abdominal pain/gastric pain
Allergic dermatitis
Angioedema
Bronchospasm/wheezing
Diarrhea
Dizziness
Edema
Erythema
Erythematous eruptions
Flatulence
Headache
Heartburn
Hyperkeratosis
Irritation
Nausea
Nervousness
Numbness
Parathesia
Photosensitivity
Pityroid desquamation
Pruritus
Rash
Skin discoloration/staining
Skin inflammation
Tingling
Vesiculation

However, clinically significant differences in toxicity among NSAIDs have been reported in a prospective long-term study conducted by the Arthritis and Aging Medical Information System (121). The most toxic NSAIDS were indomethacin, tolmetin, and meclofenamic acid, whereas aspirin, salsalate, and ibuprofen were the least toxic. In 1984, Stern and Bigby published a summary of cutaneous adverse reactions to oral NSAIDs (122). They reported numerous NSAIDs were associated with photosensitivity reactions following oral administration including the newer NSAIDs, benoxaprofen, piroxicam, meclofenamate, zomepirac, and sulindac.

Roujeau has reported that the most common skin eruptions attributed to NSAIDs are pruritus, morbilliform rashes, urticaria, and photosensitivity (123). In general, these reactions are mild and non–life-threatening.

Although one might expect the incidence of photosensitivity to be higher following topical application (because of the higher concentration in the skin), the number of instances of photosensitivity associated with topical NSAID treatment appears to be less than reported with oral administration. This may simply be due to the limited use of topical NSAIDs in skin disorders, but could also be related to intrinsic factors such as photosensitivity reactions being induced by NSAID metabolites, or application of topical NSAIDs being confined to non–sun-exposed areas or sun-exposed areas covered with opaque bandage dressings.

Because of the much lower plasma levels of NSAIDs attained by topical administration, one might expect that such administration may eliminate gastrointestinal side effects. However, such intolerance has been reported after topical administration of piroxicam gel (94).

Adverse reactions associated with the use of topical NSAIDs are listed in Table 8. This list has been complied from the adverse reactions in published clinical studies or other sources (65).

VI. FUTURE TOPICAL NONSTEROIDAL ANTI-INFLAMMATORY DRUGS

Several NSAIDs that are under development may be beneficial in the treatment of dermatological disorders. These include 5-lipoxygenase and cyclooxygenase lipoxygenase inhibitors, cell adhesion molecule inhibitors, and free-radical scavengers (Table 9). One very promising class of anti-inflammatory agents is the leumedins, compounds that block leukocyte attachment to adhesion molecules and also prevent the release of leukocytes from blood vessels. A topical leumedin compound is currently being tested in contact dermatitis, and an oral formulation is currently undergoing clinical trials in rheumatoid arthritis (124,125).

Table 9 Topical NSAIDs Under Development

NSAID	Primary mode of action	Company
WY-50295	5-Lipoxygenase inhibitor	American Home Products (US)
TMK 688	5-Lipoxygenase inhibitor	Terumo (Japan)
E6080	5-Lipoxygenase inhibitor	Eisai (Japan)
Lonapalene (RS 43179)	5-Lipoxygenase inhibitor	Syntex/Astra (US)
MK-886	5-Lipoxygenase inhibitor	Merck & Co (US)
SC-45662	5-Lipoxygenase inhibitor	Searle/Monsanto (US)
A-78773	5-Lipoxygenase inhibitor	Abbott (US)
L-651,392	5-Lipoxygenase inhibitor	Merck-Frosst (Canada)
Masoprocol	5-Lipoxygenase inhibitor	Chemex (US)
L-651,896	5-Lipoxygenase inhibitor	Merck-Frosst (Canada)
BRL 20459	Anti-inflammatory	Beecham (UK)
TN873R	Anti-inflammatory	Taiyo (Japan)
GM 7050	Cell adhesion molecule inhibitor	Glycomed (US)
NPC-15199	Cell adhesion molecule inhibitor	Nova (US)
OZP	Cyclooxygenase inhibitor	Merck, Sharp & Dohme (US)
FPL 62064	Cyclooxygenase/lipoxygenase inhibitor	Fisons (UK)
P-8977	Cyclooxygenase/lipoxygenase inhibitor	Hoescht-Roussel (US)
P-8892	Cyclooxygenase/lipoxygenase inhibitor	Hoescht-Roussel (US)
Tenidap	Cyclooxygenase/lipoxygenase inhibitor	Pfizer (US)
R68151	Cyclooxygenase/lipoxygenase inhibitor	Janssen (Belgium/US)
R70795	Cyclooxygenase/lipoxygenase inhibitor	Janssen (Belgium/US)
Flunoxaprofen	Cyclooxygenase/lipoxygenase inhibitor	Ravizza (Italy)
BMY 30094	Cyclooxygenase/lipoxygenase inhibitor	Bristol-Myers Squibb (US)
Superoxide dismutase	Free radical scavenger	Takeda (Japan)
UR 10324	PAF antagonist	Uriach (Spain)

REFERENCES

1. Arthritis Drugs Advisory Committee Meeting, Food and Drug Administration, December 6, 1990. NDA Pipeline 1990; V-18.
2. White S. Topical non-steroidal anti-inflammatory drugs (NSAIDs) in the treatment of inflammatory musculoskeletal disorders. Prostaglandins Leukotrienes Essential Fatty Acids 1991; 43:209–22.
3. Gruber CM, Ridolfo AS, Nickander R, Mikulaschek WM. Delay of erythema of human skin by anti-inflammatory drugs after ultraviolet irradiation. Clin Pharmacol Ther 1972; 13:109–13.
4. Gupta N, Levy L. Delayed manifestation of ultraviolet reaction in the guinea-pig caused by anti-inflammatory drugs. Br J Pharmacol 1973; 47:240–8.
5. Snyder DS, Eagelstein WH. Topical indomethacin and sunburn. Br J Dermatol 1974; 90:91–3.
6. Snyder DS. Cutaneous effects of topical indomethacin, an inhibitor of prostaglandin synthesis on UV-damaged skin. J Invest Dermatol 1975; 64:322–5.
7. Gomez EC, Trancik RJ. Effect of topical diflumidone on ultraviolet-light-induced erythema. Dermatologica 1981; 162:175–182.
8. Farr PM, Diffey B. A quantitative study of the effects of topical indomethacin on cutaneous erythema induced by UVB and UVC radiation. Br J Dermatol 1986; 115:453–66.
9. Tan P, Flowers Fp, Araujo OE, Doering P. Effect of topically applied flurbiprofen on ultraviolet-induced erythema. Drug Intell Clin Pharm 1986; 20:496–9.
10. Torrent J, Izquierdo I, Barbanjo MJ, Moreno J, Laurado J, Jane F. UV-induced erythema model: a tool in dermatopharmacology for testing the topical activity of non-steroidal anti-inflammatory agents in man. Methods Find Exp Clin Pharmacol 1988; 10:341–5.
11. Bauer J, Wendelberger A, Schweiberer L, Wurster K, Conzen P. Effect of BW 755C and etofenamate on wound healing and arachidonic acid metabolism in a pig scald burn injury model [abstract]. Presented at the second world conference on inflammation; antirheumatics, analgesics, immuno-modulators, March 1986, Monte-Carlo, Monaco.
12. Bauer JA, Wendelberger A, Felix W. A new sonographic model for effective quantification of antioedematous and anti-inflammatory drugs in burns. Lipid Mediators Immunol Shock 1987; 139:523–36.
13. Sauer T, Lehn N, Eitel F, Bauer JA. Der einfluβ von etofenamat auf das fruhe verbruhungsodem. Unfallchirurg 1987; 90:391–3.
14. Johansson J, Lahti A. Topical non-steroidal anti-inflammatory drugs inhibit nonimmunologic immediate contact reactions. Contact Derm 1988; 19:161–5.
15. Poelman MC, Piot B, Guyon F, Deroni M, Leveque JL. Assessment of topical non-steroidal anti-inflammatory drugs. J Pharm Pharmacol 1989; 41:720–2.
16. Duteil L, Queille C, Poncet M, Ortonne JP, Czerneiewski J. Objective assessment of topical corticosteroids and non-steroidal anti-inflammatory drugs in methylnicotinate-induced skin inflammation. Clin Exp Dermatol 1990; 15:195–9.
17. Lawrence CM, Shuster S. Mechanism of anthralin inflammation. I. Dissociation of response to clobetasol and indomethacin. Br J Dermatol 1985; 113:107–15.
18. Kaidbey KH, Kurban A. The influence of corticosteroids and topical indomethacin on sunburn erythema. J Invest Dermatol 1976; 66:153–6.
19. Kook HI, Han JY. A study on the effect of topical non-steroidal anti-inflammatory drugs and corticoids on ultraviolet light induced erythema. Korean J Dermatol 1980; 18:115–20.
20. Snyder DS, Eaglestein WH. Intradermal anti-prostaglandin agents and sunburn. J Invest Dermatol 1974; 62:47–50.
21. Black AK, Greaves MW, Hensby CN, Plumber NA, Warin AP. The effects of indomethacin on arachidonic acid and prostaglandin E_2 and $F_{2\alpha}$ levels in human skin 24 hours after UVB and UVC irradiation. Br J Dermatol 1978; 6:261–6.
22. Voorhees JJ. Leukotrienes and other lipoxygenase products in the pathogenesis and therapy of psoriasis and other dermatoses [editorial]. Arch Dermatol 1983; 119:541–7.

23. Kragballe K, Voorhees JJ. Arachidonic acid in psoriasis. Pathogenic role and pharmacological regulation. Acta Derm Venereol [Suppl] 1985; 120:12–17.
24. Greaves MW. Neutrophil polymorphonuclears, mediators, and the pathogenesis of psoriasis. Br J Dermatol 1983; 109:115–8.
25. Hammarstrom S, Hamberg M, Samuelsson B, et al. Increased concentrations of nonesterified arachidonic acid, 12-L-hydroxy-5,8,10,14-eicosatetraenoic acid, prostaglandin E_2, and prostaglandin $F_{2\alpha}$ in epidermis of psoriasis. Proc Natl Acad Sci USA 1975; 72:5130–4.
26. Hensby C, Juhlin L, Civier A, et al. Arachidonic acid and prostanoids in suction blister fluid for psoriatic lesions and unaffected skin. Arch Dermatol Res 1983; 275:350–2.
27. Brain SD, Camp RDR, Dowd PM, et al. Psoriasis and leukotriene B_4. Lancet 1982; 2:762–3.
28. Brain SD, Camp RD, Charleson S, et al. The release of LTC_4-like material from the involved lesional skin in psoriasis. Br J Clin Pharmacol 1984; 17:650P.
29. Ziboh VA, Casebolt TL, Marcelo CL, Voorhees JJ. Biosynthesis of lipoxygenase products by enzyme preparations from normal and psoriatic skin. J Invest Dermatol 1984; 10:426–30.
30. Grabbe J, Czarnetzki BM, Rosenbach T, Mardin M. Identification of chemotactic lipoxygenase products of arachidonate metabolism in psoriatic skin. J Invest Dermatol 1984; 82:477–9.
31. Dowd PM, Greaves MW. Cutaneous responses to lipoxygenase products of arachidonic acid. Acta Dermvenereol [suppl] 1985; 120:18–22.
32. Kragballe K, Duell EA, Voorhees JJ. Selective decrease of 15-hydroxyeicosatetraenoic acid (15-HETE) formation in uninvolved psoriatic dermis. Arch Dermatol 1986; 122:877–80.
33. Green CA, Shuster S. Lack of effect of topical indomethacin on psoriasis. Br J Clin Pharmacol 1987; 24:381–4.
34. Knopf B, Barta U. Lokale wirking des nichtsteroidalen antipholgistikums indomethacin auf die psoriasis. Dermatol Monatsschr 1987; 173:454–7.
35. van der Meersch J. Comparative study of bufexamac (Droxaryl) ointment and of its recipient on psoriasis cases; a double-blind test. Curr Ther Res 1974; 16:904–8.
36. Meyerhoff JO. Exacerbation of psoriasis with meclofenamate. N Engl J Med 1983; 309:496.
37. Paller AS, Wisher A, Roenigk HH. Meclofenamate for psoriasis. Arch Dermatol 1984; 120:438.
38. Reshad H, Hargreaves GK, Vickers CFH. Generalized pustular psoriasis precipitated by phenbutazone and oxyphenbutazone. Br J Dermatol. 1983; 109:111–3.
39. Shelley WB. Birch pollen and aspirin in psoriasis. JAMA 1964; 189:985–8.
40. Katayama H, Kawada A. Exacerbation of psoriasis induced by indomethacin. J Dermatol (Tokyo) 1981; 8:323–7.
41. Powles AV, Griffiths CEM, Seifert MH, Fry I. Exacerbation of psoriasis by indomethacin. Br J Dermatol 1987; 117:799–800.
42. Winthrop GJ. Does meclofenamate help psoriasis and arthritis? N Engl J Med 1982; 307:1528.
43. Kragballe K, Herlin T. Benoxaprofen improves psoriasis. A double-blind study. Arch Dermatol 1983; 119:548–52.
44. Shall L, Marks, R. The effects of concomitant administration of oral indomethacin with topical dithranol treatment in psoriasis. Br J Dermatol 1987; 116:739–44.
45. Sheehan-Dare RA, Goodfield MJD, Rowell NR. The effect of oral indomethacin on psoriasis treated with the Ingram regime. Br J Dermatol 1991; 125:253–5.
46. Fogh K. Lipoxygenase products of arachidonic acid in psoriasis, atopic dermatitis and experimental arthritis. Dan Med J 1990; 37:289–308.
47. Dale HH. Progress in autopharmacology: a survey of present knowledge of the chemical regulation of certain functions by natural constituents of the tissues. Bull John Hopkins Hosp 1933; 53:293–347.
48. Vane JR. Prostaglandins in the inflammatory response. In: Lepow IH, Ward PA, eds. Inflammation; mechanisms and control. Academic Press, New York, 1972; 261–79.
49. Ternowitz T, Fogh K, Kragballe K. 15-hydroxyeicosatetraenoic acid (15-HETE) specifically

inhibits LTB4-induced chemotaxis of polymophonuclear leukocytes. Skin Pharmacol 1988; 1:93–9.
50. Ellis CN, Fallon JD, Kang S, Vanderveen EE, Voorhees JJ. Topical application of nonsteroidal anti-inflammatory drugs prevents vehicle-induced improvement in psoriasis. J Am Acad Dermatol 1986; 14:39–43.
51. Garland LG, Salmon JA. Hydroxamic acids and hydroxyureas as inhibitors of arachidonate 5-lipoxygenase. Drugs Future 1991; 16:547–58.
52. Ford-Hutchinson AW. Potential and therapeutic value of development of novel 5-lipoxygenase inhibitors. In: Crooke ST, Wong A, eds. Lipoxygenases and their products. New York: Academic Press, 1991:137–160.
53. Camp R, Jones RR, Brain S, Woollard P, Greaves M. Production of intraepidermal microabscesses by topical application of leukotriene B_4. J Invest Dermatol 1984; 82:200–4.
54. Cunningham FM, Woollard PM, Camp RDR. Proinflammatory properties of unsaturated fatty acids and their monohydroxy metabolites. Prostaglandins 1985; 30:497–510.
55. Duell EA, Ellis CN, Voorhees JJ. Determination of 5, 12, and 15- lipoxygenase products in the keratomed biopsies of normal and psoriatic skin. J Invest Dermatol 1989; 91:446–50.
56. Miyazawa K, Iimori Y, Makino M, Mikami T, Miyasaka K. Effect of some nonsteroidal anti-inflammatory drugs and other agents on cyclooxygenase and lipoxygenase activities in some enzyme preparations. Jpn J Pharmacol 1985; 39:199–205.
57. Salmon JA, Tiling LC, Moncada S. Evaluations of inhibitors of eicosanoid synthesis in leucocytes; possible pitfall of using the calcium ionophore A23187 to stimulate 5-lipoxygenase. Prostaglandins 1985; 29:377–85.
58. Camp R, Black A, Cunningham F, Mallet A, Greaves M. Pharmacologic effects of topical lonapalene in psoriasis. J Invest Dermatol 1988; 90:550.
59. Lassus A, Forsstrom S. A dimethoxynaphthalene derivative (RS-43179 gel) compared with 0.025% fluocinolone acetonide gel in the treatment of psoriasis. Br J Dermatol 1985; 113:103–6.
60. Jansen CT, Lammintausta K, Bullingham RES, Forsstrom S. A clinical trial of lonapalene, fluocinolone acetonide gel in the treatment of psoriasis. J Invest Dermatol 1986; 86:483.
61. Black AK, Camp RDR, Mallet AI, Cunningham FM, Hofbauer M, Greaves MW. Pharmacologic and clinical effects of lonapalene (RS 43179), a 5-lipoxygenase inhibitor, in psoriasis. J Invest Dermatol 1990; 95:50–4.
62. deDoncker P, Cauwenbergh G. The therapeutic potential of 5-lipoxygenase inhibitors in dermatological conditions. Poster presentation P-191, American Academy of Dermatology, Dallas, 1991.
63. deJong EMGJ, van Vlijmen IMMJ, Scholte JCM, Buntinx A, Friedman B, Tanaka, W, van de Kerkhof PCM. Clinical and biochemical effects of an oral leukotriene biosynthesis inhibitor (MK886) in psoriasis. Skin Pharmacol 1991; 4:278–85.
64. Achten G, Bourland A, Haven E, Lapiere CHM, Pierard J, Reynaers H. A study of the activity of bufexamac cream and ointment in various dermatoses. Dermatologica 1973; 146:1–7.
65. Schlesser JL. Drugs available abroad; a guide to therapeutic drugs available and approved outside the U.S. London: Derwent Publications, 1991.
66. de Gregorio M, Meneghelli PL. Clinical evaluation of bendazac (AF-893); a non-steroidal topical anti-inflammatory agent. Acta Dermvenereol 1970; 50:466–8.
67. Washington DC Dermatologic Society Meeting, Children's Hospital, March 1983.
68. Fine JD, Johnson L. Evaluation of the efficacy of topical bufexamac in epidermolysis bullosa simplex. Arch Dermatol 1988; 124:1669–72.
69. Leyden JJ, Shalita AR, Saatjian GD, Sefton J. Erythromycin 2% in comparison with clindamycin phosphate 1% solution in acne vulgaris. J Am Acad Dermatol 1987; 16:822–27.
70. Katsambas A, Towarky A, Stratigos J. Topical clindamycin phosphate compared with oral tetracycline in the treatment of acne vulgaris. Br J Dermatol 1987; 116:387–91.
71. Chalker DK, Lesher JI, Smith JG, et al. Efficacy of topical isotretinoin 0.05% gel in acne

vulgaris; results of a multicenter, double-blind investigation. J Am Acad Dermatol 1987; 17:251–4.
72. Hensby C, Cavey D, Bouchier M, et al. The in vivo and in vitro anti-inflammatory activity of CD 271, a new retinoid like modulator of cell differentiation. In: Shroot B, et al., eds. Pharmacology of retinoids in the skin. vol 3. Basel: S Karger 1989:160–2.
73. Chatelus A, Caron JC, Shroot B, et al. Structure–activity relationships between different retinoids using the topical rhino mouse comedolytic model. In: Shroot B, et al., eds. Pharmacology of retinoids in the skin. vol 3. Basel: S Karger 1989:144–8.
74. Smith Kurtz E, Maddalena ME, Hellyer L, Ortega-Nanos M, Hanel H, Abrams B. Evaluation and comparison of the anti-inflammatory activity of antimycotic agents. Poster presentation, American Academy of Dermatology Meeting, Dallas, 1991.
75. Lee WL, Shalita AR. Naftifine; an anti-inflammatory agent. Clin Res 1989; 352A.
76. Miller WS, Ruderman FR, Smith JG. Aspirin and ultraviolet light-induced erythema in man. Arch Dermatol 1967; 95:357–8.
77. Edwards EK, Horwitz SN, Frost P. Reduction of the erythemal response to ultraviolet by non-steroidal anti-inflammatory agents. Arch Dermatol Res 1982; 272:263–7.
78. Stern RS, Dodson TB. Ibuprofen in the treatment of UV-B-induced inflammation. Arch Dermatol 1985; 121:508–12.
79. Bissett DL, Chatterjee R, Hannon DP. Chronic ultraviolet radiation-induced increase in skin iron and the photoprotective effect of topically applied iron chelators. Photobiol Photochem 1991; 54:215–23.
80. Bissett DL, Oelrich DM, Hannon DP. Clinical evaluation of a topical iron chelating compound; 2-furildioxime prevents acute photodamage. Poster presentation, American Academy of Dermatology, Dallas, 1991.
81. Brogden RN, Pinder RM, Sawyer PR, Speight TM, Avery GS. Bufexamac; a review of its pharmacological properties and therapeutic efficacy in inflammatory dermatoses. Drugs 1975; 10:351–6.
82. Valle-Jones JC. Bufexamac in the treatment of skin diseases in general practice. Practitioner 1974; 213:383–6.
83. Achten G, Bourland A, Haven E, Lapiere CM, Pierard J, Reynaers H. Bufexamac; a non-steroidal anti-inflammatory agent suitable for topical application in clinical dermatology. Arch Belg Dermatol Syphilign 1970; 26:509–10.
84. Kohnosu M. Results of clinical application of bufexamac cream. Clin Rep 1972; 6:258.
85. Grigoriu D. Comparative study of the action of *p*-butoxyphenylacethydroxamic acid and betamethasone 17-valerate in topical applications in various inflammatory skin disorders. Med Hyg 1972; 30:491.
86. Diamant F, Santillian I. A clinical trial of topical bufexamac—a non-steroidal anti-inflammatory agent. Clin Ther 1980; 2:427–32.
87. Mackey JD. A double-blind clinical study of bufexamac and fluocinolone acetonide in dermatitis. J Ir Med Assoc 1974; 67:214–16.
88. Wheatley D. A non-steroidal anti-inflammatory cream; a report from the General Practitioner Research Group. Practitioner 1975; 214:689–92.
89. Chrishansen JV, et al. Efficacy of bufexamac (NFN) cream in skin diseases. A double blind multicentre trial. Dermatologica 1977; 154:177–84.
90. Michelson AM. Medical aspects of superoxide dismutase. Life Chem Rep 1987; 6:1.
91. Mizushima Y, Hoshi K, Yanagawa A, Takano K. Topical application of superoxide dismutase cream. Drugs Exp Clin Res 1991; 17:127–31.
92. Aoki T, Numajiri M, Yamamoto M, et al. Comparative study of piroxicam gel with indomethacin gel and piroxicam placebo gel in the treatment of pain from orthopaedic trauma. Jpn J Pharmacol Ther 1984; 12:145–7.
93. Russell AL. Piroxicam 0.5% topical gel compared to placebo in the treatment of acute soft tissue injuries; a double-blind study comparing efficacy and safety. Clin Invest Med 1991; 14:35–43.

94. Dickson DJ. A double-blind evaluation of topical piroxicam gel with oral ibuprofen in osteoarthritis of the knee. Curr Ther Res 1991; 49:199–207.
95. Kroll MP, Wiseman RL, Guttadauria M. A clinical evaluation of piroxicam gel; an open comparative trial with diclofenac gel in the treatment of acute musculoskeletal disorders. Clin Ther 1989; 11:382–91.
96. Fujimaki E, Ohno M, Nagashima K, et al. Clinical evaluation of piroxicam gel versus indomethacin gel and placebo gel in the treatment of muscle pain; a double blind, multicenter study. Jpn J Pharmacol Ther 1984; 12:119–37.
97. Kageyama T. A double blind placebo controlled multicenter study of piroxicam 0.5% gel in osteoarthritis of the knee. Eur J Rheumatol Inflamm 1987; 8:114–5.
98. El-Hadidi T, El-Garf A. Double-blind study comparing the use of Voltaren Emulgel versus regular gel during ultrasonic sessions in the localized treatment of traumatic and rheumatic painful conditions. J Int Med Res 1991; 19:219–27.
99. Schapira D, Linn S, Scharf Y. A placebo-controlled evaluation of diclofenac diethylamine salt in the treatment of lateral epicondylitis of the elbow. Curr Ther Res 1991; 49:162–8.
100. Diebschlag W, Nocker W, Bullingham R. A double-blind study of the efficacy of topical ketorolac tromethamine gel in the treatment of ankle sprain in comparison to placebo and etofenamate. J Clin Pharmacol 1990; 30:82–9.
101. Matucci-Cerinic M, Casini A. Ketoprofen vs etofenamate in a controlled double-blind study: evidence of topical effectiveness in soft tissue rheumatic pain. Int J Clin Pharmacol Res 1988; 7:157–60.
102. Elswood R, McLeod DA. Treatment of ankle sprains with benzydamine. Practitioner 1985; 229:70–1.
103. Haig G. Potable thermogram technique for topically applied benzydamine cream in acute soft tissue injuries. Int J Tiss React 1986; 7:145–7.
104. Chatterjee DS. A double-blind clinical study with benzydamine 3% cream on soft tissue injuries in an occupational health centre. J Int Med Res 1977; 5:450–8.
105. Fantanto S, de Gregorio M. Clinical evaluation of topical benzydamine in traumatology. Arzneimittelforschung 1971; 21:1530–3.
106. Te CV, Seares V. An open label non-randomized, safety and efficacy trial of felbinac gel applied three times daily in patients with soft tissue trauma in the Philippines. J Int Med 1991; 29:45–52.
107. McLatchie GR, Lawrence GF, Rogmans D, Lisai P. Soft tissue trauma; a controlled trial of the topical application of felbinac, a new NSAID. Br J Clin Pharmacol 1989; 43:277–80.
108. Bolten W. Felbinac gel for the treatment of localized extra-articular rheumatic diseases—a multicenter, placebo-controlled, randomized study. Rheumatol 1991; 50:109–13.
109. Sanguinetti C. Treatment of soft tissue trauma with BPAA gel 3% (Traxam)—results of an Italian multicentre study against placebo. Clin Ter 1989; 130:255–8.
110. Bolten W, McDonald M, Lawrence GF, Williams JPG, Rossi F, Miehlke K. A multi-centre randomized double-blind placebo (P) controlled trial of topical felbinac (F) (biphenylacetic acid 3% gel) in extra-articular rheumatic conditions. EULAR symposium, Rome October, 1986.
111. Dreiser RL, Ditisheim A, Charlot J, Lopez A. A double-blind, placebo controlled study of niflumic acid gel in the treatment of acute tendonitis. Eur J Rheumatol Inflamm 1991; 11:38–45.
112. Ginsberg F, Famaey JP. Double-blind, randomized crossover study of the percutaneous efficacy and tolerability of a topical indomethacin spray versus placebo in the treatment of tendonitis. J Int Med Res 1991; 19:131–36.
113. Sinniger M, Blanchard P. Controlled clinical trial with fentizac cream in sports injuries. J Med Res 1981; 9:300–2.
114. Ramesh NK, Steuber U. Dolgit Creme bei unfallund sportverletzungen. Theraiewoche 1983; 33:4563–70.

115. Vanderstraeten G, Schuermans P. Study of the effect of etofenamate 10% gel in comparison with an oral NSAID in strains and sprains due to sports injuries. Med Phys 1990; 13:139–41.
116. Thorling J, Linden B, Berg R, Sandahl A. Curr Med Res Opin 1990; 12:242–8.
117. Sugarawa S, Ohno H, Ueda R, et al. Studies of the percutaneous absorption and tissue distribution of piroxicam gel. J Med Pharm Sci 1984; 12:1233–8.
118. MeReC on topical NSAIs. Scrip Aug 7, 1991; 1640:26.
119. Topical NSAIDs; a gimmick or a godsend? Lancet 1989; 2:779–80.
120. Greaves MW. Pharmacology and significance of non-steroidal anti-inflammatory drugs in the treatment of skin diseases. J. Am Acad Dermatol 1987; 16:751–64.
121. Fries JF, Williams CA, Block DA. The relative toxicity of non-steroidal anti-inflammatory drugs. Arthritis Rheum 1991; 34:1353–60.
122. Stern RS, Rigby M. An expanded profile of cutaneous reactions to non-steroidal anti-inflammatory drugs. JAMA 1984; 252:1433–7.
123. Roujeau JC. Clinical aspects of skin reactions to NSAIDs. Scand J Rheumatol [suppl] 1987; 65:131–4.
124. Leumedins hold promise for treating rheumatoid arthritis. Am Pharm 1991; 31:21.
125. Nova's novel anti-inflammatories. Scrip Jan 25 1991; 1585:24.

6

The Over-the-Counter Use of Nonsteroidal Anti-Inflammatory Drugs and Other Antipyretic Analgesics

KAY BRUNE
The University of Erlangen
Erlangen, Germany

KEITH McCORMACK
McCormack Ltd.
Leighton Buzzard, Bedfordshire, England

I. HISTORICAL ASPECTS

A. The Discovery of Salicylic Acid, Aspirin, Phenazone, and Acetaminophen

All prototypes of modern antipyretic analgesics in over-the-counter (OTC) use worldwide were discovered in central Europe during the last century. From Roman and Greek reports concerning the use of willow bark in painful joint and muscle diseases; the descriptions of Hildegard of Bingen (Germany) and Reverend Stone (England) of the use of concoctions from willow bark, spirea, and poplar leaves as analgesic remedies; Piria in Italy, Kolbe in Germany, and many others, have defined the active principle as salicylic acid (1). Chemical synthesis of salicylic acid and large-scale production of this compound by V. Heyden in Dresden made possible the clinical application of large doses of pure salicylic acid or its salts. This, in turn, led to the discovery of the anti-inflammatory, antipyretic, and analgesic properties of this naturally, and then synthetically, produced compound.

An attempt to substitute another natural product (quinine) by a synthetic analogue led the chemist, Knorr, and the pharmacologist and physician, Filehne, in Erlangen to synthesize and test phenazone (3). It was antipyretic, although it was later shown not to be chemically related to quinine. Phenazone (initially called antipyrine) proved effective as an antipyretic agent. This led to the widespread clinical use of this first pure chemical compound in Europe and North America. Slightly later, Cahn and Hepp (1–3), in Strasbourg, administered acetanilide instead of naphthalene to a patient suffering from infection and fever. Acetanilide was inactive against the infection (probably worms), but showed antipyretic activity and, hence, was used as an antipyretic (Antifebrine). These three prototypic compounds were later synthetically modified to yield products that were easier to manufacture, better tolerated, or had other advantages. Hoffmann at Bayer made salicylic acid and sodium salicylate more amenable to his father's taste by adding an acetyl group (2). The result, aspirin, made both Bayer and aspirin well-known. Chemists at Hoechst produced another prodrug, the water-soluble ester of 4-methyl-amino-phenazone, dipyrone (metamizole). The active principle, 4-methylaminophenazone (4-MAP) was more active than phenazone, but less water-soluble. Dipyrone, the parent compound of 4-MAP, was the sulfate ester and was more soluble in aqueous solution than 4-MAP. Phenazone, dipyrone, and other phenazone derivatives laid the foundation for the worldwide success of Hoechst.

Finally, Bayer found it easier to produce the (antipyretic) phenacetin than acetanilide or its metabolite *p*-aminophenol. Consequently, this company marketed phenacetin as a less-expensive, better-tolerated, antipyretic analgesic. It was only recently that phenacetin was supplanted by its active (but less toxic) metabolite acetaminophen, which does not produce the toxic metabolite *p*-phenetidine.

These prototypes of our present-day OTC antipyretic analgesics were found by serendipity (3). They were introduced onto the pharmaceutical market without requiring any governmental approval and without any toxicological testing or animal experimentation. As a matter of fact, until this century, most countries did not have any regulatory body in a position to control the pharmaceutical and medical use of drugs, to guarantee their quality, or to take action on the consumer's behalf.

B. The Development of Regulatory Authorities

Interestingly enough, and contrary to common belief, it was industry who approached the Department of the Interior of the former German Kaiserreich to request cooperation for the sake of the patient and to guarantee the quality of the product (Fig. 1). The separation of medications into OTC and non-OTC categories is a development of recent decades. It resulted from the political interplay among authorities, industry, the medical and pharmaceutical organizations, and the consumers. Historically, the uncontrolled OTC use was the normal event.

Traveling around the world one is quite frequently surprised that the uncontrolled use of drugs still prevails in many large countries. Any available antipyretic analgesics and NSAIDs may easily be bought OTC in many countries in South America, the Middle East, and Asia. Consequently, this chapter could just as well comprise the content of the whole book. For the sake of clarity we shall limit this chapter to OTC NSAIDs and antipyretic analgesics used in those countries with stringent governmental-sponsored control of the drug market.

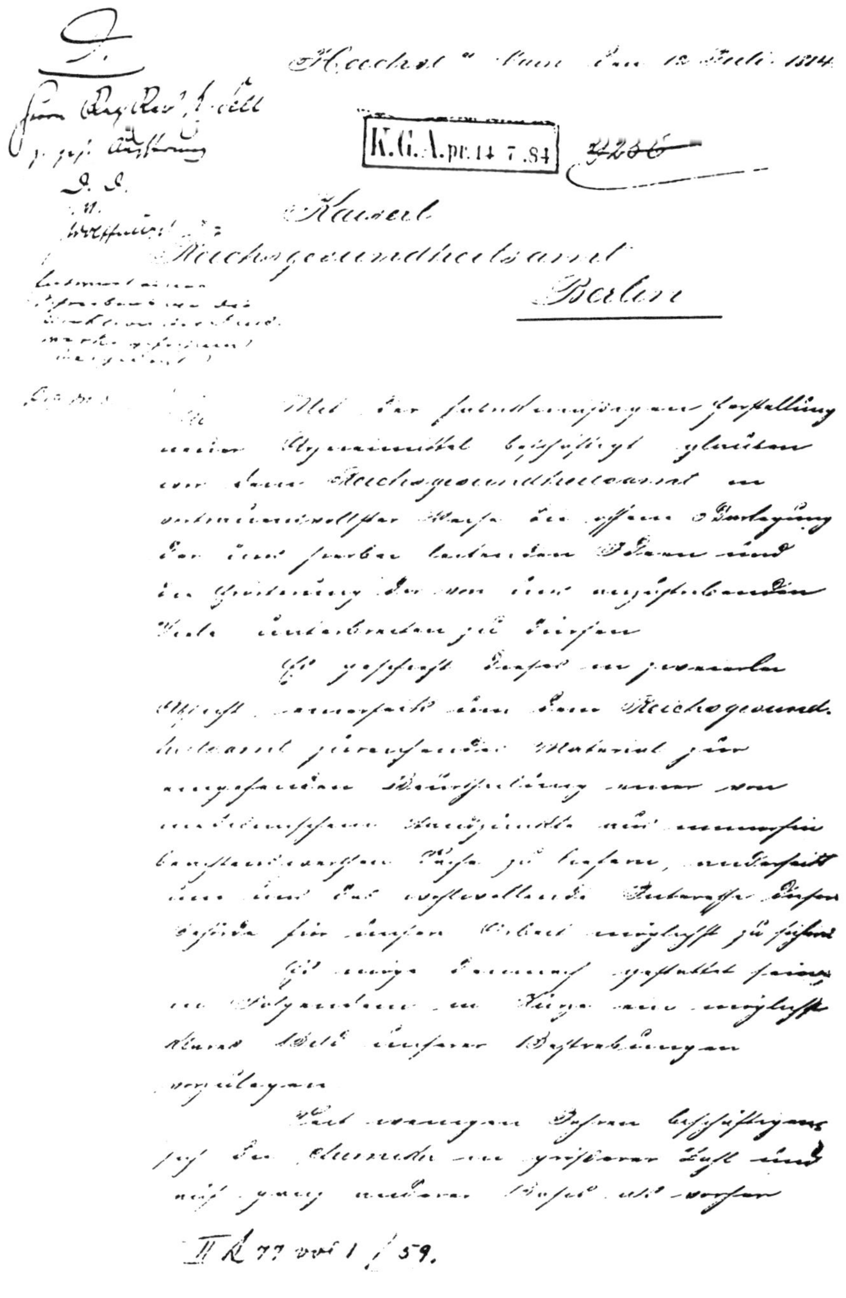

K.G.A. pr. 14 7 .84

Kaiserl.
Reichsgesundheitsamt
Berlin

Figure 1 Text of request for governmental regulatory oversight from industry to the Department of Interior of the former German Kaiserreich:

"Being engaged in the industrial production of drugs we believe we should openly disclose our intentions and trustfully discuss our goals with the Reichsgesundheitsamt (NIH).

This is to be done for two reasons. Firstly, to furnish the Reichsgesundheitsamt with sufficient information for indepth evaluation of matters which are at least of some importance from the medical point of view. On the other hand we intend by so doing to secure the benevolent interest of this governmental agency for our work.

For these reasons it may be permitted to give as complete as possible a description of our intentions."

C. Current Status

Within the last 100 years, the use of some antipyretic analgesics for self-medication (i.e., OTC use) has become accepted practice. Their use in most Western countries is limited to the following indications: transient, mild-to-moderate pain, fever, and inflammation that are most likely of transient quality and within the usual intensity. Self-medication appears to be permitted only if pain, fever, and inflammation occur in children and adults between the ages of 7 and 75 years who are generally otherwise healthy. At least, they should not be suffering from serious diseases, such as chronic allergic reactions (including asthma), liver or kidney damage, coagulopathy, or hematopoietic dysfunction. Furthermore, the patients should not be pregnant or mentally disabled. Previous experience with the drug is also preferred. Excluded from self-medication in most industrialized countries are chronic inflammatory or painful diseases, as well as intense or chronic pain and fever, where physician consultation is recommended. On a historical basis leading to the foregoing criteria, plus the influence of both industry and consumers, aspirin, acetaminophen, and within the last decade, ibuprofen, are OTC in almost all industrialized countries. Phenazone and its derivatives are not OTC in most Anglo-Saxon and Scandinavian countries. These compounds are also widely used in central and eastern Europe, Asia, and South America. Recently, mefenamic acid and naproxen have been made OTC in New Zealand, and ketoprofen has been proposed for OTC use in a few countries (4). The reader should judge the wisdom of the present OTC conditions worldwide compared with the pharmacological and toxicological knowledge of the drugs, which will be outlined as follows.

II. PHARMACOKINETIC REQUIREMENTS

According to the accepted indications, as outlined under Section I (present basis of decisions of the BGA; i.e., comparable with the American FDA), certain pharmacokinetic qualities for the OTC use of NSAIDs and other antipyretic analgesics appear desirable, at least from the pharmacologist's point of view. These comprise

1. Fast absorption, to guarantee rapid onset of action.
2. A short elimination half-life, to guarantee timely limited presence of any active ingredient in the body just sufficient to remedy transient pain conditions and fever. Also, the elimination should be rapid in young and elderly patients, as well as in those possibly suffering from mild, as yet, undiscovered liver and kidney dysfunction to avoid unwanted drug accumulation.
3. No dangerous pharmacokinetic interactions of drugs in OTC use with widely used compounds, such as antihypertensive agents, antidiabetic agents, or other drugs in broad clinical use.

We have attempted to compile the major pharmacokinetic characteristics of widely used NSAIDs, acetaminophen, and some phenazone derivatives in Table 1. It is obvious from this table that none of the compounds suit the foregoing pharmacokinetic requirements perfectly.

A. Salicylates and Fenamates

Aspirin, itself, is a prodrug, and its metabolite, salicylic acid, has a dose-dependent elimination half-life ($t_{1/2}$). Diflunisal, a more modern salicylate, is characterized by an unnecessary slow elimination ($t_{1/2}$ about 12 h) and a dose-dependent increase in elimination half-life with higher doses. The fenamates, a still-used class of drugs, developed in the early 1960s have not been carefully investigated. Most pharmacokinetic data have not been defined according to modern standards of specificity and quality (see Table 1).

These compounds, therefore, may not be considered suitable for OTC use under the foregoing definition, despite that they have been in medical use for more than a decade, and mefenamic acid has recently been made OTC in New Zealand (4).

B. Aryl Acetic Acid Derivatives

The aryl acidic acid derivatives are among the most widely used compounds worldwide. Indomethacin was the first new NSAID to be marketed (after aspirin and phenylbutazone) for the treatment of rheumatic diseases (5). Nevertheless, many later members of this group (e.g., tolmetin, zomepirac, and others) have not been adequately investigated or have been proved toxic in early clinical use (see Table 1). Indomethacin, itself, shows a variable elimination, a complex enterohepatic circulation, and many side effects (e.g., central nervous system disturbances) that would disqualify this compound from OTC use, according to the characteristics outlined under Section I (6).

Diclofenac, finally, although now being the most widely used NSAID worldwide, appears not ideal for OTC use because the usual formulations of diclofenac, containing diclofenac enclosed in an acid-resisting coating, are not absorbed fast enough to guarantee adequate and reliable pain relief within approximately 1–2 h (8,80). This drawback could, however, probably be remedied by galenic modifications. A more serious drawback is the limited and variable bioavailability of diclofenac, which appears particularly low at lower doses otherwise suitable for analgesic and antipyretic effects in OTC use (8). This characteristic of diclofenac appears to be related to its high lipophilicity and high potency, which cause both low-dosage ranges, but also relatively high drug extraction during the first liver passage (9). Obviously, this second drawback is related to the chemistry of the compound and cannot easily be remedied by pharmaceutical measures.

C. 2-Arylpropionic Acid Derivatives

On the other hand, the group of 2-arylpropionic acids appears to offer several candidates for OTC use. In principle, most 2-arylpropionic acids in clinical use show a relatively fast elimination, which is only marginally influenced by age, liver or kidney diseases, particularly if these defects are not too prominent (e.g., ibuprofen) (7). Moreover, at least four compounds, fenoprofen, ibuprofen, ketoprofen, and naproxen, show a complete oral bioavailability. The only pharmacokinetic drawback of this group of compounds may consist in its relatively slow absorption owing to the relatively high degree of lipophilicity (exception: ketoprofen). It has been shown that, for example, ibuprofen, given as sugar-coated tablets containing ibuprofen acids, may be absorbed only with major retardation causing individual t_{max} values of up to 6 h (11). Obviously, such retarded absorption would not be acceptable for a compound swallowed for acute relief of pain or fever. The development of new galenic forms of 2-arylpropionic acids, containing either more soluble salts or consisting of syrups or effervescent tablets, has shown that, even with these drugs, fast and reliable absorption is possible. Further improvement in the use of these compounds may come from investigation of the enantiomers of this group of NSAIDs. The different degrees of inversion, the different handling of both enantiomers in the human body and, finally, the different profile of effects and side effects are likely

Table 1 Pharmakokinetic Parameters NSAIDs, Phenazone Derivatives and Acetaminophen

Drugs	Time to peak (t_{max}) (h)	Bioavailability (%)	Elimination half-life ($t_{1/2}$) (h)	Extended in patients with (disease)	Comments: Suitability for OTC-use on the basis of *pharmacokinetics*	Refs.
Benzoic acid der.						
Salicylates						
Aspirin	0.5–1.5	~30 (100[b])	0.2 (2–30[b,d])	Renal dis[b]	Basically not suitable: slow and dose-dependent elimination of the active drug	61–66
Diflunisal	1–5	80–100	10–16[d]	Renal dis[f]		67–74
Salicylic a.	0.5–1.5	~100	2–30[d]	Renal dis		61–66
Fenamates						
Flufenamic a.	1–4[a]	?[a]	?[a]	?[a]	Not suitable, lack of data	75–78
Meclofenamic a.	1–4	?[a]	?[a]	?[a]		
Mefenamic a.	1–4	?[a]	?[a]	?[a]		
Acetic acid der.						
Diclofenac	1–12	30–70	1–2	–[e]	Not suitable, variable t_{max} and bioavail.	8,79–90
Fenbufen	1–2(8[b])	?[b]	~12[b]	?[a,b]	Not suitable, prodrug, lack of data	91–98
Indomethacin	1–4	~100	2–10	–[e]	Not suitable, variable $t_{1/2}$	99–109
Tolmetin	1–4	?[a]	4–6	?[a]	Not *yet* suitable, lack of data	110–116

Propionic acid der.						
Fenoprofen	1–4	?[a]	2–4	–[e]	Possibly suitable, data lacking	117–123
Flurbiprofen	1–4	?[a]	2–4	–[e]	Possibly suitable, data lacking	124–132
Ibuprofen	1–4[c]	~100	1–3	–[e]	Suitable	11,13,14,133–139
Ketoprofen	1–4	~100	2–4	–[e]	Suitable	140–155
Naproxen	1–4[c]	~100	10–15	–[e]	Not fully suitable, slow elimination	156–173
Tiaprofen	1–4	~100	–2	Renal dis.	Possibly suitable, data lacking	174–193
Ketoenolic acids						
Azapropazone	3–4[c]	80–90[c]	12–25	Renal dis.	}	194–201
Phenylbutazone	2–5[b]	~100	24–120	–[e]	} Not suitable	202–207
Piroxicam	1–4[c]	~100	14–150	–[e]	} Slow and variable $t_{1/2}$	208–215
Tenoxicam	1–4	~100	30–160	–[e]	}	216–234
Acetaminophen	1–2	80–100	2–4	Renal dis; liver dis.	Suitable	17,235–242
Phenazone der.						
Dipyrone	0.5–2[c]	~100[b]	2–4[b]	Renal dis; liver dis.	Suitable	18,243–251
Phenazone	0.5–1.5	~100[d]	5–25	Liver dis.	Not suitable, variable t_{50}	252–256
Propyphenazone	0.5–1.5	~100[d]	2–3	?[a]	Suitable	257

[a]Exact data are not available.
[b](For the) active metabolite.
[c]Depending on the galenic form.
[d]Dose-dependent.
[e]Appears of no clinical relevance.
[f]Appears of little clinical relevance.

to lead to the use of pure enantiomer in both clinical (high-dose) antirheumatic and OTC (low-dose) use (12–14).

D. Ketoenolic Acids

Since the accidental discovery of the anti-inflammatory, analgesic, and antipyretic effects of phenylbutazone, this compound, its major metabolite oxyphenbutazone, its pharmacologically different chemical relative azapropazone, and the more modern oxicams, have been widely used as anti-inflammatory (antirheumatic) compounds. As may be seen from Table 1, all ketoenolic NSAIDs now in long-term human use are eliminated relatively (azapropazone) or extremely slowly (phenylbutazone, tenoxicam). These elimination characteristics are based, in part, on intensive and variable enterohepatic circulation (16). They disqualify all well-investigated and widely used ketoenolic acids from OTC use, in our opinion. Slow elimination should, however, not be considered a general characteristic of ketoenolic acids. Some other oxicams (e.g., meloxicam) are eliminated relatively rapidly and, after long-term, postmarketing experience, such compounds may also be interesting candidates for OTC use. One advantage of the ketoenolic acids might be their relatively amenable taste, allowing easy production of effervescent preparations, solutions, and other suitable galenic forms. Their high potency may make them even suitable for transcutaneous pain relief.

E. Nonacidic Antipyretic Analgesics

Aside from the NSAIDs mentioned so far, acetaminophen, the successor of phenacetin, and pyrazole drugs, such as phenazone, propyphenazone, 4-methylaminophenazone, and others, have been, and are, widely used as antipyretic OTC analgesics. They lack anti-inflammatory effects at therapeutic doses. From the point of pharmacokinetics, acetaminophen, as well as dipyrone and propyphenazone, appear well-suited for OTC use. They are absorbed and eliminated quickly. The somewhat retarded elimination of acetaminophen (17) and the active metabolite of dipyrone, 4-methylaminophenazone (18), in patients suffering from liver dysfunctions appear of limited clinical importance, since even in these patients, acetaminophen shows elimination half-lives of only up to 6 h, and dipyrone (4-methylaminophenazone) of up to 10 h, still less than naproxen or salicylic acid released from high-doses of aspirin (7). Also, these nonacidic antipyretic analgesics may be given in forms of solutions, effervescents, and suppositories, because the taste is acceptable and the compounds are devoid of local irritant activity, in contrast with many NSAIDs.

III. PHARMACODYNAMIC ASPECTS

A. Differences in the Mode of Action

Many textbooks proclaim that the mode of action of all nonopioid analgesics is related to the inhibition of prostaglandin synthesis. There is no doubt that most of the classic (acidic) NSAIDs (as acetic acid derivatives, propionic acid derivatives, and oxicams) do inhibit prostaglandin synthesis in a dose-related manner, and that the relative potency of prostaglandin synthesis inhibition correlates with their analgesic and anti-inflammatory effects. On the other hand, neither salicylic acid nor acetaminophen nor phenazone is likely to block prostaglandin synthesis at analgesic and antipyretic doses, at least not in inflamed tissue and to a degree comparable with the other NSAIDs (19–21). Recently, clinical results and experimental data involving $S(+)$ and $R(-)$ enantiomers of 2-arylpropionic acids (13,24,25) also challenge the concept of the sole role of prostaglandin synthesis inhibition as the only mechanism of analgesic effects. Other hypotheses explaining the analgesic action of the latter ones have been put forward. They do include predominant effects in the spinal cord or the central nervous system (CNS) (22) and additional cyclooxygenase-unrelated effects in inflamed tissue as well as the CNS (23). The gastrointestinal toxicity, as well as the acute kidney toxicity, appears to be related to prostaglandin (PG) synthesis inhibition by all of these compounds. Since acetaminophen and phenazone, at analgesic doses, do not inhibit PG-synthesis in the gastrointestinal tract, the kidney, or the damaged tissue, these compounds appear to exert their effects particularly in noninflammatory pain and they are practically devoid of GI-tract and kidney toxicity at therapeutic doses. Therefore, there are different population groups at risk for NSAIDs, compared with acetaminophen, phenazone, dipyrone, and propyphenazone.

B. Differences in Clinical Effects

The anti-inflammatory and antirheumatic effects, as well as the analgesic and antipyretic properties, of all modern NSAIDs have been investigated. Consequently, it may be taken as proved that all of them are effective in inflammatory pain such as injury pain, dysmenorrhea, many forms of headache (including tension headache, vascular headache, and headache as a consequence of osteoarthrosis of the neck; 26,27). Moreover, some reports indicate analgesic effects in spastic pain, including biliary colic and gastrointestinal tract and genitourinary colic (28). The situation is less clear for acetaminophen and the phenazone derivatives. Acetaminophen is most widely used in combination with acetylsalicylic acid. Despite claims of sufficient activity of acetaminophen alone in posttraumatic and other pain conditions (29,30), there is doubt concerning the value of acetaminophen for these indications (36). Interestingly, a recent investigation involving children with fever and volunteers with traumatic pain indicated that the effect of different doses of acetaminophen was not so much the inhibition of pain, but rather, an improvement in the retrospective rating of the experienced intensity of the discomfort (31,32). It appears possible that acetaminophen is not an analgesic, per se, but rather, a centrally acting drug that improves the sense of patient well-being during pain (31). Phenazone and its derivatives are clearly of relatively low anti-inflammatory activity (33). Similar to acetaminophen, these compounds, in analgesic doses, do not significantly reduce prostaglandin production in inflamed tissue (see foregoing). However, in addition to more than 100 years of clinical experience, there are controlled studies that prove that metamizole is analgesic (36), and that indicate that, in addition, the phenazone derivatives may have some spasmolytic effects (37).

The NSAIDs and the antipyretic analgesics (acetaminophen, dipyrone, phenazone, and propyphenazone) appear to be used most successfully for treating different clinical pain conditions. On the basis of experimental and clinical findings, it may be suggested that NSAIDs (which have been adequately characterized kinetically) could be used for treatment of occasionally inflammation-related pain, including some forms of headache, posttraumatic pain (e.g., toothache), or dysmenorrhea. Suitable compounds for OTC use could be ibuprofen (displaying a particularly wide dose range for OTC and clinical use), ketoprofen, and possibly also fenoprofen, flurbiprofen, and naproxen. The latter NSAIDs may be less suitable owing to the lack of adequate pharmacokinetic or pharmacodynamic data (flurbiprofen), renal toxicity (fenoprofen; see Sect. IV.B) or slow elimination (naproxen). Acetaminophen can be (and is) used as an antipyretic agent that may improve the well-being of the patient suffering from the common cold. Propyphenazone and dipyrone appear well-suited for pain related to spasms of the gastrointestinal tract, the urogenital tract, and the bile duct (37). However, these spastic conditions are rarely mild enough to be treated by OTC medications. The high potency and relatively benign adverse effect profile of phenazone, which in contrast with that of NSAIDs (see Sect. IV), may qualify these compounds for painful conditions in which NSAIDs should not be used or in which (e.g., high fever) acetaminophen is insufficient.

IV. UNWANTED DRUG EFFECTS

A. Safety and Side Effects

A most important issue in the OTC use of drugs is their safety. The OTC compounds should not be toxic if used properly. They should, however, also be relatively safe if used under unusual circumstances or by patients basically not eligible for OTC treatment. Currently, there is no analgesic or antipyretic that is reliably active and is without any risks (38–40). On the other hand, there *are* differences in safety. Consequently, drugs that are defined "too dangerous" should be excluded from OTC use.

The major unwanted drug effects (together with estimates of their incidence and the populations at particular risk) are compiled in Tables 2 and 3 for those drugs that, on the basis of their pharmacokinetic and pharmacodynamic characteristics, appear possible candidates for OTC use. Aspirin, even at low doses, causes bleeding owing to its long-term inhibition of platelet aggregation (40). Moreover, recent epidemiological data on the incidence and association of Reye's syndrome (41) with aspirin use (39,40) indicate that the rationale for large-scale OTC use of this compound as an analgesic is fading. Experimental data and limited clinical experience with salicylic acid indicate that this metabolite of aspirin may be better suited as an analgesic and antipyretic drug than aspirin (42). This contention is supported by the fact that a superior analgesic or antipyretic effect of aspirin has neither been proved nor does it appear likely, since aspirin is cleaved before, during, and shortly after absorption, to yield salicylic acid (7,42). However, this suggestion is not yet supported by sufficient clinical data. Perhaps economic factors prohibit the reinvestigation of salicylic acid and its salts, an otherwise worthwhile topic. All the other NSAIDs of potential OTC use or in OTC use (ibuprofen, ketoprofen, flurbiprofen) also display clear-cut drawbacks in that they cause unwanted drug effects. These are mainly in the gastrointestinal tract, but include allergic and pseudoallergic reactions, (rare) renal dysfunction, and possible aseptic meningitis and visual disturbances (44). In our opinion, some (unique) side effects, such as aseptic meningitis, appear too rare to be of proved relevance to the use of these compounds (this also holds for some surprising benefits as, e.g., a lower incidence of colon carcinoma; 45). The other unwanted drug effects are more common to the whole group and, consequently, cannot be avoided totally. They do, however, occur preponderantly in groups of patients at risk (see Table 2) and might be avoided by adequate labeling and physician education, at least in theory.

On the other hand, the different spectra of side effects of acetaminophen on the one side, and dipyrone, propyphenazone, and phenazone on the other (see tables 2 and 3), as well as the different groups of patients at risk, suggest the possibility that the latter compounds could remain in OTC use, on the basis of their adverse effect profile. The patient subgroups suffering from pain and fever who are not eligible for the use of NSAIDs,

Table 2 Unwanted Drug Effects of NSAIDs, Phenazone Derivatives, and Acetaminophen

Drugs	Often (>1%)	Occasional (1%>but>1%	Single events (<1%oo)	Patients excluded from (OTC) use	Comments: Suitability for OTC-use on the basis of unwanted drug effects	Refs.
Benzoic acid der.						
Salicylates						
Aspirin	G_f	A,C,G_u,K	B	a,b,c,k,p,u	Basically not suitable	39,40,258–279,
Diflunisal	G_f	A,G_u,K	B,C,L	Not OTC	Not suitable, lack of data	287–290, 312,
Salicylic acid	?	?	?	(a,b,c,d,p.u)	Not suitable, lack of data	315, 331, 336
Acetic acid der.						
Diclofenac	G_f	A,G_u,K,L	B,C	Not OTC	Probably not, liver damage	258–289, 291–303, 305–309, 312
Propionic acid der.						
Fenoprofen	G_f	A,G_u,K	B,C,L	Not OTC	Not suitable, kidney damage	
Flurbiprofen	G_f	A,G_u,K	B,C,L	Not OTC	Not (yet) suitable, no epid. data	
Ibuprofen	G_f	A,G_u,K	B,C,L	a,b,k,p,u	Relatively suitable	
Ketoprofen	G_f	A,G_u,K	B,C,L	a,b,k,p,u	Relatively suitable	
Naproxen	G_f	A,G_u,K	B,C,L	a,b,k,p,u	Relatively suitable	
Acetaminophen	O	A	B,C,L(K?)	a,b,l	Relatively suitable (?) Unresolved risk of kidney tumors	4,31,46,47,317–326, 331
Phenazone der.						
Dipyrone	O	A	B,L	a,b,l	Relatively suitable	18,22, 37,53
Phenazone	O	A	B,C	a,b,l	Relatively suitable	54, 303–316
Propyphenazone	O	A	B,C	a,b,l(?)	Relatively suitable	327–330

Symbols used:

A, allergic reactions
B, blood and bone marrow damage
C, CNS disturbances
G_f, gastrointestinal damage, functional or mild
G_u, gastrointestinal damage, ulcers blood loss
K, kidney damage
L, liver damage
?, No valid data available

a, allergie
b, blood and bone marrow impairment
c, children >7 yr of age
e, elderly >65 yr of age
k, impaired kidney function
l, impaired liver function
p, pregnant women
u, ulcers of the GI-tract

Table 3 Epidemiological and Toxicological Risks Associated with the Use, Abuse, and Overdose of NSAIDs: Phenazone Derivatives, and Acetaminophen

Drugs	Acute toxicity (overdose)	Acute toxicity (relative risk)[1]	Chronic toxicity (abuse)	Comments: suitability for OTC use on the basis of toxicity	Refs.
NSAIDs					
Benzoic acid der.					
Salicylates					
Aspirin	Coma, death	B(1.8),G_u(7),C	K(?)	Risk of G_u and Reye's syndrome could be held against OTC use of aspirin	40,41,331–334,336
Propionic acid der.					
Ibuprofen	CNS symptoms; recovery (Ibuprofen, Ketoprofen, Naproxen)	B(?),G_u(1)	K(?)	Good epidemiological data on the incidence of serious side effects are lacking (except naproxen) (Ibuprofen, Ketoprofen, Naproxen)	40,287,291,303,305, 307,308,331,332 (Ibuprofen, Ketoprofen, Naproxen)
Ketoprofen		B(?),G_u(?)	K(?)		
Naproxen		B(?)[1],G_u (6.5,12)	K(?)		
Acetaminophen	Coma, death	B(Ø),G_u(Ø)	L,K(?)	Epidemiological data on the risk of kidney and liver damage are lacking; kidney damage appears likely	40,47,317–326,337
Phenazone der.					
Dipyrone	CNS symptoms; full recovery with dipyrone, Death reported after aminophenazone (Dipyrone, Phenazone, Propyphenazone)	B (2–23),G_u(Ø)	?	Good epidemiological data on the risk of bone marrow damage and GI toxicity (for dipyrone) (mild) (Dipyrone, Phenazone, Propyphenazone)	40,38,50,303–305,327–330,335 (Dipyrone, Phenazone, Propyphenazone)
Phenazone		?	?		
Propyphenazone		?	?		

Symbols used:
A, allergic reactions
B, blood and bone marrow damage
C, CNS disturbances
G_f, gastrointestinal damage, functional
G_u, gastrointestinal damage, ulcers blood loss
K, kidney damage
L, liver damage
?, no epidemiological data available
1, defined as odds ratio (i.e., increase of incidence above background); for details compare literature cited

because they have blood-clotting disorders, ulcers, kidney dysfunction, or other, could benefit from the nonacidic antipyretic analgesics. The latter contention, although relatively unpopular, is also based on the fact that the widely feared liver damage caused by acetaminophen (46) and the agranulocytosis on the basis of phenazone drugs (38) are relatively rare events. The risk ratios are well defined. From the published data it appears that dipyrone is more dangerous relative to agranulocytosis (risk ratio 1:22) than NSAIDs, but the latter are causing bleeding ulcers, in contrast with the former (risk ratio of serious gastrointestinal bleeding, approximately 1:7). A sevenfold increase of life-threatening bleeds could cause more deaths per treatment period than a 22-fold increase in a rare condition, agranulocytosis, since both events show a lethality of 2–10% but the normal incidence of bleeding ulcers is 1:10,000 inhabitants while the incidence of agranulocytosis is 1:100,000 in the populations surveyed (39,40).

B. Toxicity with Overdose or with Chronic Use

An additional factor qualifying or disqualifying a drug from OTC use is its acute or chronic toxicity, leading to either acute life-threatening conditions or chronic diseases. It is well documented (see Table 3) that the worldwide OTC drugs, aspirin and acetaminophen, can kill people after overdose. Particularly acetaminophen causes lethal liver and kidney damage at doses above 6 g/day in adults (47). The toxic effects of acetaminophen in children are less dramatic, apparently depending on the speed of metabolization of acetaminophen and also the somewhat larger stores of glutathion in the liver of children. Aspirin also is responsible for many death cases per year, particularly in children (48). Although adults, particularly in Anglo-Saxon countries, use acetaminophen for suicide, children may find aspirin in the household, mistake it for sweets, and die of coma resulting from aspirin overdose. Moreover, literature indicates that the fenamates may cause seizure-type CNS effects with overdose, occasionally leading to convulsions and coma (48,49). Quite in contrast, neither the 2-arylpropionic acids nor dipyrone appear of comparable acute toxicity with overdose. There are very few reports of lethal events resulting from accidental or planned overdose with these drugs (50). In these cases, it often remains unclear if the analgesic or a comedication, such as barbiturates, sedatives, or other tranquilizers, was the main reason for the lethal outcome (50).

Chronic toxicity resulting from abuse of OTC analgesics has become a major concern within the last 30 years. The observation of Spuehler and Zollinger that the chronic use of high doses of mixtures containing aspirin, phenazone, and caffeine leads to chronic kidney damage and early death (51) has led to the elimination of phenacetin from OTC use in most countries. This risk may, however, not be eliminated, particularly because analgesic mixtures now containing acetaminophen and caffeine (52) are still abused in many countries. The resulting concern includes worries about chronic kidney damage and the risk of carcinoma of the kidney or bladder (probably related to the chronic use of phenacetin or acetaminophen). It is probable that the chronic use of acetaminophen will carry the same risk as its prodrug phenacetin. Acetaminophen yields almost all of the metabolites of phenacetin, and it appears overly optimistic to believe that carcinomata of the kidney, the ureters, and the bladder will not result from the long-term use of acetaminophen (338). Other concerns relate to the long-term use of NSAIDs (aplastic anaemias; 38) and dipyrone (stomach carcinomata; 53, 54). In general, these concerns argue against the long-term use of any analgesic. Recent reports on the beneficial events of the long-term administration of, for example, 2-arylpropionic acids such as ibuprofen, resulting in a reduced rate of rectum carcinomata (45), will not outbalance, according to our present knowledge, the arguments brought forward against any long-term use of these compounds. From these data, one wonders why the relatively toxic drugs, aspirin and acetaminophen, are OTC worldwide, whereas the less toxic drugs of the phenazone type and the 2-arylpropionic acids are regarded as being less well-suited for OTC use.

Finally, we do not find any valid arguments in favor of combining together different types of OTC analgesics and adding other ingredients such as caffeine (54). The abuse liability may be enhanced by these measures (55), the analgesic effect is not (clearly) enhanced (56), and the risk is not measurably reduced (57).

C. Dangerous Drug Interactions

As one might expect, major or frequent dangerous drug interactions would preclude the use of NSAIDs or other drugs as OTC medications. Some drugs of this group, particularly aspirin, may cause dangerous drug interactions. They are typical only at higher doses (i.e., beyond those permitted for OTC use). The other compounds suitable for OTC use appear less prone in that respect. Aspirin does increase the effectiveness of all compounds that reduce the clotting capacity of blood. Moreover, at high doses, aspirin can increase the free fraction of some oral antidiabetics and, thereby, cause an abrupt fall in blood sugar concentration. Acetaminophen and phenazone may, in principle, interfere with the cytochrome P-450 enzyme systems (58). Recently, it has become likely that acetaminophen may exhaust the same glutathion stores as do other drugs which, in turn, could increase the toxicity of acetaminophen (58). Ibuprofen, as for all NSAIDs, does interact with the absorption and elimination of other drugs of the same type. It may reduce the effectiveness of diuretic compounds and influence the excretion of lithium. Moreover, single cases of interference with vitamin K antagonists have been described. These effects (59) are well documented and, in our opinion, are of minor importance if these drugs are used occasionally at low doses in otherwise healthy patients.

V. FUTURE DEVELOPMENT

Obviously, any extrapolations on the future development of OTC use of analgesics and antipyretic drugs are highly speculative. National preferences, local traditions, and unexpected findings may influence public opinion and the decisions of regulatory authorities. The following conclusions are possible, although they must be regarded as personally biased.

Aspirin will probably remain an OTC preparation to prevent myocardial infarction and selected thromboembolic diseases. However, the accumulating evidence that aspirin should not be taken in pregnancy; by children up to the age of puberty; by patients with allergic conditions, including asthmatics, patients with inadequate blood coagulation, significant kidney dysfunction, and gastrointestinal tract ulcers, will, in the long run, make aspirin an OTC drug for preventing cardiac infarctions and other thrombaembolic diseases but not to remedy pain.

Acetaminophen is neither a potent analgesic nor a reliable pain reliever under all clinical conditions. Despite public opinion, acute toxicity, chronic toxicity, and the risk of drug interactions argue against the use of this compound as an "every-day" OTC analgesic. In our view, its use should be restricted to fever in children and some forms of headache.

Despite some public turmoil concerning the OTC use of ibuprofen, particularly the risk of ibuprofen in patients with kidney dysfunction and the occasional occurrence of aseptic meningitis, overall, this drug appears the least dangerous of the NSAIDs. In our opinion, its OTC use will increase. Of the other NSAIDs only ketoprofen and possibly flurbiprofen appear likely to achieve OTC standard. Additional data, particularly concerning the safety and effectiveness at low doses should be provided in the near future. Moreover, these three 2-arylpropionic acids will soon be available in chirally pure form, and it appears possible that the *S*-forms should be used for the indication "inflammation," whereas the *R*-forms may achieve OTC standards as analgesics in pain conditions showing little inflammation (25).

We believe that phenazone, propyphenazone and dipyrone are useful analgesics. Phenazone appears to have a somewhat variable and lengthy elimination half-life. Consequently, this compound should be withdrawn from OTC use. On the other hand, propyphenazone and also possibly dipyrone offer more suitable pharmacokinetic characteristics. The risk of agranulocytosis is low, although not vanishingly so. The risk of shock reactions is similar to that seen with other antipyretic analgesics. Moreover, these compounds do not damage the gastrointestinal tract, do not appear toxic to the kidney, and do not influence the blood-clotting system (at low analgesic doses). If the incidence of agranulocytosis is not considered serious, the lack of other unwanted drug effects should argue in favor of these compounds, particularly for those groups who should not take aspirin or ibuprofen because of gastrointestinal tract problems, kidney diseases, or blood coagulation problems.

It is not to be expected that new OTC analgesics from the group of fenamates, arylacetic acids or ketoenolic compounds will emerge soon. Diclofenac could prove suitable. However, its dose-dependent oral bioavailability and the risk of liver damage (8,60) may be used against it.

This chapter has presented currently available data on the pros and cons of the available compounds for OTC markets. Certainly, there is no "miracle drug" in the pipeline that will be impressively superior to those available at present. Consequently we recommend cautious evaluation and reconsideration of the drugs known and available.

REFERENCES

1. Collier HOJ. The story of aspirin. In: Parnham MJ, Bruinvels J, eds. Discoveries in pharmacology. Haemodynamics, hormones and inflammation. Amsterdam: Elsevier, 1984:555–94.
2. Erhart G, Ruschig H. Arzneimittel, Entwicklung, Wirkung, Darstellung. Weinheim: Verlag Chemie, 1972.
3. Haas H. History of analgesic therapy. In: Zimmermann M, Long DM eds. Antipyretic analgesic therapy. Am J Med 1983; 1–3.
4. Clark DWJ. OTC analgesic availability and use in New Zealand. In: Brune K, Santoso B, eds. Antipyretic analgesics: new insights. Basel: Birkhä◇△r , 1992:89–94.
5. Buchanan WW, Kean WF. Current non-steroidal anti-inflammatory drug therapy in rheumatoid arthritis, with emphasis on use in the elderly. In: Lewis AJ, Furst DE, eds. Nonsteroidal anti-inflammatory drugs. New York: Marcel Dekker, 1987:9–30.
6. Brune K, Fenner H, Kurowski M, Lanz R. Adverse reactions to NSAIDs: consecutive evaluation of 30,000 patients in rheumatology. In: Rainsford KD, Velo GP, eds. Side-effects of anti-inflammatory drugs, 3, Inflammation and drug therapy series, vol 5. London: Kluwer, 1992:33–42.
7. Brune K, Lanz R. Pharmacokinetics of nonsteroidal anti-inflammatory drugs. In: Bonta IL, Bray MA, Parnham MJ, eds. Handbook of inflammation. vol 5. Amsterdam: Elsevier, 1985;413–49.

8. Heinze F. Darstellung und galenische Optimierung kleindimensionierter Retardformkörper durch ein spezielles Extrusionsverfahren am Beispiel von Diclofenac-natrium. Thesis, Erlangen, 1987.
9. Willis JV, Kendall MJ, Flinn, RM, Thornhill DP, Welling PG. The pharmacokinetics of diclofenac sodium following intravenous and oral administration. Eur J Pharmacol 1979; 16:405–10.
10. Fini A, Laus M, Orienti I, Zecchi V. Dissolution and partition thermodynamic functions of some nonsteroidal and anti-inflammatory drugs. J Pharm Sci 1986; 75:23–5.
11. Geisslinger G, Dietzel K, Bezler H, Nuernberg B, Brune K. Therapeutically relevant differences in the pharmacokinetic and pharmaceutical behavior of ibuprofen lysinate as compared to ibuprofen acid. Int J Clin Pharmacol Ther Toxicol 1989; 29:324–8.
12. Jamali F. Pharmacokinetics of enantiomers of chiral nonsteroidal anti-inflammatory drugs. Eur J Drug Metab Pharmacokinet 1988; 13:1–9.
13. Geisslinger G, Schuster O, Stock KP, Loew D, Bach GL, Brune K. Pharmacokinetics of *S*(+)- and *R*(–)-ibuprofen in volunteers and first clinical experience of *S*(+)-ibuprofen in rheumatoid arthritis. Eur J Clin Pharmacol 1990; 38:493–7.
14. Knihinicki RD, Day RO, Graham GG, Williams KM. Stereoselective disposition of ibuprofen and flurbiprofen in rats. Chirality 1990; 2:134–40.
15. Lee EJD, Williams KM, Graham GG, Day RO, Champion GD. Liquid chromatographic determination and plasma concentration profile of optical isomers of ibuprofen in humans. J Pharm Sci 1984; 73:1542–4.
16. Schneider H-T, Nuernberg B, Dietzel K, Brune K. Biliary elimination of nonsteroidal anti-inflammatory drugs in patients. Br J Clin Pharamacol 1990; 29:127-31.
17. Bonkowsky HL, Mudge GH, McMurty RJ. Chronic hepatic inflammation and fibrosis due to low doses of paracetamol. Lancet 1978; 1:1016–8.
18. Schade R, Bien E, Skorka G. Hepatotoxicological studies of pyrazolone derivatives on rats. Pharmazie 1981; 36:H9.
19. Glatt M, Peskar B, Brune K. Leucocytes and prostaglandins in acute inflammation. Experientia 1974; 30:1257–9.
20. Graf P, Glatt M, Brune K. Acidic nonsteroid anti-inflammatory drugs accumulating in inflamed tissue. Experientia 1975; 31:951–4.
21. Morris HG, Sherman NA, McQuain C, Goldlust MB, Chang SF, Harrison LI. Effects of salsalate (nonacetylated salicylate) and aspirin on serum prostaglandins in humans. Ther Drug Monit 1985; 7:435–8.
22. He X, Neugebauer V, Schaible HG, Schmidt RF. New aspects of the mode of action of dipyrone. In: Brune K, ed. New pharmacological and epidemiological data in analgesics research. Basel: Birkhäuser, 1990:9–18.
23. Menzel-Soglowek S, Geisslinger G, Beck W, Brune K. Variability of inversion of *R*-flurbiprofen in different species. J Pharm Sci 1992; 81:888–891.
24. Yamaguchi T, Hirose K, Nakamura Y, Sugeno K. The inhibitory activities of 480156-S and its related compounds on prostaglandin synthetase. Nippon Yakurigaku Zasshi 1987; 90:295–302.
25. Brune K, Beck WS, Geisslinger G, Menzel-Soglowek S, Peskar BM, Peskar BA. Aspirin-like drugs may block pain independently of prostaglandin synthesis inhibition. Experientia 1991; 47:257–61.
26. Dubinsky B, Gebre-Mariam S, Capetola RJ, Rosenthale ME. The antialgesic drugs: human therapeutic correlates of their potency in laboratory animal models of hyperalgesia. Agents Actions 1987; 20:50–60.
27. McCormack K, Brune K. Dissociation between the antinociceptive and anti-inflammatory effects of the nonsteroidal anti-inflammatory drugs. Drugs 1991; 41:533–47.
28. Patel CV, Koppikar MG, Patel MS, Parulkar GB, Pinto Pereira LM. Management of pain after abdominal surgery: dipyrone compared with pethidine. Br J Clin Pharmacol 1980; 10:351S–354S.

29. Cooper SA. The relative efficacy of ibuprofen in dental pain. Article 6, Compend Contin Educ Dent 1986; 7/8:587.
30. Mehlisch DR. Review of the comparative analgesic efficacy of salicylates, acetaminophen and pyrazolones. In: Zimmermann M, Long DM, eds. Antipyretic analgesics therapy. Am J Med 1983; 47–52.
31. Kramer MS, Naimark LE. Risks and benefits of paracetamol antipyresis in young children with fever of presumed viral origin. Lancet 1991; 337:591–4.
32. Graham GG, Champion GD, Day RO, Kaski AL, Hills LG, Paull PD. Salicylates in rheumatoid arthritis: pharmacokinetics and analgesic response. In: Rainsford KD, Brune K, Whitehouse MW, eds. Aspirin and related drugs: their actions and uses. Agents Actions 1977; Suppl 1:37–42.
33. Brune K, Aehringhaus U, Peskar BA. Pharmacological control of leukotriene and prostaglandin production from mouse peritoneal macrophages. Agents Actions 1984; 14:729–34.
34. Similae S, Kousalainen K, Kainanen S. Oral antipyretic therapeutic therapy. Arzneimittelforschung 1977; 27:687–8.
35. Gomez-Jimenez I, Franco-Patino R, Chargoy-Vera J, Olivares-Sosa R. Clinical efficacy of mild analgesics in pain following gynaecological or dental surgery. Br J Clin Pharmacol 1980; 10:355S–362S.
36. Forster C, Magerl W, Beck A. Geisslinger G, Gall T, Brune K, Handwerker HO. Differential effects of dipyrone, ibuprofen, and paracetamol on experimentally induced pain in man. Agents Actions 1992; 35:112–21.
37. Schroth HJ, Steinstrasser A, Berberich R, Kloss G. Investigations on the effect of metamizol on ureteral motility. Agents Actions 1980; Suppl 19:177–88.
38. International agranulocytosis and aplastic anemia study: Risks of agranulocytosis and aplastic anemia. A first report of their relation to drug use with special reference to analgesics. JAMA 1986; 256:1749–57.
39. Levy M, Miller DR, Kaufman DW, et al. Major upper gastrointestinal bleeding. Relation to the use of aspirin and other non-narcotic analgesics. Arch Intern Med 1988; 148:281–5.
40. Laporte JR, Carne X, Vidal X, Moreno V, Juan J. Upper gastrointestinal bleeding in relation to previous use of analgesics and nonsteroidal anti-inflammatory drugs. Lancet 1991; 337:85–9.
41. Hurwitz ES, Barret MJ, Bergman D, et al. Public Health Service study on Reye's syndrome and medications: the main study. JAMA 1987; 257:1905–11.
42. Preston SJ, Arnold MH, Beller EM, Brooks PM, Buchanan WW. Comparative analgesic and anti-inflammatory properties of sodium salicylate and acetylsalicylic acid (aspirin) in rheumatoid arthritis. Br J Clin Pharmacol 1989; 27:607–11.
43. Pedersen AK, FitzGerald GA. Dose-related kinetics of aspirin. Presystemic acetylation of platelet cyclooxygenase. N Engl J Med 1984; 311:1206–11.
44. Mifsud AJ. Drug-related recurrent meningitis. J Infect 1988; 17:151–3.
45. Rosenberg L, Palmer JR, Zauber AG, Warshauer ME, Stolley PD, Shapiro S. A hypothesis: nonsteroidal anti-inflammatory drugs reduce the incidence of large-bowel cancer. JNCI 1991; 83:355–8.
46. Seeff LB, Cuccerini BA, Zimmermann HJ, Alder E, Benjamin S. Acetaminophen hepatotoxicity in alcoholics—a therapeutic misadventure. Ann Intern Med 1986; 104:399–404.
47. Meredith TJ, Vale JA, Goulding R. The epidemiology of acute acetaminophen poisoning in England and Wales. Arch Intern Med 1981; 141:397–409.
48. Vale JA, Meredith TJ. Acute poisoning due to nonsteroidal anti-inflammatory drugs. Clinical features and management. Med Toxicol 1986; 1:12–31.
49. Hendrickse MT. Mefenamic acid overdose mimicking brainstem stroke. Lancet 1988; 2:1019–20.
50. Wolhoff H, Altrogge G, Pola W, Sistovaris N. Metamizole—a case of acute overdosage with suicidal intent. Dtsch Med Wochenschr 1983; 108:1761–4.
51. Spuhler O, Zollinger HU. Die chronisch interstitielle Nephritis. Z Klin Med 1953; 151:1.

52. Pommer W, Glaeske G, Molzahn M. The analgesic problem in the Federal Republic of Germany: analgesic consumption, frequency of analgesic nephropathy and regional differences. Clin Nephrol 1986; 26:273–8.
53. Kumagai H, Kawaura A, Shibata M, Otsuka H. Carcinogenicity of dipyrone in (C57BL/6 x C3H)F1 Mice 1.2. JNCI 1983; 71:1295–7.
54. Donaubauer HH, Kief H, Kramer M, Krieg K, Mayer D, Scheutz E. Investigations on the carcinogenicity of dipyrone in rats. Toxicol Appl Pharmacol 1985; 81:443–51.
55. Diener H-C, Buhler K-U, Dichgans J, Geiselhart S, Gerber D, Scholz E. Analgetikainduzierter dauerkopfschmerz. Arzneimittelther 1988; 6:156–63.
56. Lee P, Anderson JA, Miller J, Webb J, Buchanan WW. Evaluation of analgesic action and efficacy of antirheumatic drugs. J Rheumatol 1976; 3:283–93.
57. Sato C, Izumi N. Mechanism of increased hepatotoxicity of acetaminophen by the simultaneous administration of caffeine in the rat. J Pharmacol Exp Ther 1989; 248:1243–47.
58. Brune K, Lindner J. Increased liver toxicity of diclofenac by paracetamol: results and possible mechanisms. In: Rainsford KD, Velo GP, eds. Side-effects of anti-inflammatory drugs 3. London: Kluwer, 1992:198–203.
59. Schulmannoff S, Henriksson K, Johnsson M. Interaction between ibuprofen and warfarin with influence on primary homeostasis. Scand J Rheumatol 1987; 16:456.
60. Helfgott SM, Sandberg-Cook J, Zakim D, Nestler J. Diclofenac-associated hepatotoxicity. JAMA. 1990; 264:2660–2.
61. Levy G. Pharmacokinetics of salicylate in man. Drug Metab Rev 1979; 9:3–19.
62. Levy G. Clinical pharmacokinetics of salicylates: a reassessment. Br J Clin Pharmacol 1980; 10:2855–2905.
63. Levy G, Tsuchiya T. Salicylate accumulation kinetics in man. New Engl J Med 1972; 287:430–2.
64. Dromgoole SH, Furst DE. Salicylates. In: Evans MA, ed. Applied pharmacokinetics. San Francisco: Applied Therapeutics 1980:486–517.
65. Rowland M, Riegelman S, Harris PA, Sholkoff SD. Absorption of aspirin in man following oral administration of an aqueous solution. J Pharm Sci 1972; 61:379–85.
66. Tocco DH, Breault GO, Zacchei AG, Steelman SL, Perrier CV. Physiological disposition and metabolism of 5-(2′,4′-difluorphenyl) salicylic acid, a new salicylate. Drug Metab Dispos 1975; 3:453–66.
67. Verbeeck R, Tjandramaga TB, Mullie A, Verbesselt R, De Schepper PJ. Effect of aluminium hydroxide on diflunisal absorption. Br J Clin Pharmacol 1979; 7:519–22.
68. De Schepper PJ, Mullie A, Tjandramaga TG, Verbeeck R, Verberckmoes R. Pharmacokinetics of diflunisal elimination in patients with renal insufficiency. Br J Clin Pharmacol 1977; 4:645–6.
69. Holmes GI, Irvin JD, Schrogie JJ, Davies RO, Breault GO, Rogers JD, Huber PB, Zinny MA. Effects of Maalox on the bioavailability of diflunisal. Clin Pharmacol Ther 1979; 25:229.
70. Levy G. Decreased body clearance of diflunisal in renal insufficiency—an alternative explanation. Br J Clin Pharmacol 1979; 8:601.
71. Winter CA, Shen TY, Tocco DJ, Robertson RT, Shackleford RW. Diflunisal. In: Goldberg ME, ed. Pharmacological and chemical properties of drug substances. vol 3. Washington DC: American Pharmaceutical Assoc, 1981:291–323.
72. Steelman SL, Breault GO, Tocco D, Besselaar GH, Tempero KF, Lutterbeck PM, Perrier CV, Gribnau FW, Hinselmann M. Pharmacokinetics of MK-647, a novel salicylate. Clin Pharmacol Ther 1975; 17:245.
73. Tempero KF, Cirillo VJ, Steelman SL. Diflunisal: a review of pharmacokinetic and pharmacodynamic properties, drug interactions, and special tolerability studies in humans. Br J Clin Pharmacol 1977; 4:31S
74. Verbeeck R, Tjandramaga TB, Mullie A, Verbesselt R, Verberckmoes R, De Schepper PJ. Biotransformation of diflunisal and renal excretion of its glucuronides in renal insufficiency. Br J Clin Pharmacol 1979; 7:273–82.

75. Glazko AJ. Pharmacology of the fenamates. III Metabolic disposition. Ann Phys Med 1967; 9:23–6.
76. Glazko AJ, Chang T, Borondy PE, Dill WA, Young R, Croskey L. Metabolic disposition of meclofenamic acid (Meclomen) in laboratory animals and in man. Curr Ther Res 1978; 23:522–41.
77. Kaniwa N, Ogata H, Aoyagi N, Ejima A. The bioavailability of flufenamic acid from aluminium flufenamate tablet and flufenamic acid capsule, and the influence of food and aluminium hydroxide gel. J Pharmacobiodyn 1982; 5:187–92.
78. Winder CV, Kaump DJ, Glazko AJ, Holmes EL. Pharmacology of the fenamates. Experimental observations on flufenamic, mefenamic and meclofenamic acids. Ann Phys Med 1967; Suppl 7:49.
79. Willis JV, Jack DB, Kendall MJ, John VA. The influence of food on the absorption as determined by the urinary excretion of the unchanged drug and its major metabolites during chronic administration. Eur J Clin Pharmacol 1981; 19:39–44.
80. Willis JV, Kendall MJ. Pharmacokinetic studies on diclofenac sodium in young and old volunteers. Scand J Rheumatol [Suppl] 1978; 22:36–41.
81. Willis JV, Kendall MK, Flinn RM, Thornhill DP, Welling PG. The pharmacokinetics of diclofenac sodium following intravenous and oral administration. Eur J Clin Pharmacol 1979; 16:405–10.
82. Willis JV, Kendall MJ, Jack DB. A study of the effect of aspirin on the pharmacokinetics of oral and intravenous diclofenac sodium. Eur J Clin Pharmacol 1980; 18:415–8.
83. Willis JV, Kendall MJ, Jack DB. The influence of food on the absorption of diclofenac after single and multiple oral doses. Eur J Clin Pharmacol 1981; 19:33–7.
84. Geiger UP, Degen PH, Sioufi A. Quantitative assay of diclofenac in biological material by gas–liquid chromatography. J Chromatogr 1975; 111:293–8.
85. John VA. The pharmacokinetics and metabolism of diclofenac sodium (Voltarol) in animals and man. Rheumatol Rehabil 1979; 18 (Suppl 2): 22–37.
86. Menasse R, Hedwall PR, Kraetz J, Pericin C, Riesterer L, Sallmann A, Ziel R, Jacques R. Pharmacological properties of diclofenac sodium and its metabolites. Scand J Rheumatol [Suppl] 1989; 22:5–16.
87. Riess W, Stierlin H, Faigle JW, Geiger UP, Gerardin A, Schmid K, Sulc M, Wagner J, Theobald W. Kinetik und Biotransformation von Diclofenac in Tier und Mensch. Therapiewoche 1976; 26:2891–2907.
88. Riess W. Stierlin H, Degen P, Faigle JW, Gerardin A, Moppert J, Sallmann A, Schmid K, Schweizer K, Sulc M, Theobald W, Wagner J. Pharmacokinetics and metabolism of the anti-inflammatory agent Voltaren. Scand J Rheumatol [Suppl] 1978; 22:17–29.
89. Stierlin H, Faigle JW, Colombi A. Pharmacokinetics of diclofenac sodium (Voltaren) and metabolites in patients with impaired renal function. Scand J Rheumatol [Suppl] 1978; 22:30–5.
90. Zimmerer J, Tittor W, Degen P. Rheuma-therapie bei Leberkranken, Plasmaspiegel von Diclofenac und Urinausscheidung von Diclofenac und Metaboliten bei Leberkranken Patienten. Fortschr Med 1982; 100:1683–8.
91. Chiccarelli FS, Eisner HJ, Van Lear GE. Metabolic and pharmacokinetic studies with fenbufen in man. Arzneimittelforschung 1980; 30:728–35.
92. Cuisinaud G, Legheand J, Belkahia C, Sassard J. Gas chromatographic determination of 3-(4-biphenylylcarbonyl)propionic acid (fenbufen) and two metabolites in human plasma. J Chromatogr 1989; 148:509–13.
93. Cuisinaud G, Legheand J, Llorca G, Belkahia C, Lejeune E, Sassard J. Pharmacokinetics of fenbufen in man. Eur J Clin Pharmacol 1979; 16:59–61.
94. Spector RG, Armstrong R, Bradbrook I, Gibson TJ, Morrison P, Rogers H. A study of repeated administration of fenbufen in patients with chronic rheumatic disorders and renal impairment. Pharmacology 1982; 25:46–50.
95. Greenberg BP. Fenbufen. In: Huskisson EC, ed. Anti-rheumatic drugs. New York: Praeger Publishers, 1983:183–99.

96. Rogers HJ, Savitsky JP, Glenn P, Spector RG. Kinetics of single doses of fenbufen in patients with renal insufficiency. Clin Pharmacol Ther 1981; 29:74–80.
97. Sloboda AE, Tolman EL, Osterberg AC, Panagides J. The pharmacological properties of fenbufen: a review. Arzneimittelforschung 1980; 30:716–21.
98. Verbeeck RK, Walbace SM. Does fenbufen have a large distribution volume or is it subject to extensive presystemic elimation? Eur J Clin Pharmacol 1983; 24:137–8.
99. Wallusch WW, Nowak H, Leopold G, Netter KJ. Comparative bioavailability: influence of various diets on the bioavailability of indomethacin. Int J Clin Pharmacol Biopharm 1978; 16:40–4.
100. Kwan KC, Beault GO, Umbenhauer ER, McMahon RG, Duggan DE. Kinetics of indomethacin absorption, elimination and enterohepatic circulation in man. J Pharmacokinet Biopharm 1975; 4:255–80.
101. Kwan KC, Beault GO, Davis RL, Lei BW, Czerwinski AW, Besselaar GH, Duggan DE. Effects of concomitant aspirin administration on the pharmacokinetics of indomethacin in man. J Pharmacokinet Biopharm 1978; 6:451–76.
102. Turakka H, Airaksinen MM. Biopharmaceutical assessment of phenylbutazone and indomethacin preparations. Ann Clin Res 1974; 6(suppl):34–41.
103. Emori HW, Champion GD, Bluestone R, Paulus HE. Simultaneous pharmacokinetics of indomethacin in serum and synovial fluid. Ann Rheum Dis 1973; 32:433–5.
104. Emori HW, Paulus HE, Bluestone R, Champion GD, Pearson C. Indomethacin serum concentrations in man. Effects of dosage, food and antacid. Ann Rheum Dis 1976; 35:333–8.
105. Duggan DE, Hogans AF, Kwan KC, McMahon FG. The metabolism of indomethacin in man. J Pharmacol Exp Ther 1972; 181:563–75.
106. Duggan DE, Hooke KF, Noll RM, Kwan KC. Enterohepatic circulation of indomethacin and its role in intestinal irritation. Biochem Pharmacol 1975; 25:1749–54.
107. Helleberg L. Clinical pharmacokinetics of indomethacin. Clin Pharmacokinet 1981; 6:245–58.
108. Skeith MD, Simkin PA, Healey LA. The renal excretion of indomethacin and its inhibition by probenecid. Clin Pharmacol Ther 1968; 9:89–93.
109. Stein G, Kunze M, Zaumseil J, Trager A. Pharmacokinetics of indomethazine and metabolites of indomethazine continuously applied in patients with healthy and damaged kidneys. Int J Clin Pharmacol Biopharm 1977; 15:470–3.
110. Sumner DD, Dayton PG, Cucinell SA, Plostnieks J. Metabolism of tolmetin in rat, monkey and man. Drug Metab Dispos 1975; 3:283–6.
111. Selley ML, Glass J, Triggs EJ, Thomas J. Pharmacokinetic studies of tolmetin in man. Clin Pharmacol Ther 1975; 17:599–605.
112. Cressman WA, Wortham F, Plostnieks J. Absorption and excretion of tolmetin in man. Clin Pharmacol Ther 1976; 19:224–33.
113. Ayres JW, Weidler DJ, Mackichan J, Sakmar E. Hallmark MR, Lemanowicz EF, Wagner JG. Pharmacokinetics of tolmetin with and without concomitant administration of antacid in man. Eur J Clin Pharmacol 1977; 12:421–8.
114. Ehrlich GE. Tolmetin sodium: meeting the clinical challenge. Clin Rheum Dis 1979; 5:481–97.
115. Grindel JM, Migdalof BH, Plostnieks J. Absorption and excretion of tolmetin in arthritic patients. Clin Pharmacol Ther 1979; 26:122–8.
116. Plostnieks J, Cressman WA, Lemanowicz EF, Migdalof BH, Tam JJS. Human metabolism of tolmetin. In: Ward JR, ed. Tolmetin, a new nonsteroidal anti-inflammatory agent. Princeton: Excerpta Medica, 1975: 23–33.
117. Rubin A, Chernish SM, Crabtree R. Gruber CM Jr, Helleberg L, Rodda BE, Warrick P, Wolen RL, Ridolfo AS. A profile of the physiological disposition and gastrointestinal effects of fenoprofen in man. Curr Med Res Opin 1974; 2:529–44.
118. Rubin A, Rodda BE, Warrick P, Ridolfo AS, Gruber CM Jr. Physiological disposition of fenoprofen in man. I. Pharmacokinetic comparison of calcium and sodium salts administered orally. J Pharm Sci 1971; 60:1797–1801.

119. Rubin A, Rodda BE, Warrick P, Ridolfo AS, Gruber CM Jr. Physiological disposition of fenoprofen in man. II. Plasma and urine pharmacokinetics after oral and intravenous administration. J Pharm Sci 1972; 61:739–45.
120. Rubin A, Warrick P, Wolen RL, Chernish SM, Ridolfo AS, Gruber CM. Physiological disposition of fenoprofen in man. III. Metabolism and protein binding of fenoprofen. J Pharmacol Exp Ther 1972; 183:449–57.
121. Rubin A, Warrick P. Wolen RL, Ridolfo AS, Gruber CM. The metabolism of fenoprofen in man. Clin Pharmacol Ther 1972; 13:151.
122. Chernish SM, Rubin A, Rodda BE, Ridolfo AS, Gruber CM Jr. The physiological disposition of fenoprofen in man. IV. The effects of position of subject, food ingestion and antacid ingestion on the plasma levels of orally administered fenoprofen. J Med Exp Clin 1972; 3:249–57.
123. Ridolfo AS, Nichander R, Mikulasckek WM. Fenoprofen and benoxaprofen. Clin Rheum Dis 1979; 5:393–410.
124. Kaiser DG, Shaw SR, Vangiesen GJ. GLC determination of *dl*-2(2-fluoro-4-biphenylyl) propionic acid (flurbiprofen) in plasma. J Pharm Sci 1974; 63:567–70.
125. Kozma C, Daffner R. Pharmacokinetics of flurbiprofen taken fasting and after food [abstract]. Presented at the 9th European congress of rheumatology. Wiesbaden, 1979.
126. Risdall PC, Adams SS, Crampton EL, Marchant B. The disposition and metabolism of flurbiprofen in several species including man. Xenobiotica 1978; 8:691–704.
127. Chalmers LM, Bell MA, Buchanan WW. Effects of flubiprofen on the metabolism of antipyrine in man. Ann Rheum Dis 1973; 32:58–61.
128. Chalmers TM, Glass RC, Risdall PC. Concentrations of flubiprofen in serum and synovial fluid from patients with active rheumatoid disease. Some preliminary observations. Curr Med Res Opin 1977; 5:17–20.
129. Cardoe N, de Silva M, Glass RC, Risdall PC. Serum concentrations of flurbiprofen in rheumatoid patients receiving flurbiprofen over long periods of time. Curr Med Res Opin 1977; 5:21–5.
130. Adams SS, Crampton EL, Nicholson JS, Risdall PC. Metabolism of flurbiprofen in man. XIIIth International Congress of Rheumatology, Kyoto, Japan, 1973.
131. Adams SS, Buckler JW. Ibuprofen and flubiprofen. Clin Rheum Dis 1979; 5:359–79.
132. Rogers HJ, Spector RG, Morrison PJ, Bradbrook ID. Comparative steady state pharmacokinetic study of piroxicam and flurbiprofen in normal subjects. Eur J Rheumatol Rehabil 1981; 4:303–8.
133. Grennan DM, Aarons L, Siddiqui M, Richards M, Thompson R, Higham C. Dose-response study with ibuprofen in rheumatoid arthritis: clinical and pharmacokinetic findings. Br J Clin Pharmacol 1983; 15:311–6.
134. Grennan DM, Ferry DG, Ashworth ME, Kenney RE, MacKinnon M. The aspirin–ibuprofen interaction in rheumatoid arthritis. Br J Clin Pharmacol 1979; 8:497–503.
135. Kantor GT. Ibuprofen. Ann Intern Med 1979; 91:877–882.
135a. Glass RC, Swannell AJ. Concentrations of ibuprofen in serum and synovial fluid from patients with arthritis. Br J Clin Pharmacol 1978; 6:453–4.
136. Lockwood GF, Albert KS, Gillespie WR, Bole GG, Harkcom TM, Szpunar GJ, Wagner JG. Pharmacokinetics of ibuprofen in man. I. Free and total area/dose relationships. Clin Pharmacol Ther 1983; 34:97–103.
137. Mills RFN, Adams SS, Cliffe EE, Dickinson W, Nicholson JS. The metabolism of ibuprofen. Xenobiotica 1973; 3:589–98.
138. Whitlam JB, Brown KF, Crooks MJ, Room GFW. Trans-synovial distribution of ibuprofen in arthritis patients. Clin Pharmacol Ther 1981; 29:487–92.
139. Whitlam JB, Vine JH. Quantitation of ibuprofen in biological fluids by gas chromatography–mass spectometry. J Chromatogr 1980; 181:463–8.
140. Brune K. Bioavailability of ketoprofen. Unpublished data, 1990.
141. Tamisier JN, Brazier JL, Ambert D, Bannier A. Study of bioavailability of oral ketoprofen (Profenid) given in association with a gastric protector (aluminium phosphate, Phosphalugel). Sem Hop Paris 1983; 59:3214–7.

142. Delbarre F, Roucayroll JJ, Amor B, et al. pharmacokinetic study of ketoprofen (19.583 RP) in man using the tritiated compound. Scand J Rheumatol [Suppl] 1976; 14:45–52.
143. Populaire P, Terlain B, Pascal S, et al. Comportement biologique: taux seriques, excretion et biotransformation de l'acide (benzoyl-3-phenyl)-2 propionique ou ketoprofene chez l'animal et chez l'homme. Ann Pharm Fr 1973; 31:735–49.
144. Queneau P, Decousus H, Ollagnier M, et al. Chronokinetics of ketoprofen administered orally and by continuous intravenous infusion. Rev Rheum 1985; 52:403–8.
145. Advenier C, Roux A, Gobert C, et al. Pharmacokinetics of ketoprofen in the elderly. Br J Clin Pharmacol 1983; 16:65–70.
146. Banwarth B, Lapicque F, Netter P, et al. The effect of food on the systemic availability of ketoprofen. Eur J Clin Pharmacol 1988; 33:643–5.
147. Ishizaki T, Sasaki T, Suganuma T, et al. Pharmacokinetics of ketoprofen following single oral, intramuscular and rectal doses and after repeated administration. Eur J Clin Pharmacol 1980; 18:407–14.
148. Stafanger G, Larsen HW, Hansen H, Sorensen K. Pharmacokinetics of ketoprofen in patients with chronic renal failure. Scand J Rheumatol 1981; 10:189–92.
149. Houghton GW, Dennis MJ, Rigler ED. Comparative pharmacokinetics of ketoprofen derived from single oral doses of ketoprofen capsules or a novel sustained pellet formulation. Biopharm Drug Dispos 1984; 5:203–9.
150. Lempianinen M, Makela AL. Determination of ketoprofen by high performance liquid chromatography from serum and urine: clinical application from serum and urine in children with juvenile rheumatoid arthritis. Int J Clin Pharmacol 1987; 7:265–71.
151. Lewellen ORW, Templeton R. The pharmacokinetics of ketoprofen in man during and after repeated oral dosing (50 mg qid) with Orudis. Scand J Rheumatol 1976; 14:53–62.
152. Upton RA, Buskin JN, Williams RL, Holford NHG, Riegelman S. Negligible excretion of unchanged ketoprofen, naproxen and probenecid in urine. J Pharm Sci 1980; 69:1254–7.
153. Upton RA, Busin JN, Guentert TW, Williams RL, Riegelman S. Convenient and sensitive high-performance liquid chromatographic assay for ketoprofen, naproxen and other allied drugs in plasma or urine. J Chromatogr 1980; 190:119–28.
154. Upton RA, Williams RL, Buskin JN, Jones RM. Effects of probenecid on ketoprofen pharmacokinetics. Clin Pharmacol Ther 1982; 31:705–12.
155. Upton RA, Williams RL, Guentert TW, Buskin JN, Riegelman S. Ketoprofen pharmacokinetics and bioavailability based on an improved sensitive and specific assay. Eur J Clin Pharmacol 1981; 20:127–33.
156. Kiang C-H, Lee C, Kushusky S. Isolation and identification of 6-desmethylnaproxen sulfate as a new metabolite of naproxen in human plasma. Drug Metab Dispos 1989; 17:43–8.
157. Weber SS, Bankhurst AD, Mroszczak E, Ding TL. Effect of Mylanta on naproxen bioavailability. Ther Drug Monit 1981; 3:75–83.
158. Williams RL, Upton RA, Cello JP, et al. Naproxen disposition in patients with alcoholic cirrhosis. Eur J Clin Pharmacol 1984; 27:291–6.
159. Ling TL, Yee JP, Cohen A, et al. A multiple-dose pharmacokinetic comparison of naproxen as a once-daily controlled-release tablet and a twice-daily conventional tablet. J Clin Pharmacol 1987; 27:325–9.
160. Cohen A, Basch C. Steady state pharmacokinetics of naproxen in young and elderly healthy volunteers. Semin Arthritis Rheum 1988; 17(suppl):7–11.
161. Ryley NJ, Lingam G. A pharmacokinetic comparison of controlled-release and standard naproxen tablets. Curr Med Res Opin 1988; 11:10–27.
162. Shah J, Mroszczak E, Bynum L, Fratis A, Kiang C. Bioequivalence comparison of enteric-coated (EC) naproxen versus standard naproxen tablets [abstract]. Pharm Res 1989; 6(suppl):S232.
163. Gamst ON. Oral naproxen formulations. Scand J Gastroenterol 1989; 24(suppl 163):44–7.
164. Calvo MV, Dominguez-Gil A, Macias JG, Diez JL. Naproxen disposition in hepatic and biliary disorders. Int J Clin Pharmacol Ther Toxicol 1980; 18:242–6.

165. Moyer S. Pharmacokinetics of naproxen sodium. Cephalalgia 1986; 6(suppl 4):77–80.
166. Mroszczak E, Runkel R, Roe R, Ortega E, Segre E. Naproxen pharmacokinetics and metabolism in renal failure [abstract]. Presented at the world conference in clinical pharmacology and therapeutics. London, Aug 3–9, 1988:0544.
167. Wibell L. The metabolism of naproxen in renal insufficiency. Scan J Rheumatol 1977; 6:71–2.
168. Dahl H. Naproxen (Naproxyn). Pharmacokinetics: therapeutical relevance and tolerance profile. Cephalalgia 1986; 6(suppl 4):69–75.
169. Runkell RA, Chaplin M, Boost G, Segre E, Forchielli E. Absorption, distribution, metabolism and excretion of naproxen in various laboratory animals and human subjects. J Pharm Sci 1972; 61:703–8.
170. Runkel R, Chaplin MD, Sevelius H, Ortega E, Segre E. Pharmacokinetics of naproxen overdose. Clin Pharmacol Ther 1976; 20:269–77.
171. Runkel R, Forchielli E, Boost G, Chaplin M, Hill R, Sevelius H, Thompson G, Segre E. Naproxen metabolism, excretion and comparative pharmacokinetics. Scand J Rheumatol [Suppl] 1973; 2:39–46.
172. Runkel RA, Forchielli E, Sevelius H, Chaplin M, Segre E. Nonlinear plasma level response to high doses of naproxen. Clin Pharmacol Ther 1974; 15:261–6.
173. Runkel RA, Kraft KS, Boost G, Sevelius H, Forchielli E, Hill R, Mogoun R, Szakacs JB, Segre E. Naproxen oral absorption characteristics. Chem Pharm Bull 1972; 20:1457–66.
174. Daymond TJ, Herbert R. Simultaneous bioavailability of tiaprofenic acid (Surgam) in serum and synovial fluid in patients with rheumatoid arthritis. Rheumatology 1982; 7:188–93.
175. Lucker PW, Perth B, Wetzelsberger K. Pharmacokinetic interaction between tiaprofenic acid and several other compounds for chronic use. Rheumatology 1982; 7:99–106.
176. Pottier J, Cousty-Berlin D, Busigny M. Human pharmacokinetics of tiaprofenic acid. Rheumatology 1982; 7:70–7.
177. Daymond TJ, Herbert R. Pharmacokinetic studies of tiaprofenic acid in patients suffering from rheumatoid arthritis. Ann Rheum Dis 1981; 40:622–6.
178. Marecek N. Pharmacokinetics of tiaprofenic acid and possible interactions with acetylsalicylic acid and aluminium hydroxide [translation]. Arzneimittelforschung 1981; 31:116–20.
179. Hosie J, Hosie G. The pharmacokinetics of tiaprofenic acid in elderly arthritis patients—evidence for nonaccumulation. In: Nilsen OG, ed. New trends in rheumatology. vol 3. Amsterdam: Excerpta Medica, 1985:87–95.
180. Strusberg AM, Arroyo SR, Meirovich CI, Montrull HI, Salgado R. Pharmacokinetics of tiaprofenic acid in rheumatoid arthritis and osteoarthritis [translation]. Prens Med Arg 1984; 71:79–86.
181. Nilsen OG, Jacobsen G, Walstad RA. Steady state pharmacokinetics of tiaprofenic acid in elderly patients. Arzneimittelforschung 1985; 35:875–9.
182. Swainson CP. The chronic effects of tiaprofenic acid on renal haemodynamics and hormones in patient with chronic renal disease. In: Berry M, ed. New trends in rheumatology. vol 4. (16th International congress of rheumatology. Sydney, 19–25 May 1985). Amsterdam: Excerpta Medica, 1985:111.
183. Nilsen OG, Wessel-Aas T, Walset F. Single dose pharmacokinetics of tiaprofenic acid: effects of food and severe renal insufficiency. Arzneimittelforschung 1985; 35:871–5.
184. Jones RW, Tremblay D, Stead JA. Comparative pharmacokinetics of standard and controlled-release forms of tiaprofenic acid following repeated administration under clinically relevant conditions. In: Nilsen OG, ed. New trends in rheumatology. vol 3. (16th International congress of rheumatology. Sydney, 19–25 May 1985). Amsterdam: Excerpta Medica, 1985:122.
185. Nilsen OG. Steady state pharmacokinetics and serum protein binding of tiaprofenic acid in old people. In: Nilsen OG, ed. New trends in rheumatology. vol 3. (16th International congress of rheumatology. Sydney, 19–25 May 1985). Amsterdam: Excerpta Medica, 1985:122.
186. Jones RW, McLean AEM. The comparative pharmacokinetics of different preparations of tiaprofenic acid [abstract]. J Clin Pharmacol 1984; 24:402.

187. Hosie G. Drug kinetics in the elderly. Rheumatology—which way? Symposium held in Oxford, September 1984. 10–1.
188. Jamali F, Russell AS, Lehmann C, Berry BW. Pharmacokinetics of tiaprofenic acid in healthy and arthritic subjects. J Pharm Sci 1985; 74:953–6.
189. Platt D, Eicher H, Rieck W. Hilgert D. Pharmacokinetics of tiaprofenic acid in elderly patients. Drugs 1988; 35(suppl 1):53–56. (11th European congress of rheumatology. Athens, 28th June–4th July, 1987).
190. Hosie J, Hosie GAC. The pharmacokinetics of single and multiple doses of tiaprofenic acid in elderly patients with arthritis. Eur J Clin Pharmacol 1987; 32:93–5.
191. Nilsen OG. Is the kinetic profile of tiaprofenic acid favourable for use in the elderly? In Huskisson EC, Shiokawa Y, eds. New trends in rheumatology. vol 5. (Proceedings of the international symposium on rheumatology. Tokyo, 23–24 January, 1987). Amsterdam: Excerpta Medica, 1987:98–102.
192. Cerretani D. Fiaschi AI, Micheli L, Runci FM, Giorgi G, Bozzo M. Pharmacokinetic study on tiaprofenic acid in elderly. Arch Gerontol Geriatr 1991; 52:539–43.
193. Bertin L, Rey E, Pons G, Mathiot JL, Richard MO, Chretien P, Saint-Maurice C, Moran C, Ginisty D. Pharmacokinetics of tiaprofenic acid in children after a single oral dose. Eur J Clin Pharmacol 1991; 41:251–3.
194. Maggon KK, Lam GM. Aspects of clinical pharmacology and bioavailability of azapropazone. In: Rainsford KD, ed. Azapropazone—20 years of clinical use. Lancaster, UK: Kluwer Academic, 1989:123–50.
195. McElnay JC, Walker FS. The pharmacokinetics of azapropazone. In: Rainsford KD, ed. Azapropazone—20 years of clinical use. Lancaster, UK: Kluwer Academic, 1989:63–80.
196. Ritch AES, Perera WNR, Jones CJ. Pharmacokinetics of azapropazone in the elderly. Br J Clin Pharmcol 1982; 14:116–9.
197. Breuing KH, Gilfrich HJ, Meinertz T, Jahnchen E. Pharmacokinetics of azapropazone following single oral and intravenous doses. Arzneimittelforschung 1979; 29(suppl 6):971–2.
198. Breuing KH, Gilfrich HJ, Meinertz T, Wiegand UW, Jahnchen E. Disposition of azapropazone in chronic renal and hepatic failure. Eur J Clin Pharmacol 1981; 20:147–55.
199. Klatt VL, Koss FW. Humanpharmakokinetische Untersuchungen mit 14C-Azapropazon-dihydrat. Arzneimittelforschung 1973; 23:920–1.
200. Schatz F, Adrian RW, Mixich G, Molnarova M, Reller J, Jahn U. Pharmakokinetische Untersuchungen mit dem Antiphlogistikum azapropazon (Prolixan 300) am Menschen. Therapiewoche 1970; 20:2327–33.
201. Leach H. The determination of azapropazone in blood plasma. Curr Med Res Opin 1976; 4:35–43.
202. Sioufi A, Caudal F, Marfil F. GLC determination of phenylbutazone in human plasma. J Pharm Sci 1978; 67:243–5.
203. Sioufi A, Colussi D, Caudal F, Schoeller JP, Massias P. Pharmacokinetics of phenylbutzone in healthy subjects after oral administration of single and multiple doses. J Pharm Sci 1980; 69:1413–6.
204. Higham C, Aarons L, Holt PJL, Lynch M, Rowland M. A chronic dose-ranging study of the pharmacokinetics of phenylbutazone in rheumatoid arthritis patients. Br J Clin Pharmacol 1981; 12:123–9.
205. Dayton PG, Israeli ZH, Perel JM. Influence of binding on drug metabolism and distribution. Ann NY Acad Sci 1973; 226:172–94.
206. Dieterle W, Faigle JW, Fruh F, Mory H, Theobald W, Alt KO, Richter WJ. Metabolism of phenylbutzone in man. Arzneimittelforschung 1976; 26:572–7.
207. Aarbakke J. Clinical pharmacokinetics of phenylbutazone. Clin Pharm 1978; 3:369–80.
208. Dupont D, Dayer P, Balant L, Gorgia A, Fabre J. Variations interet intraindividuelle du comportement du piroxicam. Pharmacocinetique chez l'homme en bonne sante et chez le malade en insuffisance renale. Pharm Acta Helv 1982; 57:20–6.
209. Ishizaki T, Nomura T, Abe T. Pharmacokinetics of piroxicam a new nonsteroidal anti-in-

flammatory agent, under fasting and postprandial states in man. J Pharmacokinet Biopharm 1979; 7:369–81.
210. Schiantarelli, P, Acerbi D, Bovis B. Some pharmacokinetic properties and bioavailability by oral and rectal route of piroxicam in rodents and in man. Arzneimittelforschung 1981; 31:92–7.
211. Hobbs DC, Twomey TM. Piroxicam pharmacokinetics in man. Aspirin and antacid interaction studies. J Clin Pharmacol 1979; 19:270–81.
212. Hobbs DC. Pharmacokinetics of piroxicam in man. Eur J Rheumatol Inflamm 1983; 6:46–55.
213. Twomey TM, Hobbs DC. Biotransformation of piroxicam by man. Fed Proc 1978; 37:271.
214. Wiseman EH, Hobbs DC. Review of pharmacokinetic studies with piroxicam. Am J Med 1982; 72(suppl): 9–17.
215. Woolf AD, Rogers HJ, Bradbrook ID, Corless D. Pharmacokinetic observations in piroxicam in young adult, middle-aged and elderly patients. Br J Clin Pharmacol 1983; 16:433–7.
216. Bird HA, Allen JG, Dixon JS, Wright VA. Pharmacokinetics comparison of tenoxicam in plasma and synovial fluid. Br J Rheumatol 1985; 24:351–6.
217. Bird HA, Clarke AK, Fowler PD, Little S, Podgorski MR. An assessment of tenoxican, a nonsteroidal anti-inflammatory drug of long half-life, in patients with impaired renal function suffering from osteoarthritis or rheumatoid arthritis. Clin Rheumatol 1989; 4:453–60.
218. Bird HA, Francis RJ, Gallez P, Hill J, Dixon JS. Single and multiple oral dose pharmacokinetics of tenoxicam in the elderly. Eur J Rheumatol Inflamm 1985; 8:60–9.
219. Crevoisier C, Gerber N, Ott H, Meyer J, Heizmann P. Simultaneous pharmacokinetics of tenoxicam in plasma and synovial fluid. Presented at the 1st world conference on inflammation, antirheumatics, analgesia and immunomodulators. Venice, 16–18 April, 1984.
220. Crevoisier C, Heizmann P, Forgo I, Dubach UC. Plasma tenoxicam concentrations after single and multiple oral doses. Eur J Drug Metab Pharmacokinet 1989; 14:23–7.
221. Crevoisier C, Zaugg PY, Heizmann P, Meyer J. Influence of liver cirrhosis upon the pharmacokinetics of tenoxicam. Int J Clin Pharmacol Res 1989; 9:327–34.
222. Day RO, Lam S, Paull P, Wade D. Effect of food and various antacids on the absorption of tenoxicam. Br J Clin Pharmacol 1987; 24:323–8.
223. Francis RJ, Allen JG, Looi D, Dixon JS, Bird MA. Pharmacokinetics of tenoxicam after oral administration in healthy human subjects of various single doses. Eur J Drug Metab Pharmacokinet 1987; 12:59–63.
224. Francis RJ, Dixon JS, Lower JR, Harris PS. The effects of food and of antacid on the single oral dose pharmacokinetics of tenoxicam. Eur J Drug Metab Pharmacokinet 1985; 10:309–14.
225. Guenter TW, Heintz RC, Joly R. Overview of the pharmacokinetics of tenoxicam. Eur J Rheumatol Inflamm 1987; 9:15–25.
226. Heintz RC, Ducarre JM, Blouin RA, Guenzi A. Influence of oral dose escalation on the pharmacokinetics of tenoxicam (Tilcotil) in healthy male subjects, Lit Rheumatol 1988; 10:9–15.
227. Heintz RC, Guentert TW, Crevoisier C, Jeunei F. Influence of age, sex and disease on the pharmacokinetics of tenoxicam, a new nonsteroidal anti-inflammatory drug. Presented at the EULAR symposium. Rome, 16–18, 1986.
228. Horber FF, Guentert TW, Weidekamm E, Heizmann O, Descoedres C. Pharmacokinetics of tenoxicam in patients with impaired renal function. Eur J Clin Pharmacol 1986; 29:697–701.
229. Kobayashi S, Oba T, Oguchi K, et al. Pharmacokinetics of tenoxicam in healthy volunteers and geriatric patients. Rinsho Yakuri 1984; 15:399–405.
230. Kwon K. Bourne DWA. Physiological pharmacokinetic model for the distribution and elimination of tenoxicam. Int J Pharm 1987; 37:219–26.
231. Nilsen OG, Walstad RA, Eckert M, et al. Single and multiple dose pharmacokinetics of tenoxicam in the elderly. Eur J Clin Pharmacol 1988; 35:563–6.
232. Schmitt M, Guentert TW. Effect of age on the pharmacokinetics of tenoxicam in comparison to other nonsteroidal anti-inflammatory drugs (NSAIDs). Scand J Rheumatol [Suppl] 1989; 80:86–9.

233. Schmitt M, Kolle V, Stockel K, et al. Pharmacokinetic profile of tenoxicam in elderly patients with rheumatoid arthritis. Lit Rheumatol 1988; 10:25–31.
234. Williams KM, Day RO, Murphy BR, Curranti F. The pharmacokinetics of total and unbound concentrations of tenoxicam in synovial fluid and plasma. Presented at the 6th South East Asia and Pacific league against rheumatism congress of rheumatology. 5–10 September, 1988.
235. Pedraz JL, Alonso E, Calvo MB, Lanao JM, Dominguez-Gil A. Bioequivalence study of two oral formulations of paracetamol. Int J Clin Pharmacol Ther Toxicol 1988; 26:232–6.
236. Perlik F, Janko I, Kordac V. The effect of guaiaphenesin on absorption and bioavailability of paracetamol from composite analgesic preparations. Int J Clin Pharmacol Ther Toxicol 1988; 26:413–6.
237. Aoki FY, Sitar DS. Effects of chronic amantadine hydrochloride ingestion on its and acetaminophen pharmacokinetics in young adults. J Clin Pharmacol 1992; 32:24–7.
238. Hopkins CS, Underhill S, Booker PD. Pharmacokinetics of paracetamol after cardiac surgery. Arch Dis Child 1990; 65:971–6.
239. Baraka OZ, Truman CA, Ford JM, Roberts CJ. The effect of propranolol on paracetamol metabolism in man. Br J Clin Pharmacol 1990; 29:261–4.
240. Prescott LF, Speirs GC, Critchley JA, Temple RM, Winney RJ. Paracetamol disposition and metabolite kinetics in patients with chronic renal failure. Eur J Clin Pharmacol 1989; 36:291–7.
241. Bennett WM, Aronoff GR, Morrison G, Golper TA, Pulliam J, Wolfson M, Singer I. Drug prescribing in renal failure: dosing guidelines for adults. Am J Kidney Dis 1983; 3:155
242. Benson GD. Acetaminophen in chronic liver disease. Clin Pharmacol Ther 1983; 33:95–101.
243. Zylber-Katz E, Granit L, Stessman J, Levy M. Effect of age on the pharmacokinetics of dipyrone. Eur J Clin Pharmacol 1989; 36:513–6.
244. Asmardi G, Jamali F. Pharmacokinetics of dipyrone in man; role of the administration route. Eur J Drug Metab Pharmacokinet 1985; 10:121–5.
245. Vlahov V, Badian M, Verho M, Bacracheva N. Pharmacokinetics of metamizol metabolites in healthy subjects after a single oral dose of metamizol sodium. Eur J Clin Pharmacol 1990; 38:61–5.
246. Badian MJ, Eckert HG. Kinetics of radiolabelled dipyrone (metamizol) after oral and intravenous administration to healthy men. (III World conference on clinical pharmacology and therapeutics. Stockholm). Acta Pharmacol Toxicol 1986;59(suppl 5 Pt 2):310, abstr 1591.
247. Kampf D, Roots I. Kinetics of dipyrone (Novalgin) and its major metabolites in patients with renal insufficiency. Naunyn Schmiedebergs Arch Pharmacol 1982; 319(suppl):R87.
248. Roots I, Kampf D, Heinemeyer G, Gramm HJ, Dennhardt R. Changes in metamizol kinetics and metabolism during chronic and acute renal failure as compared to healthy volunteers. Naunyn Schmiedebergs Arch Pharmacol 1985; 330(suppl):R81.
249. Gramm HJ, Heinemeyer G, Roots I, Dennhardt R. Delayed elimination of metamizol (Novalgin) in intensive care patients with sepsis and acute renal failure. Naunyn Schmiedebergs Arch Pharmacol 1983; 324(suppl):R80.
250. Balogh A, Simon HJ, Reinhardt M, Splinter FK, Traeger A. Zum einfluss von verschiedenen lebererkrankungen auf die aktivitat zweier subtypen des cytochrom P-450. Dtsch Z Verdau Stoffwechsel kr 1987; 47:1–13.
251. Ortweiler W, Peiker G, Siegert C, Splinter FK, Traeger A. Der einfluss der intrahepatischen schwangerschaftscholestase auf verschiedene cytochrom P-450-abhangige biotransformationsreaktionen. Pharmazie 1987; 42:329–31.
252. Vestal RE, Norris AH, Tobin JD, Cohen BH, Shock NW, Andres R. Antipyrine metabolism in man: influence of age, alcohol, caffeine and smoking. Clin Pharmacol Ther 1975; 18:425–32.
253. Branch RA, Herbert CM, Read AE. Determinants of serum antipyrine half-lives in patients with liver disease. Gut 1973; 14:569–73.
254. Scavone JM, Blyden GT, Greenblatt DJ. Lack of effect of influenza vaccine on the

pharmacokinetics of antipyrine, alprazolam, paracetamol (acetaminophen) and lorazepam. Clin Pharmacokinet 1989; 16:180–5.

255. Nayak VK, Desai NK, Kshirsagar NA, Bhandarkar SD, Satoskar RS. Antipyrine and doxycycline pharmacokinetics in patients with thyroid disorders. J Postgrad Med (India) 1991; 37:5–8.
256. Greenblatt DJ, Divoll MK, Marmatz JS, Shader RL. Antipyrine absorption and disposition in the elderly. Pharmacology 1988; 36:125–33.
257. Brune K. The pharmacological basis for the rational use of non-opioid OTC analgesics: aspirin, paracetamol (acetaminophen), ibuprofen, and phenazones. In: Brune K, Santoso B, eds. Antipyretic analgesics: new insights. Basel: Birkäuser Verlag, 1990:33–40.
258. Bardare M, Cislaghi GV, Mandeli M, Sereni F. Value of monitoring plasma salicylate levels in treating juvenile rheumatoid arthritis. Arch Dis Child 1978; 53:381–5.
259. Morassut P, Yang W, Karsh J. Aspirin intolerance. Semin Arthritis Rheum 1989; 19:22–30.
260. Fenner H. Skin reactions to nonsteroidal anti-inflammatory drugs. EULAR Bull 1986; 3:92–6.
261. Clark DWJ. Allergic and pseudoallergic reactions to antipyretic analgesics. In: Brune K, Santoso B, eds. Antipyretic analgesics: new insights. Basel: Birkhäuser Verlag, 1990:33–40.
262. Kimberly RR, Plotz PH, Aspirin-induced depression of renal function. N Engl J Med 1977; 926:418–24.
263. New Zealand Rheumatism Association. Aspirin and the kidney. Br Med J 1974; 1:593–6.
264. Levy M. Unwanted drug effects of antipyretic analgesics: epidemiological data. In: Brune K, Santoso B, eds. Antipyretic analgesics: new insights. Basel: Birkhäuser Verlag, 1990:57–65.
265. Editorial CSM Update. Non-steroidal anti-inflammatory drugs and serious gastrointestinal adverse reactions—2. Br Med J 1986; 292:1190–1.
266. Zeidler H. Epidemiology of NSAID induced gastropathy. J Rheumatol 1991; 18(suppl 28):2–5.
267. Somerville K, Faulkner G, Langman M. Non-steroidal anti-inflammatory drugs and bleeding peptic ulcer. Lancet 1986; 1:462–4.
268. Walt R, Katschinski B, Logan R, Ashley J, Langman M. Rising frequency of ulcer perforation in elderly people in the United Kingdom. Lancet 1986; 1:489–92.
269. Langman M. Epidemiologic evidence on the association between peptic ulceration and anti-inflammatory drug use. Gastroenterology 1989; 96:640–6.
270. Weber JCP. Epidemiology of adverse reactions to nonsteroidal anti-inflammatory drugs. In: Rainsford KD, Velo GP, eds. Advances in inflammation research. vol 6. New York: Raven Press, 1984:1–7.
271. Carson JL, Strom BL, Morse L, West SL, Soper KA, Stolley PD, Jones JK. The relative gastrointestinal toxicity of the nonsteroidal anti-inflammatory drugs. Arch Intern Med 1987; 147:1054–9.
272. Strandberg K, Wiholm BE. Regulatory decisions: emphasis on safety issues. In: Brune K, Santoso B, eds. Nonnarcotic analgesics today: an update of benefits and risks. Med Toxicol 1986; 1(suppl 1):137–49.
273. Levy M, Miller DR, Kaufman DW, Siskind V, Schwingl P, Rosenberg L, Strom B, Shapiro S. Major upper gastrointestinal tract bleeding. Relation to the use of aspirin and other non-narcotic analgesics. Arch Intern Med 1988; 148:281–5.
274. Langman MJ, Brooks P, Hawkey CJ, Silverstien F, Yeomans N. Nonsteroid anti-inflammatory drug associated ulcer: epidemiology, causation and treatment. J Gastroenterol Hepatol 1991; 6:442–9.
275. Langman MJ. Ulcer and ulcer complications from non-steroidal anti-inflammatory drugs: what is the risk? Aliment Pharmacol Ther 1988; 2:27–31.
276. Thiefin G. Epidemiology and treatment of gastroduodenal lesions caused by nonsteroidal anti-inflammatory agents. Rev Med Interne 1991 May–June; 12:227–36.
277. Pincus T, Griffin M. Gastrointestinal disease associated with nonsteroidal anti-inflammatory drugs: new insights from observational studies and functional status questionnaires [editorial: comment]. Am J Med 1991; 91:209–12.

278. Simon LS. Toxicity of the nonsteroidal anti-inflammatory drugs. Curr Opin Rheumatol 1991; 3:341–7.
279. Laine L. NSAID-induced gastroduodenal injury: what's the score? Gastroenterology 1991; 101:555–7.
280. Banerjee AK. Enteropathy induced by nonsteroidal anti-inflammatory drugs. Br Med J 1989; 298:1539–40.
281. Langman MJS, Morgan L, Worrall A. Use of anti-inflammatory drugs by patients admitted with small or large bowl perforations and haemorrhage. Br Med J 1985; 298:347–9.
282. Hawkey CJ. Nonsteroidal anti-inflammatory drugs and peptic ulcers. Facts and figures multiply, but do they add up? Br Med J 1990; 300:278–84.
283. Upadhyay R, Torley HI, McKinlay AW, Sturrock RD, Russell RI. Iron deficiency in patients with rheumatic disease receiving nonsteroidal anti-inflammatory drugs; the role of upper gastrointestinal lesions. Ann Rheum Dis 1990; 49:359–62.
284. Jenkins RT, Rooney PJ, Jones DB, Bienenstock J, Goodacre RL. Increased intestinal permeability in patients with rheumatoid arthritis: a side-effect of oral nonsteroidal anti-inflammatory drug therapy. Br J Rheumatol 1987; 26:103–7.
285. Bjarnsason I, Zanelli G, Prouse P, Williams P, Gumpel MJ, Levi AJ. Effect of nonsteroidal anti-inflammatory drugs on the human small intestine. Drugs 1986; 32(suppl 1):35–41.
286. Bjarnason I, So A, Levi AJ, Williams P, Zanelli GD, Gumpell JM, Ansell B, Intestinal permeability and inflammation in rheumatoid arthritis: effects of nonsteroidal anti-inflammatory drugs. Lancet 1984; 2:1171–4.
287. Rainsford KD. Side-effects of anti-inflammatory analgesic drugs: epidemiology and gastrointestinal tract. Trends Pharmacol Sci 1984; 5:156–9.
288. Fries JF, Williams CA, Block DA. The relative toxicity of nonsteroidal anti-inflammatory drugs. Arthritis Rheum 1991; 34:1353–60.
289. Needs CJ, Brooks PM. Occasional review—1. Antirheumatic medication in pregnancy. Br J Rheumatol 1985; 24:282–90.
290. Levy G, Garrettson LK. Kinetics of salicylate elimination by newborn infants of mothers who ingested aspirin before delivery. Pediatrics 1974; 53:201–10.
291. Levy M. Unwanted drug effects of antipyretic analgesics: epidemiological data. In: Brune K, Santoso B, eds. Antipyretic analgesics: new insights. Basel: Birkhäuser Verlag, 1990:57–65.
292. Jamali F, Stevens DRS. Naproxen excretion in milk and its uptake by the infant. Drug Intell Clin Pharm 1983; 17:910–1.
293. Todd PA, Clossold SP. Naproxen: a reappraisal of its pharmacology and therapeutic use in rheumatic diseases and pain states. Drugs 1990; 40:91–137.
294. Pavelka K, Vojtisek O, Kankova D. The occurrence of adverse side-effects during controlled clinical trials of nonsteroidal anti-rheumatic agents. Rheumatol Rehabil 1980; 19:109–12.
295. Rainsford KD. Toxicity of currently used anti-inflammatory and antirheumatic drugs. In: Lewis AJ, Furst DE, eds. Nonsteroidal anti-inflammatory drugs. Mechanisms and clinical use. New York: Marcel Dekker, 1987:215–44.
296. Brezin JH, Katz SM, Schwartz AB, Chinitz HL. Reversible renal failure and nephrotic syndrome associated with nonsteroidal, anti-inflammatory drugs. N Engl J Med 1979; 301: 1271–3.
297. Cartwright KC, Trotter TL, Cohen MC. Naproxen nephrotoxicity. Ariz Med 1979; 36:124–6.
298. Grennan DM, Jolly J, Hollowat CJ, Palmer DG. Vasculitis in a patient receiving naproxen. NZ Med J 1979; 89:48–9.
299. Segre ES. Naproxen. Clin Rheum Dis 1979; 411–26.
300. Liaus L, Moxcaritola JD, Burcher J. Diclofenac. In: Lewis AJ, Furst DE, eds. Nonsteroidal anti-inflammatory drugs. Mechanisms and clinical use. New York: Marcel Dekker, 1987:215–44.
301. Smith RJ, Lomen PL, Kaiser DG. Flurbiprofen. In: Lewis AJ, Furst DE, eds. Nonsteroidal anti-inflammatory drugs. Mechanisms and clinical use. New York: Marcel Dekker, 1987:393–418.

302. Vavra I. Ketoprofen. In: Lewis AJ, Furst DE, eds. Nonsteroidal anti-inflammatory drugs. Mechanisms and clinical use. New York: Marcel Dekker, 1987:419–38.
303. Levy M. Unwanted drug effects of antipyretic analgesics. epidemiological data. (World congress on pain. Adelaide 4/1990). In: Brune K, ed. New pharmacological and epidemiological data in analgesics research. Basel: Birkhäuser Verlag, 1990:39–47.
304. International agranulocytosis and aplastic anemia study. The design of a study of the drug etiology of agranulocytosis and aplastic anaemia. Eur J Clin Pharmacol 1983; 24:833–6.
305. Vlahov V. Quantitative evaluation of adverse drug reaction's risks: epidemiological methods. Zentralbl Pharm Pharmakother Lab Diagn 1990; 129:300–2.
306. Pommer W, Bronder E. Grieser E, Helmert U, Jesdinsky HJ, Klimpel A, Borner K, Molzahn M. Regular analgesic intake and the risk of end-stage renal failure. Am J Nephrol 1989; 9:403–12.
307. Miescher PA, Pola W. Hematological effects of non-narcotic analgesics. Drugs 1986; 32(suppl 4):90–108.
308. Heit W. Hematologic effects of anti-pyretic analgesics—drug-induced agranulocytosis. Am J Med 1983; 75:65–9.
309. Szczeklik A, Gryglewski RJ, Czerniawska-Mysik G. Clinical patterns of hypersensitivity to nonsteroidal anti-inflammatory drugs and their pathogenesis. J Allergy Clin Immunol 1977; 60:276–84.
310. Czerniawska-Mysik G, Szczeklik A. Idiosyncrasy to pyrazolone drugs. Allergy 1981; 36:381–4.
311. Szczeklik A, Czerniawska-Mysik G, Nizankowska E. Allergische und pseudoallergische reaktionen auf pyrazolonpraparate. In: Brune K, Lanz R, eds. 100 jahre pyrazolone—eine bestandsaufnahme. Baltimore: Urban & Schwarzenberg, 1985:247–52.
312. Szczeklik A. Analgesics, allergy and asthma. Drugs 1986; 32(suppl 4):148–63.
313. Voigtlander V. Dermatologische nebenwirkungen von pyrazolonen. In: Brune K, Lanz R, eds. 100 jahre pyrazolone—eine bestandsaufnahme. Baltimore: Urban & Schwarzenberg, 1985:261–6.
314. Virchow C, Schmitz-Schumann M, Juhl-Schaub E. Pyrazolone und analgetika-asthma syndrome. In: Brune K, Lanz R eds. 100 jahre pyrazolone—eine bestandsaufnahme. Baltimore: Urban & Schwartzenberg, 1985; 253–360.
315. Fabro L, Wuetrich B, Walti M. Acetylsalicylic acid allergy and pyrazone allergy and pseudoallergy? Results of the skin tests and antibody determinations in a multicentre study. Z Hautkr Z 1987; 62:470–8 [in German].
316. Schneider CH, Kasper MF, De Weck AL, Rolli H, Angst BD. Diagnosis of antibody-mediated drug allergy. Pyrazolinone and pyrazolidine-dione cross-reactivity relationship. Allergy 1987; 42:597–603.
317. Rosenberg DM, Neelon FA. Acetaminophen and liver disease. Ann Intern Med 1978; 88:129.
318. Maddrey WC. Hepatic effects of acetaminophen. Enhanced toxicity in alcoholics. J Clin Gastroenterol 1987; 9:180–5.
319. Wilson HTH. A fixed drug eruption due to paracetamol. Br J Dermatol 1975; 92:213–4.
320. Thomas RHM, Munro DD. Fixed drug eruption due to paracetamol. Br J Dermatol 1986; 115:357–9.
321. Lloyd TW. Agranulocytosis associated with paracetamol [letter]. Lancet 1961; 1:114–5.
322. Manor E, Marmor A, Kaufman S, Lieba H. Hemolysis caused by acetaminophen: positive determination by direct Coombs test. JAMA 1976; 236:2777–8.
323. Datta SB. Fatal pancytopenia after administration of Fortagesic [letter]. Br Med J 1973; 3:173.
324. Fernandez E, Fernandez-Brito AC. Acetaminophen toxicity [letter]. New Engl J Med 1977; 296:577.
325. Olsson R. Increased hepatic sensitivity to paracetamol [letter]. Lancet 1978; 2:152–3.
326. Neuberger J, Davis M, Williams R. Long term ingestion of paracetamol and liver disease. J R Soc Med 1980; 73:701–7.

327. Kadar D, Kalow W. Acute and latent leukopenic reaction to antipyrine. Clin Pharmacol Ther 1980; 28:820–2.
328. Prankerd TAJ. Hemolytic effects of drugs and chemical agents. Clin Pharmacol 1963; 4:334–50.
329. Ortuno J, Botella J. Recurrent acute kidney failure induced by phenazone hypersensitivity. Lancet 1973; 2:1473–6.
330. Altmann HW. Morphological changes in the liver due to phenazone and its derivatives. Agents Actions [Suppl] 1986; 19:267–79.
331. Fowler PD. Aspirin, paracetamol and nonsteroidal anti-inflammatory drugs. A comparative review of side effects. Med Toxicol Adverse Drug Exp 1987; 2:338–66.
332. Smolinske SC, Hall AH, Vandenberg SA, Spoerke DG, McBridge PV. Toxic effects of nonsteroidal anti-inflammatory drugs in overdose. An overview of recent evidence on clinical effects and dose–response relationships. Drug Safety 1990; 5:252–74.
333. Divry P. Reye's syndrome and inborn errors of metabolism. In: Brune K, Santoso B, eds. Antipyretic analgesics: new insights. Basel: Birkhäuser Verlag, 1990: 67–74.
334. Braun J. Analgesic drug use and Reye's syndrome. An analysis of the Yale Reye's syndrome study. In: Brune K, Santoso B, eds. Antipyretic analgesics: new insights. Basel: Birkhäuser Verlag, 1990:75–8.
335. Dipyrone: An assessment of the risk of agranulocytosis. Summary handguide to the international agranulocytosis and aplastic anaemia study. Hoechst AG, 1992.
336. Bannwarth B, Netter P, Pourel J, Royer RJ, Gaucher A. Clinical pharmacokinetics of nonsteroidal anti-inflammatory drugs in the cerebrospinal fluid. Biomed Pharmacother 1989; 43:121–6.
337. Rumack BH. Acetaminophen overdose. In: Zimmermann M, Long DM, eds. Proceedings of a symposium. Antipyretic analgesic therapy. Current worldwide status. Mainz, May 28–29, 1982. Am J Med 1983; (Special Issue): 104–12.
338. Poriaczy P, Schramek P. Analgesic nephropathy and phenacetin-induced transitional cell carcinoma—analysis of 300 patients with long-term consumption of phenacetin-containing drugs. Eur Urol 1981; 7:349–54.
339. Kaufman DW, Kelly JP, Sheehan JE, Laszlo A, Wilholm B-E, Alfredsson L, Koff RS, Shapiro S. Nonsteroidal anti-inflammatory drug use in relation to major upper gastrointestinal bleeding. Clin Pharmacol Ther 1993; 53:485–94.

7

Nonsteroidal Anti-Inflammatory Drugs and Their Enantiomers

KENNETH M. WILLIAMS, IRIS HALL, and RICHARD DAY
University of New South Wales
and St. Vincents Hospital
Sydney, Australia

FRANZISKA LÖHRER
University of Basel
Basel, Switzerland

I. INTRODUCTION

Between 1815 and 1818 Biot discovered that some natural liquids (oil of turpentine, oil of lemon) and solutions of some natural products (camphor, sugar) exhibited optical activity (1) (i.e., they were able to rotate the plane of polarized light). Pasteur further noticed (1848) that the ammonium sodium salt of tartaric acid crystalized in two forms, differing slightly in the arrangement of the crystal faces, and that a solution of the right-handed crystals deviated plane polarized light to the right [denoted (+)], whereas a solution of left-handed crystals resulted in an equal deviation, but to the left [denoted (–)]. Pasteur also noted that mixing equal weights of the two forms of crystal resulted in an optically inactive solution. It was not until 1874, that the theories of Van't Hoff and Le Bel led to a better understanding of this phenomenon of optical activity. They proposed, independently, that the four valences of the carbon atom are directed toward the corners of a tetrahedron. When a carbon atom has four different groups attached to it, the resulting molecule generally exists as two nonsuperimposable mirror images (termed *enantiomers*) and the molecule is dissymmetric or *chiral*. The nonsteroidal anti-inflammatory drugs (NSAIDs), such as ibuprofen (Fig. 1), commonly have this biologically important, structural characteristic.

The actual spacial orientation of the groups around the chiral carbon, as distinct from the effect on polarized light, is termed the *absolute configuration*. The reader will be most familiar with the D- and L-nomenclature for absolute configuration, as used for amino acids and sugars. It is important to note that the lower-case symbols [*d*, dextrorotatory = (+); *l*, levorotatory = (–)] denote the effects on polarized light and give no information concerning absolute configuration. Indeed, these are dependent parameters and vary with concentration, temperature, pH, and the wavelength of light used to determine the rotation.

A more universal system for designating absolute configuration is that proposed by

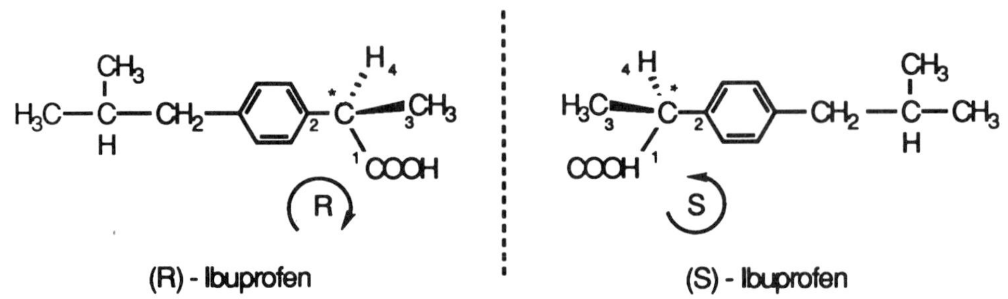

Figure 1 The structures of the enantiomers of ibuprofen, a 2-arylpropionic acid. The absolute configuration, either (*R*)- or (*S*)-, is assigned to the chiral carbon (C*) after the method of Cahn et al. (2) (see text).

Cahn et al. (2). It assigns a priority to groups attached to the chiral carbon (see Fig. 1). The molecule is viewed with the lowest priority atom or group distal to the viewer, and the direction of rotation in decreasing order of priority for the other three groups is then determined. If the direction is clockwise, it is assigned the symbol (*R*) (rectus), if anticlockwise, it is assigned the symbol (*S*) (sinister). Each chiral center in a molecule can be assigned an absolute configuration (see Fig. 1). Such data are based on x-ray crystallographic information. Again, there is no fixed relation between the symbols (*R*) and (*S*), and D and L. Some L-amino acids are designated (*S*), whereas some are designated (*R*) according to this scheme.

Pairs of enantiomers have identical chemical and physical properties in an achiral environment. However, importantly, their biological properties differ because living organisms provide a chiral environment and, thus, have the ability to distinguish between stereoisomers. For instance, L-asparagine is tasteless, whereas D-asparagine is sweet (1). The dominance of L-amino acids and D-sugars within living systems is well known, as is the stereoselectivity of enzymes. Within the body, a drug exists in a chiral environment where it is exposed to a variety of potentially stereoselective reactions. It is not surprising, therefore, that the enantiomers of xenobiotics such as the NSAIDs exhibit different biological activities.

Most nonsteroidal anti-inflammatory drugs are chiral compounds and, with the exception of naproxen and, more recently, flunoxaprofen, are marketed as racemates (i.e., equal proportions of enantiomers). The 2-arylpropionates constitute the most important subset of this group and have been the most intensively studied relative to stereochemical factors. The focus of this chapter is on the disposition of chiral NSAIDs in humans.

II. STEREOSELECTIVE PHARMACODYNAMICS

The primary anti-inflammatory action of the NSAIDs is mediated by inhibition of the prostaglandin cascade, although other mechanisms may be of interest (3). It is clear that, for the 2-arylpropionates, the most important structural feature for antiprostaglandin activity is the stereochemistry at the α-carbon. All studies have shown that the (*S*)-enantiomers are many times more potent anti-inflammatory agents than the (*R*)-enantiomers. Ratios of activities of *S*/*R* in in vitro systems range from 16 (clidanac, minimum ratio) to 880 (flurbiprofen). At these ratio values, the data may actually reflect the chiral purity of the enantiomers used for the studies.

There have been studies contrasting the antiplatelet activity of the enantiomers. Consistent with the inactivity of the (*R*)-enantiomers in inhibiting prostaglandin synthesis in vitro, the (*R*)-2-arylpropionates have little effect on platelet aggregation, whereas the (*S*)-enantiomers are active (4–9). The reversible action of (*S*)-ibuprofen on platelet thromboxane B_2 production has been demonstrated with the unbound IC_{50} being 9.8 ± 1.0 μg/L (10).

The recent interesting finding that (*R*)-flurbiprofen has analgesic activity of similar potency to (*S*)-flurbiprofen has reopened the question of the role of prostaglandin inhibition in the analgesic activity of aspirinlike drugs (11). It is also a confounding factor in the question of whether single enantiomers are superior to racemates (see later discussion).

III. STEREOSELECTIVE PHARMACOKINETICS

The relatively limited human pharmacokinetic data for the enantiomers of the 2-arylpropionates (Table 1) illustrate several points. The clearances of enantiomeric pairs are generally low and are not substantially different, with the exception of etodolac, for which the (*S*)-enantiomer is much more rapidly eliminated. In this particular instance, measurement of total racemic drug is particularly misleading relative to the amount of active enantiomer present in plasma at any given time (contrary to an incorrect previous statement concerning these data; 38). The distribution of these drugs, as measured by the volume of distribution, is not particularly different for the enantiomers, again with the exception of etodolac, and distribution is relatively low, a reflection of the avid binding of these drugs to albumin (see later discussion). Although there are some suggestions of pharmacokinetic interactions between the enantiomers (27), these do not appear to be substantial, although there are insufficient data to be certain of the extent and importance of this consideration in humans. Similarly, although there are some differences between the pharmacokinetics in different groups of people, the data do not allow a conclusion to be made concerning the effects of factors such as age, gender, and disease, on the pharmacokinetics and, in particular, the degree of inversion of the enantiomers.

The half-lives of enantiomeric pairs are, in general, not very different, although after administration of the racemate the (*S*)-enantiomers may have a greater apparent half-life because of continued formation from the (*R*)-enantiomers after absorption is complete. This phenomenon may tend to prolong the action of the racemate, compared with the (*S*)-enantiomer alone, akin to a slow-release formulation, although it is unlikely that this has any great clinical value. The half-lives of the enantiomers are generally short (2–4 h; see Table 1) such that there is little accumulation of the drug enantiomers in plasma after long-term dosing (i.e., extended plasma concentration profiles are essentially those of repetitive single doses). This is because these drugs are often dosed at a frequency much less than their half-lives, twice-daily administration often giving satisfactory symptomatic relief.

Pharmacokinetic studies of the disposition of the enantiomers in synovial fluid are also of interest, as it is a reasonable hypothesis that these concentrations may better reflect the time course of action of the NSAIDs. Studies of ibuprofen (22,39) demonstrated that the active (*S*)-enantiomers were present in higher concentrations than the (*R*)-enantiomers (approximately twofold) and, consistent with the duration of action of this drug, the active enantiomers fluctuated to a much smaller degree in synovial fluid than did the

Table 1 Pharmacokinetic Data for the Enantiomers of NSAIDs in Humans

		Dosage		$t_{1/2}$(h)		CL/F (ml/min)[a]		V/F (L)			
NSAID	Ref.	Form	(mg)	*R*	*S*	*R*	*S*	*R*	*S*	Inversion[b]	Subjects
Carprofen	12	(*RS*)	150			38.3	29.3			No	3 healthy
	13	(*RS*)	50	14.4	13.4	39.8	33.6	49.6	39.0	No	2 healthy
	13	(*R*)	25	14.4		28.8		35.9		No	1 healthy
	13	(*S*)	25		13.4		35.2		40.8	No	2 healthy
Etodolac	14	(*RS*)	200/12 h	3.5/5.0	2.35/2.35	108/112[c]	1328/998[c]	16.5/24.4	135/101	No	2 healthy
Fenoprofen	4									High	4 male
Flunoxaprofen	15,16	(*RS*)	100	7.8	7.6	27.4[d]	17.8[d]	18.2	11.9	No	6 healthy
	15,16	(*R*)	100	8.1		23.5[d]		16.1		No	6 healthy
	17	(*S*)	200		6.3		20.0[d]		10.9[d]	No	6 healthy
Flurbiprofen	18,19	(*RS*)	100/12 h	2.3	2.6	75[c]	57[c]	12.5	12.8	No	15 arthritic
	20	(*RS*)	100	4.2	4.2	24.5	20.5	8.41	7.23	No	6 healthy
	21[e]	(*RS*)	100	6.0	6.9	43.2	37.3	22.4	22.2	No	23 healthy
	21[f]	(*RS*)	100	6.2	6.8	40.7	34.6	21.7	20.5	No	23 healthy
Ibuprofen	22–24	(*RS*)	400,800/8,12 h	1.6	2.3	78[g]	99[g]	11.2	—[h]	Mod	8 arthritic
	25	(*RS*)	400	2.0	3.1	87.9	—[h]	15.7	—[h]	Mod	24 healthy
	25	(*RS*)	200	1.7	2.3	74.8	—[h]	11.1	—[h]	Mod	24 healthy
	25	(*RS*)	800	1.6	2.5	90.5	—[h]	12.5	—[h]	Mod	24 healthy
	26	(*RS*)	600	2.3	2.3	94.4	—[h]	18.8	—[h]	Mod	11 healthy
	26	(*R*)	300	2.1	2.2	99.3		18.1		Mod	11 healthy
	26	(*S*)	300		2.1		80.1		14.6	Mod	11 healthy
	26	(*S*)	150		1.9		68.6		11.3	Mod	4 healthy
	26	(*S*)	500		2.2		76.5		14.6	Mod	4 healthy
	27	(*RS*)	800	1.7	2.5	87.6	—[h]	11.5	—[h]	Mod	4 healthy
	27	(*R*)	400	2.0		67.9		9.9		Mod	4 healthy
	27	(*S*)	400		1.7		74.4		10.5	Mod	4 healthy
	28	(*RS*)[i]	800	2.5	2.5	114	87.4	24.1	18.6	Mod	8 healthy
	28	(*R*)[i]	600	2.5	2.5	130	86.4	27.5	18.4	Mod	8 healthy
	28	(*S*)	600		2.5		82.2	—	17.5	Mod	8 healthy

Indoprofen	29	(*RS*)	200	2.3	2.8	72.0	41.0	14.6	9.8	No	4 healthy
	29	(*S*)	100		2.9		40.6		10.2	No	4 healthy
	30	(*RS*)	400	3.4/2.9	3.9/3.1	52.5/48.2	34.0/34.1	15.4/12.2	11.2/8.7	No	2 surgical
	31	(*RS*)	400	3.1	3.4	48.8	32.2	12.6	9.0	No	10 surgical
Ketoprofen	32	(*RS*)	50	3.8	2.5	62.2	—[j]	19.1	—[j]	V. low	8 healthy
	32	(*RS*)	50/6 h	3.8	3.2	81.5		21.5		V. low	8 healthy
	33	(*RS*)	50	2.1	2.4	105	110	16.6	19.5	V. low	4 healthy
	33	(*R*)	25	1.5		90.3		13.5		V. low	4 healthy
	33	(*S*)	25		2.7		104		17.3	V. low	4 health
	34	(*RS*)	50	3.2	2.6	78.5		21.0		V. low	9 young arthritic
	34	(*RS*)	50/6 h	3.1	3.2	80.5		20.8		V. low	9 young arthritic
	34	(*RS*)	50	3.1	3.3	59.8		15.8		V. low	9 old arthritic
	34	(*RS*)	50/6 h	3.8	3.8	65.8		21.0		V. low	9 old arthritic
	35	(*RS*)	50	1.8	1.8	80.7	—[j]	12.8	—[j]	V. low	5 surgical
Suprofen	36	(*RS*)[h]	200	1.1	1.1	80.7	130	7.45[i]	12.7[i]	V. low	3 healthy
Tiaprofenic acid	37	(*RS*)	200/8 h	2.6	2.6	45.3	46.9	10.5	10.7	No	4 arthritic

Note: In the cases in which only two subjects were involved, values for each person mentioned are included.

[a]Clearance values are expressed as CL/F and assume zero metabolic chiral inversion unless otherwise stated.

[b]The extent of inversion is indicated by No (no inversion), V. low (very low inversion of 5–12%), Mod (moderate inversion of 30–60%) and High (extensive inversion of >60%).

[c]Steady-state clearance.

[d]Normalized to an average mass of 70 kg/person.

[e,f]These pharmacokinetic parameters were measured during a comparative bioavailability study, using Ansaid[e] and Froben[f].

[g]CL/F calculated assuming 60% inversion of (*R*)-ibuprofen to (*S*)-ibuprofen.

[h]Due to metabolic chiral inversion, these values were not calculated.

[i]This study was performed after oral administration of a pseudoracemate, using deuterium-labeled enantiomers.

[j]Values were not calculated for (*S*)-ketoprofen, because the authors felt that the possibility of (*R*)- to (*S*)-ketoprofen inversion could not be ruled out; hence, the fraction of the dose, F, entering the systemic circulation as (*S*)-ketoprofen remained unknown.

corresponding plasma concentrations over a dosage interval. In contrast, the concentrations of the enantiomers of ketoprofen (40) and tiaprofenic acid (37) were similar in synovial fluid, whereas (*R*)-etodolac was the preponderant species in synovial fluid (4). These data parallel the respective ratios of the enantiomers in plasma. Interestingly, there was evidence that (*S*)-etodolac conjugates were also present in synovial fluid (41).

IV. STEREOSELECTIVE PROTEIN BINDING

The 2-arylpropionates, such as naproxen and ibuprofen, are very highly bound to plasma proteins (in many cases exceeding 99%), primarily human serum albumin (HSA) and, therefore, even small stereospecific differences in protein binding of these drugs will result in significant differences in the unbound concentrations of the enantiomers. Because the unbound drug is the pharmacologically active species which, furthermore, determines the clearance of this group of drugs, the significance of stereoselective protein binding is evident.

The major drug-binding sites on albumin have been identified and characterized as site I (warfarin- and azopropazone-binding area) and site II (indole- and benzodiazapine-binding area; 42). The specific-binding site for the "profens" has been identified as site II (42–46), which is a low-capacity, high-affinity site. Interactions with this site account for the observation that the binding of the profens is commonly stereoselective. Binding generally favors the (*S*)-enantiomers (with the exception of etodolac; 41), is dependent on HSA concentration, and becomes nonstereoselective at high plasma concentrations of the drug when the weaker, high-capacity, low-affinity interactions predominate (44,45, 47,48). Interindividual variability is evident in protein-binding interactions such that, for example, (*R*)-flurbiprofen was more avidly bound than the (*S*)-enantiomer in some subjects. Such interindividual variations may contribute to variability in the disposition of the racemic drug (47).

Other factors found to affect binding include uremia, which preferentially decreases the binding of (*R*)-flurbiprofen (47); and fatty acids, for which, for example, (*R*)-carprofen is more avidly bound in the presence of fatty acids, whereas (*S*)-carprofen is more strongly bound by fatty acid-free HSA. Fatty acids are known to play a major role in determining the binding characteristics of ligands to the HSA molecule (46), possibly by inducing conformational changes within the albumin molecule (43).

Surprisingly, the glucuronides of some 2-arylpropionates (e.g., carprofen; 43) may also be highly bound to human serum albumin (99%), and this may reduce the renal clearance of carprofen glucuronides in humans. (*S*)-Carprofen glucuronide is bound more strongly than (*R*)-carprofen glucuronide both in the presence and absence of fatty acids. Interestingly, whereas the carprofen enantiomers, similar to the other profens, bind to site II, their glucuronide conjugates bind to site I. It is perhaps not surprising then that fatty acids affect the stereospecific binding of carprofen and its glucuronides differently.

Enantiomer–enantiomer interactions at the protein-binding sites have been described for ibuprofen (27,48) and flurbiprofen (20,47). The kinetics of the racemate may thus not be the simple sum of the disposition of the individual enantiomers.

V. STEREOSELECTIVE METABOLISM

There is evidence of stereoselective conjugation pathways of the 2-arylpropionates, such as with glucuronic acid (27,28), and also stereoselective oxidation of (*S*)-ibuprofen to the pharmacologically inactive metabolites, hydroxyibuprofen and carboxyibuprofen (28). It is not known whether metabolic oxidation displays polymorphic metabolism, although this is an interesting hypothesis that requires investigation.

There may be some interest in the glucuronides, as these have the potential to covalently bind to biological macromolecules to form potential antigens (49–52). Reactivity with plasma proteins and biological degradation demonstrate stereoselective differences (52). Hydrolysis of the glucuronides releases parent drug, and this "futile cycling" (53), may be of particular interest in renal failure. Effects of renal dysfunction have not been studied in humans, but are of potential interest and importance, particularly for those drugs for which clearance is highly dependent on this mode of metabolism, such as ketoprofen and naproxen.

A. Chiral Inversion of 2-Arylpropionic Acids

One reason the 2-arylpropionates have come under particular scrutiny has been because of the intriguing chiral inversion whereby the "inactive" (*R*)-enantiomers are converted to the "active" (*S*)-enantiomers in vivo. The mechanism of this inversion, the stereoselective pharmacokinetics and pharmacodynamics of the enantiomers, the variability of inversion both in terms of substrate and species, and the potential therapeutic consequences have been a focus of activity (see other reviews; Refs. 38,54–56).

1. Interspecies Differences

Although the focus of this chapter is on human studies, much of our current understanding comes from animal studies. Inversion is substrate- and species-dependent (56,57). The rat has been the most extensively studies species, and the data generally seem to be more relevant to the disposition in humans than, for example, that of the guinea pig, in which inversion appears to occur with greater avidity (58), or the rabbit, in which the clearances of the enantiomers are substantially different from those in humans (59), although fractional inversion may not be dissimilar. Even so, there may be differences even between strains of rats (60); hence, it is imperative that detailed human studies be undertaken.

2. Mechanism of Inversion

Studies of the mechanism of inversion have been of particular interest, and some controversy, and have raised interesting questions with potential clinical consequences. The following is a brief outline of the putative mechanism of inversion and the reader may refer to several reviews for more detailed discussion (38,54,56,61).

Central to inversion is the initial formation of CoA thioester intermediates (62; Fig. 2). These activated species are formed by synthetases yet to be characterized in humans, although in rats, long-chain acyl-CoA synthetase has been implicated, and this enzyme has been demonstrated to be stereospecific for the (*R*)-enantiomers of ibuprofen and fenoprofen (63,64).

Several studies have now validated the proposition that the CoA thioester intermediates are then inverted enzymatically (62,64; see Fig. 2), and importantly, that if the CoA thioesters of the (*S*)-enantiomers are synthesized, these are also inverted in in vitro preparations (60,65). These data further validate the thesis that the stereochemical outcome of inversion is determined by the stereoselectivity of the CoA synthetase(s).

The final hydrolase(s), which complete the overall inversion (see Fig. 2), have not

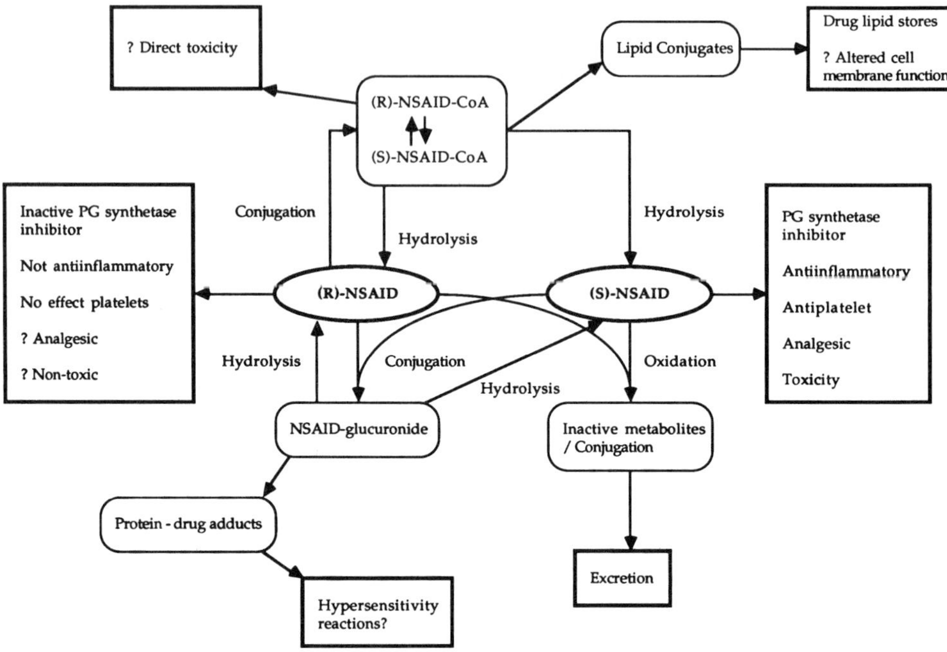

Figure 2 The NSAIDs of the 2-arylpropionate class, may undergo simple oxidative metabolism, leading to termination of pharmacological action. Alternatively, several scenarios may occur. They may undero stereoselective chiral inversion from the "inactive" (*R*)-enantiomer [(*R*)-NSAID] to the "active" (*S*)-enantiomer [(*S*)-NSAID] in vivo. Inversion is dependent on stereoselective formation of a CoA thioester intermediate [(R)-NSAID-CoA], which is racemized to give (*S*)-NSAID-CoA. Subsequent hydrolysis of the CoA thioesters yields either the (*S*)-enantiomer (i.e., inversion is complete), or reformation of the (*R*)-enantiomer. The activated CoA thioester intermediates are putative reactive species that may exert direct pharmacological activity, or allow incorporation of drug into "hybrid" lipid products, again with uncertain consequences. Other conjugates with glucuronic acid also provide the possibility of formation of protein–drug conjugates, putatively associated with the occasional hypersensitivity reactions associated with this class of drug.

been characterized. There may be one for each of the CoA thioesters of the enantiomers, or one that is not stereoselective. There are animal data suggesting that there is more than one hydrolase involved (60,66). Highly stereoselective hydrolases have been identified for the enantiomers of the related CoA thioesters of methylmalonic acid (67).

3. *Consequences of Chiral Inversion*

There are few hard data to demonstrate important clinical consequences of the inversion of the 2-arylpropionates; thus, most considerations remain speculative. Naproxen, which as noted is formulated as the enantiomerically pure (*S*)-form, is not clearly different from other racemic NSAIDs in either efficacy or toxicity. The activated CoA thioesters may modulate biochemical parameters, such as occurs for other endogenous and xenobiotic CoA thioesters (68), or may be overtly toxic by analogy to the toxic CoA thioester formed after ingestion of the Jamaican ackee fruit (69).

4. *Interrelationship Between the Stereoselective Metabolism of 2-Arylpropionates and Lipids*

The CoA thioesters allow the 2-arylpropionates to become involved in the metabolic pathways of lipids (see Fig. 2). (*R*)-Ibuprofen is stereoselectively incorporated into hybrid triglycerides (70,71). Furthermore, recent data have suggested a relation between the occasional incidence of microvesicular steatosis associated with pirprofen administration and the inhibition of fatty acid oxidation (72). It was hypothesized that this adverse event was stereoselectively mediated by the (*R*)-enantiomer after activation to the CoA thioester. However, studies have demonstrated that this inhibition of fatty acid oxidation is primarily through a nonstereoselective CoA-independent mechanism (73,74), although there may be a secondary stereoselective component, which may become evident when there is reduced availability of CoA (73).

5. *Implications for Variability in Response*

Variability in the stereoselective disposition of the NSAIDs, in particular inversion, has been proposed as one of the factors contributing to the commonly observed interpatient variability in response to this class of drugs (54,75). This is an hypothesis that still requires testing. Thus, a single 400-mg dose of racemic ibuprofen may, at the two extremes, represent either 400 mg of active drug (i.e., 100% inversion), or 200 mg (i.e., no inversion). In a recent study of the enantiomeric disposition of ibuprofen in healthy volunteers administered racemate, there was surprisingly little variability in the ratio of the areas under the concentration curve (AUCs) for (*S*)- to (*R*)-ibuprofen (25). In a further elegant study of the stereoselective disposition of ibuprofen, the clearance by inversion varied approximately twofold, with the fractional inversion moderately variable, ranging from 40 to 63% (28), in agreement with other data (27). These data also contrasted the differences in fractional inversion, depending on the method of estimation of this parameter. Calculations based on determination of the chirality of the excreted urinary products may be superior, but assume that there is no inversion of metabolites after their formation. It has yet to be demonstrated that in a larger group in which factors, such as age, disease, and concomitant drug intake, are important, variability in inversion may be a more important factor. Surprisingly, although the collective data in animals and humans imply that inversion is relatively common, it appears, on the basis of the available data (see Table 1), that inversion in humans is more the exception than the rule.

Administration of other drugs may also be a consideration. Recent data in rats demonstrated induction of the inversion of ibuprofen by clofibrate by induction of CoA thioester formation and differential effects on fatty acyl-CoA hydrolases (66). The data illustrate the potential for further variability in the availability of active drug from racemic preparations and the potential diversion of drug into other pathways, such as the formation of hybrid lipids (see Fig. 2).

B. Metabolism of Other Chiral Nonsteroidal Anti-Inflammatory Drugs

The 2-arylpropionates are the most important and widely used group of chiral NSAIDs. There are several other chiral NSAIDs that are administered as their racemates, but for which there are little data (61). These include sulindac, oxyphenbutazone, etodolac, and azapropazone.

1. Sulindac

Sulindac, a sulfoxide, is a prodrug, with its activity attributable to reduction to the sulfide in vivo. As such, sulindac is potentially less toxic to the gastric mucosa than other NSAIDs, although most data throw doubt on this claim (76). The contention that sulindac has renal-sparing effects is also controversial. The relative activities of the enantiomers are unknown, with the claim that they are equally active (77) being in some question because of the apparent lack of purity of the enantiomers used in this report (61,78).

2. Oxyphenbutazone

Oxyphenbutazone is a minor metabolite of phenylbutazone, but is rarely used because of its tendency to cause bone marrow suppression. Rapid interconversion of the enantiomers means that there is little chance of detecting pharmacological differences between the enantiomers and no benefit to be attained by administering one of the enantiomers alone (61).

3. Etodolac

Etodolac is an interesting chiral drug, again administered as the racemate. The (*S*)-enantiomer is much more potent than the (*R*)-enantiomer (79). Particular interest arises from the large differences in the concentrations of the enantiomers generated in vivo such that the inactive (*R*)-enantiomer is by far the preponderant enantiomer in plasma after oral administration of the drug in humans (20). The interesting data on the synovial fluid distribution of the enantiomers (41) were discussed earlier.

4. Azapropazone

Although a racemic drug, it is rarely used, and there are no data on the relative activities of the enantiomers.

VI. CLINICAL STUDIES OF ENANTIOMERS

There is an increasing interest in the potential for marketing single enantiomers of the 2-arylpropionates, with possible advantages such as reduced dose, fewer side effects, and more rapid onset of analgesic action. Over the short term (2 weeks) patients ($n = 5$) with rheumatoid arthritis responded well to therapy with (*S*)-ibuprofen (500 mg bid or tds) with clear clinical improvement and no side effects (26). It also appeared that there was a more rapid onset of analgesic action of (*S*)-ibuprofen compared with the racemate, perhaps because of solubility differences between the two dosage forms. (In contrast to the enantiomers, which have identical solubility characteristics, the racemic drug may not have the same solubility as the enantiomers). The onset rate of analgesia is not as important a consideration for management of rheumatoid arthritis, but may be of interest when these drugs are used as simple analgesics. The reader should be reminded of the potential analgesic activity of the (*R*)-enantiomers in this context (11).

It is a reasonable hypothesis that plasma concentrations of the (*S*)-enantiomer ought to correlate better with therapeutic outcome than if only the racemic drug is measured. It has been proposed that this is one factor contributing to the difficulty in establishing plasma concentration–effect relations for this group of drugs (54,75). In a recent short-term study of the response to treatment of osteoarthritis of the hip and knee with racemic ibuprofen, there was a correlation between plasma trough concentrations of (*S*)-ibuprofen and overall disability (Stanford Health Assessment Questionnaire Disability Scale), and with physician's global assessment (80). However, these correlations were no stronger than those obtained when outcome was correlated with concentrations of racemic drug, despite the large variability in the trough concentrations and AUCs for (*S*)-ibuprofen. The failure to detect statistically significant correlations with other clinical outcome measures may reflect the general imprecision of these methods and other difficulties such as the limited dose range noted in this study.

An alternate approach is to use the (*R*)-enantiomers as prodrugs when there is significant inversion in vivo (75). This would reduce the direct exposure of the gastrointestinal tract to the active drug and, thereby, reduce the inhibition of the cytoprotective prostaglandins in the gastric mucosa. There would still be indirect effects of the (*S*)-enantiomer after drug distribution and the potential direct physical effects of acidic (*R*)-enantiomers. Clearly, larger numbers and longer chronicity studies are required to validate the use of pure (*S*)-enantiomers and their potential advantages over the corresponding racemic preparations. Similarly clinical studies with (*R*)-ibuprofen and (*R*)-fenoprofen, for example, would be of interest. Additionally, the report that (*R*)-flurbiprofen is equianalgesic to (*S*)-flurbiprofen (11) further increases the complexity of the issues. For example, there may be advantages in terms of analgesic efficacy in the use of (*R,S*)-flurbiprofen in arthritic conditions because of the potential contribution of the (*R*)-enantiomer to analgesic efficacy by a nonprostaglandin-mediated mechanism. For simple analgesia, (*R*)-flurbiprofen may have advantage over the (*S*)-enantiomer because of its lack of ulcerogenic activity (11).

There has also been a move to measuring the enantiomers of racemic preparations in bioavailability studies. Two studies have found that the availability of the respective formulations were not equivalent on the basis of pharmacokinetic parameters for the (*S*)-enantiomers (39,81). However, it would be unlikely that *clinical* inequivalence could be demonstrated for such preparations.

VII. CONCLUSIONS

In summary, most of the nonsteroidal anti-inflammatory drugs are chiral compounds and are administered as racemates, despite the fact that the anti-inflammatory activity appears to reside only in the (*S*)-enantiomers. Although analgesic activity is similarly believed to be due to the (*S*)-enantiomers, recent data suggesting that (*R*)-flurbiprofen is analgesic requires careful reassessment of this assumption. Clearly, pharmacokinetic studies need to identify the dispositional characteristics of the active enantiomer to facilitate understanding of concentration–effect relations. The stereoselective chiral inversion of 2-arylpropionates has been of mechanistic interest, leading to an investigation of the role of CoA thioesters as intermediates in drug metabolism, but as yet to be demonstrated to be of clinical importance. Surprisingly, few 2-arylpropionates appear to be inverted to any great degree in humans. Understanding the reason for this will provide further useful insights. Administration of the single (*S*)-enantiomer, rather than the racemate, is intuitively more reasonable, but again, the therapeutic benefit to be attained is uncertain.

ACKNOWLEDGMENTS

Financial support from the Swiss National Science Foundation and Stiftung zur Förderung des pharmazeutischen Nachwuchses in Basel to F. L. and from the Australian National Health and Medical Research Council to K. W. and R. D. is gratefully acknowledged.

REFERENCES

1. Bertrand Ramsay O. Stereochemistry. In: van Spronsen JW, ed. London: Heyden, 1981.
2. Cahn RS, Ingold CK, Prelog V. The specification of asymmetric configuration in organic chemistry. Experientia 1956; 12:81–124.
3. Williams KM, Day RO, Breit SN. Biochemical actions and clinical pharmacology of anti-inflammatory drugs. Adv Drug Res 1993; 24:121–98.
4. Rubin A, Knadler MP, Ho PPK, Bechtol LD, Wolen RL. Stereoselective inversion of (*R*)-fenoprofen to (*S*)-fenoprofen in humans. J Pharm Sci 1985; 74:82–4.
5. Kulmacz RJ, Lands WEM. Stoichiometry and kinetics of the interaction of prostaglandin H synthetase with anti-inflammatory agents. J Biol Chem 1985; 260:12572–8.
6. Kean WF, Lock CJ, Rischke J, Butt R, Buchanan WW, Howard-Lock H. Effect of *R* and *S* enantiomers of naproxen on aggregation and thromboxane production in human platelets. J Pharm Sci 1989; 78:324–7.
7. Cerletti C, Manarini S, Colombo M, Tavani A. The (+)-enantiomer is responsible for the antiplatelet and anti-inflammatory activity of (+/–)-indobufen. J Pharm Pharmacol 1990; 42:885–7.
8. Patrignani P, Volpi D, Ferrario R, Romanzini L, Di Somma M, Patrono C. Effects of racemic *S*- and *R*-indobufen on cyclooxygenase and lipoxygenase activities in human whole blood. Eur J Pharmacol 1990; 191:83–8.
9. Strolin Benedetti M, Frigerio E, Tamassia V, Noseda G, Caldwell J. The dispositional enantioselectivity of indobufen in man. Biochem Pharmacol 1992; 9:2032–4.
10. Evans AM, Nation RL, Sansom LN, Bochner F, Somogyi AA. Effect of racemic ibuprofen dose on the magnitude and duration of platelet cyclo-oxygenase inhibition: relationship between inhibition of thromboxane production and the plasma unbound concentration of *S*(+)-ibuprofen. Br J Clin Pharmacol 1991; 31:131–8.
11. Brune K, Beck WS, Geisslinger G, Menzel-Soglowek S, Pekar BM, Peskar BA. Aspirin-like drugs may block pain independently of prostaglandin synthesis inhibition. Experientia 1991; 47:257–61.
12. Spahn H, Spahn I, Benet LZ. Probenecid-induced changes in the clearance of carprofen enantiomers: a preliminary study. Clin Pharmacol Ther 1989; 45:500–5.
13. Iwakawa S, Suganuma T, Lee S-F, Spahn H, Benet LZ, Lin ET. Direct determination of carprofen glucuronides in human plasma and urine and preliminary measurements of stereoselective metabolic and renal elimination after oral administration of carprofen in man. Drug Metab Dispos 1989; 17:414–9.
14. Jamali F, Mehvar R, Lemko C, Eradiri O. Application of a stereospecific high-performance liquid chromatography assay to a pharmacokinetic study of etodolac enantiomers in humans. J Pharm Sci 1988; 77:963–6.
15. Pedrazzini S, De Angelis M, Zanoboni Muciaccia W, Sacchi C, Forgione A. Stereochemical pharmacokinetics of the 2-arylpropionic acid nonsteroidal anti-inflammatory drug flunoxaprofen in rats and in man. Arzneimittelforschung 1988; 38:1170–5.
16. Palatini P, Montanari G, Perosa A, Forgione A, Pedrazzini S, Furlanut M. Stereospecific disposition of flunoxaprofen enantiomers in human beings. Int J Clin Pharm Res 1988; 8:161–7.
17. Bareggi SR, Pedrazzini S, De Angelis M. Pharmacokinetic study in man with the non-steroidal anti-inflammatory drug flunoxaprofen. Arzneimittelforschung 1988; 38:574–7.
18. Young MA, Aarons L, Toon S. The pharmacokinetics of the enantiomers of flurbiprofen in patients with rheumatoid arthritis. Br J Clin Pharmacol 1991; 31:102–4.
19. Jamali F. Pharmacokinetics of enantiomers of chiral non-steroidal anti-inflammatory drugs. Eur J Drug Metab Pharmacokinet 1988; 13:1–9.
20. Jamali F, Berry BW, Tehrani MR, Russel AS. Stereoselective pharmacokinetics of flurbiprofen in humans and rats. J Pharm Sci 1988; 77:666–9.
21. Jamali F, Collins DS, Berry BW, Molder S, Cheung R, McColl K, Cheung H. Comparative

bioavailability of two flurbiprofen products: stereospecific versus conventional approach. Biopharm Drug Dispos 1991; 12:435–45.

22. Day RO, Williams KM, Graham GG, Lee EJ, Knihinicki RD, Champion GD. Stereoselective disposition of ibuprofen enantiomers in synovial fluid. Clin Pharmacol Ther 1988; 43:480–7.
23. Kaiser DG, Vangiessen GJ, Reischer RJ, Wechter WJ. Isomeric inversion of ibuprofen (*R*)-enantiomer in humans. J Pharm Sci 1976; 65:269–73.
24. Geisslinger G, Stock K-P, Bach GL, Loew D, Brune K. Pharmacological differences between *R*(–)- and *S*(+)-ibuprofen. Agents Actions 1989; 27:455–7.
25. Avgerinos A, Hutt AJ. Interindividual variability in the enantiomeric disposition of ibuprofen following the oral administration of the racemic drug to healthy volunteers. Chirality 1990; 2:249–56.
26. Geisslinger G, Schuster O, Stock K-P, Loew D, Bach GL, Brune K. Pharmacokinetics of *S*(+)- and *R*(–)-ibuprofen in volunteers and first clinical experience of *S*(+)-ibuprofen in rheumatoid arthritis. Eur J Clin Pharmacol 1990; 38:493–7.
27. Lee EJD, Williams K, Day R, Graham G, Champion D. Stereoselective disposition of ibuprofen enantiomers in man. Br J Clin Pharmacol 1985; 19:669–74.
28. Rudy AC, Knight PM, Brater C, Hall SD. Stereoselective metabolism of ibuprofen in human: administration of *R*-, *S*- and racemic ibuprofen. J Pharmacol Exp Ther 1991; 259:1133–9.
29. Tamassia V, Jannuzzo MG, Moro E, Stegnjaich S, Groppi W. Pharmacokinetics of the enantiomers of indoprofen in man. Int J Clin Pharm Res 1984; 4:223–30.
30. Björkman S. Determination of the enantiomers of indoprofen in blood plasma by high-performance liquid chromatography after rapid derivatization by means of ethyl chloroformate. J Chromatogr 1985; 339:339–46.
31. Björkman S. Stereoselective disposition of indoprofen in surgical patients. Br J Clin Pharmacol 1985; 20:463–7.
32. Foster RT, Jamali F, Russel AS, Alballa SR. Pharmacokinetics of ketoprofen enantiomers in healthy subjects following single and multiple doses. J Pharm Sci 1988; 77:70–3.
33. Jamali F, Russel AS, Foster RT, Lemko C. Ketoprofen pharmacokinetics in humans: evidence of enantiomeric inversion and lack of interaction. J Pharm Sci 1990; 79:460–1.
34. Foster RT, Jamali F, Russel AS, Alballa SR. Pharmacokinetics of ketoprofen enantiomers in young and elderly arthritic patients following single and multiple doses. J Pharm Sci 1988; 77:191–5.
35. Foster RT, Jamali F, Russel AS. Pharmacokinetics of ketoprofen enantiomers in cholecystectomy patients: influence of probenecid. Eur J Clin Pharmacol 1989; 37:589–94.
36. Shinohara Y, Magara H, Baba S. Stereoselective pharmacokinetics and inversion of suprofen enantiomers in humans. J Pharm Sci 1991; 80:1075–8.
37. Singh NN, Jamali F, Pasutto FM, Russel AS, Coutts RT, Drader KS. Pharmacokinetics of the enantiomers of tiaprofenic acid in humans. J Pharm Sci 1986; 75:439–42.
38. Williams KM. Enantiomers in arthritic disorders. Pharmacol Ther 1990; 46:273–95.
39. Cox SR, Gall EP, Forbes KK, Gresham M, Goris G. Pharmacokinetics of the *R*(–) and *S*(+) enantiomers of ibuprofen in the serum and synovial fluid of arthritis patients. J Clin Pharmacol 1991; 31:88–94.
40. Foster RT, Jamali F, Russell, AS, Ketoprofen enantiomers in synovial fluid. J Pharm Sci 1989; 78:881–2.
41. Brocks DR, Jamali F, Russell AS. Stereoselective disposition of etodolac enantiomers in synovial fluid. J Clin Pharmacol 1991; 31:741–6.
42. Fehske KJ, Müller WE, Woller U. The location of drug binding sites in human serum albumin. Biochem Pharmacol 1981; 30:687–92.
43. Iwakawa S, Spahn H, Benet LZ, Lin ET. Stereospecific binding of the glucuronide conjugates of carprofen enantiomers to human serum albumin. Biochem Pharmacol 1990; 39:949–53.
44. Oravcová J, Mlynárik V, Bystricky S, Soltés L, Szalay P, Bohácik L, Trnovec T. Interaction of pirprofen enantiomers with human serum albumin. Chirality 1991; 3:412–7.
45. Otagiri M, Masuda K, Imai T, Imamura Y, Yamasuki M. Binding of pirprofen to human

serum albumin studied by dialysis and spectroscopy techniques. Biochem Pharmacol 1989; 38:1–7.
46. Oida T. Proton nuclear magnetic resonance study on the multimode interactions of human serum albumin with drug molecules. J Biochem 1986; 100:99–113.
47. Knadler MP, Brater DC, Hall SD. Plasma protein binding of flurbiprofen: enantioselectivity and influence of pathophysiological status. J Pharmacol Exp Ther 1989; 249:378–85.
48. Evans AM, Nation RL, Sansom LN, Bochner F, Somogyi AA. Stereoselective plasma protein binding of ibuprofen enantiomers. Eur J Clin Pharmacol 1989; 36:283–90.
49. Hyneck ML, Smith PC, Munafo A, McDonagh AF, Benet LZ. Disposition and irreversible plasma protein binding of tolmetin in humans. Clin Pharmacol Ther 1988; 44:107–14.
50. Van Breeman R, Fenselau C. Acylation of albumin by 1-*O*-acyl glucuronides. Drug Metab Dispos 1985; 13:318 20.
51. McKinnon GE, Dickinson RG. Covalent binding of diflunisal and probenecid to plasma proteins in humans: persistence of the adducts in the circulation. Res Commun Chem Pathol Pharmacol 1989; 66:339–54.
52. Volland C, Sun H, Dammeyer J, Benet LZ. Stereoselective degradation of the fenoprofen acyl glucuronide enantiomers and irreversible binding to plasma protein. Drug Metab Dis 1991; 19:1080–6.
53. Meffin PJ. The effect of renal dysfunction on the disposition of nonsteroidal anti-inflammatory drugs forming acylglucuronides. Agents Actions [Suppl] 1985; 17:85–7.
54. Hutt AJ, Caldwell, J. The metabolic chiral inversion of 2-arylpropionic acids. A novel route with pharmacological consequences. J Pharm Pharmacol 1983; 35:693–704.
55. Caldwell J, Hutt AJ, Fournel-Gigleux S. The metabolic chiral inversion and dispositional enantioselectivity of the 2-arylpropionic acids and their biological consequences. Biochem Pharmacol 1988; 37:105–14.
56. Williams KM. Metabolic chiral inversion. In: Simonyi M, ed. Problems and wonders of chiral molecules. Budapest: Akademiai Kiado, 1990:181–204.
57. Fournel S, Caldwell J. The metabolic chiral inversion of 2-phenylpropionic acid in rat, mouse and rabbit. Biochem Pharmacol 1986; 35:4153–9.
58. Tamura S, Kuzuna S, Kawai K, Kishimoto S. Optical isomerization of *R*(–)-clidanac to the biologically active *S*(+)-isomer in guinea pigs. J Pharm Pharmacol 1981; 33:701–6.
59. Williams KM, Knihinicki RD, Day RO. Pharmacokinetics of the enantiomers of ibuprofen in the rabbit. Agents Actions 1991; 34:381–6.
60. Knihinicki RD, Day RO, Williams KM. Chiral inversion of 2-arylpropionic acid non-steroidal anti-inflammatory drugs—II. Biochem Pharmacol 1991; 10:1905–11.
61. Williams KM. Molecular asymmetry and its pharmacological consequences. Adv Pharmacol 1991; 22:57–135.
62. Nakamura Y, Yamaguchi T, Takahashi S, Hashimoto S, Iwatani K, Nakagawa Y. Optical isomerization mechanism of *R*(–)-hydratropic acid derivatives. J Pharmacobiodyn 1981; 4:S-1.
63. Knights KM, Drew R, Meffin PM. Enantiospecific formation of fenoprofen coenzyme A thioester in vitro. Biochem Pharmacol 1988; 37:3539–42.
64. Knihinicki R, Williams KM, Day RO. Chiral inversion of 2-arylpropionic acid non steroidal anti-inflammatory drugs—1. Biochem Pharmacol 1989; 38:4389–95.
65. Knadler MP, Hall SD. Stereoselective arylpropionyl-CoA thioester formation in vitro. Chirality 1990; 2:67–73.
66. Knights KM, Addinall TF, Roberts BJ. Enhanced chiral inversion of *R*-ibuprofen in liver from rats treated with clofibric acid. Biochem Pharmacol 1991; 41:1775–7.
67. Kovachy RJ, Copley SD, Allen RH. Recognition, isolation and characterization of rat liver D-methylmalonyl coenzyme A hydrolase. J Biol Chem 1983; 258:11415–21.
68. Krahenbuhl S, Brass EP. Inhibition of hepatic propionyl-CoA synthetase activity by organic acids. Biochem Pharmacol 1991; 41:1015–23.
69. Sherratt HSA. Hypoglycin, the famous toxin of the unripe Jamaican ackee fruit. Trends Pharmacol Sci 1986; 7:186–91.

70. Williams KM, Day RO, Knihinicki R, Duffield A. The stereoselective uptake of ibuprofen enantiomers into adipose tissue. Biochem Pharmacol 1986; 35:3403–5.
71. Sallustio BC, Meffin PJ, Knights KM. The stereospecific incorporation of fenoprofen into rat hepatocyte and adipocytes triacylglycerols. Biochem Pharmacol 1988; 37:1919–23.
72. Geneve J, Hayat-Bonan B, Labbe G, Degott C, Letteron P, Freneaux E, Dinh TL, Larrey D, Pessayre D. Inhibition of mitochondrial β-oxidation of fatty acids by pirprofen. Role in microvesicular steatosis due to this non-steroidal anti-inflammatory drug. J Pharmacol Exp Ther 1987; 242:1133–7.
73. Freneaux E, Fromenty B, Berson A, Labbe G, Degott C, Letteron P, Larrey D, Pessayre D. Stereoselective and nonstereoselective effects of ibuprofen enantiomers on mitochondrial β-oxidation of fatty acids. J Pharmacol Exp Ther 1990; 2:529–35.
74. Zhao B, Geisslinger G, Hall I, Day RO, Williams KM. The effect of the enantiomers of ibuprofen and flurbiprofen on the β-oxidation of palmitate in the rat. Chirality 1992; 4:137–41.
75. Williams KM, Day RO. Stereoselective disposition—basis for variability in response to NSAID's. Agents Actions [Suppl] 1985; 17:119–26.
76. Carson JL, Strom BL, Morse ML, West SL, Soper KA, Stolley PD, Jones JK. The relative gastrointestinal toxicity of the nonsteroidal anti-inflammatory drugs. Arch Intern Med 1987; 147:1054–9.
77. Shen TY, Winter CA. Chemical and biological studies on indomethacin, sulindac and their analogs. Adv Drug Res 1977; 12:89–245.
78. Light DR, Waxman DJ, Walsh C. Studies on the chirality of sulphoxidation catalysed by bacterial flavoenzyme cyclohexanone monooxygenase and hog liver flavin adenine dinucleotide containing monooxygenase. Biochemistry 1982; 21:2490–8.
79. Demerson CA, Humber LG, Abraham NA, Schilling G, Martel RR, Pace-Asciak C. Resolution of etodolac and anti-inflammatory and prostaglandin synthetase inhibition properties of the enantiomers. J Med Chem 1983; 26:1778–80.
80. Bradley JD, Rudy AC, Katz BP, Ryan SI, Kalasinski LA, Brater DC, Hall SD, Brandt KD. Correlation of serum concentrations of ibuprofen stereoisomers with clinical response in the treatment of hip and knee osteoarthritis. J Rheumatol 1992; 19:130–4.
81. Cox SR, Brown MA, Squires DJ, Murrill EA, Lednicer D, Knuth DW. Comparative human study of ibuprofen enantiomer plasma concentrations produced by two commercially available ibuprofen tablets. Biopharm Drug Dispos 1988; 9:539–49.

II

Toxicity of Nonsteroidal Anti-Inflammatory Drugs

8

Lower Bowel Toxicity of Nonsteroidal Anti-Inflammatory Drugs

INGVAR BJARNASON, ANDREW MACPHERSON,
and SIVAGURUNATHAN SOMASUNDARAM
King's College Hospital
London, England

JEREMY HAYLLAR
Mt. Isa Base Hospital
Queensland, Australia

I. INTRODUCTION

The ingestion of nonsteroidal anti-inflammatory drugs (NSAIDs) is associated with significant morbidity and mortality resulting from adverse effects throughout the gastrointestinal tract (1–5). Most attention has been given to the gastroduodenal side effects, for which the magnitude of the problem has recently been clarified. There is a 10–30% point prevalence of ulcers in patients taking NSAIDs which, like any other ulcer, have the potential to bleed and perforate. For every 500–800 prescriptions of NSAIDs, one patient may experience a major complication that has a 10% mortality risk (6–9). The Food and Drug Administration (FDA) estimates that there are 200,000 major complications in the United States annually (10) and, in the United Kingdom, the corresponding figure is 30,000 (8). There is little relation between symptoms and damage (11–14), and a proportion of cases are asymptomatic. It has been suggested that NSAIDs are an important cause of sudden apparently unexplained deaths in elderly patients (15).

The gastroduodenal complications, because they are easily documented, have overshadowed the fact that the small and large intestine may be adversely affected even more often by NSAIDs than the gastroduodenal mucosa (4,5,16–22). The lower bowel toxicity of NSAIDs contributes significantly to many management problems in patients with chronic arthritides. It affects their quality of life and, at times, may lead to life-threatening complications. A systematic approach to the elucidation of the side effects of NSAIDs on the small intestine has been possible only because of the development and application of highly specific and sensitive investigational techniques (23). Widespread acceptance of the results has been confounded by the belief that the intestine plays a pathogenic role in rheumatoid arthritis and other arthropathies (24–33).

II. THE INTESTINE IN RHEUMATIC DISEASES

It is important to consider the possible effects of age on intestinal function. Although age alone has not been implicated in major alterations of gastrointestinal function, there may be subtle changes in villus architecture, but these are insufficient to cause malabsorption (34–39). The intestinal barrier function is preserved (40,41), but other age-related diseases, such as atherosclerosis, diverticulosis, motility disturbances, bacterial overgrowth, or concomitant medication, may enhance any potentially noxious effects of NSAIDs.

The possible interactions between joint disease and the intestine form a subject of great interest (24–33). Although osteoarthritis is confined to the joints, it has long been suspected that the intestine plays a pathogenic role in rheumatoid arthritis. Historically, this goes back to the 19th century when William Hunter's theory of "focal sepsis" led to the practice of tonsillectomy and even colectomy in the vain search for a cure and, when unsuccessful, to vaccine therapy (42). Enthusiasm was flamed when Svartz discovered that sulfasalazine was an effective form of treatment for rheumatoid arthritis (43,44). It now appears, however, that the beneficial effect is mediated through the immunological action of systemically absorbed sulfapyridine, rather than its antimicrobial properties (45,46).

There have been no large studies of intestinal function in patients with rheumatoid arthritis untreated by NSAIDs, and such studies are now hampered by these agents' early and widespread use. Current limited evidence does, however, suggest that the small and large intestine are morphologically and functionally normal in patients with untreated rheumatoid arthritis (16,17,23,24).

The situation in ankylosing spondylitis is clearly different. A proportion of patients (30–70%) have histological evidence of a terminal ileitis (24,27,47). It is suggested that this may be acute or chronic, according to the genetic background. Although considered subclinical, ileal inflammation may correlate with joint disease activity. Although the correlation appears to have sound basis, there is little evidence of a cause-and-effect relation between the two, despite widespread speculation. The other importance of the terminal ileitis in ankylosing spondylitis and reactive arthropathies is that it is easily confused with the effect of NSAIDs on the small intestine by the uninitiated. As far as we know, NSAIDs do not affect the terminal ileum (in either rheumatoid arthritis or the reactive arthropathies).

III. SPECIFIC SMALL-INTESTINAL DAMAGE

A. Nonsteroidal Anti-Inflammatory Drug Enteropathy

Four different groups have independently and unequivocally shown that ingestion of NSAIDs causes small-intestinal inflammation in 60–70% of patients receiving the drugs long-term (16,20,48,49). Initially, the inflammation was demonstrated with the use of indium 111-labeled autologous leukocytes. The technique involves taking 60 ml of the patient's blood, isolating the neutrophils by sedimentation and centrifugation, and incubating the cells with indium 111 together with an ionophore such as tropolone. If done properly, the neutrophils maintain their function so that on reinjection they migrate to the sites of acute inflammation. Abdominal scintigrams are obtained for localization of disease and a 40-day fecal collection is done to quantitate the indium 111 excretion, and this correlates with detailed histological disease activity assessment in patients with classic inflammatory bowel disease (50). The technique is currently thought to be the method of choice to assess disease activity in Crohn's disease, for which it gives information that is unobtainable by other means.

Patients with rheumatoid or osteoarthritis untreated by NSAIDs have entirely normal indium 111 fecal excretion. Fifty percent of those receiving NSAIDs regularly for more than 6 months have scintigraphic evidence of small-intestinal inflammation, and 65–70% are clearly abnormal when the stools are analyzed (Fig. 1). The inflammation is usually low-grade, comparable with that found in quiescent inflammatory bowel disease and may take up to 18 months to clear on discontinuing the NSAID (17). All NSAIDs appear to be equally associated with the inflammation in the small number of patients examined, and quantitatively, to a similar extent, apart from aspirin, which does so only rarely. This is of interest, as aspirin is clearly quite toxic to the gastroduodenal mucosa. The importance of individual drugs and dose, the patients compliance, whether ingested with food or not, and the particular drug delivery system is, however, difficult to assess, and it should be emphasized that the foregoing information is deduced from a patient group that has received a variety of NSAIDs in the past. The precise localization of the inflammation is not easily obtained from the scintigrams, although kinetic studies suggested that the main damage was in the mid-small intestine, similar to that seen in experimental animals. More recently, this has been further substantiated at enteroscopy with direct visualization of a range of lesions from hemorrhagic blebs, to frank ulceration, in the mid-small intestine of patients receiving NSAIDs (20).

The inflammation caused by NSAIDs is of theoretical importance because of the similarities with that of classic inflammatory bowel disease, but the practical importance lies in the associated complications.

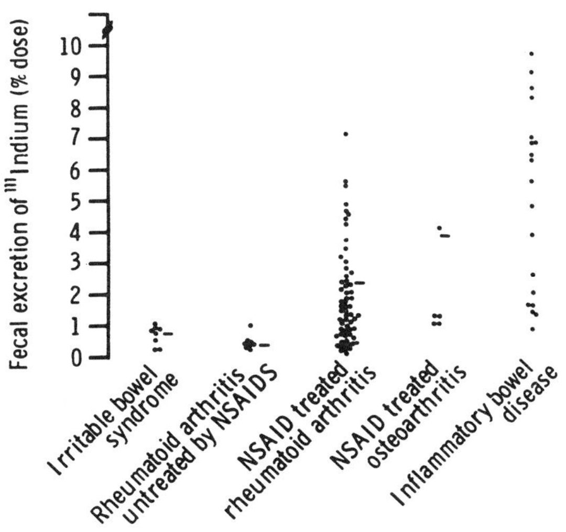

Figure 1 Intestinal inflammation, as assessed by the 4-day fecal excretion of indium 111-labeled autologous neutrophils, showing that patients with the irritable bowel syndrome and patients with rheumatoid arthritis untreated by NSAIDs have no significant intestinal inflammation (normal<1% of the administered dose). Patients treated with NSAIDs for over 6 months often (70%) have small-intestinal inflammation, at times, comparable with that of patients with active inflammatory bowel disease.

B. Complications

1. *Bleeding*

More than 50% of rheumatoid patients taking NSAIDs who have anemia of chronic disease have coexisting iron deficiency, and a significant number of patients will develop a pure iron-deficiency anemia (51–53). The pathogenesis of the iron deficiency is clearly multifactorial and involves reduced food intake, reduced gastric acid secretion, and an inability to increase iron absorption from the small intestine. Furthermore, there is evidence of increased intestinal blood loss, but its origin is often uncertain (54–56). Certainly, a satisfactory explanation is found only rarely at gastroscopy or at colonoscopy. Two lines of evidence suggests that the small intestine is the main site of bleeding in patients taking NSAIDs. Thirty-two patients underwent dual labeling of neutrophils with indium 111 and of red cells with technetium 99m, followed by abdominal scintigraphy to localize the inflammation and the blood loss. All 19 patients with NSAID-induced small-intestinal inflammation had identical abnormal localization of red cells, indicating that they were bleeding from the inflammatory site (21). Second, inflammation and blood loss was quantitated by a 5-day stool collection in 32 patients taking NSAIDs. There was a significant correlation ($R = 0.59$, $P < 0.01$) between inflammation and bleeding. These patients also underwent gastroscopy, but neither macro- nor microscopic damage correlated with the inflammation or the blood loss. Indeed, patients with gastric or duodenal ulcers had blood loss similar to those who were normal (57).

These studies have established that patients with NSAID enteropathy bleed from the small bowel, and this is a major site of chronic, mild (2–10 ml/day) blood loss in patients taking NSAIDs. The clinical importance is that the blood loss contributes to the iron deficiency that is so common in these patients. There are also practical financial implications. It is often a matter of routine to test stools for occult blood in patients with an iron-deficiency anemia. When positive it gives rise to a gastroenterological opinion, followed by normal gastroscopy in 70% of patients taking NSAIDs, who will then often be subjected to colonoscopy or a barium enema to exclude polyps or malignancy. The expense encountered is not trivial because of the sheer number of patients, and a more cost-effective approach is needed.

2. *Protein Loss*

Ten percent of patients with rheumatoid arthritis who require hospitalization have hypoalbuminemia. An early study described a protein-losing enteropathy in such patients that was attributed to intestinal amyloidosis (58). Reduced hepatic synthesis was also sometimes held responsible, but the evidence, at best, was circumstantial. The relation between NSAID-induced small-intestinal inflammation and protein loss was studied, in nine patients, by the simultaneous use of indium 111 leukocytes and chromium 51 labeling of proteins (21). All six patients with NSAID enteropathy had a protein-losing enteropathy. One had hypoalbuminemia and was losing over 300 ml of plasma into the intestine a day. These studies establish the small intestine as a possible important site of protein loss in patients taking NSAIDs and suggest a potentially treatable cause for severe hypoalbuminemia, which can be so troublesome in these patients.

3. *Ileal Dysfunction*

Ileal dysfunction was specifically sought in 20 patients with the most severe enteropathy, using a new dual radioisotope technique (17,59). This involved whole-body retention measurement of simultaneously administered ^{58}Co-vitamin B_{12} and ^{75}Se-HCAT (selena

25-labeled homocholic acid, a stabile synthetic bile acid), both of which are absorbed selectively from the ileum. The vitamin B_{12} absorption was normal, but 13 of 20 had bile acid malabsorption. The clinical implications are less important because the patients were asymptomatic (although ileal dysfunction may predispose to gallstones) (60).

4. *Small-Intestinal Strictures*

The most striking complication of NSAID enteropathy is the intestinal stricture. The pathology varies from relatively nonspecific fibrous ulceration to "diaphragm disease," which is pathognomonic of NSAID damage (61–68). Diaphragm disease of the small intestine consist of multiple (*N*, 3–70), symmetric, concentric septatelike narrowings. Their thickness is 2–4 mm and, histologically, they are composed of submucosal fibrosis, with a normal overlying mucosa, except at the villus tip, where there may be some inflammation. The strictures are located mainly in the mid–small intestine and are notoriously difficult to diagnose. The symptoms of subacute intestinal obstruction are intermittent and difficult to elicit, particularly if the patient has dyspepsia or other nonspecific abdominal discomfort. Unlike the strictures of Crohn's disease, intestinal lymphoma, or following potassium supplements, diaphragm disease does not distort the bowel wall. Accordingly, small-intestinal radiology is often thought to be normal, but with hindsight, slitlike narrowings are evident. The strictures may even be missed at surgery unless specifically sought. In the future, enteroscopy may prove the most sensitive investigation.

C. Pathogenesis of Nonsteroidal Anti-Inflammatory Drug Enteropathy

The foregoing studies show that the small intestine is an important site of NSAID-related damage to the gastrointestinal tract. The NSAID-induced enteropathy is a disease in its own right, affecting 60–70% of patients taking these drugs long-term (using indium III scanning). The pathogenesis is not fully understood, but there is sufficient data to propose a multistep mechanism. Thus, it can be simplified to early metabolic or biochemical effects, which are specific to NSAIDs, and the late effects, which are relatively nonspecific, but account for most of the macroscopic damage.

During drug absorption, there is a high local concentration of NSAID, which exerts its full metabolic effect. The earliest damage in rats is evident biochemically and on electron microscopy within hours of administration (69,70). Mitochondria seem to be the principal organelles involved, showing increased activities of succinate dehydrogenase. On electron microscopy, there is striking ballooning and vacuolization of the mitochondria. This is indicative of a heightened respiratory chain activity. Endoplasmic reticulum is also affected, but at a later stage. Although these changes are seen in the stomach, as well as throughout the small intestine, they are most pronounced in the mid-small intestine. It has been suggested that the main biochemical effect, accounting for these changes, may be a combination of NSAID-induced uncoupling of oxidative phosphorylation and inhibition of cytochrome *C* oxidase, the main mitochondrial peroxidase (71). This may lead to a heightened activity of the tricarboxylic acid cycle, with an increased flow of electrons down the respiratory chain, forming oxygen-reactive species that would ordinarily be channeled through cytochrome *C* oxidase.

There are several ways that secondary cytosolic damage could occur as a consequence. In any event, the cell becomes depleted of ATP and loses control over its intercellular junctions. Repair of the damaged mucosal cells is hampered by NSAID inhibition of cyclooxygenase. The lack of prostaglandins generation, with their effects on mucus production, blood flow, and reepithelization, may be particularly important for persistence of the ultrastructural damage. The final consequence of these biochemical alterations is that the mucosa is compromised on an ultrastructural level, which manifests itself as loss of mucosal integrity or increased intestinal permeability. What follows is a nonspecific interplay between the luminal aggressive factors and the response of the compromised mucosa. The consequence of increased permeability is that the mucosa is exposed to luminal toxins. In the small intestine these are bile acids, pancreatic juices, bacteria and their degradation products, and others, and in the stomach, acid and pepsin. In humans the loss of the integrity of the intercellular junctions in the small intestine is evident within 12 h of NSAID administration as increased intestinal permeability to ^{51}Cr-EDTA (72–77). The increased permeability relates to the potency of NSAID inhibition of cyclooxygenase and is partially prevented by concomitant prostaglandin administration. Pro-NSAID do not increase intestinal permeability and a glucose–citrate formulation of indomethacin is almost completely protective, but the mechanism is unknown (78,79). There is now compelling evidence that a metronidazole-sensitive bacteria is the main neutrophil chemoattractant in NSAID enteropathy (80). Once the neutrophils are in contact with the chemoattractant, there is immediate tissue damage from oxygen-reactive species and lysosomal enzyme release, and it seems likely that the complications of blood and protein loss are a direct result of the neutrophil-mediated damage. The same mechanism appears to be responsible in the stomach, but the neutrophil chemoattractant has not been characterized here. It follows that if neutrophils can be prevented from responding to the chemoattractant, the damage would be reduced. However, this is a late event in the pathogenesis of NSAID-related damage to the intestinal mucosa, and it may be more profitable to focus on means to prevent the earlier damage.

Prevention and Treatment

There is now no proved way of preventing NSAID enteropathy, although in theory, it may be that concomitant prostaglandins, pro-NSAID, or formulations with micronutrients, all of which minimize the initial changes in permeability, may reduce the prevalence and severity of the lesions (73,74,78,79).

Treating established cases of NSAID enteropathy is more straightforward. Sulfasalazine reduces both the inflammation and blood loss in most patients, but rarely normalizes the intestine (81). Metronidazole is equally, if not more, effective, but the frequency of neuropathy limits its long-term use (80). In the patient with problematic hypoalbuminemia it is certainly worth trying, as there is currently no other effective treatment.

IV. NONSPECIFIC SMALL-INTESTINAL DAMAGE

There are a few individual case reports of sulindac and mefenamic acid causing malabsorption, with subtotal villus atrophy resembling celiac disease (82–84). Others have found a high prevalence of malabsorption in patients with rheumatoid arthritis who are taking NSAIDs (85,86). The relation to the enteropathy is unclear, as in the short-term, NSAIDs do not appear to alter active or passive carrier-mediated transport (87). The severity of the malabsorption, however, is insufficient by itself to cause malnutrition.

Indomethacin has caused small-intestinal perforations in infants when used to close a patent ductus arteriosus (88–90). Several perforations were reported with the indomethacin sodium salt trihydrate (Osmosin), since withdrawn from the market (91–94). This preparation used potassium bicarbonate to release indomethacin. It is thought that the capsules may have stuck to the mucosa, and the high local concentration of either indomethacin or potassium could have caused the damage. The magnitude of these problems is uncertain. Langman et al. found, in a retrospective review, that a significant proportion of patients with small-intestinal perforations and bleeding were taking NSAIDs (95). By the nature of the study, the mechanisms are unclear, and it is not known whether these events are the consequence of the enteropathy. By analogy with peptic ulcer disease, it would seem likely that small-bowel ulceration is a prerequisite for these life-threatening events. These serious complications arising from the small intestine, however, are uncommon (96,97).

V. NONSTEROIDAL ANTI-INFLAMMATORY DRUG–INDUCED COLONIC DAMAGE

The large intestine is, by comparison, only rarely affected by NSAIDs. Inflammation, as found in the small intestine, does not occur, possibly because of the low concentration of NSAID reaching the colon.

Some publications suggest that NSAIDs may cause an aggressive form of diverticulitis, with fistulas and perforation (98–104). The mechanism is unclear, but in early reports, undissolved tablets were found in or near the perforated diverticula. Most episodes of diverticulitis are not caused by NSAIDs; similarly, a proportion of patients with colonic bleeding are taking NSAIDs, but most are not. Patients taking NSAIDs may rarely develop isolated colonic ulcers, with nonspecific histological findings (105–109). These resemble the more common benign idiopathic colonic ulcers (110), but both conditions remain so rare that they are a medical curiosity. Rectal administration of NSAIDs is attractive because, in theory, it avoids exposing the gastroduodenal mucosa to high concentrations of NSAID. This is not, however, the case in practice, as a significant amount of most circulating NSAID is excreted in bile. Rectal administration of NSAID is also associated with local irritation. Up to 50% of patients stop treatment because of difficulties in retaining the suppositories, pain and irritation, loose movements, and bleeding (111). On average 10–30% of patients have distressing side effects (112,113). Locally administered NSAID may cause a nonspecific proctitis with bleeding, and a recent report describes eight cases of rectal ulceration and strictures following aspirin and acetaminophen (paracetamol) suppositories (114,115).

The NSAIDs may cause more specific damage. Fenemates (mefenamic and flufenamic acid) frequently cause diarrhea. When this occurs early in the treatment, the patient may be aware of the termporal relationship and discontinue the drugs. More often diarrhea occurs after months of treatment, and it is under these circumstances that the patient continues treatment and develops a colitis. In the reported cases, the extent of disease has ranged from a proctitis to a pancolitis (116–121).

Histologically it may resemble ulcerative colitis, but more often, the picture is of a nonspecific colitis. There is full symptomatic and histological recovery on stopping the fenemates, and patients tolerate other NSAIDs, suggesting that the inflammation occurs by an action of the drug that is not common to all NSAIDs.

Four patients have developed a colitis after other NSAIDs (ibuprofen, naproxen, and two piroxicam) (121). The rarity of colitis is also shown by Mielants et al., who found no colitis on colonoscopic biopsy in over 250 patients taking NSAIDs (24,27,47).

Patients with rheumatoid arthritis, taking NSAIDs with a coexisting colitis, often have continuous chronic active colitis, which is difficult to control without the use of corticosteroids. The NSAIDs have now also been implicated in the relapse of inflammatory bowel disease (122–126). The mechanism is uncertain, but it seems that most of the factors that do cause relapse of inflammatory bowel disease (alcohol, NSAID, infections, and such) share an action to increase intestinal permeability. This may allow mucosal exposure to luminal antigens and neutrophil chemoattractants (127). In normal subjects this leads to low-grade inflammation, but in inflammatory bowel disease, a major relapse occurs because of the heightened immunological response, which may indeed be the primary abnormality in patients with ulcerative colitis and with Crohn's disease (128).

In summary, the idea of site-specific gastric and duodenal damage caused by NSAIDs is misleading and incorrect. Indeed, the small intestine appears to be more frequently adversely affected by ingestion of NSAIDs than the stomach. The complacency concerning the lower bowel damage stems from several factors. The inflammation in the small intestine contributes to the morbidity of patients with rheumatoid arthritis and other arthropathies, but the complications are not usually life-threatening. Pharmaceutical companies, many of whom have made a significant contribution in identifying the problem in the upper gastrointestinal tract, have not been particularly interested in the prevention: and treatment of small-intestinal inflammation is not as simple or straightforward as in the stomach and certainly not as profitable. Finally, the investigation of the small intestine is expensive and demanding. Nevertheless, the realization of NSAIDs enteropathy and the potential side effects of NSAIDs on the large bowel may lead to better patient care in the long term.

REFERENCES

1. CMS Update. Non-steroidal anti-inflammatory drugs and serious gastrointestinal adverse reactions. Br Med J 1986; 292:614.
2. Kurata JH, Elashoff JD, Grossman MI. Inadequacy of the literature on the relationship between drugs, ulcers, and gastrointestinal bleeding. Gastroenterology 1982; 82:373–82.
3. Langman MJS. Epidemiologic evidence on the association between peptic ulceration and antiinflammatory drugs. Gastroenterology 1989; 96:640–6.
4. Rampton D. Non-steroidal anti-inflammatory drugs and the lower gastrointestinal tract. Scand J Gastroenterol 1987;22:1–4.
5. Bjarnason I, Price AB. The effects of non-steroidal anti-inflammatory drugs on the large intestine. GI Futures Cln Pract 1988; 3:7–10.
6. Walt R, Katschinsky B, Logan R, Ashley J, Langman M. Rising frequency of ulcer perforation in elderly people in the United Kingdom. Lancet 1986; 1:489–92.
7. Somerville K, Faulkner G, Langman M. Non-steroidal anti-inflammatory drugs and bleeding peptic ulcer. Lancet 1986; 1:462–4.
8. Beardon PHG, Brown SV, Mcdevitt DG. Gastrointestinal events in patients prescribed NSAID's: a controlled study using record linkage in Tayside. Q J Med 1989; 71:497–505.
9. Cockel R. NSAIDs—should every prescription carry a government health warning? Gut 1987; 28:515–8.
10. Armstrong CP, Blower AC. Non-steroidal anti-inflammatory drugs and life threatening complications of peptic ulceration. Gut 1987; 28:527–32.
11. Rooney P, Bjarnason I. NSAID enteropathy: not just a pain in the stomach. J Rheumatol 1991; 18:796–8.
12. Quinn CM, Price AB, Bjarnason I. Endoscopic and microscopic findings in symptomatic and asymptomatic patients on long term non-steroidal anti-inflammatory drugs. Gastroenterology 1990; 98:A109.

13. Mellem R, Stave R, Myren J, Osnes M, Hansen LE. Symptoms in patients with peptic ulcer and haematemesis and/or melena related to the use of NSAIDs. Scand J Gastroenterol 1985; 20:1246–8.
14. Collins AJ, Davies J, Dixon A St J. Contrasting presentation and findings between patients with rheumatic complaints taking NSAIDs and general population referred for endoscopy. Br J Rheumatol 1986; 25:50–3.
15. FDC Reports. November 29, 1987:8–9.
16. Bjarnason I, Williams P, So A, Zanelli G, Levi AJ, Gumpel MJ, Peters TJ, Ansell B. Intestinal permeability and inflammation in rheumatoid arthritis; effects of nonsteroidal anti-inflammatory drugs. Lancet 1984; 2:1171–4.
17. Bjarnason I, Zanelli G, Smith T, Prouse, P, De Lacey G, Gumpel MJ, Levi AJ. Nonsteroidal antiinflammatory drug induced inflammation in humans. Gastroenterology 1987; 93:480–9.
18. Bjarnason I, Macpherson A. The changing gastrointestinal side effect profile of non-steroidal anti-inflammatory drugs. A new approach for the prevention of a new problem. Scand J Gastroenterol 1989; 24 (suppl 163):56–64.
19. Bjarnason I, Smethurst P, Hayllar J, Levi AJ. NSAID enteropathy; the main site of chronic blood loss in patients on NSAIDs. Gut 1990; 91:A1203.
20. Morris J, Madhok R, Sturrock RD, Capell HA, Mackenzie JF. Enteroscopic diagnosis of small bowel ulceration in patients receiving non steroidal anti-inflammatory drugs. Lancet 1991; 337:520.
21. Bjarnason I, Zanelli G, Prouse P, Smethurst P, Smith T, Levi S, Gumpel MJ, Levi AJ. Blood and protein loss via small intestinal inflammation induced by nonsteroidal anti-inflammatory drugs. Lancet. 1987; 2:711–4.
22. Lang J, Price AB, Levi AJ, Burk M, Gumpel JM, Bjarnason I. Diaphragm disease: the pathology of non-steroidal anti-inflammatory drug induced small intestinal strictures. J Clin Pathol 1988; 41:516–26.
23. Bjarnason I. Non-steroidal anti-inflammatory drug induced small intestinal inflammation in man. In: Pounder R, ed. Recent advances in gastroenterology—7. London: Churchill-Livingstone, 1988:23–46.
24. Mielants H, Veys EM, Cuvelier C, De Vos M, Botelberge L. HLA-B27 related arthritis and bowel inflammation. Part 2. Ileocolonoscopy and bowel histology in patients with HLA-B27 related arthritis. J Rheumatol 1984; 12:294–8.
25. Walker AW, Isselbacher KJ. Uptake and transport of macromolecules by the intestine. Possible role in clinical disorders. Gastroenterology 1974; 67:531–50.
26. Svartz N. Sulphasalazine II. Some notes on the discovery and development of salazopyrin. Am J Gastroenterol 1988; 83:497–503.
27. Mielants H, Veys EM, Cuvelier C, De Vos M. Ileocolonoscopic findings in seronegative spondylarthropathies. Br J Rheumatol 1988; 27(suppl 11):95–105.
28. Editorial. Rheumatoid arthritis and the gut. Br Med J 1979; 278:1104.
29. Zaphiropoulus GC. Rheumatoid arthritis and the gut. Br J Rheumatol 1986; 15:138–9.
30. Bjarnason I, Peters TJ. Helping the mucosa make sense of macromolecules. Gut 1987; 28:1057–61.
31. Prendergast JH, Sullivan JS, Csczy A, Upfold LI, Edmunds JP, Bashir HV, Reiss-Levy E. Possible role of enteric organisms in the pathogenesis of ankylosing spondylitis and other seronegative arthropathies. Infect Immun 1983; 41:935–41.
32. Ebringer A. The cross tolerance hypothesis, HLA-B27 and ankylosing spondylitis. Br J Rheumatol 1983; 22 (suppl 2):53–66.
33. Keat A. Reiter's syndrome and reactive arthritis in perspective. N Engl J Med 1983; 309:1605–15.
34. Corazza GR, Frazzoni M, Gatto MR, Gasbarrini O. Ageing and small bowel mucosa: a morphometric study. Gerontology 1986; 32:60–5.
35. Webster SGP. Small bowel morphology and function. In: Hellemans J, Vantrappen G, eds. Gastrointestinal tract disorders in the elderly. Edinburgh: Churchill-Livingstone, 1984; 85–95.

36. Webster SGP, Leeming JT. The appearance of the small bowel mucosa in old age. Age Aging 1975; 4:168–74.
37. Warren PM, Pepperman MA, Montgomery RD. Age changes in small-intestinal mucosa. Lancet 1978; 2:849–50.
38. Haeny MR, Cluank LS, Montgomery RD, Sammonds HG. Evaluation of xylose absorption as measured in blood and urine; a one-hour blood xylose screening test in malabsorption. Gastroenterology 1978; 75:393–400.
39. McEvoy AN, Fenwick JD, Boddy K, James OFW. Vitamin B_{12} absorption from the gut does not decline with age in normal elderly humans. Age Ageing 1982; 11:180–3.
40. Saweirs WM, Andrews DJ, Low-Beer TS. The double sugar test of intestinal permeability in the elderly. Age Ageing 1985; 14:312–5.
41. Black DA. Intestinal permeability in the elderly. Dig Dis Sci 1988; 33:382.
42. Bywaters ELG. Historical aspects of the aetiology of rheumatoid arthritis. Br J Rheumatol 1988; 27(suppl 2):110–5.
43. Svartz N. Salazopyrin, a new sulfonamide preparation. Acta Med Scand 1942; 110:577–98.
44. Svartz N. The treatment of rheumatoid poly-arthritis with azo compounds. Rheumatism 1948; 4:56–60.
45. Pullar T, Hunter JA, Capell HA. Which component of sulphasalazine is active in rheumatoid arthritis? Br Med J 1985; 290:1535–8.
46. Taggart AJ, Neuman VC, Hill J, Astbury C, Gallez PL, Dixon JS. 5-Aminosalicylic acid or sulphapyridine. Which is the active moiety of sulphasalazine in rheumatoid arthritis? Drugs 1986; 32(suppl 1):27–34.
47. Mielants H, Veys EM, DeVos M, Cuvelier C. Gut inflammation in the pathogenesis of idiopathic forms of reactive arthritis and in the peripheral joint involvement of ankylosing spondylitis. In: Mielants H, Veys EM, eds. Spondylarthropathies. Involvement of the gut. Amsterdam: Excerpta Medica, 1987:11–21.
48. Segal AW, Isenberg DA, Hajirousow V, Toffree S, Clark J, Snaith SM. Preliminary evidence for gut involvement in the pathogenesis of rheumatoid arthritis? Br J Rheumatol. 1986; 25:162–6.
49. Rooney PJ, Jenkins RT, Smith KM, Coates G. 111-Indium–labelled polymorphonuclear leucocyte scans in rheumatoid arthritis—an important clinical cause of false positive results. Br J Rheumatol 1986; 25:167–70.
50. Saverymuttu SH, Camillery M, Rees H, Lavender JP, Hodgson HJF. 111-Indium granulocyte scanning with colonoscopy, histology and faecal 111-indium excretion in assessing disease extent and activity in colitis. Gastroenterology 1986; 90:1121–8.
51. Cartwright GE, Lee GR. The anaemia of chronic disorders. Br J Haematol 1972; 21:147–52.
52. Hansen TM, Hansen NE, Birgens HS, Holund B, Lorenzen I. Serum ferritin and the assessment of iron deficiency in rheumatoid arthritis. Scand J Gastroenterol 1983; 12:353–9.
53. Vreugdenhill G, Wognum AW, Van Eijk HG, Swaak AJ. Anaemia in rheumatoid arthritis: the role of iron, vitamin B_{12}, for folic acid deficiency, and erythropoietin responsiveness. Ann Rheum Dis 1990; 49:93–8.
54. Collins AJ, Davies J, Dixon ASJ. Contrasting presentation and findings between patients with rheumatic complaints taking non-steroidal anti-inflammatory drugs and a general population referred for endoscopy. Br J Rheumatol 1986; 25:50–3.
55. Weber G, Werre JM, Julius HW, Marx JM. Decreased iron absorption in patients with active rheumatoid arthritis, with and without iron deficiency. Ann Rheum Dis 1988; 47:404–9.
56. Boddy K, Will G. Iron absorption in rheumatoid arthritis. Ann Rheum Dis 1969; 28:537–70.
57. Bjarnason I, Smethurst P, Hayllar J, Levi AJ. NSAID enteropathy; the main site of chronic blood loss in patients on NSAIDs. Gut 1990; 91:A1203.
58. Plantini LO, Strandberg O. Gastrointestinal protein loss in rheumatoid arthritis, studied with 51-chromic chloride and 125-I albumin. Scand J Rheumatol 1974; 3:169–73.
59. Smith T, Bjarnason I, Hesp R. Critical analysis of a combined test (^{75}SeHCAT and ^{58}CoVit B_{12}) of ileal function using whole body counter. J Clin Phys Physiol Meas 1987; 8:159–71.

60. Carey MC, Leighton LS. Formation of cholesterol gallstones. In: Boucher IAD, Allan RN, Hodgson HJF, Keighley MRB, eds. Textbook of gastroenterology. London: Bailliere Tindall, 1988; 1389–400.
61. Sturges HF, Krone CL. Ulcers and strictures of the jejunum in a patient on long term indomethacin therapy. Am J Gastroenterol 1973; 59:162–9.
62. Venturatos SG, Hines C, Blalock JB. Ulceration of the small intestine in a patient with coeliac disease. South Med J 1984; 77:520–2.
63. Neoptolemos JP, Locke TJ. Recurrent small bowel obstruction associated with phenylbutazone. Br J Surg 1983; 70:244–5.
64. Madhok R, Mackenzie JA, Lee FD, Bruckner FE, Terry TR, Sturrock RD. Small bowel ulceration in patients receiving NSAIDs for rheumatoid arthritis. Q J Med 1986; 58:53–8.
65. Saverymuttu SH, Thomas A, Grundy A, Maxwell JD. Ileal stricturing after long term indomethacin treatment. Postgrad Med J 1986; 62:267–8.
66. Sukumar L. Recurrent small bowel obstruction with piroxicam. Br J Surg 1987; 74:186.
67. Johnson F. Recurrent small bowel obstruction with piroxicam. Br J Surg 1987;74:654.
68. Bjarnason I, Price AB, Zanelli G, Smethurst P, Burke M, Gumpel MJ, Levi AJ. Clinico-pathological features of NSAID induced small intestinal strictures. Gastroenterology 1988; 94:1070–74.
69. Hayllar J, Somasundaram S, Sarathchandra P, Levi AJ, Bjarnason I. Early cellular events in the pathogenesis of NSAID enteropathy in the rat. Gastroenterology 1991; 100:A216.
70. Hayllar J, Somasundaram S, Sarathchandra P, Levi AJ, Bjarnason I. The effect of synthetic prostaglandins, a glucose citrate formulation of indomethacin and other agents in preventing NSAID enteropathy in the rat. Gastroenterology 1991; 100:A586.
71. Somasundaram S, Hayllar J, Macpherson A, Bjarnason I. The biochemical basis of intestinal damage due to NSAIDs. A review and a hypothesis. (submitted).
72. Bjarnason I, Williams P, Smethurst P, Peters TJ, Lewis AJ. The effects of NSAID and prostaglandins on the permeability of the human small bowel. Gut 1986; 27:1292–7.
73. Bjarnason I, Smethurst P, Clarke P, Menzies IS, Levi AJ, Peters TJ. Effect of prostaglandins on indomethacin induced increased intestinal permeability in man. Scand J Gastroenterol 1989; 29 (suppl 164):97–103.
74. Bjarnason I, Smethurst P, Fenn CG, Lee CF, Menzies IS, Levi AJ. Misoprostol reduces indomethacin induced changes in human small intestinal permeability. Dig Dis Sci 1989; 34:407–11.
75. Jenkins RT, Rooney PJ, Jones DB, Bienenstock J, Goodacre RC. Increased intestinal permeability in patients with rheumatoid arthritis: a side effect of oral NSAID therapy? Br J Rheumatol 1987; 26:103–7.
76. Auer IO, Habscheid W, Hiller S, Gerhards W, Eilles C. Nicht-steroidale antiphlogistika erohen die darmpermeabilitat. Dsch Med Wochenschr 1987; 112:1032–7.
77. Aabakken C, Osnes M. 51-Cr ethylenediaminetetraacetic acid absorption test. Effects of naproxen, a NSAID. Scand J Gastroenterol 1990; 25:917–24.
78. Bjarnason I, Fehilly B, Smethurst P, Menzies IS, Levi AJ. The importance of local versus systemic effects of NSAID to increase small intestinal permeability in man. Gut 1991; 32:275–7.
79. Bjarnason I, Smethurst P, Walker F, Macpherson A, McElnay SC, Pearson P, Menzies IS. Glucose and citrate reduce the permeability changes caused by indomethacin. Gastroenterology (in press).
80. Bjarnason I, Turner-Stokes L, Smethurst P, Levi AJ, Gumpel MJ. Metronidazole reduces inflammation in NSAID enteropathy. Gastroenterology 1990; 98:A439.
81. Bjarnason I, Hopkinson N, Zanelli G, Prouse P, Snethurst P, Gumpel MJ, Jevi AJ. The treatment of NSAID induced enteropathy. Gut 1990; 31:777–80.
82. Freeman HJ. Sulindac-associated small bowel lesion. J Clin Gastroenterol 1986; 8:569–71.
83. Hall RI, Petty AH, Cobden I, Lendrum R. Enteritis and colitis associated with mefenamic acid. Br Med J 1983; 287:1182.

84. Isaacs PET, Sladen GE, Filpie I. Mefenamic acid enteropathy. J Clin Pathol 1987; 40:121–7.
85. Kendall MJ, Hawkins CF. Xylose test; effects of aspirin and indomethacin. Br Med J 1971; i:533–5.
86. Dyer NH, Kendall MJ, Hawkins CF. Malabsorption in rheumatoid arthritis. Ann Rheum Dis 1971; 30:626–30.
87. Bjarnason I, Smethurst P, Menzies IS, Peters TJ. The effect of polyacrylic acid polymers (carbacol) on small intestinal function and permeability changes caused by indomethacin. Scand J Gastroenterol 1991; 26:685–8.
88. Nagaraj HS, Sandhu AS, Cook LN, Buchuno JT, Groff DB. Gastrointestinal perforation following indomethacin in very low birth weight infants. J Paedriatr Surg 1981; 16:1003–7.
89. Alpan G, Eyal F, Vinograd I, Udassin R, Amir G, Mogle P, Glick B. Localized intestinal perforation after enteral administration of indomethacin in premature infants. J Pediatr 1985; 106:277–81.
90. Marshall TA. Intestinal perforation following enteral administration of indomethacin. J Pediatr 1985; 107:484–5.
91. Day TK. Intestinal perforation associated with slow release indomethacin capsules. Br Med J 1983; 287:1671–2.
92. Cree IA, Walker MA, Wright M, Forrester JS. Osmosin and ileal ulceration: a case report. Scot Med J 1985; 30:40–1.
93. Laidler P, Maslin SC, Gilhome RW. What's new in Osmosin and intestinal perforation? Pathol Res Pract 1985; 180:74–6.
94. Florence AT, Salole EG, Al-Dujaili H. Osmosin tablets. Pharm J 1984; March 17:308.
95. Langman MJS, Morgan L, Worrall A. Use of anti-inflammatory drugs by patients with small or large bowel perforation and haemorrhage. Br Med J 1985; 290:347–9.
96. Saw KC, Quick CRG, Higgins AF. Ileocaecal perforation and bleeding—are NSAID responsible? J R Soc Med 1990; 83:114–5.
97. Shack ME. Drug induced ulceration and perforation of the small bowel. Ariz Med 1966; 23:517–23.
98. Coutrot S, Roland D, Barbier J, Marq PVD, Matuchansky C. Acute perforation of colonic diverticula associated with short term indomethacin. Lancet 1978; 2:1055–6.
99. Stewart JT, Pennington CR, Pringle R. Br Med J. 1985; 290:787–8.
100. Tancer ML, Zahiruddin S. Diagnosis of sigmoidovaginal fistula by vaginogram. Obstet Gynecol 1966; 28:815–9.
101. Corder A. Steroids, NSAID and serious septic complications of diverticular disease. Br Med J 1987; 295:1238.
102. Finkelstein JA, Jamieson CG. An association between anti-inflammatory medication and internal pelvic fistulas. Dis Colon Rectum 1987; 30:168–70.
103. Wilson RG, Smith AN, Macintyre IMC. Complications of diverticular disease and NSAID: a prospective study. Br J Surg 1990; 77:1103–4.
104. Campbell K, Steele RJC. NSAID and complicated diverticular disease; a case controlled study. Br J Surg 1990; 77:1418.
105. Debenham GP. Ulcer of the caecum during oxyphenylbutazone (Tanderil) therapy. Can Med Assoc J 1966; 94:1182–4.
106. Charuzi I, Ovnat A, Zirkin H, Peiser J, Sukewik S. Ibuprofen and benign cecal ulcer. J Rheumatol 1985; 12:188–9.
107. Uribe A, Johansson C, Scezak P, Rubio C. Ulceration of the colon associated with naproxen and acetylsalicylic acid treatment. Gastrointest Endosc 1986; 32:242–4.
108. Bravo AC, Lowman RM. Benign ulcer of sigmoid colon. Radiology 1968; 90:113–5.
109. Carson J, Notis WM, Orris ES. Colonic ulceration and bleeding during diclofenac therapy. N Engl J Med 1990; 323:135.
110. Shallman RW, Kuehner M, Williams GH, Sajjad S, Sautter R. Benign cecal ulcers. Dis Colon Rectum 1985; 28:732–7.
111. Woolf DL. Indomethacin suppositories. Br Med J 1965; 1:1497.

112. Berryl H, Seinson D, Jones H, Hamilton EBD. Indomethacin and naproxen suppositories in the treatment of rheumatoid arthritis. Ann Rheum Dis 1978; 37:370–2.
113. Wright V, Hopkins R. A note on indomethacin suppositories in rheumatic conditions. Rheumatol Rehabil 1979; 18:186–7.
114. Levy N, Gaspar E. Rectal bleeding and indomethacin suppositories. Lancet 1975; 1:577.
115. Lanthier P, Detry R, Debongnie JC, Mahieu P, Vanheuverzwyn R. Solitary rectal lesions due to suppositories containing acetylsalicylic acid and paracetamol. Gastroenterol Clin Biol 1987; 11:250–3.
116. Phillips MS, Fehilly B, Stewart S, Dronfield WM Enteritis and colitis associated with mefenamic acid. Br Med J 1983; 287:1626–7.
117. Edwards AL, Heagerty AM, Bing RF. Enteritis and colitis associated with mefenamic acid. Br Med J 1983; 287:1627.
118. Rampton DS, Trapping PJ. Enteritis and colitis associated with mefenamic acid. Br. Med J 1983; 287:1627.
119. Williams R, Glazier G. Enteritis and colitis associated with mefenamic acid. Br Med J 1983; 287:1627.
120. Ravi S, Keat AC, Keat ECB. Colitis caused by NSAID. Postgrad Med J 1986; 62:773–6.
121. Tanner AR, Raghunat H. Colonic inflammation and NSAID administration. Digestion 1988; 41:116–20.
122. Kaufman HJ, Taubin. NSAID activate quiescent inflammatory bowel disease. Ann Intern Med 1987; 107:513–6.
123. Rampton DS, Sladen GE. Relapse of ulcerative protocolitis during treatment with NSAID. Postgrad Med J 1981; 57:297–9.
124. Rampton DS, McNeil NI, Sarner M. Analgesic ingestion and other factors preceding relapse in ulcerative colitis. Gut 1983; 24:187–9.
125. Schwartz HA. Lower gastrointestinal side effects of NSAID. J Rheumatol 1981; 8:952–4.
126. Walt RP, Hawkey CJ, Langman, MJ. Colitis associated with NSAID. Br Med J 1984; 288:238.
127. Teahon K, Smethurst P, Levi AJ, Bjarnason I. The effect of elemental diet on intestinal permeability and inflammation in Crohn's disease. Gastroenterology 1991; 101:84–9.
128. Duane P, Teahon K, Crabtree JE, Levi AJ, Heatley RV, Bjarnason I. The relationship between nutritional status and serum soluble interleukin-2 receptor concentration in patients with Crohn's disease treated with elemental diet. Clin Nutr 1991; 10:222–7.

9

Prevention and Treatment of Gastric and Duodenal Ulcers Induced by Nonsteroidal Anti-Inflammatory Drugs

ESAM Z. DAJANI*
G. D. Searle & Co.
and Northwestern University School of Medicine
Chicago, Illinois
and University of California at Los Angeles
Los Angeles, California

NAURANG M. AGRAWAL
Ochsner Clinic
New Orleans, Louisiana

I. INTRODUCTION

Nonsteroidal anti-inflammatory drugs (NSAIDs) are the most widely used therapy in rheumatic diseases. These drugs are known to cause gastrointestinal (GI) damage and have been implicated as a cause of peptic ulceration and life-threatening GI bleeding and perforation (1–4). Recent studies indicated that increased NSAID dosage results in clinically significant increased risk for serious ulcer disease (5). Meta-analysis of clinical trials that examined the risks of serious GI complication among NSAID users showed a three times greater relative risk among these users for developing serious adverse GI complication than for nonusers (6).

The NSAIDs must be used prudently to limit this toxicity. However, in many clinical situations, the reduction of NSAID dosages or use of only analgesic drugs are not helpful. Concomitant antiulcer agents with NSAID therapy is an important option that needs to be considered. This review covers the data derived from well-designed studies employed for the prevention and treatment of NSAID-induced GI toxicity.

II. PREVENTION OF NONSTEROIDAL ANTI-INFLAMMATORY DRUG-INDUCED ULCERS

The following discussion focuses on the prevention of NSAID-associated ulcers with various antiulcer drugs in patients maintained on NSAIDs. Only prospective, double-blind,

---

The opinions expressed by the authors represent their view on the subject. These are not official statements of either Ochsner Clinic, G. D. Searle & Co., Northwestern University, or the University of California at Los Angeles.

This chapter was adapted with permission from a recent report (40).

* Present affiliation: International Drug Development Consultants, A Division of Mid Gulf U.S.A., Inc. Long Grove, Illinois.

randomized studies will be reviewed. In all of these studies, an initial esophagogastroduodenal endoscopy must have shown the absence of esophageal, gastric, or duodenal ulcers.

A. Histamine (H_2) Receptor Antagonists

Two major prospective, placebo-controlled, double-blind studies examined the effect of ranitidine in the prevention of NSAID-induced gastric and duodenal ulcers (7,8). Since these two trials had similar study design, only one trial will be discussed in depth. Ehsanullah et al. conducted a study in 263 patients with various types of arthritis and normal upper GI endoscopies (7). The patients were treated with an NSAID and ranitidine (150 mg bid) or its matching placebo for 8 weeks. The NSAIDs administered included naproxen, ibuprofen, diclofenac, and indomethacin. Endoscopies were repeated at 4 and 8 weeks, and symptoms of dyspepsia were also recorded during 8 weeks of observation. The incidence of duodenal ulcer in patients receiving ranitidine plus NSAIDs was 1.5%, compared with 8% in the placebo group; ranitidine was more effective than placebo in preventing the development of duodenal ulcer ($p = 0.024$; Table 1). At 4 weeks, fewer ranitidine patients had developed a gastric ulcer compared with those receiving placebo (3 and 5%, respectively); however, at 8 weeks the percentages of gastric ulcer were similar (Table 2). The study did not support the efficacy of ranitidine in preventing NSAID-induced gastric ulcer. This study also examined the effect of ranitidine or placebo on GI symptoms; there were no significant differences between the two treatment groups in the relief of either dyspeptic symptoms or withdrawal because of GI symptoms. An unusual feature of this study was that the incidence of gastric ulcers was less than that of duodenal ulcer, which is inconsistent with other published studies. In general, the literature suggests a ratio of about 2:1 between gastric ulcers and duodenal ulcers secondary to NSAIDs (3). One reason for the increased incidence of duodenal ulcer in this study may be that a disproportionately large number of patients had a history of previous duodenal ulcer. The foregoing

Table 1 Prevention of NSAID-Induced Duodenal Ulcers in Controlled Clinical Trials. Values Represent Percentage Incidence of Ulcerations

Trials	Misoprostol (200 μg qid)	Misoprostol (200 μg bid/qid)	Ranitidine (150 mg bid)	Placebo
Graham et al. (10) (misoprostol vs placebo)	1.0%[a]			6.3%
Geis et al. (11) (misoprostol vs placebo)		0.0%[a]		8.2%
Raskin et al. (13) (misoprostol vs ranitidine)		1.1%[b]	1.1%[a]	
Ehsanullah et al. (7) (ranitidine vs placebo)			1.5%[a]	8.0%
Robinson et al. (8) (ranitidine vs placebo)			0.0%[a]	8.0%

[a]Misoprostol and ranitidine were significantly ($p < 0.05$) effective in preventing NSAID-induced ulcers when compared with placebo.
[b]Misoprostol and ranitidine did not significantly differ from each other in preventing NSAID-induced duodenal ulcers.

Table 2 Prevention of NSAID-Induced Gastric Ulcers in Controlled Clinical Trials. Values Represent Percentage Incidence of Ulcerations

Trials	Misoprostol (100 μg qid)	Misoprostol (200 μg qid)	Misoprostol (200 μg bid/tid)	Sucralfate (1 g qid)	Ranitidine 150 mg bid)	Placebo
Graham et al. (9) (misoprostol vs placebo)	5.6%[a]	1.4%[a]				21.7%
Graham et al. (10) (misoprostol vs placebo)			1.5%[a]			9.0%
Geis et al. (11) (misoprostol vs placebo)			3.0%[a]			15.0%
Agrawal et al. (12) (sucralfate vs misoprostol)		1.6%[a]		16.0%		
Ehsanullah et al. (7) (ranitidine vs placebo)					6.0%	6.0%
Robinson et al. (8) (ranitidine vs placebo)					12.0%	10.0%
Raskin et al. (13) (ranitidine vs misoprostol)		1.1%[a]			5.2%	

[a]Misoprostol in all dosages was significantly ($p < 0.05$) superior to placebo and to ranitidine in the prevention of NSAID-induced gastric ulcers.

findings concerning the lack of beneficial effect of ranitidine in the prevention of gastric ulcer induced by NSAIDs have been confirmed by Robinson et al. (8; see Table 2).

B. Prostaglandins

Although several synthetic E-prostaglandins have been studied in a preliminary manner, the bulk of the clinical evidence, to date, exists only for misoprostol. The studies supporting the efficacy of this prostaglandin will be discussed in detail.

Graham et al. (9) conducted a double-blind, placebo-controlled study to determine the effect of misoprostol in preventing gastric ulcer induced by NSAIDs, and its effect on the relief of abdominal pain caused by this group of drugs. Four hundred twenty patients with osteoarthritis and NSAID-associated abdominal pain were included. The NSAID therapy included ibuprofen, piroxicam, or naproxen. Demographic characteristics relating to age, sex, and duration of osteoarthritis were similar in all patients. Patients were endoscoped, and if they were found to have an ulcer, they were excluded. Only patients with normal endoscopic findings or erosions and intramucosal hemorrhages were randomized into the three treatment groups: 100 μg misoprostol qid, 200 μg misoprostol qid, or placebo qid for a subsequent 12 weeks, while the patients continued to take their NSAIDs. Patients were examined endoscopically at 4-week intervals for the subsequent 12 weeks. The principal outcome measurement was the number of patients in each treatment group who developed a gastric ulcer (at least 3 mm in diameter) during the 3-month follow-up period. The NSAID-associated abdominal pain was assessed independently from the patient's daily rating (as recorded on a diary card) and the investigator's monthly ratings of abdominal pain.

Of the patients who received misoprostol, 100 μg qid, while continuing to receive their NSAIDS, 94% were ulcer-free at the end of 12 weeks (see Table 2). Of those who received misoprostol, 200 μg qid, 99% were ulcer-free at the end of 12 weeks while they concurrently received NSAIDs for treatment of osteoarthritis (see Table 2). Of the placebo-treated patients, only 78% were ulcer-free. The difference between the two misoprostol groups, compared with the placebo group, was statistically significant ($p < 0.001$).

By the end of 12 weeks, 57% of the patients in the placebo group had relief of abdominal pain compared with 70% of the patients in each misoprostol group. This difference between placebo and misoprostol group for relief of pain was not statistically significant. However, it should be noted that all patients at the time of entry had abdominal pain.

The most common adverse effects encountered in this trial were abdominal pain, diarrhea, dyspepsia, flatulence, and nausea. Withdrawals resulting from diarrhea occurred in 2.8% of patients in the 100-μg misoprostol group and 6.4% of patients in the 200-μg misoprostol group. From this study one concludes that misoprostol in dosages of 100 μg and 200 μg qid, when given with therapeutic dosages of NSAIDs, is well-tolerated and effective in preventing NSAID-induced gastric ulcers in patients with osteoarthritis, and it does not increase abdominal pain or induce other GI symptoms.

A second double-blind, placebo-controlled study performed by Graham et al., in patients with osteoarthritis and rheumatoid arthritis, compared the efficacy of misoprostol (200 μg qid) and placebo in the prevention of NSAID-induced duodenal ulcers (10) (see Table 1). Patients without evidence of gastric or duodenal ulcer were randomized into the two groups. All patients were expected to receive NSAIDs of choice for treatment of arthritis for 12 weeks. Endoscopic examinations were performed at 4-, 8-, and 12-week intervals. There were no demographic differences between the two treatment groups in age, sex, and type of arthritis The development of duodenal ulcer occurred in 6.3% of patients receiving placebo, compared with 1% in the misoprostol group ($p \leq 0.01$, see Table 1). In the same study, the incidence of gastric ulcer development in the placebo group was 9% compared with 1.5% in the misoprostol group ($p \leq 0.01$; see Table 2). The result of this study provides evidence that misoprostol prevents NSAID-induced gastric as well as duodenal ulcers. A third major trial (11) also supports the efficacy of misoprostol in preventing NSAID-induced gastroduodenal ulcer formation (see Tables 1 and 2). Misoprostol was superior to sucralfate (12) and to ranitidine (13) for preventing NSAID-induced gastric ulcers (see Table 2). However, misoprostol had an efficacy similar to ranitidine for preventing NSAID-induced duodenal ulcers (13; see Table 1).

III. TREATMENT OF NONSTEROIDAL ANTI-INFLAMMATORY DRUG-INDUCED ULCERS

The ensuing discussion will focus on the treatment of NSAID-associated ulcer with various antiulcer therapies, especially for patients who must continue the use of NSAIDs in the presence of ulcer disease. Although many studies have examined the efficacy of histamine (H_2) antagonists in healing NSAID-induced mucosal erosions or ulcers (14–31), unfortunately, most of these studies were either uncontrolled or did not particularly specify whether NSAIDs were continued or discontinued. In addition, several studies were retrospective. In some nonrandomized, nonblinded, open-label trials, it has been reported that 75–100% of gastric ulcers heal within 12 weeks, despite continued use of NSAIDs during antiulcer therapy with H_2-antagonists (14). This review will examine only the results of prospective, randomized, double-blind studies in patients who must continue to use NSAIDs.

A. Histamine (H_2) Antagonists

The bulk of the evidence exists only for cimetidine. Two major double-blind placebo-controlled trials, involving numerous patients, were carried out with cimetidine during which NSAID therapy was continued (15,32). A third double-blind study, conducted with a small number of patients, will also be discussed to clarify the role of gastric acid in the pathogenesis of NSAID-induced gastric ulcers. The largest study was reported in an abstract form in 1988 by Wallin et al. (15), in which rheumatic patients with one or more endoscopically proved gastric or duodenal erosions or ulcers of at least 4 mm in diameter were randomized to one of two regimens of cimetidine (400 mg bid or 800 mg hs) or placebo. The NSAID treatment was continued throughout the 8-week study period, and repeat endoscopies were carried out at 4, 6, and 8 weeks. Healing was defined as complete reepithelialization of all original lesions. The cumulative healing rates are shown in Table 3. Mucosal healing rates associated with cimetidine were slightly higher than placebo. Only one group (cimetidine, 400 mg bid, at 8 weeks) achieved a statistical significance when compared with placebo by only the intent-to-treat cohort analysis. There are three major shortcomings in this trial: (a) there were no subgroup analyses to look at the rate of ulcer healing of gastric versus duodenal ulcers, despite the large number of patients; (b) there were no subgroup analyses to examine healing of erosions versus ulcers; (c) the statistical significance between cimetidine and placebo was achieved only in one cohort

Table 3 Efficacy of Cimetidine in the Healing of NSAID-Induced Gastric and Duodenal Erosions or Ulcers in Rheumatic Patients Receiving Continuous NSAID Therapy[a]

	% Ulcer healing at specified intervals		
Treatment arm	4 wk	6 wk	8 wk
Placebo	17	43	52
Cimetidine 800 mg hs	31	51	60
Cimetidine 400 mg bid	30	49	66[b]

[a]Patients with one or more endoscopically proved gastric or duodenal erosions or ulcers were randomized by either cimetidine (400 mg bid or 800 mg hs) or placebo. The NSAID therapy was continued. Endoscopy was repeated at 4, 6, and 8 weeks.
[b]Cimetidine was statistically ($p = 0.01$) superior to placebo only in the intent-to-treat cohort analysis.
Source: Data adapted from Ref. 15.

analysis. It would have been more assuring if statistical superiority of cimetidine over placebo was also confirmed in the evaluable cohort analysis.

The second double-blind, placebo-controlled, randomized trial examined the efficacy of cimetidine for the treatment of NSAID-induced mucosal injury in 104 patients with rheumatoid arthritis who continued the use of NSAIDs (32). Of these, 94 patients had submucosal hemorrhages or erosions upon initial screening endoscopy and were enrolled. Patients were allowed to take cimetidine (300 mg) four times a day or placebo concurrently with their NSAIDs. Mucosal damage was evaluated by endoscopy after 8 weeks of treatment. Of the patients who received cimetidine, 56% had erosions or submucosal hemorrhages, as compared with 52% of the placebo-treated patients. This indicates that short-term treatment with cimetidine was not effective in the healing of submucosal hemorrhages and erosions in patients with rheumatoid arthritis who continued on NSAIDs. Further observations were made on a group of patients who did show improvement and recovery from gastrointestinal damage. These patients were then followed for an additional 10 months and were continued on cimetidine (400 mg) or placebo given at bedtime as well as their NSAIDs. At the end of 10 months, endoscopic evaluation revealed that 42% of those receiving cimetidine and 50% of those receiving placebo showed endoscopic lesions. Thus, cimetidine failed to demonstrate efficacy for either the treatment or the prevention of NSAID-related gastric mucosal injury.

A third double-blind, placebo-controlled study conducted in 18 rheumatic patients compared the efficacy of cimetidine plus antacid as needed versus placebo plus antacids in the healing of aspirin-associated gastric ulcers during continued salicylate ingestion over a 2-month period (25). Healing occurred in 44% of the placebo and 56% of the cimetidine-treated patients ($p > 0.05$). Subjects in both groups ingested potentially therapeutic dose of antacids. The lack of efficacy of cimetidine and antacids in healing aspirin-induced gastric ulcers suggests that gastric acid may not be of crucial importance for the pathogenesis of NSAID-induced gastric ulcer. In contrast, the reduction of gastric acidity is important for the healing of non-NSAID or idiopathic gastric ulcers.

No meaningful major placebo-controlled, randomized studies were conducted with other H_2-receptor antagonists (ranitidine, famotidine, nizatidine) in which NSAID-induced erosions or ulcers were effectively treated in patients who continued the use of NSAIDs for the symptomatic control of their rheumatic disease.

B. Omeprazole

In a double-blind, placebo-controlled trial that compared the efficacy of omeprazole with ranitidine for the treatment of gastric ulcer (33) Walan et al. found a subgroup of patients taking NSAIDs during antiulcer drug therapy. The results of gastric ulcer healing with omeprazole was substantially superior to those achieved with ranitidine. There was no difference in ulcer-healing rates in the omeprazole group, whether or not the patients were taking NSAIDs. In the ranitidine group, a one-third decrease in the healing rate of gastric ulcer was observed in patients taking NSAIDs. This promising preliminary data with omeprazole needs to be confirmed in future large trials.

C. Sucralfate

Sucralfate, which is effective for the treatment of gastric and duodenal ulcer, has also been studied extensively for treatment of NSAID-induced mucosal damage. The exact mechanism by which sucralfate either prevents or heals gastric mucosal damage is unknown. Caldwell et al. carried out a double-blind, placebo-controlled, randomized trial in 143 patients with rheumatoid arthritis who were on a fixed regimen of NSAIDs, for 2 weeks (34). When examined by endoscopy before initiation of double-blind treatment, 60 of these patients had significant mucosal damage (erosions or ulcer). Sucralfate, 1 g qid, or placebo was added to their therapeutic regimen for a period of 4 weeks. Repeat endoscopy after 4 weeks of treatment with either sucralfate (30 patients) or placebo (30 patients) plus NSAIDs revealed no significant difference between the two groups in the amelioration of mucosal damage. Thus, sucralfate was not effective for the treatment of NSAID-induced gastric erosions and ulcers.

D. Prostaglandins

Roth et al. conducted a multicenter, double-blind, placebo-controlled, randomized study to determine the effects of misoprostol in reducing aspirin-induced gastroduodenal lesions in patients with active rheumatoid arthritis (35). Since prostaglandins have inflammatory properties that may interfere with the analgesic/antirheumatic effect of aspirin, the effect of misoprostol on the antirheumatic activity of aspirin was also studied. The patients had definite or classic rheumatoid arthritis, as defined by the criteria of the American Rheumatism Association (currently recognized as the American College of Rheumatology), a functional capacity classification of state I–III, and onset of rheumatoid arthritis after aged 16. At entry into the study, all patients received aspirin alone four times daily for 4 weeks, with an average daily dose of 3.9 g/day (pretreatment phase). After 4 weeks of aspirin monotherapy, the patients underwent endoscopy for evaluation of gastrointestinal damage. Endoscopic findings were graded on an 8-point scale (0 = normal mucosa; 7 = well-defined ulcer craters). Those with endoscopic scores of 3 or more were randomly assigned to receive 8 additional weeks of therapy with a fixed dose of aspirin plus either misoprostol, 200 μg qid, or placebo qid (treatment segment). During this segment of the study, patients were evaluated for rheumatoid arthritis disease activity every 2 weeks and were endoscoped every 4 weeks.

The criteria for treatment success in this study were based on changes in the endoscopic score, as follows: for patients with pretreatment scores of 7 or 6, a decrease of at least 1 grade point was required, indicating disappearance of ulcer or erosion; for patients with pretreatment scores of 5, 4, or 3, a decrease of at least 2 grade points was required, indicating significant improvement in mucosal damage. After 4 weeks of aspirin alone (before randomization), 22% of patients had ulcers, 50% had erosions, and 18% had various types of mucosal hemorrhages. Only 10% of the patients did not experience sufficient damage to qualify for randomization. Thus, in this set of patients with rheumatoid arthritis, there is little question that chronic high-dose aspirin therapy for relief of signs and symptoms of rheumatoid arthritis did cause significant mucosal damage.

Of 326 patients who entered the study, 270 were endoscoped, and 239 patients with endoscopic scores of 3–7 were randomly assigned to receive either misoprostol or placebo, in addition to the fixed dose of aspirin. The demographic characteristics of each group were similar. One hundred ninety-eight patients completed the study and were evaluated for treatment successes and rheumatoid arthritis disease activity.

After 4 weeks of concomitant treatment, 69% of patients receiving misoprostol and 31% of patients receiving placebo were treatment successes ($p = 0.0001$). After 8 weeks, the therapeutic success rate remained constant at 70% in the misoprostol group, but decreased to 25% in the placebo group ($p = 0.0001$).

When the effects of combined treatment of aspirin and misoprostol or aspirin and placebo were evaluated on duodenal mucosal injury, at both week 4 as well as week 8, significantly more improvement in duodenal mucosal injury occurred among patients who received misoprostol than among those who received placebo (84 vs 47%, $p < 0.002$; 86 vs 53%, $p < 0.001$, respectively).

In this study, 36 patients assigned to the misoprostol group and 34 patients assigned to the placebo group had gastric or duodenal ulcer at randomization. Of particular importance, in the presence of on-going aspirin use, 56% of misoprostol patients with initial gastroduodenal ulcers versus 24% of the placebo patients, were ulcer-free after 4 weeks ($p = 0.0056$), and 67 versus 26% (misoprostol vs placebo) were ulcer-free after 8 weeks ($p = 0.0006$).

There were no clinically significant differences in rheumatic disease activity between patients receiving misoprostol and those receiving placebo. Thus, misoprostol did not interfere with the antirheumatic efficacy of aspirin, but it provided significant healing of aspirin-induced mucosal damage.

In examining the incidence of adverse reactions, the only important difference between the two treatment groups was the incidence of diarrhea, which was seen in 14% of patients who received misoprostol versus 6% of patients who received placebo. However, in most patients, the diarrhea was short-lived, mild, and self-limiting. Only 4% of patients had to be withdrawn from the study as a consequence of diarrhea.

Several conclusions can be drawn from this study. Misoprostol was found to be effective in healing aspirin-induced mucosal damage, well tolerated, and did not interfere with the antirheumatic activity of aspirin. Four additional controlled trials unequivocally support the efficacy of misoprostol in healing NSAID-induced gastric or duodenal ulcers in rheumatic patients who continued the use of NSAIDs (36–39; Table 4).

E. Conclusions

Obviously, the most important step in healing NSAID-induced ulcers is discontinuation of these drugs, if feasible. Multiple, double-blind, placebo-controlled trials of reasonable

Table 4 Misoprostol (200 μg qid) vs Placebo in the Healing of Gastroduodenal Mucosal Injury in Rheumatic Patients Receiving Continuous NSAID Therapy: A Statistical Summary of Four Trials

Author	No. patients	Efficacy in healing in comparison with placebo: Duodenal	Gastric
Roth et al. (35)	238	$p < 0.0022$	$p < 0.0001$
Bolten (36,37)	462	$p < 0.05$[a]	$p < 0.05$
Saggioro (38)	106	$p < 0.05$	$p < 0.05$
Henriksson et al. (39)	40	$p < 0.05$	$p < 0.05$

[a]At a total daily dose of 600–800 μg.

duration are conclusive that misoprostol is currently the only agent that is effective in both the prevention and treatment of NSAID-induced gastric and duodenal ulcers. Subset analysis of one study with omeprazole shows promise in healing gastric ulcers while NSAIDs are continued. These data require further confirmation. Histamine (H_2) antagonists have not been effective for the treatment of gastric and duodenal ulcers if NSAIDs are continued. Furthermore, the histamine (H_2) antagonist ranitidine does not prevent NSAID-induced gastric ulcer development. However, ranitidine is effective in preventing NSAID-induced duodenal ulcers. Sucralfate therapy is ineffective in treatment or prevention of NSAID-related, gastric and duodenal ulcers.

REFERENCES

1. Griffin MR, Ray WA, Schaffner W. Nonsteroidal anti-inflammatory drug use and death from peptic ulcer in elderly persons. Ann Intern Med 1988; 109:359–63.
2. Armstrong CP, Blower AL. Nonsteroidal anti-inflammatory drugs and life threatening complications of peptic ulceration. Gut 1987; 28:527–32.
3. Graham DY, Smith JL. Gastroduodenal complications of chronic NSAID therapy. Am J Gastroenterol 1988; 83:1081–4.
4. Fries JF, Miller SR, Spitz PW, Williams CA, Hubert HB, Bloch DA. Toward an epidemiology of gastropathy associated with nonsteroidal anti-inflammatory drug use. Gastroenterology 1989; 96:647–55.
5. Dajani EZ, Agrawal NM. Protective and therapeutic effects of prostaglandins. Clin Pharmacol Res 1989; 9:359–69.
6. Gabriel SE, Jaakkimainen L, Bombardier C. Risk for serious gastrointestinal complications related to use nonsteroidal anti-inflammatory drugs—a meta-analysis. Ann Intern Med 1991; 115:787–96.
7. Ehsanullah RSB, Page MC, Tildesley G, Wood R. Prevention of gastroduodenal damage induced by nonsteroidal anti-inflammatory drugs: controlled trial of ranitidine. Br Med J 1988; 297:1017–21.
8. Robinson MG, Griffin JW Jr, Bowers J, Kogan FJ, Kogut DG, Lanza FL, Warner CW. Effect of ranitidine on gastroduodenal mucosal damage induced by nonsteroidal anti-inflammatory drugs. Dig Dis Sci 1989; 34:424–8.
9. Graham DY, Agrawal NM, Roth SH. Prevention of NSAID-induced gastric ulcer with misoprostol: multi-center, double-blind, placebo-controlled trial. Lancet 1988; 2:1277–80.
10. Graham DY, Stromatt SC, Jaszewski R, White RH, Triadafilopoulos G. Prevention of duodenal ulcer in arthritics who are chronic NSAID users: a multi-center trial of the role misoprostol [abstract]. Gastroenterology 1991; 100:A-75.

11. Gies GS, Stead H, Wallemark C-B, Nicholson PA. Prevalence of mucosal lesions in the stomach and duodenum due to chronic use of NSAIDs in patients with RA or OA, an interim report on prevention by misoprostol of diclofenac associated lesions. J Rheumatol 1991; 18 (suppl 28):11–4.
12. Agrawal NM, Roth S, Graham D, White RH, Germain B, Brown J, Stromatt S. Misoprostol compared with sucralfate in the prevention of non-steroidal anti-inflammatory drug-induced gastric ulcer. Ann Intern Med 1991; 115:195–200.
13. Raskin JB, White R, Jaszewski R, Teoh LS, Sue SD. Misoprostol and ranitidine in the prevention of NSAID-induced gastric and duodenal ulcer disease: a multi-center trial [abstract]. Gastroenterology 1992; 102:A151.
14. Soll AH, Weinstein WM, Kurata J, McCarthy D. Nonsteroidal anti-inflammatory drugs and peptic ulcer disease. Ann Intern Med 1991; 114:407–19.
15. Wallin BA, Frank WO, Fox MJ, McCafferty JP, McDevitt JT, Seibert GB, Arias LF, Young MD. The effects of cimetidine on the healing of nonsteroidal anti-inflammatory drug-induced gastroduodenal damage while continuing NSAID therapy [abstract]. Am J Gastroenterol 1988; 83:1076.
16. Davis J, Collins AJ, Dixon A St J. The influence of cimetidine on peptic ulcer in patients with arthritis taking anti-inflammatory drugs. Br J Rheumatol 1986; 25:54–8.
17. O'Laughlin JC, Silvoso GK, Ivey KJ. Resistance to medical therapy of gastric ulcers in rheumatic disease patients taking aspirin. A double-blind study with cimetidine and follow-up. Dig Dis Sci 1982; 27:976–80.
18. Loludice TA, Saleem T, Lang JA. Cimetidine in the treatment of gastric ulcer induced by steroidal and nonsteroidal anti-inflammatory agents. Am J Gastroenterol 1981; 75:104–10.
19. Petrillo M, Ardizzone S, Bianchi Porro G. Cimetidine versus colloidal bismuth subcitrate (De-Nol) in peptic ulcer therapy of patients with rheumatoid arthritis undergoing chronic nonsteroidal anti-inflammatory drug treatment. Eur J Gastroenterol Hepatol 1990; 2(suppl 1):S82–3.
20. Biachi Porro G, Pace F, Caruso I. Why are nonsteroidal anti-inflammatory drugs important in peptic ulceration? Aliment Pharmacol Ther 1987; 1:540S–47S.
21. Bijlsma JWJ. Treatment of NSAID-induced gastrointestinal lesions with cimetidine: an international multicentre collaborative study. Aliment Pharmacol Ther 1988; 2S:85–96.
22. Gierckskу KE, Husby G, Rugstad HE, Revhaug A. Epidemiology of NSAID-induced gastrointestinal problems and the role of cimetidine in their prevention. Aliment Pharmacol Ther 1988; 2S:33–41.
23. Rainer F, Petritsch W. The influence of cimetidine on gastrointestinal lesions in patients with rheumatoid arthritis taking nonsteroidal antirheumatic drugs. Clin Exp Rheumatol 1987; 5:55.
24. Croker JR, Cotton PB, Boyle AC, Kinsella P. Cimetidine for peptic ulcer in patients with arthritis. Ann Rheum Dis 1980; 39:275–8.
25. O'Laughlin JC, Silvoso GR, Ivey KJ. Healing of aspirin-associated peptic ulcer disease despite continued salicylate ingestion. Arch Intern Med 1981; 141:781–3.
26. Jaszewski R, Calzada R, Dhar R. Persistence of gastric ulcers caused by plain aspirin or nonsteroidal anti-inflammatory agents in patients treated with a combination of cimetidine, antacids, and enteric-coated aspirin. Dig Dis Sci 1989; 34:1361–4.
27. Lancaster-Smith MJ, Jaderberg ME, Jackson DA. Ranitidine in the treatment of nonsteroidal anti-inflammatory drug associated gastric and duodenal ulcers. Gut 1991; 32:252–5.
28. Stock KP, Bach GL. Ulcer healing under ranitidine and antacids despite continuous nonsteroidal anti-inflammatory therapy. Z Rheumatol 1988; 47:177–81.
29. Bank S, Greenberg RE, Magier D, Lavin PT. The efficacy and tolerability of famotidine and ranitidine on the healing of active duodenal ulcer and during six-month maintenance treatment, with special reference to NSAID/aspirin-related ulcers. Clin Ther 1991; 13:304–18.
30. Simon B, Dammann HG, Leucht U, Muller P. Ranitidine in the therapy of NSAID-induced gastroduodenal lesions. Results of a randomized, placebo-controlled, double-blind study in patients with rheumatic diseases. Scand J Gastroenterol [Suppl] 1988; 154:18–21.

31. Muller P, Damman HG, Marinis E, Weise D, Simon B. Treatment of NSAID-induced gastric and duodenal mucosal lesions with ranitidine. Comparison of two different regimens. Fortschr Med 1989; 31:667–71.
32. Roth SH, Bennett RE. Nonsteroidal anti-inflammatory drug gastropathy. Arch Intern Med 1987; 147:2093.
33. Walan A, Bader JP, Classen M, Lamers CBHW, Piper DW, Rutgersson K, Eriksson S. Effect of omeprazole and ranitidine on ulcer healing and relapse rates in patients with benign gastric ulcer. N Engl J Med 1989; 320:69–75.
34. Caldwell JR, Roth SH, Wu WC, et al. Sucralfate treatment of nonsteroidal anti-inflammatory drug-induced gastrointestinal symptoms and mucosal damage. Am J Med 1987; 83(suppl 3B):74.
35. Roth S, Agrawal N, Mahowald M, et al. Misoprostol heals gastroduodenal injury in patients with rheumatoid arthritis receiving aspirin. Arch Intern Med 1989; 149:775–79.
36. Bolten W, Brodenfeldt R. Efficacy of misoprostol in the therapy of NSAID-induced symptoms and lesions of the upper GI-tract under continued NSAID medication. Clin Exp Rheumatol 1990; 8:S-4, 59.
37. Bolten W. Treatment of NSAID-induced symptoms with the prostaglandin analogue misoprostol in rheumatoid arthritis patients. A multi-centered double-blind, placebo-controlled study. Akt Rheumatol 1989; 14:214–20.
38. Saggioro A. Efficacy of misoprostol on symptoms and lesions with NSAIDs. Italian experience. In: Cheli R, ed. Treatment and prevention of NSAID-induced gastropathy. London: RSM Services International Congress and Symposium Services International Congress and Symposium Series no. 147, 1989:63–67.
39. Henriksson AEK, Uribe A, Gullberg R, Johansson C. Effects of prostaglandin E_1 analogue on gastroduodenal mucosa in patients with rheumatoid arthritis [abstract]. Presented at 7th international conference on prostaglandins. Florence, May, 1990: 346.
40. Agrawal NW, Dajani EZ. Prevention and treatment of ulcers induced by nonsteroidal anti-inflammatory drugs. J Association for Academic Minority Physicians 1992; 3:142–8.

10

Hepatic Injury Associated with Nonsteroidal Anti-Inflammatory Drugs

HYMAN J. ZIMMERMAN*
George Washington University School of Medicine
Washington, D.C.

I. INTRODUCTION

Nonsteroidal anti-inflammatory drugs (NSAIDs) have been associated with hepatic disease for three-quarters of a century. In 1923, cinchophen, a drug once used to treat rheumatic disease and gout, introduced the medical world to the phenomenon of hepatic injury induced by an idiosyncratic reaction to a drug (1,2). Indeed, so many instances were recorded, and so complete were the descriptions of the clinical and histological features of the hepatic injury, that cinchophen-induced hepatic injury serves as a prototype of one form of drug-induced liver disease (3).

Cinchophen has long since fallen from clinical use, and its hepatotoxic threat is no longer relevant. However, the adverse effects of NSAIDs have again become the focus of attention (4), an attention in part triggered by the dramatic appearance of the hepatotoxic effects of benoxaprofen (Oroflex, Opren) and its withdrawal from use almost immediately after approval of its use in the United States (5).

The concern with the hepatic injury induced by benoxaprofen and the examination of the effects of other NSAIDs led the Food and Drug Administration (FDA) Arthritis Advisory Committee (4) to conclude that "hepatic toxicity should be considered a class characteristic of NSAIDs." The committee noted that NSAIDs can lead to biochemical abnormalities interpreted as mild hepatic injury in up to 10% of recipients, but rarely, to overt hepatic disease. This uniform characterization of the group of NSAIDs, as a whole, obscures the differences between the various members. While NSAIDs comprise a group that is fairly uniform in anti-inflammatory effects and inhibition of prostaglandin formation, the group is quite heterogeneous for adverse effects on the liver (Table 1). Types and mechanisms of hepatic injury and hepatotoxic potency differ.

A number of anti-inflammatory and minor analgesic agents have been incriminated in the causation of hepatic injury (Table 2). Reliable figures for the incidence of liver damage induced by most of these agents are not available; but there appears to be

*Professor of Medicine Emeritus and Distinguished Scientist Emeritus.

Table 1 Various Patterns of NSAID-Associated Hepatic Injury

NSAID	Hepatocellular[a]	Cholestatic[a]	Granulomas[b]	Mechanism[c]
Phenylbutazone	++	+	+	Idio-imm
Sulindac	+	++	±	Idio-imm
Ibufenac	+	0	±	Idio-met
Benoxaprofen	0	+	0	Idio-met
Aspirin	+	0	0	Tox
Diclofenac	+	0	0	Idio-met
Acetaminophen	+	0	0	Tox

[a]Relative prominence of pattern in hepatic injury.
[b]+, Relatively frequent cause of granulomas, compared with other drugs.
±, Granulomas reported but very rare.
[c]Idio-immun, Immunological idiosyncrasy (hypersensitivity); Idio-met, metabolic immunological; Tox, intrinsic toxicity.

striking variability. For phenylbutazone (PBZ), a figure of 0.25% is provided by one study (6). For ibufenac, an incidence of approximately 5% led to its abandonment (7,8). Only a few published instances of hepatic damage have been ascribed to indomethacin or ibuprofen (9). Recent attention in the literature has focused on several other agents that are discussed later. The usual injury from many of the NSAIDs is characterized in Table 2.

The *mechanism* by which these agents induce overt injury is the unusual susceptibility of individual patients (i.e., the adverse effects are idiosyncratic reactions). For some of these drugs, (e.g., sulindac), the idiosyncratic reaction appears to be immunologically mediated (hypersensitivity), as deduced from circumstances associated with development of injury and the clinical features (10). For others (e.g., diclofenac), metabolic idiosyncrasy, rather than drug allergy, may be responsible (11). For some, the data are too scanty to permit even speculation.

Several analgesic–antirheumatic agents show a dose-dependent, intrinsic toxicity. Salicylates, in high doses, can produce hepatic injury, apparently as a manifestation of intrinsic mild hepatotoxicity, rather than host idiosyncrasy (12,13). Acetaminophen, a mild analgesic, in an overdose is a potent hepatotoxin (12,13). Although phenylbutazone, in therapeutic doses, can lead to idiosyncratic hepatic injury, apparently immunologically mediated, it also can lead to liver damage in large overdose—evidence of intrinsic hepatotoxic potential (14).

The *pattern of injury* (see Table 2) induced by cinchophen, ibufenac, indomethacin, salicylates, acetaminophen, and most other NSAIDs is hepatocellular. Several (e.g., benoxaprofen, diflunisal) lead to cholestasis (3). The hepatic injury secondary to PBZ is mixed-hepatocellular in most cases, but cholestatic in some (12,14). Sulindac (10) also can lead to cholestatic or hepatocellular injury. Phenylbutazone can lead to granulomatous change (14). Clometacin (15), glafenine (16), and diclofenac (17) have been incriminated in cases of chronic active hepatitis.

Most of the drugs that produce overt hepatic injury (i.e., jaundice) in low incidence, lead to a higher incidence of mild hepatic abnormality. Although the incidence of jaundice may be as low as 0.1, 0.01%, or even lower among recipients of some NSAIDs, levels of aspartate and alanine aminotransferases [AST (GOT) and ALT (GPT)] may become abnormal in 5–15% of patients taking the respective drug. Most of the elevated levels are

Table 2 NSAIDs Used in Rheumatic Disease and as Analgesics

Agent	Incidence[a]	Mechanism[b]	Form of injury[c]	Other[d]
Acetaminophen	Dose	Tox	H-CELL	
Amphenac	L	I-M	H-CELL	
Azapropazone (apazone)	0			
Benorilate	VL/dose	Tox	H-CELL	
Benoxaprofen	L	I-M	Chol	
Carprofen	>50% tests	I-M	H-CELL	
Cinchophen	L	I-M	H-CELL	
Clometacin	L	I-M	H-CELL	CAH, GRAN
Diclofenac	L	I-M	H-CELL	
Diflunisal	VL	I?	Chol	
Etofenamic acid O				
Fenbufen	L	I-M	H-CELL	
Fenclofenamic acid	VL	I-M	H-CELL	
Fenclozic	10%	I-M[b]	Chol-M	
Fenoprofen	VL	I?	H-CELL/CHOL	
Fentiazac	10%	I-M[b]	H-CELL	
Feprazone	VL	I-M	Chol-M	GRAN
Floctafenine	0			
Flufenamic acid	0			
Flurbiprofen	VL	I-M	H-CELL	
Glafenine	L	I-M	H-CELL	CAH?
Ibufenac	5%	I-M[b]	H-CELL	
Ibuprofen	VL	I-M?	H-CELL	STEATOSIS
Idomethacin	VL	Idio?	H-CELL	
Indoprofen	0			
Isoxepac	L	I-M	H-CELL	
Isoxecam	VL	I-M	Chol-M	
Kebuzone	L	I-M	H-CELL	
Ketoprofen	0			
Meclofenamic acid	VL	I-M	TESTS	
Mefenamic acid	VL	I-M	TESTS	
Naproxen	VL	I-I	Chol-M	
Niflumic acid	VL	I?	H-CELL	
Oxaprozin	VL	I-I	H-CELL	
Oxyphenbutazone	L	I?	H-CELL-M	GRAN
Phenazone (antipyrine)	L	Idio?	TESTS	
Phenylbutazone	L	I-M (b)	H-CELL-M	GRAN
Piroxicam	VL	Idio?	H-CELL-M	
Pirprofen	L	I-M	H-CELL	
Proquazone	L	I-M	H-CELL	
Salicylates	Dose	Tox	H-CELL	STEATOSIS
Sudoxicam	<1%	I-M	H-CELL	
Sulindac	L	I-M	Chol-M	
Tolfenamic acid	VL	Idio?	H-CELL	CAH?
Tolmetin	VL	Idio?	H-CELL	

[a]L, low; VL, very low; 0, no reported cases; 50% tests, incidence of abnormal aminotransferase levels; Dose, dose-dependent.
[b]Mechanism shown is, of course, speculative. IM, metabolic idiosyncrasy; II, immunologic idiosyncrasy (i.e., hypersensitivity); I (?), too little information for useful speculation; Tox, toxic.
[c]H-CELL, Hepatocellular (cytolytic); Chol, cholestatic. H-CELL–M, Hepatocellular usually and some cholestatic cases or hepatocellular with prominent cholestatic features; Chol-M, cholestatic usually, with some hepatocellular cases also or cholestatic with some hepatocellular features; TESTS, abnormal biochemical values, but no overt liver disease.
[d]CAH, chronic active hepatitis; GRAN, granulomas.

less than threefold the upper limit of normal (ULN); a small proportion may exceed that level. In general, it is assumed that the higher the incidence of even mildly elevated aminotransferase levels (especially ALT), the more likely a drug is to lead to overt hepatic disease. This reasonable assumption remains to be substantiated.

The categorization of NSAIDs is generally based on structural character. Even though there is no clear relation between the chemical category of a NSAID and its likelihood of producing hepatic injury, the following discussion is organized according to chemical categories.

II. ANTHRANILIC ACID DERIVATIVES (FENAMATES)

Several agents in this group have seen clinical use in the United States. One of them, *cinchophen*, was the first drug to come to attention as a cause of idiosyncratic hepatic injury (1,2). Although it has long since been adandoned, this drug is described in some detail because it provided a dramatic prototype of idiosyncratic hepatic injury (3); and because a modern NSAID (glafenine), which structurally resembles cinchophen, produces similar hepatic injury (16). *Mefenamic acid* (Ponstan) has been incriminated in an instance of severe, but nonfatal, bridging necrosis (18). Mefenamic and *meclofenamic* (Meclomen) acids, as well as other agents in this group, lead to minor elevations of aminotransferase levels in fewer than 5% of recipients. This group also includes *niflumic acid*, *tolfenamic acid*, *flufenamic acid*, *floctafenine*, and *diclofenac*. Only glafenine, diclofenac, and cinchophen have provoked significant hepatic disease in sufficient numbers to be meaningful; and the injury has been hepatocellular.

Niflumic acid (Nifluril) has been reported to be responsible for a mixed hepatocellular form of hepatic injury (19). The mechanism appeared to be hypersensitivity.

Tolfenamic acid (Clotam) also has been held responsible for an instance of hepatocellular injury, with histological features resembling chronic active hepatitis (20). Hepatic injury became apparent after 6 months of taking the drug.

A. Diclofenac (Voltaren)

A recent addition to the NSAID family, diclofenac has become a popular remedy in arthritis; it also can produce hepatic injury. Abnormal aminotransferase levels develop in about 15% of patients taking the drug. It has been implicated in at least 50 published reports of hepatocellular damage (11,21–29). In addition, we have been able to analyze 181 reports of hepatic injury in recipients of diclofenac that have been submitted to the FDA and that, on analysis, seemed reasonably ascribable to the drug (11).

1. Character of Injury

The injury is consistently hepatocellular with acute disease resembling acute viral hepatitis, and chronic injury resembling chronic hepatitis (11,17,21–29). On biopsy or autopsy the main lesion has been hepatic necrosis, matching the often-marked elevation of aminotransferase levels (24,25).

2. Factors in Susceptibility

Sex, the disease being treated and, perhaps, age affect vulnerability. Females constitute two-thirds of reported cases, a disproportionate figure relative to use of the drug (11). Also, patients with osteoarthritis constitute a greater number of cases of hepatic injury than would be expected from frequency of use (11). Elevated aminotransferase levels also are more frequent in women and osteoarthritic patients taking the drug than in men and patients with rheumatoid arthritis (11). Advancing age also appears to affect vulnerability, with patients older than 60 in greater number among those with hepatic injury than among all users of the drug (11). When corrected for use, women older than 60 with osteoarthritis appear be be an especially susceptible group (11).

3. Clinical Features

Most recorded cases have presented with the syndrome of acute hepatitis characterized by jaundice and, to a varying degree, by fatigue, anorexia, nausea, and vomiting. Fever, rash, and eosinophilia are uncommon, occurring in about 10% of patients (17,25). Although these features were recorded in the report of Schapira et al. (26), other descriptions have not noted them (17), and we have been impressed by their rarity (11). As with other drug-induced hepatocellular injury, massive necrosis with fulminant hepatic failure and death is a feared development, having been noted in about 10% of icteric cases (11). Chronic hepatitis also has been described (11,17,28).

4. Biochemical Features

Aminotransferase levels have ranged from 10 to 100 times the normal in clinically overt cases. Alkaline phosphatase levels are only slightly elevated (11). Jaundice may become intense. At least 50% of the cases analyzed by us, however, have been anicteric, with aminotransferase levels more modestly elevated. For the most part, these appear to be asymptomatic individuals whose aminotransferase levels had been measured as part of a program to prevent clinically overt injury or had been discovered in routine examinations.

The mechanism is clearly idiosyncrasy. Delayed onset of injury, after long periods of taking the drug, and delayed recurrence of injury after reinstitution of administration, warrant the inference that metabolic idiosyncrasy is the mechanism (11). That inference is supported by lack of fever, rash, or eosinophilia in most of the reported cases (17,28). Schapira et al., however, have cited the presence of these clinical hallmarks of hypersensitivity in their cases as support for the presumption that hypersensitivity is the mechanism (26). Other support for that view includes blastic transformation of lymphocytes and inhibition of macrophage or lymphocyte migration on exposure to the drug in vitro (9). The issue remains unresolved.

B. Glafenine (Glifan)

Glafenine bears a structural resemblance to cinchophen according to Stricker et al. (16). They also point out that glafenine can produce hepatic injury similar to cinchophen-induced liver disease. Indeed, glafenine has been incriminated in a number of instances of severe hepatocellular injury, with a fatal outcome in about half of the reported cases (16). The necrosis appears to involve mainly zone 3 (centrolobular area) (16). At least two cases have shown chronic changes.

The mechanism is idiosyncrasy. Onset of hepatic injury 1 to several months after starting the drug suggests the idiosyncrasy to be metabolic, but the reports of fever, eosinophilia, hemolysis, and renal disease and of eosinophil aggregates in the liver point toward immunological idiosyncrasy (hypersensitivity). The issue is unclear.

Factors affecting susceptibility remain to be elucidated. Female preponderance among cases (8 of 12) reported by Stricker et al. (11) suggests disproportionate female susceptibility.

Even more important than the hepatotoxic threat of glafenine is the striking potential of this drug to provoke anaphylaxis (29a). It is 10–20 times more common with glafenine than with other NSAIDs or even the penicillins. Indeed, it is the high incidence of anaphylaxis that has led to the recommendation that glafenine be withdrawn from use in the European Community (29a).

C. Indomethacin (Indocin)

Despite wide use of this drug, an indole and acetic acid derivative, relatively few published individual instances of jaundice have been attributed to it (9). The injury that has been recorded has been mainly hepatocellular. Necrosis, massive or central (30–33), accompanied in some cases by microvesicular steatosis (30,31), has been described. The case reported by Fenech et al. (30) showed striking histological cholestasis and striking biliverdinemia as well as necrosis. Indomethacin-associated hepatic injury appears to be of low incidence, but of hepatocellular character (34). Cuthbert's analysis (34) of adverse reactions to anti-inflammatory drugs occurring during a 10-year period in the United Kingdom, showed indomethacin to be responsible for 1260 total reactions, of which 114 were fatal [Estimated from the graphic data of Cuthbert (34)]. Approximately 3% (about 40 cases) of the total indomethacin reactions appeared to involve the liver, whereas approximately 6% (about 7 cases) of fatal indomethacin reactions represented hepatic disease. (This is relatively few cases of hepatic injury for a 10-year period, but the number of fatal cases seems relatively high.) Figures provided by the FDA also show that indomethacin is less frequently reported to produce hepatic injury than most other NSAIDs, an observation in accord with the view expressed by Henrard (33). The impression that indomethacin-related injury is hepatocellular is derived from individual case reports and by the high fatality rate (approximately 15%) among cases of hepatic injury that can be estimated from the figures of Cuthbert (34). There are few hints concerning susceptibility to the hepatic injury, other than the surprising impression of greater vulnerability of children (36).

D. Clometacin

Clometacin, an isomer of indomethacin, has strikingly different effects on the liver. Apparently employed more for its analgesic than for its anti-inflammatory properties, the drug has led to several dozen cases of hepatic disease (9,37–50). Most patients have presented with the syndrome and hepatic lesions of chronic active hepatitis (CAH), but acute hepatocelluar injury has also been reported. The chronic hepatic disease has become apparent after periods of 6 months to several years after beginning the drug.

The clinical manifestations are those of very active chronic hepatitis (9,37–50), with features of cirrhosis in some patients (37,39,49), and other features typical of the CAH provoked by drugs. Levels of total globulin and gamma globulin are high, and serological markers of autoimmunity are found in about 70% of patients. Indeed, the studies of clometacin-associated CAH are among those that have led to the suggestion that the presence of antibodies to double-stranded DNA in a patient with CAH should be considered a clue to drug-induced disease (9,50). As is seen in other instances of drug-induced CAH, the level of aminotransferases and bilirubin may be high enough to suggest acute injury; and the syndrome appears to have features of both chronic and acute disease. Indeed, the syndrome and hepatic lesion resemble the "autoimmune type" of CAH to a striking degree, including the markedly disproportionate involvement of women, usually elderly.

In a few cases, the injury and associated syndrome have been that of acute hepatic disease. Disproportionate cholestasis has been reported (41). One case has been reported to have portal granulomas (15).

The mechanism of injury appears to be immunological idiosyncrasy. The striking resemblance to the autoimmune type of CAH, and the immunologically relevant serological markers, the high gamma globulin, the frequency of eosinophilia, rash, and renal injury in the acute cases, all support the view (9) that the pathogenesis is immunological. Readministration of the drug leads to recurrence of injury within several weeks.

The relevance of clometacin injury is mainly in the light that it casts on the syndrome of chronic drug-induced hepatic disease. The drug is apparently employed mainly in France, from where all of the published reports have come.

E. Sulindac (Clinoril)

Sulindac, an acetic acid derivative, resembles indomethacin structurally. Approximately 25 individual cases of sulindac-associated jaundice have been reported in the literature (51–67), and we have analyzed 91 cases reported to the FDA (10). Most of the cases appear to have had cholestatic or mixed jaundice, with appreciable parenchymal injury accompanying the cholestasis. About 20% of cases have had hepatocellular injury. Since pancreatitis also has been induced by the drug (68–71), the possibility that ductal obstruction owing to pancreatitis may have contributed to the cholestasis in some cases warrants consideration. About 5% of cases of sulindac jaundice appear to end fatally (10). Deaths appear to have been due to severe generalized hypersensitivity, rather than hepatic disease, but there have been instances of fatal hepatic necrosis (10).

The mechanism of injury seems to be hypersensitivity in most cases as deduced from the associated fever and rash (10) and even the Stevens–Johnson syndrome (59,62,66,67), seen in some patients. In several cases a challenge dose of the drug, after recovery, led to recurrence of hepatic injury within several days (10,53,54,56–58,67). Onset of illness is usually in less than 8 weeks and, in many cases, less than 4 weeks, after starting the drug.

F. Tolmetin (Tolectin)

Tolmetin, an acetic acid derivative that is also a pyrrol, has been in use in the United States for about 10 years. I am aware of only one published report of tolmetin-associated hepatic injury; that one described a syndrome and lesion resembling Reye's syndrome (72). Reports submitted to the FDA also suggest that the drug has led to instances of jaundice. The tendency to produce hepatic injury, however, appears to be less than that of several other NSAIDs analyzed by the FDA. The injury appears to be hepatocellular, and the associated characteristics suggest the mechanism to be metabolic idiosyncrasy, rather than hypersensitivity. Minor elevations of serum aminotransferase levels have been reported in about 5% of recipients (9).

G. Zomepirac (Zomax)

Zomepirac, also an acetic acid derivative, has seen more use as an analgesic than as an antirheumatic drug. Accordingly, its intake has been intermittent, rather than regular.

Furthermore, adverse hematological effects may have obscured other effects. In any event, I am aware of no reports of zomepirac-associated hepatic injury.

H. Fenclofenac (Flenac)

Fenclofenac has apparently not been incriminated in any reported instances of hepatic injury. Approximately 1% of patients in a clinical trial were reported to develop elevations of aminotransferase levels of sufficient degree to lead to withdrawal of the drug (9).

I. Fenclozic Acid (Myalex)

Fenclozic acid has seen only clinical trials. It was withdrawn from testing (9) when it led to a 10% incidence of mixed cholestatic jaundice (73,74).

J. Fentiazac (Flogene)

Fentiazac has been reported to lead to mildly elevated aminotransferase levels in over 30% of a group under study (75) and to clinically apparent injury in 10% of another group (76). *Etodolac* has been reported (77) to lead to a low incidence of minor elevations of aminotransferase levels.

III. PROPIONIC ACID DERIVATIVES

Among the multiple drugs in this category there are several agents with overt potential for producing hepatic injury and a number that do not. One of the members of the group, *benoxaprofen*, provoked the recent sharp focus on the adverse effects of NSAIDs on the liver. Other agents in this group that have drawn attention as causes of hepatic injury include *ibufenac* and *naproxen*.

A. Ibufenac (Ibunac)

Ibufenac appeared to be responsible for hepatic disease of sufficient severity and frequency to warrant removal from clinical use (7,8). The combined results of two studies (7,8), totaling 61 patients, suggested that ibufenac led to elevated aminotransferase levels in over 30% and jaundice in approximately 5% of individuals taking the drug. The jaundice was hepatocellular, with hepatic necrosis and several deaths. Indeed, ibufenac was apparently responsible for more deaths from hepatic injury than other antirheumatic agents in use during the same period (34). A slight change in the molecule converted the drug to one with very little adverse effect on the liver, ibuprofen.

B. Ibuprofen (Motrin)

A derivative of ibufenac, ibuprofen appears to produce hepatic injury very rarely. The relative scantiness of reports of hepatic injury to the British Committee on Safety of Medicines (34) and to the US FDA supports the view that ibuprofen is one of the least likely of the commonly used NSAIDs to produce hepatic injury. Indeed, Cuthbert's figures (34) suggest that adverse reactions to ibuprofen rarely include the liver (4%). Nevertheless, occasional cases of hepatic injury of hepatocellular (78–81) or mixed cholestatic pattern (82–83) have been reported. The fever and generalized hypersensitivity syndrome that may accompany the injury support the view that immunological idiosyncrasy is the mechanism of injury (9). This interpretation, however, is belied by the occurrence of fatal steatosis in one patient (79), a lesion suggesting the injury to be metabolically mediated. Furthermore, the report (83) of acute hepatocellular injury in a patient who had taken a huge overdose (20 g), suggests some intrinsic toxicity of the agent, albeit of a very low order. The issue remains unclear.

C. Naproxen (Naprosen)

Of the propionic acid derivatives, naproxen has been incriminated in a few specific cases of hepatic injury (84–90). It also has received mention with other NSAIDs as the cause of hepatic injury (91,92); and hepatic injury has been listed with other effects of naproxen (93). Hepatocellular jaundice (84–87), including a case of fulminant hepatic failure (87), cholestatic jaundice (88,89), and indeterminate jaundice (90), have been described. Fever in one case and hepatic eosinophil aggregates in another, have led to the suggestion that the mechanism is hypersensitivity. Onset of overt hepatic injury between 1 and 12 weeks after starting the drug throws little light on the mechanism, which remains unclear.

D. Fenoprofen (Nalfon)

Fenoprofen, a calcium salt of 2-(3-phenoxyphenyl)propionic acid resembles ibuprofen in its structure, effects, and metabolism. Fenoprofen also rarely leads to hepatic injury, having been incriminated in only two instances (hepatocellular injury in one), to my knowledge (86,94). One of them (86) had developed jaundice while taking naproxen. After withdrawal of naproxen and recovery from jaundice, administration of fenoprofen led to recurrence of the abnormality.

E. Fenbufen (Bufemid)

The phenylpropionic acid derivative fenbufen has been employed in other countries, but has not been approved for clinical use in the United States. Fenbufen has led to elevated aminotransferase or alkaline phosphatase levels in up to 25% of recipients (95–98), with some values in the range of overt hepatic disease (96). Although the ability of this drug to provoke hypersensitivity reactions seems demonstrated by cases that develop rash and fever, the hepatic abnormality occurring in one out of four recipients presumably reflects an element of intrinsic toxicity, albeit mild. The rare, recorded instances of overt hepatic injury apparently reflect increased susceptibility, dependent on immunological or metabolic idiosyncrasy.

F. Benoxaprofen (Oroflex)

The use of benoxaprofen has been abandoned, but the history of this drug and of its adverse effects is an important chapter in the annals of hepatotoxicology. The abrupt and surprising appearance of hepatic injury, the character of the injury, the paradoxically fatal outcome, and the presumed mechanism of injury, all compose an entity that provided an important lesson.

This NSAID was only briefly available in the United States. After 2 years of use in the United Kingdom, it was approved for use in this country in April 1982—only to be withdrawn 4 months later, after a number of reports of fatal hepatic and renal disease appeared in the British literature (4,99). During its use in the United Kingdom, one-half million patients had taken the drug (100), and approximately 3500 reports of adverse reactions were submitted to the UK Committee of Safety of Medicines (100,101). Most of these reactions involved the skin, owing to photosensitization; some were gastrointestinal; a few were of the Stevens–Johnson type (101, 102), and several were hepatic (103–109). Indeed, many of the 61 fatal reactions had hepatic and renal involvement (9). At least 14 of the cases of hepatic injury were published (103–109).

A striking feature of benoxaprofen-associated hepatic injury has been its cholestatic nature, yet its paradoxically high fatality rate (4,9,105,110). It has become a clinical axiom that acute, drug-induced cholestasis is rarely fatal (3,9,105), yet 11 of 14 cases of benoxaprofen-induced cholestasis died.

1. Histology

Morphological features consisted of severe hepatic cholestasis accompanied by slight to moderate necrosis. The cholestasis was particularly marked in zone 3 and showed strikingly inspissated bile casts in cholangioles, canaliculi, and even in portal bile ducts (111).

2. Mechanism of Injury

Clearly, the apparent rarity of overt injury demonstrates that the mechanism was idiosyncrasy. The lack of hallmarks of hypersensitivity in patients with jaundice and the prolonged exposure to the drug before development of injury suggests that the idiosyncrasy was metabolic, rather than immunological. About 50% of the drug is converted to glucuronide, and the concretions of the drug in bile canaliculi may consist of this or other, poorly soluble metabolites. The degree or rate of conversion, or the type or amount of metabolite formed, would affect precipitation in canaliculi and play a role in the causation of jaundice. In any event, benoxaprofen appeared to cause jaundice in a small proportion of recipients, as an idiosyncratic reaction, presumably dependent on abnormal metabolism or disposal of the drug.

3. Susceptibility to Injury

Factors contributing to enhanced susceptibility included age and sex. All but 1 of the 14 reported cases were women, and 11 of the 14 were older than 70 years old; only one was younger than 60 (103,109). Indeed, elderly patients appear to metabolize the drug much more slowly than younger individuals (112,113). Hamdy et al. (113) found the half-life of the drug to be almost fourfold greater in a group of patients with an average age of 82 years, than in those about half that age. Such prolongation of metabolism might lead to cumulatively higher blood levels of the drug and ultimately biliary excretion of larger amounts and higher concentrations of an apparently poorly soluble product.

4. Prognosis

The limited data base clouds the view of prognosis. Eleven of the 14 cases died, one as a complication of liver biopsy. Undoubtedly, reports of milder cases and a larger sample would yield a lower fatality rate.

5. Cause of Death

The cause of death in these patients remains an enigma. The biochemical data and morphological features suggested that parenchymal injury was insufficiently severe in most patients to lead to death. Prescott et al. (105) have offered an intriguing, hypothetical explanation for the fatal outcome. They suggested that the slowed disposition of the drug in elderly persons leads to higher blood (and tissue) levels of the drug, and that these lead to cholestasis and renal injury. The cholestasis and renal failure, according to this hypothesis, arrest drug disposal further and lead to drug levels so high that patients die of drug toxicity, not liver failure.

The withdrawal of the drug from clinical use would appear to make the issue of benoxaprofen jaundice moot. Nevertheless, the drug played in important role in views of NSAID-associated hepatic injury, and its history is pertinent.

G. Flurbiprofen (Ansaid)

There has been little evidence for hepatotoxic effects of this drug. To my knowledge, there has been only one published report of jaundice (114), although there are apparently other, unpublished cases (9). The injury has appeared to be hepatocellular and accompanied by hallmarks of hypersensitivity. Onset in the published case, however, was unusually delayed for a hypersensitivity-determined reaction, occurring 3 months after starting the drug. Flurbiprofen is not available in the United States.

H. Pirprofen (Rengasil)

Pirprofen has been reported to have led to at least 14 cases of hepatic injury, all hepatocellular (115–122). Four of the reported case were fatal. Prolonged exposure to the drug before onset of jaundice (2–6 months) and absence of hallmarks of hypersensitivity, suggest the mechanism to have been netabolic idiosyncrasy. Twelve of the 14 patients were women, all but 3 older than 60 years, suggesting that women, especially elderly ones, are particularly susceptible.

The inference that the mechanism of injury is metabolic idiosyncrasy (110), based on clinical manifestations and the delayed onset, seems borne out by experimental studies (122) demonstrating toxic effects of the drug in mice. Pirprofen was found to inhibit mitochondrial β-oxidation and to lead to microvesicular steatosis, presumably as a consequence (122).

I. Carprofen (Imadyl)

Carprofen has not seen extensive use, and no instances of overt liver disease have been attributed to it. In several controlled trials (123,124), however, the reported incidence of elevated aminotransferase and alkaline phosphatase levels was high, in one study approaching 50% (123). *Ketoprofen* (Orudis) appears not to have been incriminated in instances of hepatic injury.

J. Oxaprozin (Oxapro)

The propionic acid derivative oxaprozin has produced a 15% incidence of elevated aminotransferase levels, almost all less than threefold the ULN (125). In only 1% of recipients did the values exceed the threefold level. In two-thirds of the patients with abnormal levels, the values decreased or remained essentially unchanged, despite continuation of the drug. Overt hepatitis appears to be rare.

K. Suprofen (Suprol)

Suprofen was withdrawn from clinical use in 1987 after a brief period, because of unexplained flank pain, in some cases accompanied by renal abnormalities. The drug also had been found to lead to elevated aminotransferase levels in 15% of recipients and had been incriminated in several instances of severe hepatocellular injury (reports submitted to the FDA).

IV. PYRAZOLONE DERIVATIVES (ENOLIC NONSTEROIDAL ANTI-INFLAMMATORY DRUGS)

A. Phenylbutazone (Butazolidine)

As an extensively used prototype of the enolic β-diketone NSAIDs, phenylbutazone is the most thoroughly studied member of the group. At one time widely used in the treatment of bursitis, gout, and other musculoskeletal lesions, phenylbutazone (PBZ) has led to several instances of liver damage (3,6,9,14). During the four decades that PBZ has been in clinical use, approximately 100 patients have been reported to have developed hepatic injury. As with most drugs, it is difficult to define the incidence of hepatic injury. Kuzell et al. (6) found a 0.25% incidence of overt "hepatitis" among recipients (2 of 800).

1. Factors in Susceptibility

Vulnerability seems to be modified by age. Almost all cases involve adults. Dhatt et al. (126) reported an instance of fatal hepatitis provoked by therapeutic doses of PBZ in an 11-year-old child, but were unable to find other reports of childhood cases. Other instances of PBZ-induced liver damage in children appear to have been the result of poisoning from very large overdoses (14). There are no firm data on sex as a factor in susceptibility to injury. Although the 41 cases analyzed by Fowler et al. (127) yielded a ratio of males to females of 1:3.5, Benjamin et al. (14), found the number of males and females to be approximately equal.

2. Clinical Features

Onset of illness occurs within the first 6 weeks of treatment in over 80% of reported patients, and within the first 4 weeks in two-thirds of them (14). Approximately 10% develop overt hepatic injury only after taking the drug for at least 3 months, and about 5% do not develop liver disease until they have been taking PBZ for longer than 1 year.

The clinical characteristics are a composite of systemic manifestations, gastrointestinal complaints, and jaundice. In an estimated 50% of patients, fever, rash, and arthralgia singly or in combination, and accompanied by varying degrees of nausea, vomiting, and abdominal pain, have preceded the appearance of the jaundice (14). In about half of reported patients, gastrointestinal complaints and fatigability precede or accompany the jaundice, without antecedent fever or rash. In a few patients jaundice may be the presenting and main complaint. Fowler et al. (127) have suggested that lack of systemic factors is more characteristic of patients with the cholestatic form of PBZ jaundice than of those with the hepatocellular type of injury.

Hematological injury, another serious complication of PBZ administration, has been observed in fewer than 1% of patients taking the drug (6). Indeed, among reactions to PBZ, fatalities owing to myelotoxicity have outnumbered those caused by hepatic necrosis. The two, however, may coincide (3).

3. Form of Hepatic Injury

Both cytolytic and cholestatic forms of injury have been found (14). Approximately two-thirds of reported cases have had cytolytic injury. These have shown necrosis, with or without steatosis. In fatal cases, necrosis may be massive. Cholestatic features, in many of the patients with hepatocellular injury, may be sufficiently prominent to warrant categorizing the injury as mixed hepatocellular; and cholestasis with little parenchymal damage has been found in about 30% of patients with PBZ-induced hepatic injury. The inflammatory response accompanying the cholestatic type of injury may resemble that of chlorpromazine jaundice, and may include granulomas (129–130). Solitary giant cells without a full granulomatous lesion may also be seen in the portal areas (130). Granulomas found in the liver may be part of a systemic granulomatous reaction (sarcoidosislike) to PBZ, with or without cholestasis or parenchymal injury (131).

4. *Biochemical Features*

The biochemical features reflect the histological pattern of injury. The patients with hepatic necrosis have had moderately (5-fold) to markedly (40-fold) elevated values for the aminotransferases, and slightly or moderately elevated values for alkaline phosphatase (14). The cases of cholestatic injury have had high values for cholesterol and alkaline phosphatase, but only slightly or modestly elevated aminotransferase values (9,14, 127,129).

5. *Prognosis*

The outcome also relates to the form of injury. Fowler et al. described a case fatality rate of 12% (127). Fatalities have been in patients with hepatic necrosis. Patients with the granulomatous lesion and cholestasis recover, although the duration of the cholestasis may be as long as 4 months. More instances of a fatal reaction appear to have been the result of bone marrow injury than of hepatic damage.

6. *Mechanism of Injury*

Hypersensitivity has been judged (14) to be responsible for the hepatic injury produced by therapeutic doses of PBZ. The evidence, although circumstantial, is very suggestive. It includes the frequent presence of fever, rash and, in some cases, eosinophilia. Onset of illness, within the first 4–6 weeks of taking the drug in most of the cases (14), is also consistent with the view that hypersensitivity plays a role in the genesis of the hepatic injury. Whether the cases without clinical hallmarks of hypersensitivity result from a different mechanism is open to speculation (14).

That intrinsic toxicity of the drug may also play a role, however, is suggested by an apparent relation between dose and toxicity and by the experimental hepatotoxic effects of the drug (132–134). There is a prevailing view in the literature that hepatic injury occurred more frequently in the early years of clinical use of PBZ, when high doses were employed, than in the more recent period, during which the doses have been lower. Furthermore, at least nine instances of hepatic injury among children and young adults who had taken very large amounts of PBZ have been reported (14). Also large doses of the drug can produce steatosis, necrosis (132,133), and cholestasis (134) in experimental animals.

7. *Comment*

Hepatic injury is an important side effect of PBZ. Although rare, enough instances have occurred to characterize it. The hepatocellular form, which is the more common, is a serious lesion and accounts for the instances of fatal liver damage (14). The cholestatic form is benign. In some patients, hypersensitivity combined with mild intrinsic toxicity is presumed to be responsible. In others, aberrant metabolism with production of toxic metabolites probably leads to the hepatic injury. The hepatotoxic threat of PBZ seems largely moot, since the many NSAIDs that have been introduced have led to abandonment of long-term use of the drug.

B. Oxyphenbutazone (Tanderil)

Oxyphenbutazone, as a hydroxylated derivative of PBZ, usually receives mention in the same breath with PBZ. The side reactions of the two appear to be similar, although there is very scant information on the hepatic injury produced by oxyphenbutazone. The pattern of injury seems similar to that of PBZ. Necrosis (135) and granulomas (136) have been described.

C. Kebuzone (Ketazone)

Ketobutazone appears to have greater hepatotoxic potential than PBZ (137–139). It was found to produce hepatic injury, as reflected by elevated aminotransferase levels in 20 and jaundice in 2 of 75 patients in one study (138). Another report described 12 patients who developed jaundice accompanied by hallmarks of hypersensitivity during the first 4 weeks of taking the drug (139).

D. Azapropazone (Rheumox)

The pyrazolone derivative apazone (azapropazone) has not been incriminated in hepatic injury. It appears to have specific effects on metabolism or disposition of some drugs, in that it enhances strikingly the hypoglycemic effects of tolbutamide (140), the anticoagulant effects of warfarin (141), and neurological toxicity of phenytoin (142). Competition for binding to blood proteins, interference with metabolism, or both may be responsible (142).

V. OXICAMS

A. Piroxicam (Feldene)

Piroxicam had appeared to show little evidence other than a 1–2% incidence of elevated AST levels in early studies (143). Nevertheless, instances of hepatic injury have been described (144–150). Several have involved fatal hepatic necrosis (145–147) or required transplantation (148). Others have shown severe cholestatic or mixed jaundice (144,149, 150). As with several other drugs, elderly patients have seemed particularly susceptible. Pancreatitis has been reported (151).

B. Isoxicam

Only one report (152) has appeared of hepatic injury secondary to this drug, the latest oxicam on the scene. The injury appeared after 2 weeks of therapy and was ushered in with fever, rash, and eosinophilia. The pattern of injury was mixed cholestatic. Recovery occurred within 5 weeks. This drug is not in use in the United States.

VI. SALICYLATES

A. Aspirin

After more than a century of widespread use, aspirin joined the ranks of drugs that are known to produce hepatic injury (153–157). As recently as 1975, a leading textbook of pharmacology (158) specifically stated that salicylates, even in large doses, do not seem to damage the hepatic parenchyma. Beginning in 1971 (154), however, papers had begun to appear drawing specific attention to the hepatic injury produced by aspirin and other salicylates (153–158); and the phenomenon had been sensed earlier. A report in 1945 described hepatic damage (microvesicular steatosis) in four patients who had taken large overdoses of aspirin (159), but the suggestion that aspirin might be hepatotoxic appeared to draw little attention. With the advent of clinical enzymology, the effects of aspirin on the liver began to attract notice. Studies (160) of serum aminotransferase levels in patients with rheumatic fever (who were taking aspirin) demonstrated elevated values in 50% of them. Many reports describing aspirin-associated hepatic injury have since appeared.

1. Incidence

Hepatic damage induced by aspirin may be noted in 50% or more patients with high blood levels of the drug (13,157). Most of the patients who have developed hepatic injury had levels above 15 mg/dl of serum. The levels that lead to hepatic injury are achieved by the "full dosage" usually employed in treating rheumatic fever and active rheumatoid arthritis (13).

2. Types of Injury

The injury is manifested by values of aminotransferases that are elevated from 5- to 40-fold (13). Bilirubin levels are normal or slightly elevated, and jaundice (15) is noted in fewer than 5% of cases (13). Biopsy has shown areas of focal necrosis, with mild inflammatory response (157) in the portal areas and sinusoids, and ultrastructural changes (161) similar to those of intrinsic hepatotoxins. Lysosomes, peroxisomes, and mitochondria, all seem to be increased in number, and there is dilatation of the smooth and rough endoplasmic reticulum (SER and RER) and increase in SER concentration (161,162). Poisonous overdoses of aspirin lead to microvesicular steatosis (163).

The injury described, for the most part, has not been serious. The abnormality disappears promptly on stopping the drug. No convincing instances of fatal necrosis have been reported, although discussion of a "Cabot case" that involved a patient who had received both aspirin and acetaminophen contained the implication that the fatal hepatic necrosis was due to the aspirin (164). Suggestions (157) that aspirin can lead to chronic active hepatitis (CAH) remain to be substantiated.

3. Mechanism

The hepatic injury reflects intrinsic toxicity. It is a property, apparently, of the salicylate molecule (9,155). Not only acetylsalicylate, but also sodium and choline salicylate lead to elevated serum levels of aminotransferases (155). The effect is dose- and blood level-related (9,153), and aspirin can produce hepatic injury in several species of animals (165).

4. Susceptibility

Host factors appear to modify vulnerability. Patients with juvenile arthritis, systemic lupus erythematosus (SLE), and rheumatic fever appear to be more vulnerable than others (9,157). Furthermore, patients with SLE not only seem particularly susceptible to the hepatotoxic effects of aspirin, but also seem to show a positive correlation between activity of the underlying disease and susceptibility to the hepatic injury (13). However, patients without rheumatic disease and normal persons also can develop evidence of hepatic injury when given large doses of aspirin (13). Furthermore, there are striking individual variations in the degree of hepatic injury provoked by various blood levels of salicylates, particularly among patients in remission from rheumatic disease (13).

The apparently enhanced susceptibility of patients with SLE and the correlation between activity of the rheumatic disease and susceptibility to aspirin-related hepatic injury suggest that the underlying disease may affect the metabolism or toxicity of the drug. Indeed, adjuvant-produced arthritis leads to altered metabolism of drugs (166). One report (167) suggests that hepatic disease enhances susceptibility to salicylate injury. Gitlin has suggested that hypoalbuminemia enhances toxicity by permitting higher levels of free salicylate (168), a phenomenon that would explain the increased susceptibility of cirrhotic patients reported by Okomura (167).

5. Aspirin and Reye's Syndrome

The hepatotoxic effects of aspirin also involve its apparent role in producing Reye's syndrome. For years considered a relatively rare manifestation of several fairly common viral illnesses, Reye's syndrome is now attributed to a combination of the viral illness and toxic chemical agents (169). Although several biological and chemical agents have been suspected of being the provocative toxicants, evidence for the role of aspirin has been most compelling (170, 171), although somewhat controversial (172).

By now, however, the evidence seems even more convincing that children given aspirin during the viral illness are more likely to develop Reye's syndrome than those who are not given the drug (170,171). Furthermore, the development of Reye's syndrome in patients with rheumatoid arthritis, systemic lupus erythematosus, or related syndromes, who had been receiving regular aspirin therapy (173,174), adds convincing data of the association. Even an adult with an aspirin-treated viral syndrome has been reported to have developed Reye's syndrome (174). Additional support for the association between aspirin use and Reye's syndrome is the striking decrease in incidence of Reye's syndrome in the United States that has accompanied decreased use of aspirin (170,171).

Benorilate is an acetaminophen ester of acetylsalicylic acid. The instances of hepatic injury attributed to it have the characterictics of acetaminophen injury, namely zone 3 necrosis, rather than the degeneration or microvesicular steatosis of aspirin-induced injury. Nevertheless, the high salicylate levels (35 mg/dl) in one case suggests that salicylate toxicity may have contributed to the injury. The relevance of benorilate-induced injury does not seem great, however, since the drug appears to have limited use and offers no advantage over either component (9).

B. Acetaminophen

Acetaminophen (ACM), a weakly anti-inflammatory drug that is used mainly for its analgesic and antipyretic effects, has dose-related hepatotoxic potential. Its hepatotoxic effects have been seen mainly in gross overdose, most often suicidally motivated (13). However, several instances of hepatic necrosis have resulted from therapeutic misadventures; however, either because careless use led to a larger than normal daily dose or because of unusual susceptibility (175). Indeed, a recent report from one institution describes the number of cases caused by therapeutic use of the drug to be at least as large as the number from suicidally motivated overdoses (176). Enhanced susceptibility to toxic effects of ACM is attributable to the factors leading to enhanced conversion of ACM to its toxic metabolite and to depletion of body glutathione (GSH) stores (175). The most relevant factor has appeared to be alcoholism, which leads to induction of the cytochrome

P-450 system (175), especially the isozyme mainly involved in ACM metabolism (P450IIE1). Alcoholism also leads to depletion of GSH owing to the associated malnutrition as well as to the inhibition by alcohol of GSH synthesis (175).

VII. OTHER DRUGS USED IN RHEUMATIC DISEASE

A. Corticosteroids

Analysis of adverse effects of drugs used to treat rheumatic disease would be incomplete without reference to hepatic changes effected by corticosteroids. Large doses produce steatosis and have even been described to produce "alcoholic hyaline"-like change. Even modest doses (10–15 mg/day of prednisolone) when administered for long periods lead to fat in the liver (3).

B. Gold Compounds

During an earlier era of chrysotherapy (1925–1950), several reports seemed to indicate the potential for producing hepatic injury (177–183). At least some of the instances of liver disease can, in retrospect, be judged to have been viral hepatitis transmitted by contaminated needles, as was observed in diabetes and syphilis clinics during that period. Instances of hepatic injury include both hepatocellular and cholestatic injury. Although most of the individually reported cases of gold-induced hepatic injury, have shown mainly cholestasis (177–183), cases of hepatic necrosis, some fatal, have been reported (181–183).

C. Penicillamine

Best known for its use in the treatment of Wilson's disease, penicillamine also has been employed in the treatment of rheumatoid arthritis and related syndromes. By now, about 20 cases of jaundice have been described, almost all mainly cholestatic (184–189). The uniformity of the syndrome, almost all cases starting within the first 2–4 weeks of taking the drug, accompanied by rash, fever, eosinophilia, abdominal pain and nausea, and consistently cholestatic jaundice, demonstrates penicillamine jaundice to be a definable entity.

D. Methotrexate

Treatment of rheumatoid arthritis and related conditions with low doses of methotrexate (MTX) has become increasingly popular. The injury attributed in the past to MTX in patients who received the drug for treatment of psoriasis or leukemia, for the most part, has not been matched by changes in the patients with rheumatic disease (191,192). [Even in patients with psoriasis the risk of MTX-induced hepatic injury seems to be a less serious threat than formerly regarded; and there is general agreement that hepatotoxic effects are reduced by maintenance of weekly intervals between doses, and avoiding patients with increased susceptibility to injury (alcoholics and obese diabetics; (196)].

In the patients with rheumatoid arthritis, the low doses of MTX given according to this schedule appear even less likely to produce hepatic injury. Nevertheless, even in them, steatosis, fibrosis, and even cirrhosis can appear during treatment (193,194). Accordingly, monitoring effects of treatment by liver biopsy continues to be recommended (193).

VIII. CONCLUDING COMMENTS

Liver damage caused by most of the nonsteroidal anti-inflammatory drugs (NSAIDs), tends to be hepatocellular. A few of the NSAIDs, penicillamine, and gold compounds tend to lead to cholestatic injury.

Several of the NSAIDs can lead to hepatic granulomas. The mechanism for injury, for some of the NSAIDs, appears to be hypersensitivity; for others metabolic idiosyncrasy; and, for several of the drugs, intrinsic toxicity appears to play a role.

REFERENCES

1. Hueper WE. Cinchophen (Atophan): a critical review. Medicine 1948; 27:43.
2. Palmer WL, Woodall PS. Cinchophen—is there a safe method of administration? JAMA 1936; 107:760.
3. Zimmerman HJ, Maddrey WC. Toxic and drug-induced hepatitis. In: Schiff L, Schiff ER, eds. Diseases of the liver. 6th ed. Philadelphia: JB Lippincott, 1987:591–668.
4. Paulus HE. FDA Arthritis Advisory Committee meeting. Arthritis Rheum 1982; 25:1124.
5. Arthritis drug withdrawn. FDA Consum 1982; 16 (Nov):4.
6. Kuzell WC, Schaffarzick RW, Naugler WE, et al. Phenylbutazone, further clinical evaluation. Arch Intern Med 1953; 92:603.
7. Thompson M, Stephenson P, Percy JS. Ibufenac in the treatment of arthritis. Ann Rheumat Dis 1964; 23:397.
8. Hart FD, Boardman PL. Ibufenac (4-isobutylphenyl acetic acid). Ann Rheumat Dis 1965; 24:61.
9. Stricker BHC, Spoelstra P. Drug-induced liver injury. Amsterdam: Elsevier, 1985:45–76.
10. Tarazi E, Harter JG, Zimmerman HJ, et al. Sulindac-associated hepatic injury. Analysis of 91 cases reported to the FDA. Gastroenterology 1993; 104:569–574.
11. Banks T, Zimmerman HJ, Harter J, Ishak KG. Diclofenac-associated hepatic injury analysis of 181 cases. (in press).
12. Prescott LF. Effects of non-narcotic analgesics on the liver. Drugs 1986; 32 (suppl 4):129.
13. Zimmerman HJ. Effects of aspirin and acetaminophen on the liver. Arch Intern Med 1981; 141:33.
14. Benjamin SB, Ishak KG, Zimmerman HJ, Grushka A. Phenylbutazone liver injury: a clinical pathologic survey of 23 cases and review of the literature. Hepatology 1981; 1:255.
15. Chagnon JP, Barge J. Hepatite chronique active a la clometacine et antigene HLA. B8. Gastroenterol Clin Biol 1983; 7:556.
16. Stricker BHC, Blok AP, Bronkhorst FB. Glafenine-associated hepatic injury: analysis of 38 cases and review of the literature. Liver 1986; 6:63.
17. Iveson TJ, Ryley NA, Kelly PMA, et al. Diclofenac associated hepatitis. J Hepatol 1990; 10:585.
18. Imoto S, Matsumoto H, Fujii M. Drug-related hepatitis. Ann Intern Med 1979; 91:129.
19. Van Berge-Henegouwen GP, Hartman AP, Werre JM, Brandt KH. Icterus door niflumine (Inflaryl). Ned T Geneskd 1974; 118:1229.
20. Mickley H, Amtrap F. Leverpavirkning unter tolfenamsyrebehandling. Ugeskr Laeger 1981; 143:2036.
21. Dunk AA, Walt RP, Jenkins WJ, Sherlock SS. Diclofenac hepatitis. Br Med J 1982; 284:1605.
22. Babany G, Pessayre D, Benhamou JP. Hepatite au diclofenac. Gastroenterol Clin Biol 1983; 7:316.
23. Deshayes P, Leloet X, Bercoff E, Fouin-Fortunet H. Diclofenac hepatitis. Nouv Presse Med 1984; 13:1847.
24. Lascar G, Grippon P, Levy VG. Hepatite aigue mortelle au cours d'un traitment par le diclofenac (Voltarene). Gastroenterol Clin Biol 1984; 8:881.

25. Breen EG, McNicholl J, Cosgrove E, et al. Fatal hepatitis associated with diclofenac. Gut 1986; 27:1390.
26. Schapira D, Bassan L, Nahir AM, Scharf Y. Diclofenac-induced hepatotoxicity. Postgrad Med J 1986; 62:63.
27. Helfgott SM, Sanberg-Cook J, Zakimr D, Nestler J. Diclofenac-associated hepatotoxicity. JAMA 1990; 264:2660.
28. Purcell P, Henry D, Melville G. Diclofenac hepatitis. Gut 1991; 32:1381.
29. Ouellette GS, Stitsky BE, Gates JA, et al. Reversible hepatitis associated with diclofenac. J Clin Gastroenterol 1991; 13:205.
29a. Withdrawal of glafenine. Lancet 1992; 339:357.
30. Fenech FF, Bannister WH, Grech JL. Hepatitis with biliverdinaemia in association with indomethacin therapy. Br Med J 1967; 3:155.
31. Kelsey WM, Scharyi M. Fatal hepatitis probably due to indomethacin. JAMA 1967; 199:154.
32. Opolon P, Cartron P, Chicot D, Carole J. Application due test de transformation lymphoblastique (TTL) diagnostic de certaines hepatitis medicamenteuses. Presse Med 1969; 77:2041.
33. Dekicker-Sangster M, Bronkhorstst FB, Brandt KH, Boersa JW. Massive hepatocellular necrosis after administration of indomethacin in combination with aminophenazone. Med T 1981; 125:1825.
34. Cuthbert MG. Adverse reactions to nonsteroidal antiinflammatory drugs. Curr Med Res Opin 1974; 2:12.
35. Henrard JC. Les medications anti-inflammatories analgiques courantes. Presse Med 1970; 78:1205.
36. Boardman PL, Hart FD. Side effects of indomethacin. Ann Rheum Dis 1967; 26:127.
37. Lenoir C, Labayle D, Buffet C. Hepatite au clometacine. Nouv Presse Med 1978; 7:3035.
38. Goldfarb G, Pessayre D, Boisseau C, et al. Hepatite a la clometacine. Gastroenterol Clin Biol 1979; 3:537.
39. Manigand G, Pointud P, Taillandier J, et al. Hepatite a la clometacine. Nouv Presse Med 1979; 8:213.
40. Mamou P, Levy VG. Atteintes hepatiques apres clometacine 6 cas dont 2 mortels. Nouv Presse Med 1981; 10:2719.
41. Hillion D, Filsenheld C, Oberlin P, et al. Pericholiangitie chez in adulta traite par clometacine. Gastroenterol Clin Biol 1983; 7:1038.
42. Tassou JJ, Bretagne JF, Marion J. Hepatite a la clometacine. Concours Med 1981; 103:679.
43. Chavenet P, Blettery B, Aube H, et al. Hepatonephrite decours d'un traitement a la cholmetacive. Lyon Med 1983; 250:407.
44. Pessayre D, Degros P, Feldman G, Degott C. Chronic active hepatitis and giant multinucleated hepatocytes in adults treated with clometacin. Digestion 1981; 22:66.
45. Parini M, Benevent D, Leroux-Robert C. Insuffisance renale aigue et hepatite lors d'un traitement par clometacine. Nouv Presse Med 1982; 11:2641.
46. Poitrine A, Poynard T, Naveu S, et al. Clometacine-induced hepatitis: a fatal crisis. Gastroenterol Clin Biol 1983; 7:99.
47. Braillon A, Capron JP, Quichaud J. Hepatite aique a la clometacine. Interet du dosage des anticorps anti-noyaux et anti-muscle lisse. Gastroenterol Clin Biol 1983; 7:318.
48. Caruana A, Andre C, Zafrani ES, et al. Serum antibodies against double-stranded DNA in chronic active hepatitis: an index of drug-induced liver disease? Lancet 1983; 1:776.
49. Meyer C, Chassagnon C. Un noueau cas mortel de cirrhose du a la clometacine. J Med Lyon 1984; 65:139.
50. Metreau JM, Andre C, Zafrani ES, et al. Hepatites chroniques actives associees a des anticorps anti-DNA natif: frequence de l'etiologie medicamenteuse. Gastroenterol Clin Biol 1984; 8:883.
51. Anderson RJ. Severe reaction associated with sulindac administration. N Engl J. Med 1979; 300:735.

52. Wolfe, PB. Sulindac and jaundice. Ann Intern Med 1979; 91:656.
53. Smith FE, Lindberg PJ. Life-threatening hypersensitivity to sulindac. JAMA 1980; 244: 269.
54. Kaul A, Reddy JC, Fagman E, Smith GF. Hepatitis associated with use of sulindac in a child. J Pediatr 1981; 99:650.
55. McIndoe GAJ, Menzies KW, Reddy J. Sulindac (Clinoril) and cholestatic jaundice. NZ Med J 1981; 94:430.
56. Dhand AK, LaBreque DR, Metzger J. Sulindac (Clinoril) hepatitis. Gastroenterology 1981; 80:585.
57. Whittaker SJ, Amar JN, Wanless IR, Heathcote J. Sulindac hepatotoxicity. Gut 1982; 23:875.
58. Giroux Y, Moreau M, Kass TG. Cholestatic jaundice caused by sulindac. Can J Surg 1982; 25:334.
59. Park GD, Spector R, Headstream T, Goldberg M. Serious adverse reactions associated with sulindac. Arch Intern Med 1982; 142:1292.
60. Kammerer J, Sabaardeil S, Rumeau J-L, et al. Hepatite au sulindac; une observation avec revue des trois precedents. Gastroenterol Clin Biol 1982; 6:712.
61. Klein SM, Muhammad AK. Hepatitis, toxic epidermal neurolysis and pancreatitis in association with sulindac therapy. J Rheumatol 1983; 10:512.
62. Fagan EA, Walford N, Hodgson HJF. Sulindac hepatotoxicity. Gut 1983; 24:1199.
63. Wood LJ, Searle J, Mundo F, Powell LW. Sulindac hepatotoxicity: effects of acute and chronic exposure. Aust NZ J Med 1985; 15:397.
64. Gallanosa AG. Sulindac hepatotoxicity: a case report and review. Clin Toxicol 1985; 23:205.
65. Neufeld MY, Karczyn AD. Encephalopathy associated with sulindac. Hum Toxicol 1986; 5:55.
66. Levitt L, Pearson RW. Sulindac-induced Stevens Johnson toxic epidermal neurolysis syndrome. JAMA 1980; 243:1262.
67. Bodin F, Habibi B, Legendre C, et al. L'hepatotoxicite du sulindac: une nouvelle observation. Gastroenterol Clin Biol 1985; 9:546.
68. Goldstein J, Laskin DA, Ginsberg GH. Sulindac-associated pancreatitis [letter]. Ann Intern Med 1980; 93:151.
69. Siefkin AD. Sulindac and pancreatitis. Ann Intern Med 1980; 93:932.
70. Lilly EL. Pncreatitis after administration of sulindac [letter]. JAMA 1981; 246:2680.
71. Zygmunt DJ, Williams HJ, Bienz SR. Acute pancreatitis associated with long-term sulindac therapy. West J Med 1986; 144:461.
72. Shaw GR, Anderson WR. Multisystem failure and hepatic multivesicular metamorphosis associated with tolmetin ingestion. Arch Lab Med 1991; 15:818.
73. Editorial. Fenclozic acid. Lancet 1970; 1:662.
74. Hart FD, Bain LB, Huskisson EC, et al. Hepatic effects of fenclozic acid. Ann Rheum Dis 1970; 29:684.
75. Katona G, Bondani A. Efficacy and tolerability of fentiazac in rheumatoid arthritis: double blind study versus indomethacin. Curr Med Res Opin 1979; 6(suppl 2):71.
76. Bunde B, Deckers Y, Dequeker J. Fentiazac in rheumatoid arthritis: comparison with sulindac and long-term tolerance. Curr Med Res Opin 1983; 8:310.
77. Ryder S, Salom I, Jacob G. Etodolac (Ultradol): the safety profile of a new structurally novel nonsteroidal anti-inflammatory drug. Curr Ther Res 1983; 33:948.
78. Sonnenblick M, Abraham AS. Ibuprofen hypersensitivity in systemic lupus erythematosus. Br Med J 1978; 1:619.
79. Bravo JF, Jacobson MP, Mertens BF. Fatty liver and pleural effusion with ibuprofen therapy. Ann Intern Med 1977; 87:200.
80. Stempel DA, Miller JJ III. Lymphopenia and hepatic toxicity with ibuprofen. J Pediatr 1977; 90:651.
81. Gasparetto P. Un caso di ittero epatocellulare in corso di trattamento con ibuprofen. Minerva Pediatr 1974; 26:531.

82. Sternleib P, Robinson RM. Stevens–Johnson syndrome plus toxic hepatitis due to ibuprofen. NY State J Med 1978; 87:200.
83. Lee CY, Finkler A. Acute intoxication due to ibuprofen overdose. Arch Pathol Lab Med 1986; 110:747.
84. Law JP, Knight H. Jaundice associated with naproxen. N Engl J Med 1976; 295:1201.
85. Victorino RMM, Silveira JCB, Baptista A, et al. Jaundice associated with naproxen. Postgrad Med J 1980; 56:368.
86. Andrejak M, Davion T, Gineston JL, Capron JP. Cross hepatotoxicity between non-steroidal anti-inflammatory drugs. Br Med J 1987; 295:180.
87. Giarelli L, Falcomari G, Delender M. Fulminant hepatitis following naproxan administration. Hum Pathol 1986; 17:1079.
88. Bass BH. Jaundice associated with naproxen [letter]. Lancet 1974; 1:998.
89. Krogsgaard K, Harcht F, Malchow-Miller A. Liver involvement after treatment with naproxen. Ugesker Laeger 1980; 142:450.
90. Lagarriga J. Naproxen e icterica. Rev Sanid Milit 1975; 29:250.
91. Jick H, Derby LE, Garcia Rodriquez LA, et al. Liver disease associated with diclofenac, naproxen and peroxicam. Pharmacotherapy 1992; 12:207.
92. Bell H, Raknered N. Fulminating hepatitis after treatment with naproxen and/or disulfiram. Tiddskr Nort Laegefuran 1991; 111:322.
93. Johnson AG, Day RO. The problems and pitfalls of NSAID therapy in the elderly. Drugs Aging 1991; 1:130.
94. Stenett DJ, Simonson W, Hall CA. Fenoprofen-induced hepatotoxicity. Am J Hosp Pharm 1978; 35:901.
95. Buxton R, Grennan DM, Palmer DG. Fenbufen compared with indomethacin in osteoarthritis. Curr Med Res Opin 1978; 5:682.
96. Becker A, Hoffmeister RT. Fenbufen, a new non-steroidal anti-inflammatory agent in rheumatoid arthritis, its efficacy and toxicity. J Int Med Res 1980; 8:333.
97. Roth SH, Cryan WS, Harris BK, et al. Long-term double-blind comparison of fenbufen with aspirin in the treatment of rheumatoid arthritis. Pharmacology 1982; 25:63.
98. Kawamura J, Kani I, Hasegawa O, et al. Clinical effect of fenbufen in periarthritis of the shoulder. Kiso to Rinsho 1977; 11:171.
99. Arthritis drug under fire. Sci News 1982; 122:104.
100. Editorial. Benoxaprofen. Br Med J 1982; 285:249.
101. Halsey JP, Cardoe N. Benoxaprofen: side effects profile in 300 patients. Br Med J 1982; 284:1365.
102. Hindson C, Daymond T, Diffey B, et al. Side effects of benoxaprofen. Br Med J 1982; 284:1368.
103. Taggart HM, Alderdice JM. Fatal cholestatic jaundice in elderly patients taking benoxaprofen. Br Med J 1982; 284:1372.
104. Goudie BM, Birnie GF, Wathinson G, et al. Jaundice associated with the use of benoxaprofen. Lancet 1982; 1:959.
105. Prescott LP, Leslie PJ, Padfield P. Side effects of benoxaprofen. Br Med J 1982; 284:1783.
106. Firth H, Wilcock GK, Esiri M, et al. Side effects of benoxaprofen. Br Med J 1982; 284:1784.
107. Fisher BM, McArthur JD. Side effects of benoxaprofen. Br Med J 1982; 284:1783.
108. Duthie A. Fatal cholestatic jaundice in elderly patients taking benoxaprofen. Br Med J 1982; 285:62.
109. Diffey B, Hindson C. Side effects of benoxaprofen. Br Med J 1982; 284:1630.
110. Lewis JH. Hepatic toxicity of nonsteroidal anti-inflammatory drugs. Clin Pharm 1984; 3: 128.
111. MacSween RMN. Personal communication.
112. Nash JF, Carmichael RH, Ridolfo AS, Spradin CT. Pharmacokinetics studies of benoxaprofen after therapeutic doses with a review of related pharmacokinetics metabolic studies. J Rheumatol [Suppl] 1980; 7:12.

113. Hamdy RC, Murnang B, Perera N, et al. The pharmacokinetics of benoxaprofen in elderly subjects. Eur J Rheumatol Inflamm 1982; 5:69.
114. Kotowski KE, Grayson MF. Side effects of non-steroidal anti-inflammatory drugs. Br Med J 1982; 285:377.
115. Fouin-Fortunet H, Lerebours E, Bernet J, et al. Hepatite au pirprofene. Ann Gastroenterol Hepatol 1986; 22:23.
116. Danan G, Trunet P, Bernuau J, et al. Pirprofen-induced fulminant hepatitis. Gastroenterology 1985; 89:210.
117. Castot A, Netter P, Arnaudo J-P, et al. Hépatites au pirproféne d'évolution favorable. Thérapie 1984; 39:297.
118. DeHerder WW, Schröder P, Purnode A, et al. Pirprofen-associated hepatic injury. J Hepatol 1987; 4:127.
119. Reid RT. Pirprofen and aspirin in rheumatoid arthritis: a double blind comparison study. J Clin Pharmacol 1980; 20:145.
120. Saykaly RJ, Love DW, Simon JA, et al. Comparative efficacy of pirprofen and aspirin in rheumatoid arthritis. J Clin Pharmacol 1979; 19:56.
121. Singleton CM, Wild JH. A double-blind comparison of aspirin and pirprofen in the treatment of rheumatoid arthritis. J Rheumatol 1980; 7:865.
122. Geneve J, Hayat-Bonan B, Labbe G, et al. Inhibition of mitochondrial β-oxidation of fatty acids by pirprofen. Role in microvesicular steatosis due to this nonsteroidal anti-inflammatory drug. J Pharmacol Exp Ther 1987; 1:242
123. Jensen EM, Fossgreen J, Kirchheiner B, et al. Treatment of rheumatoid arthritis with car- profen (Imadyl) or indomethacin: a randomized multicentre trial. Curr Ther Res 1980; 28: 882.
124. Stein GH, Dickey RA, Cohn PD, Goldstein MK. Controlled comparison of carprofen and aspirin in osteoarthritis of the knee. Curr Ther Res 1983; 33:415.
125. Zimmerman HJ. Hepatic effects of oxaprozin. Semin Arthritis Rheum 1986; 15:35.
126. Dhatt PS, Singh H, Gupta HL, Arya RK. Fatal hepatitis due to phenylbutazone in a child. Indian J Pediatr 1973; 40:293.
127. Fowler PD, Woolf D, Alexander S. Phenylbutazone and hepatitis. Rheum Rehabil 1975; 14:71.
128. van de Merwe JP, van Blankenstein M, Wilson JH. Intrahepatic cholestasis induced by phenylbutazone. Digestion 1981; 22:317.
129. Ishak KG, Kirchner JP, Dhar JK. Granuloma and cholestatic hepatocellular injury associated with phenylbutazone. Report of two cases. Am J Dig Dis 1977; 22:611.
130. Scheuer P. Liver biopsy interpretation. 4th ed. London: Bailliere Tindall, 1988: 99–112.
131. Goldstein C. Sarcoid reaction associated with phenylbutazone hypersensitivity. Ann Intern Med 1963; 59:97.
132. Carlisle RH, Penny C, Prescott CW, Davidson H. Toxic effects of phenylbutazone on the cat. Br Vet J 1968; 124:560.
133. Zicha M. The protective effect of L-ornithine-*L*-aspartate on the liver in rats with drug-induced liver damage. Z Gastroenterol 1968; 6:423.
134. Klinger W, Elger J, Franke H, et al. Untersuchungen zum mechanisms der enzyminduktion. XV. Induktionmuster und submikroskopische veranderung in der leber nach applikation von phenylbutazone bei unter-scheidliche alter ratten. Acta Biol Med Germ 1970; 24:263.
135. Gaisford W. Fatality after oxyphenbutazone in Still's disease. Br Med J 1962; 2:1517.
136. Ludwig JR, Axelsen R. Drug effects on the liver. An updated tabular compilation of drugs and drug-related hepatic disease. Dig Dis Sci 1983; 28:651.
137. Nyfos L, Lunding NC. Clinical trial of ketazone versus phenylbutazone in rheumatoid arthritis. Acta Rheumatol Scand 1968; 14:148.
138. Gibson TJ, Burry HC. Ketophenylbutazone: a clinical trial. Clin Trials J 1971; 8:27.
139. Porst VH, Roschlau G, Schentke U, Weise L. Leberschaden durch ketophenylbutazone (ketazon). Dtsch Gesundheitsw 1978; 33:1181.
140. Andreasen PB, Simonsen K, Brocks K, et al. Hypoglycemia induced by azapropazone–tolbutamide interaction [letter]. Br J Clin Pharmacol 1981; 12:583.

141. Green AE, Hort JF, Korn HE, et al. Potentiation of warfarin by azapropazone [letter]. Br Med J 1977; 1:1532.
142. Roberts CJ, Daneshmenp TK, Macfarland ED, Dieppe PA. Anticonvulsant intoxication precipitate by azapropazone. Postgrad Med J 1981; 57:191.
143. Brogden RN, Heel RC, Speight TM, Avery GS. Piroxicam. A reappraisal of its pharmacology and therapeutic efficacy. Drugs 1984; 28:292.
144. Hartmann H, Fischer G, Janning G. Prolonged cholestatic jaundice and leukopenia associated with piroxicam. Z Gastroenterol 1984; 22:343.
145. Lee SM, O'Brien CJ, Williams R, et al. Subacute hepatic necrosis induced by piroxicam. Br Med J 1986; 30:293.
146. Zarski J-P, Aubert H, Dentani L, Rachail I. Les hepatities dues aux anti-inflammatoires non-steroidiens: un nouvelle molecule impligee, le piroxicam (Feldene). Gastroenterol Clin Biol 1984; 8:980.
147. Planas R, Leon RD, Quer JC, et al. Fatal submassive necrosis of the liver associated with piroxicam. Am J Gastroenterol 1990; 5:468.
148. Bismuth H, Samuel D, Gugenheim J, et al. Emergency liver transplantation for fulminant hepatitis. Ann Intern Med 1987; 107:337.
149. Caballeria E, Masso RM, Arago IV, Sanchis A. Piroxican hepatotoxicity. Am J Gastroenterol 1990; 85:898.
150. Hepps KS, Maliha GM, Estrada R, Goodgame RW. Severe cholestatic jaundice associated with piroxicam. Gastroenterology 1991; 101:1737.
151. Haye O. Piroxicam and pancreatitis [letter]. Ann Intern Med 1986; 104:895.
152. Ollagnon HO, Perpoint B, Decousus H, et al. Hepatitis induced by isoxicam. Hepatogastroenterology 1986; 33:109.
153. Zimmerman HJ. Aspirin-induced hepatic injury. Ann Intern Med 1974; 80:103.
154. Russell AS, Sturge RA, Smith MA. Serum transaminases during salicylate therapy. Br Med J 1971; 2:428.
155. Rich RR, Johnson JS. Salicylate hepatotoxicity in patients with juvenile rheumatoid arthritis. Arthritis Rheum 1973; 16:1.
156. Athreya BH, Gorske AL, Meyers AR. Aspirin-induced abnormalities of liver function. Am J Dis Child 1973; 126:638.
157. Seaman WE, Ishak KG, Plotz PH. Aspirin-induced hepatotoxicity in patients with systemic lupus erythematosus. Ann Intern Med 1974; 80:1.
158. Woodbury DM, Fingl E. Analgesic–antipyretics, anti-inflammatory agents, and drugs employed in the therapy of gout. In: Goodman LS, Gilman A, Koelle GB, eds. The pharmacological basis of therapeutics. 5th ed. New York: Macmilliam Publishing, 1975:325–58.
159. Troll MM, Menten ML. Salicylate poisoning: report of four cases. Am J Dis Child 1945; 69:37.
160. Manso C, Taranta A, Nydick I. Effect of aspirin administration on serum glutamic oxalacetic and glutamic pyruvic transaminase in children. Proc Soc Exp Biol Med 1956; 93:84.
161. Phillips MJ, Poucell S, Patterson J, Valencia P. The liver. An atlas and text of ultrastructural pathology. New York: Raven Press, 19XX.
162. Iamcu T, Elian E. Ultrastructural changes in aspirin hepatotoxicity. Am J Clin Pathol 1976; 66:570.
163. Starko KM, Mullick FG. Hepatic and cerebral pathology findings in children with fatal salicylate intoxication: further evidence for a causal relation between salicylate and Reye's syndrome. Lancet 1983; 1:326.
164. Koff RS, Galdabini JJ. Fever, myalgias and hepatic failure in a 17 year old girl. N Engl J Med 1977; 296:1337.
165. Webb WK, Jansen WH. Chronic and subacute toxicology and pathology of methyl salicylate in dogs, rats and rabbits. Toxicol Appl Pharmacol 1963; 5:576.
166. Carlson R, Ciaccio EI. Effect of benzo-*d*-pyrene induction of liver and lung metabolism in adjuvant diseased rats. Biochem Pharmacol 1975; 24:1893.

167. Okamura H, Ichikawa T, Obayashi K, Aramaki T. Studies on aspirin-induced hepatic injury. Recent Adv Gastroenterol 1967; 3:223.
168. Gitlin N. Salicylate hepatotoxicity. The potential role of hypoalbuminemia. J Clin Gastroenterol 1980; 2:281.
169. Crocker JFS, Rozee KR, Ozere RL, et al. Insecticide and viral interaction as a cause of fatty visceral changes and encephalopathy in the mouse. Lancet 1974; 2:22.
170. Hurwitz ES, Barett MJ, Bregeman D, et al. Public health service study on Reye's syndrome and mediations: report of the pilot phase. N Engl J Med 1985; 313:849.
171. Hurwitz ES, Barrett MJ, Bregman D, et al. Public health service study of Reye's syndrome and medications. Report of the main study. JAMA 1987; 257:1905.
172. Orlowski JP, Gillis J, Kilham HA. A catch in the Reye. Pediatrics 1987; 80:638.
173. Young RSK, Torretti D, Williams RH, et al. Reye's syndrome associated with long-term aspirin therapy. JAMA 1984; 251:754.
174. Peters LJ, Wiener GJ, Gilliam J, et al. Reye's syndrome in adults. A case report and review of the literature. Arch Intern Med 1986; 146:2401.
175. Seeff LB, Cuccherini BA, Zimmerman HJ, et al. Acetaminophen hepatotoxicity in alcoholics—a therapeutic misadventure. Ann Intern Med 1986; 104:399.
176. McClain CJ, Holtzman J, Allen J, et al. Clinical features of acetaminophen toxicity. J Clin Gastroenterol 1988; 10:76.
177. Schapira D, Nahir M, Scharf Y, Pollack S. Cholestatic jaundice induced by gold salts: treatment, clinical and immunological aspects. J Rheumatol 1984; 11:843.
178. Langan MN, Thomas P. Penicillamine-induced liver disease. Am J Gastroenterol 1987; 82:1318.
179. Kremer JM. Longterm methotrexate therapy in rheumatoid arthritis: a review. J Rheumatol 1985; 12:25.
180. Kevat S, Ahern M, Hall P. Hepatotoxicity of methotrexate in rheumatic diseases. Med Toxicol 1988; 3:197.
181. Lowthian PJ, Cleland LG, Vernon-Roberts B. Hepatotoxicity with aurothioglucose therapy. Arthritis Rheum 1984; 27:230.
182. Watkins PB, Scade R, Mills AS, et al. Fatal hepatic necrosis associated with parenteral gold therapy. Dig Dis Sci 1988; 33:1025.
183. Howrie DL, Gartner JC Jr. Gold-induced hepatotoxicity: case report and review of the literature. J Rhematol 1982; 9:727.
184. Jaffee IA. D-Penicillamine. Bull Rheum Dis 1978; 28:948.
185. Rau R, Weber S, Boni A. Allergisch-toxische lebershadigung durch D-penillamine. Munch Med Wochenschr 1974; 116:217.
186. Siegmund H. Intrahepatische cholestase nach einer nehandlung mit D-penicillamin und indometacin. Med Welt 1976; 27:172.
187. Sacher M, Thaler H. Toxic hepatitis after therapeutic doses of benorylate and D-penicillamine. Ann Rheum Dis 1978; 37:98.
188. Barzilai D, Dickstein G, Enat R, et al. Case report: cholestatic jaundice caused by D-penicillamin. Ann Rheum Dis 1978; 37:98.
189. Seibold JR, Lynch CJ, Medsger TA. Cholestasis associated with D-penicillamine therapy: case report and review of the literature. Arthritis Rheum 1981; 24:554.
190. Gefel D, Harats N, Lijoveetsky G, Eliakim M. Cholestatic jaundice associated with D-penicillamine therapy. Scand J Rheumatol 1985; 14:303.
191. Ward JR. Historical perspective on the use of methotrexate for the treatment of rheumatoid arthritis. J Rheumatol 1985; 12(suppl):25.
192. Hoffmeister RT. Methotrexate therapy in rheumatoid arthritis: 15 years experience. Am J Med 1983: 75:69.
193. Kevat S, Ahern M, Hall P. Hepatotoxicity of methotrexate in rheumatic diseases. Semin Arthritis Rheum 1986; 15:231.

11

Renal Toxicity of Nonsteroidal Anti-Inflammatory Drugs

ANDREW WHELTON and CINDY W. HAMILTON*
Johns Hopkins University School of Medicine
Baltimore, Maryland

I. INTRODUCTION

A wide variety of renal abnormalities have been attributed to nonsteroidal anti-inflammatory drugs (NSAIDs). The four most important abnormalities, in descending order of frequency, are (a) fluid and electrolyte disturbances, (b) acute deterioration of renal function, (c) nephrotic syndrome with interstitial nephritis, and (d) papillary necrosis (Table 1). The incidence of serious nephrotoxicity associated with NSAIDs is low, but the number of at-risk patients is high because of the widespread use of these agents as prescription and over-the-counter (OTC) drugs. Approximately 1% of persons taking an NSAID will manifest some degree of renal function abnormality. Thus, of the 50 million Americans expected to use NSAIDs intermittently or routinely each year, 500,000 are likely to develop a renal function abnormality.

In most cases, NSAID-induced renal syndromes are a direct or indirect result of prostaglandin inhibition. The role of prostaglandins is supported by extensive literature, which will be reviewed in this chapter, describing the induction of renal syndromes coincident with NSAID-mediated suppression of renal prostaglandin production. In addition, recent observations indicate that misoprostol, a prostaglandin analogue, partially protects against NSAID-induced renal toxicity (1). Under the right clinical circumstances, virtually any NSAID can produce renal complications. Fortunately, there complications are usually reversible if the diagnosis is recognized promptly and NSAID therapy is discontinued.

II. NONSTEROIDAL ANTI-INFLAMMATORY DRUG-ASSOCIATED RENAL ABNORMALITIES

A. Fluid and Electrolyte Disturbances

1. Sodium Chloride and Water Retention

Sodium chloride and water retention are the most commonly encountered renal effects of NSAID use and, to some extent, they occur in virtually all exposed persons; however,

*Present affiliation: Hamilton House®, Virginia Beach, Virginia.

Table 1 Documented Renal Effects of Nonsteroidal Anti-Inflammatory Drugs

Drug	Generic name	Brand name/manufacturer	Renal effects[a]				
			Edema	↑ K	ARF	NS	PN
Salicylates	Aspirin	(Various)	Cl		Cl		Cl
	Diflunisal	Dolobid/Merck	Cl		Cl	Cl	An
Propionic acids	Ibuprofen	Motrin/Upjohn	Cl	Cl	Cl	Cl	Cl
	Naproxen	Naprosyn/Syntex	Cl		Cl	Cl	An
	Fenoprofen calcium	Nalfon/Lilly	Cl		Cl	Cl	Cl
	Ketoprofen	Orudis/Wyeth–Ayerst	Cl		Cl	Cl	
	Flurbiprofen	Ansaid/Upjohn	Cl	Cl	Cl	Cl[b]	An
Indolacetic acids	Indomethacin	Indocin/Merck	Cl	Cl	Cl	Cl	Cl[c]
	Sulindac	Clinoril/Merck	Cl	Cl	Cl	Cl	An
	Tolmetin	Tolectin/McNeil	Cl		Cl	Cl	An
	Diclofenac	Voltaren/Ciba–Geigy	Cl		Cl	Cl	Cl
	Etodolac	Lodine/Wyeth–Ayerst	Cl		Cl	Cl	An
Anthranilic acids	Meclofenamate sodium	Meclomen/Parke–Davis	Cl		Cl	Cl	An
	Mefenamic acid	Ponstel/Parke–Davis	Cl		Cl	Cl	Cl
Pyrazolones	Phenylbutazone	Butazolidin/Ciba–Geigy	Cl		Cl	Cl	Cl
Oxicams	Piroxicam	Feldene/Pfizer	Cl	Cl	Cl	Cl	Cl

[a]ARF, acute renal failure; NS, interstitial nephritis and nephrotic syndrome; PN, papillary necrosis; ↑ K, hyperkalemia; Cl, reported in clinical studies; An, described in studies in animals (but not in humans).
[b]Causes interstitial nephritis without nephrotic syndrome.
[c]Reported in combination with phenylbutazone.
Source: Adapted from Ref. 4.

this fluid and electrolyte disturbance is often not detectable clinically. According to the prescribing information accompanying nearly all NSAIDs, edema occurs in at least 3% of patients. The incidence is probably higher in patients taking therapeutic doses over prolonged periods. The onset of fluid retention is usually early in the course of therapy and, although typically benign, can be dramatic (2). Occasionally, the patient may retain water in excess of sodium, resulting in severe, reversible hyponatremia (3). Fluid retention is reversible on discontinuation of the NSAID and easily is managed in patients requiring treatment.

The multiple mechanisms by which NSAIDs interfere with water and sodium metabolism may explain the frequency of this complication. These agents have the potential to disrupt diuresis and natriuresis by interfering with prostaglandin-mediated sodium chloride transport, antidiuretic hormone, and distribution of blood flow from cortical to juxtamedullary nephrons (4,5). By shunting arachidonic acid metabolism from prostaglandins to lipoxygenase products, NSAIDs may favor production of eicosanoid derivatives that increase capillary permeability (4).

2. *Hyperkalemia*

In the absence of known risk factors, hyperkalemia is an unusual complication of NSAIDs, presumably because of the multiplicity of factors that are capable of maintaining potassium balance, even in the absence of prostaglandins. Hyperkalemia is more likely to occur in patients with preexisting renal impairment (6), cardiac failure (7), diabetes (6), or multiple myeloma (8), or in patients receiving potassium supplementation (9), potassium-sparing diuretics (10), or angiotensin-converting enzyme (ACE) inhibitors. Indomethacin appears to be the major NSAID associated with this complication and has produced hyperkalemia in patients without apparent risk factors (11). Thus, it is conceivable that indomethacin may have a direct effect on the cellular uptake of potassium (12).

The pathophysiological events that lead to the development of hyperkalemia are likely due to a combination of changes in renal physiology, many of which are prostaglandin-dependent. These include NSAID-mediated reduction in aldosterone production, consequent to partial suppression of renin production; reduced glomerular filtration rate, secondary to prostaglandin inhibition; and decreased renal tubular delivery of sodium to distal tubular sodium–potassium exchange sites.

The NSAID-induced hyperkalemia often occurs in the setting of NSAID-induced acute renal deterioration or worsening of underlying renal impairment. However, the severity of hyperkalemia can be disproportionate to that of renal impairment (13).

B. Acute Deterioration of Renal Function

1. Pathogenesis

From the clinical point of view, the most worrisome renal side effect of NSAIDs is hemodynamically mediated acute renal failure, which occurs in individuals with preexisting reduced renal blood perfusion (Table 2). Renal prostaglandins play an important role in the maintenance of homeostasis in these patients; hence, drug-induced disruption of counterregulatory mechanisms can produce clinically important and even severe renal functional deterioration (5,14). Acute deterioration of renal function occurs in 0.5–1% of patients taking NSAIDs on a long-term basis.

Acute renal deterioration in this setting can be attributed to the interruption of the delicate balance between hormonally mediated pressor mechanisms and prostaglandin-related vasodilatory effects (Fig. 1) (15). In at-risk patients, volume contraction triggers pressor responses through adrenergic and renin–angiotensin pathways. Ordinarily, vasodilatory renal prostaglandins counterbalance the vasoconstrictive effects of norepinephrine and angiotensin II. The addition of NSAIDs increases the risk of azotemia and possibly ischemic damage to the kidney by removing the protective effects of vasodilatory prostaglandins and allowing unopposed vasoconstriction.

2. Clinical Features

Initially, this NSAID-induced renal syndrome is of moderate severity and is characterized by increasing blood urea nitrogen, serum creatinine, and serum potassium. Weight increases as urinary output decreases. The NSAID-induced acute renal failure is usually reversible over 2–7 days after discontinuation of therapy; however, morbid consequences can occur if the diagnosis is not recognized early. Continued NSAID therapy in the setting of deteriorating renal function may progress rapidly to the point wherein dialysis support

Table 2 At-Risk Patients for NSAID-Induced Acute Renal Failure

Severe heart disease (congestive heart failure)
Severe liver disease (cirrhosis)
Nephrotic syndrome (chronic renal disease)
Elderly population
Dehydration (protracted)

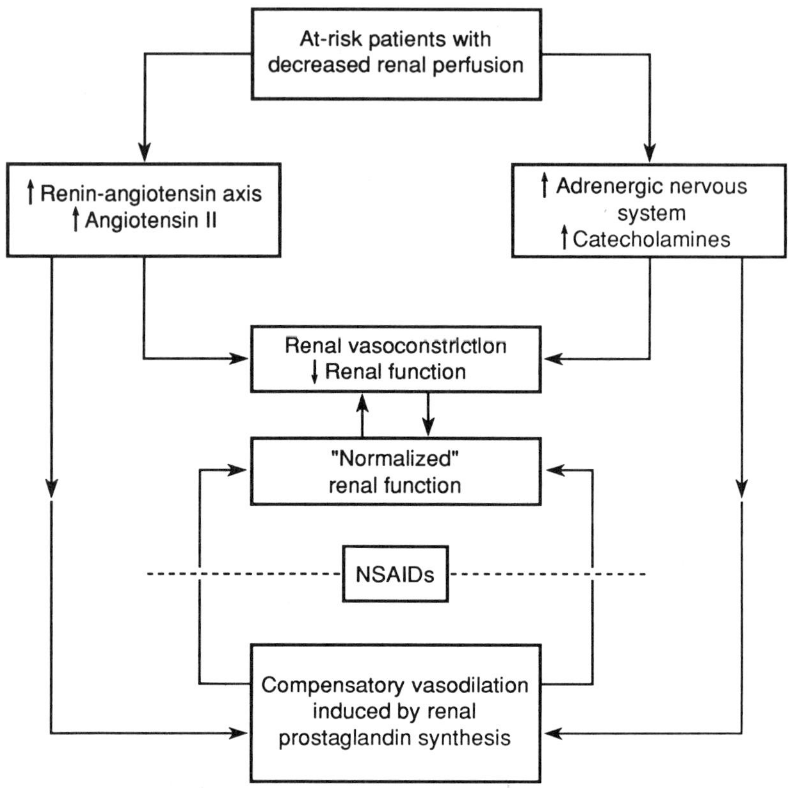

Figure 1 Mechanism by which NSAIDs disrupt the compensatory vasodilation response of renal prostaglandins to vasoconstrictor hormones in patients with prerenal conditions. A solid line (——) indicates stimulation; a dashed line (- - -) indicates inhibition. (From Ref. 15)

is required (16). Despite this profound level of renal functional impairment, the kidney will, nonetheless, recover several days to weeks following discontinuation of the NSAID. Development of this type of "total" renal failure, which is often inappropriately designated as "acute tubular necrosis," represents the extreme end of the spectrum of hemodynamic insult, rather than a separate clinical entity.

3. *Risk Factors*

The risk of acute renal deterioration is highest in patients with liver disease, preexisting renal impairment, cardiac failure, protracted volume contraction owing to diuretic therapy or intercurrent disease, or to old age. The NSAID-induced renal decompensation has been well documented in patients with cirrhosis, particularly when ascites is present (5). Urinary excretion of prostaglandin E_2, prostacyclin metabolites, and thromboxane A_2 is increased in these patients (17,18). An analogous situation exists in patients with underlying congestive heart failure (19), nephrotic syndrome (20,21), or lupus nephritis (22,23). Other predisposing factors include shock, sepsis, and third-space fluid sequestration in postoperative patients (24).

Patients with chronic renal impairment are at increased risk of NSAID-induced renal failure because of inadequate renal prostaglandin production. The NSAID-induced acute renal failure has been documented in patients with asymptomatic, mild, but chronic, renal failure (25). Baseline excretion of urinary prostaglandin E_2 and 6-keto-prostaglandin $F_{1\alpha}$ was quantitatively lower in the individuals who developed NSAID-induced renal decompensation than in those who did not; and ibuprofen proved to be more problematic than either piroxicam or sulindac. Upon initiation of ibuprofen, urinary prostaglandin excretion fell in all patients, but trough concentrations were quantitatively lower in the subset of patients who experienced acute renal failure.

Volume contraction resulting from diuretic therapy or an intercurrent disease that results in dehydration is another important risk factor for NSAID-induced acute deterioration of renal function (16,26,27). Elderly patients are also at increased risk because the physiology of aging results in a 50% loss of renal function in 50% of the population at age 80, primarily owing to the progression of arteriolonephrosclerosis.

4. *Pharmacodynamics*

The NSAID-induced acute renal decompensation is a pharmacologically predictable phenomenon that occurs in a dose-related fashion and follows a drug-specific time course (25). Ibuprofen-induced renal failure occurs within days, but piroxicam and sulindac do not cause renal deterioration as rapidly. This difference in onset may be related to pharmacokinetic factors. Ibuprofen has a short elimination half-life and reaches maximum serum concentrations quickly. In contrast, piroxicam and sulindac have longer half-lives and continue to accumulate throughout the treatment period. These findings are consistent with basic pharmacological principles and suggest that NSAIDs having short elimination half-lives will reach steady state and exert maximum pharmacologic effects before NSAIDs having longer half-lives.

Although all NSAIDs have the potential to induce acute renal impairment, there may be some quantitative differences. Sulindac has been hypothesized to be renal-sparing, possibly because of its unusual metabolic pathway (28). It has been hypothesized that, within the kidney, the active metabolite, sulindac sulfide, is oxidized back to the inactive parent compound, sulindac sulfoxide, so renal prostaglandin production is not influenced.

In clinical studies of sulindac, urinary prostaglandin levels and renal effects were unchanged in patients with normal renal function (29,30) and states of proteinuria (31). However, longer courses of sulindac in patients with slightly more severe renal impairment have been associated with statistically significant reductions in urinary prostaglandins (25) and glomerular filtration rate (32). Similar findings have been observed in patients with hepatic cirrhosis and ascites (33).

C. Nephrotic Syndrome with Interstitial Nephritis

The NSAIDs cause a renal dysfunction associated with various levels of functional impairment and characterized by the development of the nephrotic syndrome with interstitial nephritis (4,16,34,35). This syndrome is seen rarely and is reversible on discontinuation of the NSAID. The clinical features, absence of risk factors, and pathophysiology distinguish this from other NSAID-induced renal syndromes and from classic drug-induced allergic interstitial nephritis.

The features of this NSAID-induced renal syndrome are somewhat variable (36). The patient will typically present with edema and possibly oliguria. Systemic signs of allergic interstitial nephritis, such as fever, drug rash, peripheral eosinophilia, and eosinophiluria, are generaly absent (4,16,35,36). The urine sediment contains microscopic hematuria and pyuria (4,36). Proteinuria is typically in the nephrotic range (4,34). Renal functional deterioration can range from minimal to severe.

Characteristically, this form of nephrotic syndrome consists of an unusual combination of histological findings: minimal change glomerulonephritis with interstitial nephritis. The NSAID-induced nephrotic syndrome without interstitial disease is rare, but has been reported in a handful of patients taking fenoprofen, sulindac, or diclofenac. Conversely, interstitial disease without nephrosis has been reported in a few patients, but this may, in fact, represent allergic interstitial nephritis (36).

In spite of nephrotic-range proteinuria, the most impressive histopathological findings involve the interstitium and tubules. A focal diffuse inflammatory infiltrate, primarily consisting of cytotoxic T lymphocytes, but also containing other T cells, B cells, and plasma cells, can be found around the proximal and distal tubules (34). Changes in the glomeruli are minimal and resemble those of minimal change glomerulonephritis with marked epithelial foot-process fusion.

The onset of NSAID-induced nephrotic syndrome is usually delayed, having a mean time of onset of 5.4 months after initiation of NSAID therapy (35) and ranging from 2 weeks to 18 months (4). The NSAID-induced nephrotic syndrome is usually reversible 1 month to 1 year after discontinuation of NSAID therapy. During the recovery period, some patients may require dialysis. Corticosteroids have been used empirically, but it is not clear whether or not they hasten recovery (4,16,34).

Risk factors are not well understood. Underlying renal impairment does not appear to be a risk factor. Old age has been suggested as a risk factor (16,35), but this may also be a reflection of the usual candidate for chronic NSAID therapy. Of particular relevance is that the syndrome has been more commonly reported with fenoprofen than other NSAIDs; approximately two-thirds of cases have been associated with fenoprofen. Hence, the structure of the drug itself appears to be of major importance. The syndrome has been attributed, nonetheless, to virtually all NSAIDs, including those from structurally distinct classes (4,16,34–36).

The mechanism of NSAID-induced nephrotic syndrome has not been fully characterized. The association of this syndrome with structurally distinct NSAIDs suggests a common denominator. It is conceivable that T lymphocytes function as immune mediators instead of the humoral factors that are responsible for classic drug-induced allergic interstitial nephritis. In keeping with this hypothesis, NSAID-induced prostaglandin inhibition may play an indirect role. By inhibiting cyclooxygenase, NSAIDs may promote metabolism of arachidonic acid to nonprostaglandin eicosanoids. Indeed, leukotrienes, the products of the interaction between lipoxygenase and arachidonic acid, are known to recruit T lymphocytes and promote the inflammatory process. Leukotrienes may also contribute to proteinuria by increasing vascular permeability (4,35,36).

D. Papillary Necrosis

Papillary necrosis with interstitial nephritis is a well-known complication of chronic phenacetin abuse (37). It has been suggested that extended use of aspirin alone may also induce papillary necrosis (38). In preclinical studies, nearly all of the NSAIDs produced papillary necrosis in experimental animal models. Clinical toxicity is exceedingly rare, but has been reported for ibuprofen (39), phenylbutazone (40,41), fenoprofen (42), and mefenamic acid (43) and, according to prescribing information, several other NSAIDs.

Chronic (10–20 years) exposure of the kidney to high doses of analgesic combinations, such as salicylate and acetaminophen (the metabolite of phenacetin), often with the addition of caffeine, is clearly associated with chronic, progressive papillary necrosis (37). The black pigmentation found within necrotic papillae associated with phenacetin abuse (or phenacetin-containing combinations) is absent in patients ingesting aspirin alone or other NSAIDs. This black pigmentation may represent a breakdown product of phenacetin (37).

Fortunately, the incidence of NSAID-induced papillary necrosis with interstitial nephritis has diminished considerably because of patient education and a better understanding of the pathophysiology of the disease. The typical candidate for NSAID-induced papillary necrosis is a middle-aged woman, with a long history of ingesting over-the-counter, combination analgesics for headache. Renal manifestations may include flank pain, macroscopic hematuria, ureteral obstruction, and progressive uremia. Urinary tract infection and hypertension are common secondary findings. Reversibility is determined by the extent of deterioration and ability to discontinue NSAID therapy (37). Recent reports (44) of spontaneous gross hematuria associated with NSAIDs, such as ibuprofen (three cases), suggest that papillary necrosis also occurs with newer NSAIDs. These data suggest a minor degree of papillary damage, but chronic progressive deterioration of renal function is not a feature of most reports.

The mechanism of NSAID-induced papillary necrosis is unclear. It is often difficult to delineate the causative role of NSAIDs because of the presence of confounding factors, such as underlying disease, urinary tract infection, or concomitant medications. Selected NSAIDs may exert a direct toxic effect on renal papillae, particularly combinations of aspirin and acetaminophen, a major metabolite of phenacetin. Both drugs are highly concentrated in the medulla. Aspirin depletes cellular glutathione, which would otherwise neutralize the acetaminophen metabolite, *N*-acetyl-benzoquinoneimine. Without glutathione, this highly reactive metabolite could lead to cell death (37).

Prostaglandin inhibition may also play a role (4). Medullary ischemia, a possible precipitating factor in development of papillary necrosis, results from NSAID-induced reduction in blood flow to the renal medulla in experimental models (45,46).

E. Other Nonsteroidal Anti-Inflammatory Drug-Induced Renal Syndromes

Phenylbutazone, suprofen, and benoxaprofen produce unique renal syndromes that are of historical interest. These complications are now rarely encountered because phenylbutazone has been supplanted by safer NSAIDs, and suprofen and benoxaprofen have been removed from the market.

Phenylbutazone can induce acute oligoanuric renal failure by two possible mechanisms (4). First, phenylbutazone is known to inhibit uric acid reabsorption, which may cause hyperuricosuria and, ultimately, bilateral uretreral obstruction by uric acid stones (47). Second, an idiosyncratic reaction has been reported that results in acute tubular injury without uric acid precipitation (48). Underlying renal impairment is a risk factor for the latter reaction. Also, patients experiencing this reaction appear to be predisposed to subsequent renal injury from other NSAIDs. These observations suggest that prostaglandin inhibition may play a role in the development of the idiosyncratic reaction (4).

Suprofen-induced acute renal failure is characterized by acute flank or abdominal pain, occurring within 12 h after starting therapy (49). The mechanism was never conclusively identified before the drug was removed from the market. Suprofen is known to have uricosuric activity, so the suprofen flank pain syndrome may be related to acute uric acid crystal precipitation within the nephron, leading to acute urinary flow obstruction (44,49).

Benoxaprofen, an NSAID with a very long half-life, was removed from the market in 1982, within weeks after its introduction. It is best remembered for severe hepatic toxicity that occasionally resulted in death; however, renal failure also contributed to its removal. Risk factors for benoxaprofen-induced toxicity were old age and concomitant diuretic therapy, two factors known to increase the risk of acute functional renal failure.

III. MANAGEMENT OF NONSTEROIDAL ANTI-INFLAMMATORY DRUG-INDUCED RENAL TOXICITY

With an understanding of the pathophysiology involved in the development of NSAID-induced renal toxicity, preventive clinical measures can be put into operation. Risk factors have been identified for most NSAID-induced renal syndromes (Table 3). It is prudent to avoid high-dose, long-term NSAID therapy in at-risk patients (see Table 2). Unfortunately, this is not always possible. If NSAIDs are necessary in these high-risk groups, the patients should be monitored closely and receive appropriate counseling. Monitoring should begin within a week after initiation of a short-acting NSAID (e.g., ibuprofen) and continue indefinitely for signs of syndromes having delayed onset (e.g., nephrotic syndrome with interstitial nephritis).

Should NSAID-induced renal failure occur, the cornerstone of management is discontinuation of the drug, accompanied by supportive care. With the exception of those patients in whom the renal failure was precipitated by an episode of protracted dehydration, rechallenge with the offending drug or a structurally unrelated NSAID is likely to reproduce the adverse effect. If anti-inflammatory therapy is mandatory, underlying risk

Table 3 Summary of Effects of NSAIDs on Renal Function

Renal syndrome	Mechanism	Risk factors	Prevention/treatment
Sodium retention and edema	↓ Prostaglandin	NSAID therapy (most common adverse effect)	Stop NSAID
Hyperkalemia	↓ Prostaglandin, ↓ potassium to distal tubule and ↓ aldosterone/renin–angiotensin	Renal disease Heart failure Diabetes Multiple myeloma Potassium therapy K^+-sparing diuretic	Stop NSAID; avoid indomethacin in high-risk patients
Acute deterioration of renal function	↓ Prostaglandin and disruption of hemodynamic balance	Liver disease Renal disease Heart failure Dehydration Old age	Stop NSAID; avoid use in high-risk patients
Nephrotic syndrome with interstitial nephritis	↑ Lymphocyte recruitment and activation	Fenoprofen	Stop NSAID; dialysis and (?) steroids as needed
Papillary necrosis	Direct toxicity	Phenacetin abuse Aspirin–acetaminophen combination	Stop NSAID; avoid chronic analgesic use

factors should be identified and eliminated. For risk factors that cannot be eliminated, such as old age or chronic heart, kidney, or liver disease, patients may require alternative therapy (e.g., corticosteroids, acetaminophen, or colchicine, as appropriate).

REFERENCES

1. Downie WW. Prostaglandins and NSAID in the kidney. J Rheumatol 1991; 18(suppl 28):19–21.
2. Schooley RT, Wagley PF, Lietman PS. Edema associated with ibuprofen therapy. JAMA 1977; 237:1716–7.
3. Blum M, Aviram A. Ibuprofen induced hyponatremia. Rheumatol Rehabil 1980; 19:258–9.
4. Clive DM, Stoff JS. Renal syndromes associated with nonsteroidal antiinflammatory drugs. N Engl J Med 1984; 310:563–72.
5. Oates JA, FitzGerald GA, Branch RA, Jackson EK, Knapp HR, Roberts LJ II. Clinical Implications of prostaglandin and thromboxane A_2 formation (2 parts). N Engl J Med 1988; 319:689–98; 761–7.
6. Findling JW, Beckstrom D, Rawsthorne L, Kozin F, Itskovitz H. Indomethacin-induced hyperkalemia in three patients with gouty arthritis. JAMA 1980; 244:1127–8.
7. Nicholls MG, Espiner EA. Indomethacin-induced azotaemia and hyperkalaemia: a case study. NZ Med J 1981; 94:377–9.
8. Paladini G, Tonazzi C. Indomethacin-induced hyperkalemia and renal failure in multiple myeloma. Acta Heamatol (Basel) 1982; 68:256–60.
9. Akbarpour F, Afrasibi A, Vaziri ND. Severe hyperkalemia caused by indomethacin and potassium supplementation. South Med J 1985; 78:756–7.
10. Mor R, Pitlik S, Rosenfeld JB. Indomethacin- and Moduretic-induced hyperkalemia. Isr J Med Sci 1983; 19:535–7.
11. Goldszer RC, Coodley EL, Rosner MJ, Simons WM, Schwartz AB. Hyperkalemia associated with indomethacin. Arch Intern Med 1981; 141:802–4.
12. MacCarthy EP, Frost GW, Strokes GS. Indomethacin-induced hyperkalaemia. Med J Aust 1979; 1:550.
13. Tan SY, Shapiro R, Franco R, Stockard H, Mulrow PJ. Indomethacin-induced prostaglandin inhibition with hyperkalemia. Ann Intern Med 1979; 90:783–5.
14. Patrono C, Dunn MJ. The clinical significance of inhibition of renal prostaglandin synthesis. Kidney Int 1987; 32:1–12.
15. Whelton A, Hamilton CW. Nonsteroidal anti-inflammatory drugs: effects on kidney function. J Clin Pharmacol 1991; 31:588–98.
16. Blackshear JL, Napier JS, Davidman M, Stillman MT. Renal complications of nonsteroidal antiinflammatory drugs: identification and monitoring of those at risk. Semin Arthritis Rheum 1985; 14:163–75.
17. Zipser RD, Hoefs JC, Speckart PF, Zia PK, Horton R. Prostaglandins: modulators of renal function and pressor resistance in chronic liver disease. J Clin Endocrinol Metab 1979; 48:895–900.
18. Zipser RD, Radvan GH, Kronborg IJ, Duke R, Little TE. Urinary thromboxane B_2 and prostaglandin E_2 in the hepatorenal syndrome: evidence for increased vasoconstrictor and decreased vasodilator factors. Gastroenterology 1983; 84:697–703.
19. Walshe JJ, Venuto RC. Acute oliguric renal failure induced by indomethacin: possible mechanisms. Ann Intern Med 1979; 91:47–9.
20. Arisz L, Donker AJM, Brentjens JRH, van der Hem GK. The effect of indomethacin on proteinuria and kidney function in the nephrotic syndrome. Acta Med Scand 1976; 199:121–5.
21. Kleinknecht C, Broyer M, Gubler M-C, Palcoux J-B. Irreversible renal failure after indomethacin in steroid-resistant nephrosis. N Engl J Med 1980; 302:691.
22. Kimberly RP, Gill JR Jr, Bowden RE, Keiser HR, Plotz PH. Elevated urinary prostaglandins

and the effects of aspirin on renal function in lupus erythematosus. Ann Intern Med 1978; 89:336–41.
23. Fong HJ, Cohen AH. Ibuprofen-induced acute renal failure with acute tubular necrosis. Am J Nephrol 1982; 2:28–31.
24. Henrich WL. Southwestern internal medicine conference: analgesic nephropathy. Am J Med Sci 1988; 295:561–8.
25. Whelton A, Stout RL, Spilman PS, Klassen DK. Renal effects of ibuprofen, piroxicam, and sulindac in patients with asymptomatic renal failure: a prospective, randomized, crossover comparison. Ann Intern Med 1990; 112:568–76.
26. Favre L, Glasson P, Vallotton MB. Reversible acute renal failure from combined triamterene and indomethacin: a study in healthy subjects. Ann Intern Med 1982; 96:317–20.
27. McCarthy JT, Torres VE, Romero JC, Wochos DN, Velosa JA. Acute intrinsic renal failure induced by indomethacin: role of prostaglandin synthetase inhibition. Mayo Clin Proc 1982; 57:289–96.
28. Bunning RD, Barth WF. Sulindac: a potentially renal-sparing nonsteroidal anti-inflammatory drug. JAMA 1982; 248:2864–7.
29. Brater DC, Anderson S, Baird B, Campbell WB. Effects of ibuprofen, naproxen, and sulindac on prostaglandins in men. Kidney Int 1985; 27:66–73.
30. Sedor JR, Williams SL, Chremos AN, Johnson CL, Dunn MJ. Effects of sulindac and indomethacin on renal prostaglandin synthesis. Clin Pharmacol Ther 1984; 36:85–91.
31. Ciabattoni G, Cinotti GA, Pierucci A, et al. Effects of sulindac and ibuprofen in patients with chronic glomerular disease: evidence for the dependence of renal function on prostacyclin. N Engl J Med 1984; 310:279–83.
32. Mistry CD, Lote CJ, Gokal R, Currie WJ, Vandenburg M, Mallick NP. Effects of sulindac on renal function and prostaglandin synthesis in patients with moderate chronic renal insufficiency. Clin Sci 1986; 70:501–5.
33. Quintero E, Ginés P, Arroyo V, et al. Sulindac reduces the urinary excretion of prostaglandins and impairs renal function in patients with cirrhosis and ascites. Nephron 1986; 42:298–303.
34. Bender WL, Whelton A, Beschorner WE, Darwish MO, Hall-Craggs M, Solez K. Interstitial nephritis, proteinuria, and renal failure caused by nonsteroidal anti-inflammatory drugs: immunologic characterization of the inflammatory infiltrate. Am J Med 1984; 76:1006–12.
35. Abraham PA, Keane WF. Glomerular and interstitial disease induced by nonsteroidal anti-inflammatory drugs. Am J Nephrol 1984; 4:1–6.
36. Levin ML. Patterns of tubulo-interstitial damage associated with nonsteroidal antiinflammatory drugs. Semin Nephrol 1988; 8:55–61.
37. Kincaid-Smith P. Effects of non-narcotic analgesics on the kidney. Drugs 1986; 32(suppl 4):109–28.
38. Krishnaswamy S, Nanra RS. "Phenacetin" nephropathy without phenacetin [abstract]. Aust NZ J Med 1976; 6:88.
39. Shah GM, Muhalwas KK, Winer RL. Renal papillary necrosis due to ibuprofen. Arthritis Rheum 1981; 24:1208–10.
40. Lourie SH, Denman SJ, Schroeder ET. Association of renal papillary necrosis and ankylosing spondylitis. Arthritis Rheum 1977; 20:917–21.
41. Morales A, Steyn J. Papillary necrosis following phenylbutazone ingestion. Arch Surg 1971; 103:420–1.
42. Husserl FE, Lange RK, Kantrow CM Jr. Renal papillary necrosis and pyelonephritis accompanying fenoprofen therapy. JAMA 1979; 242:1896–8.
43. Robertson CE, Ford MJ, Van Someren V, Dlugolecka M, Prescott LF. Mefenamic acid nephropathy. Lancet 1980; 2:232–3.
44. Harter JG. Acute flank pain and hematuria: lessons from adverse drug reaction reporting. J Clin Pharmacol 1988; 28:560–5.
45. Kirschenbaum MA, White N, Stein JH, Ferris TF. Redistribution of renal cortical blood flow during inhibition of prostaglandin synthesis. Am J Med 1974; 227:801–5.

46. Stein JH, Fadem SZ. The renal circulation. JAMA 1978; 239:1308–12.
47. Weisman JI, Bloom B. Anuria following phenylbutazone therapy. N Engl J Med 1955; 252:1086–7.
48. Lipsett MB, Goldman R. Phenylbutazone toxicity: report of a case of acute renal failure. Ann Intern Med 1954; 41:1075–9.
49. Hart D, Ward M, Lifshitz MD. Suprofen-related nephrotoxicity. A distinct clinical syndrome. Ann Intern Med 1987; 106:235–8.

12

Nonsteroidal Anti-Inflammatory Drugs
Uses in Dermatology and Cutaneous Toxicity

MICHAEL BIGBY
Harvard Medical School
Boston, Massachusetts

I. INTRODUCTION

Any discussion of the use of nonsteroidal anti-inflammatory drugs (NSAIDs) in dermatology and their cutaneous toxicity necessarily contains both good and bad news. Part of the good news is that the pathophysiology of inflammatory responses and the mediators of inflammation that are influenced by the NSAIDs are now better understood. Many of the modes of action that the NSAIDs have on inflammatory responses have been elucidated. There are also many NSAIDs available that have differing mechanisms of action. Finally, many of the NSAIDs can be adequately formulated for sufficient topical penetration and use.

II. INFLAMMATORY MEDIATORS

The mediators that are important in understanding the role of NSAIDs in the treatment of cutaneous disorders include histamine, serotonin, bradykinin, prostaglandin E_2 (PGE_2), leukotriene B_4 (LTB_4), and leukotrienes C_4, D_4, and E_4 (reviewed in Ref. 1). Although NSAIDs have no direct effect on histamine, serotonin, or bradykinin, the actions of these products are influenced by prostaglandins, which are markedly affected by the NSAIDs. Histamine is produced by mast cells and basophils and causes an increase in vascular permeability, chemokinesis, and smooth-muscle contraction. Serotonin is produced by platelets and cells in the enterochromaffin system. Serotonin similarly increases vascular permeability and induces smooth-muscle contraction. Bradykinin is a nonapeptide produced by the proteolytic cleavage of kininogen. Bradykinin increases vascular permeability and induces smooth-muscle contraction, vasodilation, and pain.

The prostaglandins and leukotrienes are both products of arachidonic acid metabolism (reviewed in Refs. 2,3). The cyclooxygenase pathway of arachidonic acid metabolism leads to the production of prostaglandins, E_2, $F_{2\alpha}$, I_2 (prostacyclin), and thromboxanes

A_2 and B_2. Arachidonic acid may also be acted on by 5-lipoxygenase, which leads to the production of the 4 series of leukotrienes: A_4, B_4, C_4, D_4, and E_4. Both 10- and 15-lipoxygenases exist, and their metabolic pathways are currently being elucidated. The roles of the products of these pathways in inflammatory responses are not currently well understood.

Prostaglandin E_2 is a vasodilator. More importantly, it potentiates the actions of histamine, serotonin, and bradykinin. In addition, PGE_2 causes release of collagenase by monocytes and increases the production of IgE and IgG (in conjunction with interleukin-4; IL-4) by B cells (4). The roles of thromboxane, prostacyclin, and prostaglandin F in inflammatory responses are less clear (4).

Leukotriene B_4 is a potent neutrophil chemotactic factor and increases vascular permeability. The leukotrienes C_4, D_4, and E_4 collectively constitute the activity of slow-reacting substance of anaphylaxis (SRS-A). These leukotrienes cause smooth-muscle contraction and increase vascular permeability.

III. THE NONSTEROIDAL ANTI-INFLAMMATORY DRUGS

In 1973, there were only four available NSAIDs. Today, 16 NSAIDs are available by prescription in the United States (reviewed in Ref. 5). As many as 30 different NSAIDs are currently available in Europe. The availability of a wide variety of NSAIDs has led to much confusion about the choice of NSAIDs, their relative efficacy, and their toxicity. Fortunately, the NSAIDs can be organized into groups, or families, based on their structure, mechanisms of action and, in general, toxicities (Fig. 1) (6); the propionic acid NSAIDs have the lowest toxicity profile. In fact, ibuprofen has been released for over-the-counter use, and naproxen may shortly receive the same fate.

IV. MECHANISMS OF ACTION

The NSAIDs inhibit cyclooxygenase and, thereby, decrease the production of prostaglandins and thromboxanes. Because the relative order of potency in cyclooxygenase inhibition roughly parallels the anti-inflammatory potency of the NSAIDs, cyclooxygenase inhibition may be the primary anti-inflammatory mechanism of action of these agents (5). In addition to their effects on the production of prostaglandins, the NSAIDs have many other actions that may contribute to their anti-inflammatory properties. These include inhibition of monocyte chemotaxis and collagenase production and interference with neutrophil lysosomal enzyme release, aggregation, and superoxide anion production (7).

Some of the NSAIDs have additional anti-inflammatory actions. Aspirin may be a scavenger of hydroxyl radicals. Diflunisal scavenges free radicals. Anthranilic acids inhibit prostaglandin synthesis and block prostaglandin action. Phenylbutazone inhibits mucopolysaccharide biosynthesis (6).

V. TOPICAL FORMULATIONS

Topical formulations that provide adequate percutaneous absorption of NSAIDs have been produced for most of the nonsteroidal anti-inflammatory agents (reviewed in Ref. 8). Two topical nonsteroidal anti-inflammatory agents have been approved for use in Europe. These include lonapalene and bufexamec. Many of the other potent NSAIDs have been investigated for anti-inflammatory activity both in animals and humans. For a more

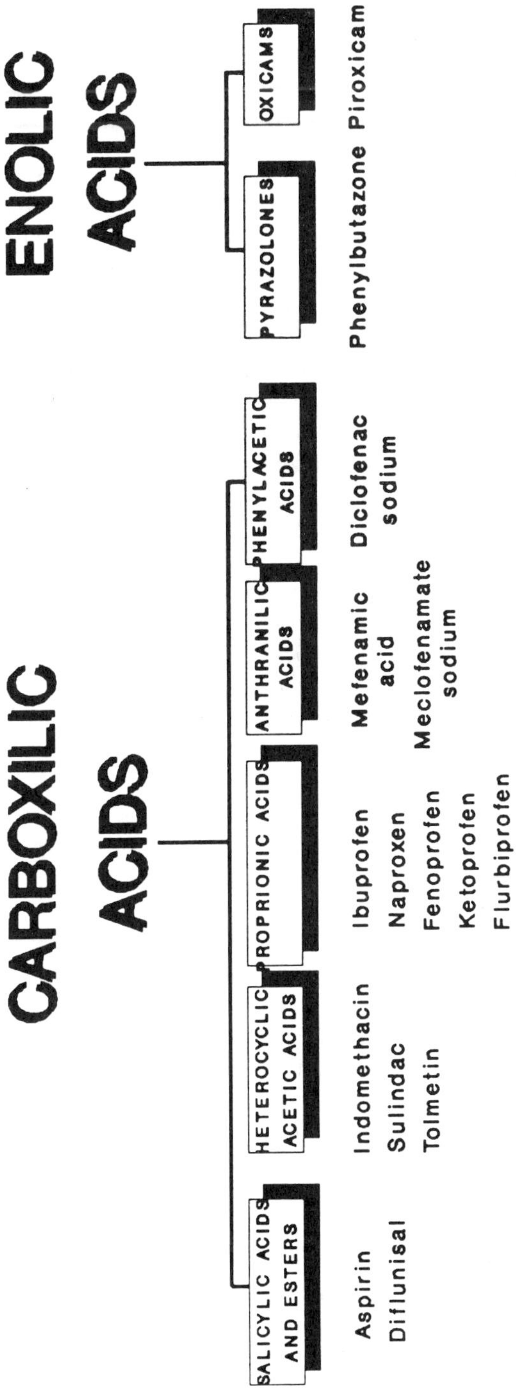

Figure 1 Groups of NSAIDs.

in-depth review of topical NSAIDs in skin diseases and musculoskeletal disorders, see Chapter 5.

VI. USE IN DERMATOLOGY

The bad news about NSAIDs and the skin is that, with very few notable exceptions, NSAIDs have not proved to be both safe and effective for the treatment of skin diseases (reviewed in Refs. 9–11). Erythermalgia (erythromelalgia) is the only cutaneous disorder for which NSAIDs are the treatment of choice. Seventy percent of patients with erythermalgia respond well to aspirin (11,12). In fact, a response to aspirin is often used as a clinical criterion for the diagnosis of this disorder.

There are very few well-designed and controlled studies that show the efficacy of NSAIDs in treating skin diseases. One of the most conclusive studies, published by Kragballe and Hurlin, demonstrated that benoxaprofen improves psoriasis. In a double-blind, placebo-controlled trial of 40 patients, 15 of 20 patients (75%) treated with benoxaprofen had excellent results versus none of 20 in the placebo group (13). Unfortunately, benoxaprofen was withdrawn from the market after it was associated with fatal hepatitis, especially in the elderly. Benoxaprofen was initially reported to be an inhibitor of 5-lipoxygenase. Subsequently, it has been shown that inhibition of 5-lipoxygenase is not a part of the action of benoxaprofen. Benoxaprofen does inhibit cyclooxygenase and chemotaxis of monocytes, and it is photosensitizer. The loss of benoxaprofen as a drug to treat psoriasis is unfortunate for several reasons. First, it may have shed some light on the pathogenesis of psoriasis. In addition, it was demonstrated in uncontrolled, open studies to be useful in treating nodular acne in young adult men and in a small number of cases of prurigo nodularis (11).

In another double-blind controlled trial, the combination of ibuprofen and tetracycline was demonstrated to be superior to either drug alone in treating papulopustular acne (14). More interestingly, ibuprofen alone was equal in efficacy to tetracycline. This study raises the possibility for using ibuprofen in combination with tetracycline in patients who have a partial, but incomplete, response to tetracycline alone and acne not severe enough to warrant retinoid therapy.

In a controlled double-blind study, lonapalene ointment was equal in efficacy to fluocinolone acetonide, 0.025%, in the treatment of psoriasis (15); lonapolene is used as a topical NSAID in Europe. Documentation of efficacy and safety are being pursued in the United States.

Reports of the efficacy of bufexamac in treating eczematous dermatitis have appeared in the literature since the 1970s. The drug has been approved for topical use in Europe. It is reported to be equal in efficacy to triamcinolone acetonide, 0.1%, in the treatment of eczematous dermatitis (16). Despite a lengthy time on the market, the drug has never been approved for use in the United States.

The NSAIDs are frequently cited as therapeutic options for the treatment of vasculitis. Very little data in the literature support this recommendation. In an open study of ten patients with urticarial vasculitis, total (six patients) or partial (three patients) resolution occurred with 75–200 mg of indomethacin. Interestingly, the disease recurred in eight patients when indomethacin was discontinued (17). The successful use of indomethacin to treat urticarial vasculitis was not confirmed in several other uncontrolled trials published in the dermatological literature. As an example, none of four patients with urticarial vasculitis had responses to indomethacin in a report of Callen and Kalbfleisch (18).

The NSAIDs are of limited effectiveness at suppressing ultraviolet (UV)B-induced erythema (19,20). In a randomized, double-blind, crossover study of 19 patients, ibuprofen was more effective than placebo in reducing technician-observed erythema, but not five other study indicators (pruritus, pain, general discomfort, restlessness, and patient-observed erythema). Ibuprofen was slightly more effective than placebo for the relief of symptoms associated with UVB-induced inflammation after high-dose UVB phototherapy of psoriasis. It is important to emphasize that the effects of ibuprofen were judged to be minimal (20).

Indomethacin has been successfully used to reduce the pain and inflammation of erythema nodosum. Several uncontrolled reports indicate that 50–150 mg of indomethacin may lead to the complete resolution of erythema nodosum (9–11). The NSAIDs, especially indomethacin, have been used with some success in the management of relapsing polychondritis (11). Of 23 patients with relapsing polychondritis 6 were controlled with NSAIDs in one reported series (21). The combination of aspirin and dipyridamole (Persantine) has been successfully used to treat atrophie blanche (10,11, 12). Aspirin has also been used in conjunction with histamine H_1 and H_2 antagonists to treat rare cases of systemic mastocytosis associated with an overproduction of prostaglandin D_2 (10,23).

Because the NSAIDs have such profound effects on inflammatory responses, one wonders why they are not more effective in treating inflammatory skin diseases. One explanation may be that the prostaglandins, in addition to proinflammatory actions, have many anti-inflammatory actions (Table 1). These inhibitory actions include inhibition of T-cell proliferation, IL-2 production, and migration (7). Prostaglandin inhibits cytotoxicity, interferon gamma, and leukotriene production, and the synthesis and secretion of IgM (7). Inhibition of PGE_2 production by the NSAIDs may, in some circumstances, enhance the immune response and, thereby, increase inflammation. This proinflammatory action of the NSAIDs has been demonstrated in an animal model of contact hypersensitivity (7). Another reason that the NSAIDs may not be as effective as assumed is that they may be used at the wrong time in the development of inflammatory skin diseases. Thus, for example, the histology of psoriasis evolves with time. The initial infiltrate may be preponderantly lymphocytic, associated with vasodilation, whereas later inflammatory responses are preponderantly by polymorphonuclear leukocytes and are associated with epidermal proliferation. The NSAIDs may be more effective as preventative therapy or early-on in the development of inflammatory skin diseases and of no use in well-established disease. Finally, the NSAIDs may be most useful in combination therapy with drugs that act by other mechanisms. This synergistic activity of the NSAIDs has been demonstrated for the treatment of acne (14).

Table 1 Inhibitory Effects of Prostaglandin E_2

T-cell proliferation and IL-2 production
Cytotoxicity
Lymphocyte migration
Interferon gamma production
Leukotriene production
IgM production

VII. GENERAL TOXICITY

Since 1981, there has been increased medical and public awareness and concern about the toxicity of the NSAIDs. Part of the reason for this concern has been the fatal adverse reactions to benoxaprofen and zomepirac sodium (6). The recognition of these reactions led to the removal of both drugs from the market. In addition, several recent reports have identified a high ratio of reported adverse reactions to prescriptions dispensed for oxyphenbutazone and phenylbutazone (fatal) and diflunisal and piroxicam (nonfatal) (24). The recognition of serious adverse effects to phenylbutazone led to a marked restriction of its use in Europe and led to the removal of oxyphenbutazone from many markets.

Major side effects of the NSAIDs include gastrointestinal bleeding and decreased renal function (reviewed in Ref. 5). Gastrointestinal ulcerations, significant bleeding, or perforations occur in 1% of patients in clinical trials for 3–6 months and in 2–4% of patients treated for 1 year. Therefore, the packaging requirements for the NSAIDs were recently changed by the Food and Drug Administration (FDA) to include specific statements concerning the risk of gastrointestinal side effects (25).

The NSAIDs produce a worsening of renal function (reviewed in Ref. 26). The mechanism is believed to be a decrease in prostaglandin E_2, which functions as a vasodilator in the kidney. Patients most at risk for developing renal complications of the NSAIDs include the elderly; patients with underlying renal, cardiac, or liver disease; patients on diuretics; and patients with hyperuricemia. The NSAIDs are associated with a wide variety of other adverse effects (Table 2; reviewed in Ref. 27). Notably, diflunisal is associated with uricosuria, headaches, cholestatic jaundice, nephritis, and exanthematous rash. Indomethacin therapy is commonly discontinued because of central nervous system side effects and headache. Phenylbutazone and sulindac are associated with blood dyscrasias and toxic hepatitis. The phenamic acids cause diarrhea and may aggravate seizures in patients with underlying seizure disorders.

Because of the wide toxicity profile of the NSAIDs, the FDA has added the following statement to the package insert for NSAIDs in this country:

> Physicians may wish to discuss with their patients the potential risks and likely benefits of NSAID treatment, particularly when the drugs are used for less serious conditions where treatment without NSAIDs may represent an acceptable alternative to both the patient and physician (25).

Table 2 Other Adverse Effects of NSAIDs[a]

Uricosuria (diflunisal, meclofenamate sodium)
Headache (diflunisal, indomethacin)
Cholestatic jaundice (diflunisal)
Nephritis (diflunisal, fenoprofen, fenamic acid)
CNS effects (indomethacin, naproxen)
Toxic hepatitis (sulindac, phenylbutazone)
Blood dyscrasias (phenylbutazone, sulindac)
Diarrhea (fenamic acids)
Seizures (fenamic acids)

[a]Specific drugs appear in parentheses if the reaction is not common to all NSAIDs.

VIII. CUTANEOUS TOXICITY

The NSAIDs are reported to cause a wide variety of adverse cutaneous reactions. Fortunately, to aid physicians in remembering which drugs are associated with which reactions, drugs in the same chemical classes (see Fig. 1) tend to cause similar cutaneous reactions. The salicylates are a common cause of acute and chronic urticaria. Aspirin is frequently associated with purpura because of its irreversible effects on platelet aggregation. Diflunisal is the only one of the salicylates frequently associated with the development of a drug exanthem.

The heterocyclic acidic acids are associated with the development of the drug exanthem and erythema multiforme. One of the heterocyclic acidic acids, sulindac, has been closely associated with the development of toxic epidermal necrolysis. Tolmetin is associated with a disproportionate number of anaphylactoid reactions.

The propionic acid derivatives are infrequently associated with the development rashes. Pruritus and erythema multiforme are uncommonly reported.

The anthranilic acids are commonly associated with the development of pruritus and the drug exanthem. Rashes are more common with meclofenamate sodium than with mefenamic acid. Diclofenac sodium, the only available phenolacidic acid, is associated with photosensitivity.

The pyrazolones are the drug class most commonly associated with the development of adverse cutaneous reactions. Phenylbutazone is the NSAID that is most closely linked to the development of toxic epidermal necrolysis and severe erythema multiforme (Stevens–Johnson syndrome). The pyrazolones also are frequently implicated as causes of the drug exanthem and pruritus. The pyrazolones are the only group of NSAIDs that have a convincing role in the induction of fixed drug reactions.

Piroxicam is the only currently available NSAID that is closely linked to the development of photosensitive eruptions. The eruption is often the vesicular bullous type and is accompanied by pruritus.

The cutaneous eruptions most closely linked to NSAID use are listed in Table 3. Each of these eruptions will be discussed in more detail.

A. Toxic Epidermal Necrolysis and Erythema Multiforme

The newer NSAIDs were the drugs most commonly implicated as the cause of toxic epidermal necrolysis (TEN) in a reported epidemiological study of 154 cases of TEN. In that report, one-third of the cases were preceded by ingestion of one of the newer NSAIDs (28). The NSAIDs most commonly implicated as the cause of TEN are phenylbutazone, sulindac, and piroxicam. Toxic epidermal necrolysis is a catastrophic illness characterized by the abrupt onset of a prodrome of fever and sore throat, followed rapidly by skin

Table 3 Cutaneous Eruptions Associated with NSAIDs[a]

Toxic epidermal necrolysis
Photosensitivity (piroxicam)
Exanthem
Urticaria
Fixed drug eruption (phenylbutazone)

[a]Specific drugs appear in parentheses if the reaction is not common to all NSAIDs.

tenderness, bullae formation, and desquamation of large sheets of full-thickness epidermis. Fifty to ninety percent of the cutaneous surface is commonly involved, and mortality rates range from 15 to 50% in various reported series. Fortunately, the incidence of TEN is quite low; it is estimated to occur once per million courses of drug therapy (29,30).

B. Photosensitivity

Piroxicam is the currently available NSAID most closely linked to the development of photosensitivity. The photosensitive eruption of piroxicam can be bullous, vesicular, or papular. The rash is commonly associated with pruritus, stinging, and burning. In more than half of the cases, the rash occurred early (within 3 days) after the patient's first exposure to the drug. Patients frequently give a history of increased sun exposure about the time the drug therapy began. Although many of these features suggest a phototoxic mechanism, the weight of recent evidence points toward a photoallergic mechanism. McKerrow and Greig reported that 6 of 11 patients with piroxicam-induced photosensitivity had demonstrable positive photopatch tests with piroxicam and cross-reacted with thimerosal (31).

C. Urticaria

Urticaria is a side effect of many of the NSAIDs. The NSAID-induced urticaria is most likely caused by direct mediator release and is not an antigen-specific immunological response. Urticaria is reported to occur in up to 20% of patients exposed to aspirin. Patients with NSAID-induced urticaria may react to many (but often not all) NSAIDs. The NSAID should be used with caution or not at all in patients with a history of aspirin "hypersensitivity" (6).

D. Drug Exanthem

Many of the NSAIDs have been associated with the development of a drug exanthem. The association has been most closely made for meclofenamate sodium, diflunisal, piroxicam, phenylbutazone, and sulindac. The rate at which the NSAIDs cause drug exanthems has not been determined accurately for most of the NSAIDs (6).

E. Fixed Drug Eruption

Oxyphenbutazone and phenylbutazone are the two NSAIDs commonly associated with the development of fixed drug eruptions. Since phenylbutazone is metabolized to oxyphenbutazone, an explanation for the link is readily available (6).

It is tempting to speculate that the wide variety of effects that the NSAIDs have on inflammatory responses is somehow related to the frequency and variety of adverse cutaneous reactions seen with these agents. There is, however, no evidence to support this hypothesis. The drug eruptions encountered in association with the NSAIDs appear not to differ from drug eruptions caused by other agents, many of which have no known or demonstrated effects on inflammation.

REFERENCES

1. Larsen GL, Henson PM. Mediators of inflammation. Annu Rev Immunol 1983; 1:335–59.
2. Davies P, Bailey PJ, Goldenberg MM. The role of arachidonic acid oxygenation products in inflammation. Annu Rev Immunol 1984; 2:335–57.
3. Goldyne ME. Eicosanoids and human skin. Prog. Dermatol. 1986; 20:1–8.

4. Goodwin JS. Immunologic effects of nonsteroidal antiinflammatory drugs. Am J Med 1984; 77(suppl 43):7–15.
5. Brooks PM, Day RO. Nonsteroidal antiinflammatory drugs—differences and similarities. N Engl J Med 1991; 324:1716–25.
6. Bigby M. Nonsteroidal anti-inflammatory drug reactions. Semin Dermatol 1989; 8:182–6.
7. Goodwin JS. Mechanism of action of nonsteroidal anti-inflammatory agents. Am J Med 1984; 77(suppl 11a):57–64.
8. Lowe NJ, Hensby CN, eds. Nonsteroidal anti-inflammatory drugs. Basel: S Karger, 1989:136–45.
9. Lichtenstein J, Flowers F, Sheretz EF. Nonsteroidal anti-inflammatory drugs in the treatment of skin diseases. Int J Dermatol 1987; 26:80–7.
10. Greaves MW. Pharmacology and significance of nonsteroidal anti-inflammatory drugs in the treatment of skin diseases. J Am Acad Dermatol 1987; 16:751–64.
11. Shelley WB, Shelley LD. Advanced dermatologic therapy. Philadelphia: WB Saunders, 1987.
12. Babb RR, Alarcon-Segovia D, Fairbairn JF. Erythermalgia: review of 51 cases. Circulation 1964; 29:136–41.
13. Kragballe K, Herlin T. Benoxaprofen improves psoriasis. Arch Dermatol 1983; 119:548–52.
14. Wong RC, Kang S, Heezen JL. Oral ibuprofen and tetracycline for the treatment of acne vulgaris. J Am Acad Dermatol 1984; 11:1076–84.
15. Lassus A, Forsstrom S. A dimethoxynapthalene derivative (RS-43179 GEL) compared with 0.025% fluocinolone acetonide gel in the treatment of psoriasis. Br J Dermatol 1985; 113:103–6.
16. Christiansen JV, Gadborg E, Kleiter I, et al. Efficacy of bufexamac (NFN) cream in skin disease. Dermatologica 1977; 154:177–84.
17. Millns JL, Randle HW, Solley GO, Dicken CH. The therapeutic response of urticarial vasculitis to indomethacin. J Am Acad Dermatol 1980; 3:349–55.
18. Callen JP, Kalbfleisch S. Urticarial vasculitis: a report of nine cases and review of the literature. Br J Dermatol 1982; 107:87–96.
19. Snyder DS, Eaglstein WH. Topical indomethacin and sunburn. Br J Dermatol 1974; 90:91–3.
20. Stern RS, Dodson TB. Ibuprofen in the treatment of UVB-induced inflammation. Arch Dermatol 1985; 121:508–12.
21. McAdam LP, O'Hanlan MA, Bluestone R, Pearson CM. Relapsing polychrondritis: prospective study of 23 patients and review of the literature. Medicine 1976; 55:193–215.
22. Drucker CR, Duncan WC. Antiplatelet therapy in atrophie blanche and livedo vasculitis. J Am Acad Dermatol 1982; 7:359–63.
23. Roberts LJ, Sweetman BJ, Lewis RA, et al. Increased production of prostaglandin D_2 in patients with systemic mastocytosis. N Engl J Med 1980; 303:1400–4.
24. Kromann-Andersen H, Pedersen A. Reported adverse reactions to and consumption of nonsteroidal anti-inflammatory drugs in Denmark over a 17-year period. Dan Med Bull 1988; 35:187–92.
25. Labeling revisions for NSAIDs. FDA Drug Bull. Feb 1989; 19:3–4.
26. Carmichael J, Shankel SW. Effects of nonsteroidal antiinflammatory drugs on prostaglandins and renal function. Am J Med 1985; 78:992–1000.
27. O'Brien WM, Bagby GF. Rare adverse reactions to nonsteroidal antiinflammatory drugs. J Rheumatol 1985; 12:13–20; 347–53; 562–7; 785–90.
28. Roujeau J-C. Clinical aspects of skin reactions to NSAIDs. Scand J Rheumatol [suppl] 1987; 65:131–4.
29. Strom BL, Carson JL, Halpern AC, et al. A population-based study of Stevens–Johnson syndrome. Arch Dermatol 1991; 127:831–8.
30. Schöpf E, Stühmer A, Rzany B, et al. Toxic epidermal necrolysis and Stevens–Johnson syndrome. Arch Dermatol 1991; 127:839–42.
31. McKerrow KJ, Greig DE. Piroxicam-induced photosensitive dermatitis. J Am Acad Dermatol 1986; 15:1237–41.

13

Rare Side Effects of Nonsteroidal Anti-Inflammatory Drugs

W. WATSON BUCHANAN and WALTER F. KEAN
McMaster University Faculty of Health Sciences
Hamilton, Ontario, Canada

> *Rare*: Of a kind, class or description seldom found, met with, or occurring; unusual, uncommon, exceptional.
>
> *Shorter Oxford English Dictionary*, 1959

I. INTRODUCTION

An *adverse drug reaction* has been defined by the World Health Organization as "one that is noxious, unintended, and occurs at doses used in man for prophylaxis, diagnosis, or therapy" (1). Although this definition is acceptable, identification is more difficult, since the incidence of adverse reactions vary according to whether a direct or indirect question is asked (2). This may explain the marked variation in the incidence of adverse reactions in different reports (3). There are, in addition, the problems of "background" symptoms occurring spontaneously (4) and the considerable differences among physicians in determining whether a patient has had an adverse drug reaction. Algorithms improve consensus among physicians (5), but have been criticized as that they merely impose the opinions of the authors of the algorithms on those of the physician assessors (6). If these difficulties exist with common side effects, how much more difficult it becomes to assess a rare adverse drug reaction (7).

Spontaneous adverse reaction-reporting systems serve as early-warning systems and do not provide an accurate assessment of risk (8). Only some 15–20% of adverse drug reactions are reported (9), and there is a tendency for physicians to report side effects with new drugs—the so-called Weber effect (10). Other factors influence spontaneous-reporting systems, including publicity of specific side effects, especially in the lay press, and overaggressive marketing by pharmaceutical companies (11). As Inman has pointed out (12), drugs have often been withdrawn because of numbers, not incidence.

Premarketing studies are performed on "squeaky-clean" patients who have participated in clinical therapeutic trials. On average, some 3000–5000 such patients are usually involved and, as a consequence, premarketing studies can be expected to identify only common adverse reactions; for example, at the 1% level (12–15). Postmarketing surveillance has been advocated to address the problem (16–18), but, as Fries et al. have pointed out (19), if the reaction is rare, say 1 in 1 million, then some 3 million patients would require to be seen to be 95% certain of finding a single case—the so-called rule of three (20). Therefore, it is doubtful whether pharmacoepidemiological studies will be helpful in identifying rare adverse drug reactions (21,22). Automated data bases may, however, help solve the problem in the future, although they will remain dependent on data quality and validity (23). Again, they will require very large numbers of patients and controls to be studied to identify rare side effects. For example, Fox and Jick failed to find one renal complication as a result of nonsteroidal anti-inflammatory drug (NSAID) therapy among 50,000 patients (24). Currently, the identification of rare adverse drug reactions depends on the clinical acumen of physicians. Nineteen of 20 adverse drug reactions that resulted in withdrawal of the drug from the market were based on published case reports (25,26).

II. HEPATOTOXICITY

Many drugs damage the liver. This may arise in one of three ways: first, as a direct cytotoxic effect of the drug or one of its metabolites on hepatic cells; second, as a result of the drug or one of its metabolites being insoluble and precipitating in the bile canaliculi; and, third, as an idiosyncratic response. Serious liver damage is uncommon with normal therapeutic use of NSAIDS, although liver damage has been reported with most of these agents. Hepatotoxicity was the reason for removal of ibufenac and benoxaprofen from the market. It is parodoxical that the two most commonly used over-the-counter analgesics, aspirin and acetaminophen, have the greatest potential for liver damage (27,28).

Salicylate liver damage usually results in asymptomatic increased concentrations of plasma transaminases, and it has been reported in acute rheumatic fever, juvenile arthritis, rheumatoid arthritis, Reiter's syndrome, and systemic lupus erythematosus (29). One of the factors common to these diseases that might be relevant is hypoalbuminemia, which would increase the serum concentration of "free" salicylate (30,31). In support of this, Tolman et al. found that lactic dehydrogenase concentrations rose in the supernatant of rat liver cells cultured in monolayers with the addition of aspirin (32), but this could be reduced if high concentrations of albumin were added to the media. On the other hand, salicylate "transaminitis" has been reported in normal subjects (33). In most patients, elevated serum transaminase concentrations return to normal when salicylate therapy is discontinued, or even when it is continued (34). Only rarely has salicylate-induced liver damage been sufficiently severe to cause prolongation of the prothrombin time (35). Hepatic biopsies have only occasionally been performed, but reported changes include centrilobular hepatocellular degeneration, with a periportal inflammatory infiltrate containing neutrophils, eosinophils, plasma cells, and lymphocytes (29,35). Similar findings have been reported in adult patients with rheumatoid arthritis, especially those with mitochondrial antibodies (36). These changes, therefore, may be associated with the immune disturbance of the disease, rather than salicylate therapy, because they are also found in patients with primary Sjögren's syndrome who have not had any drug therapy (37,38).

A. Reye's Syndrome and Aspirin

Reye's syndrome is a rare consequence of aspirin therapy, consisting of encephalopathy and fatty metamorphosis of the liver. It has been reported in children during outbreaks of influenza B and chickenpox, with a peak incidence between 5 and 15 years of age, and carrying a mortality of between 20 and 40% (29). The clinical features include an encephalopathy, varying in severity from drowsiness to deep coma, and associated with severe vomiting and hepatomegaly. Serum transaminase, lactic dehydrogenase, and ammonia concentrations are significantly elevated and, in severe cases, acid–base disturbances, hypoglycemia, and coagulation abnormalities may ensue. Surprisingly, jaundice is absent. Hepatic biopsies have been interpreted as indistinguishable or distinct from those seen in acute aspirin poisoning (29,39,40). Biochemical, histochemical, and ultrastructural changes have been consistently observed in the mitochondria. Both influenza B infection and salicylates uncouple oxidative phosphorylation in liver mitochondria in vitro, which may explain the increase in free fatty acids and ammonia and the specific inhibition of mitochondrial enzyme activity, with preservation of cytosolic enzymes (41). It has been suggested, but is as yet unconfirmed, that children who develop Reye's syndrome may have lower levels of aspirin esterases (42). Although Reye's syndrome has largely been described in children, it has also been reported in adults (43,44).

Case–control studies in the 1980s established the association between aspirin and Reye's syndrome (45–47). In some studies, patients were noted to have had higher doses of aspirin than controls (48), whereas others noted that most patients had received doses well below the upper limit of the antipyretic level, 80 mg/kg per day (29). Although the association of aspirin and Reye's syndrome was strong in most studies, a small, but significant, number of patients had not received any aspirin (29,49). One recent Australian study (49) failed to demonstrate a link between aspirin and Reye's syndrome, but aspirin use was based on chart reviews only, the patients were much younger than those who usually develop Reye's syndrome, and aspirin use was uncommon (50). Nevertheless, there has been a decline in the incidence of Reye's syndrome in parallel with the decline in the use of aspirin as an antipyretic in children (47). However, Reye's syndrome has not become an "endangered" disease, because it continues to be reported in children with juvenile arthritis and connective tissue disease (29,51,52). Surely, it is time for banning the use of aspirin in children with such diseases, and replacing it with an NSAID. Reye's syndrome will continue, however, to occur as a result of certain metabolic disorders, which usually occur in children younger than 5 years (50,54).

It is not now possible to predict which child may develop Reye's syndrome. It seems prudent not to prescribe aspirin to children as an antipyretic, especially if infected with chickenpox or influenza B. Acetaminophen is now the recommended antipyretic for children, but it is worth keeping in mind that recently hepatic impairment was observed to be more common in young adults who had received this drug during a measles epidemic (55,56).

B. Other Nonsteroidal Anti-Inflammatory Drugs

That hepatitis may rarely occur and occasionally be fatal (57) with any of the currently available NSAIDs is now well known (28,58,59,60). What is not known, however, is the true incidence of the complication (28). During prospective clinical therapeutic trials in the United States involving 1252 patients with rheumatoid arthritis, 67 (5.4%)

developed elevations of one or more liver enzymes (34). Paulus (61) opined that the elderly patient with impaired renal function, receiving prolonged therapy, especially with high doses and multiple other drugs, was particularly vulnerable, as was the patient with severe disease such as systemic lupus erythematosus. It has been recommended that monitoring of routine liver function tests be performed regularly, especially during the first 6 months of treatment (61). Whether this would prevent hepatotoxicity is unknown, and as yet, there are no ways for predicting which patients might develop the complication. As Prescott has pointed out the exact rank order of hepatotoxicity with the different nonsteroidal anti-inflammatory analgesics is unknown, since prescribing rates are not available (28). However, there have been many reports of hepatitis with phenylbutazone (62,63), but strangely, not with oxyphenbutazone (58). Hepatitis usually develops within the first few weeks of starting treatment, and recovery is the rule on discontinuation of the drug, although fatalities have been reported (58). Hepatic biopsy has shown changes consistent with a toxic hepatitis, cholestasis, and, in a few patients, granuloma formation (63). Reversible hepatitis has been reported with azapropazone, which is chemically related to phenylbutazone (28,64). In a review of the U.S. Food and Drug Administration (FDA) adverse reaction reports from 1984 to 1989, when over 439 million NSAID prescriptions were written, Katz and Love (60) found that diclofenac, phenylbutazone, and sulindac, appeared to have a slightly greater potential for liver damage than other NSAIDS, which is in agreement with other reports (65–70). However, indomethacin and tolmetin were found by Katz and Love (60) to have the highest fatality rates, whereas ketoprofen and the fenemates had the lowest number of reports of adverse drug reactions with a fatal outcome involving the liver. A Danish study of reported adverse reactions to NSAIDS, over a 17-year period, estimated that the overall average occurrence of NSAID-induced hepatotoxicity may be 3% (70). Hepatitis may occur in generalized hypersensitivity reactions to drugs, and NSAIDs are no exception (58,71), but Prescott maintains this should not be interpreted that the drug in question has specific hepatotoxicity (28).

III. OTHER GASTROINTESTINAL ADVERSE REACTIONS

Oral ulceration may occur as a result of local application of an aspirin tablet, in the mistaken belief that it will relieve toothache. Stomatitis may also occur with other NSAIDs (58), and lichenoid eruptions have been reported with fenclofenac (73).

Sialadenitis, giving rise to acute salivary gland swelling, has been reported, especially with phenylbutazone and oxyphenbutazone (74), but also with other NSAIDs, such as ibuprofen (58). However, salivary gland inflammation appears in most published reports to be part of a generalized hypersensitivity reaction, rather than an isolated event (58). It is important to differentiate this reaction from salivary gland enlargement, which may be acute and painful, in Sjögren's syndrome.

Many elderly patients, especially women, have reduced salivary flow rates and, as a consequence, have difficulty in swallowing tablets and capsules. These may occasionally remain lodged in the esophagus, leading to hemorrhage, performation, or stricture. This appears to be becoming a problem in elderly bedridden patients and could be prevented by use of liquid formulations.

The NSAIDs are being increasingly implicated in complications in both the small intestine and lower colon. Acute proctocolitis has been reported to occur as a result of aspirin hypersensitivity (75,76). This occurred in patients who suffered with asthma and recurrent nasal polyps. Baekelandt et al. have recently described rectal stenosis as a consequence of the use of suppositories containing aspirin (77).

Pancreatitis has been reported as a complication of sulindac and also other NSAIDs (58). Similar to other rare serious complications, it is difficult to be certain that the pancreatitis was drug-induced, as rechallenge would be unethical.

Acetaminophen is prescribed for approximately 40% of patients with rheumatoid arthritis, in addition to their other antirheumatic medication (78). Taking up to 4 g of acetaminophen, even over prolonged periods in otherwise healthy adults, is extremely safe, although efficacy in inflammatory joint disease has been questioned (79). In chronic liver disease, the plasma half-life of acetaminophen is slightly prolonged, but long-term administration of acetaminophen depletes liver glutathione stores, leading to an increased risk of hepatotoxicity (29). Thus, although acetaminophen can be safely prescribed over short periods to patients with stable liver disease (80), long-term use may not be so innocuous. This is particularly true in chronic alcoholics (81,82) who have reduced glutathione synthesis (83). Frail, elderly, and undernourished patients may likewise be predisposed to acetaminophen hepatotoxicity (84), and it is prudent policy to question acetaminophen intake in such patients with unexplained abnormalities in liver function tests (85).

IV. CARDIOVASCULAR SIDE EFFECTS

There have been several suggestions that NSAIDs may precipitate angina in patients with coronary artery disease (86–88) and make the myocardium more sensitive to ouabain (89). However, no untoward cardiovascular complications have been reported using large doses of indomethacin in the treatment of acute gouty arthritis in elderly patients (90) and, in a Canadian controlled clinical therapeutic trial, indomethacin, 100 mg daily, did not cause worsening of exercise-induced angina or reduce the efficacy of nitroglycerin (91). Coronary artery spasm has been suggested to occur in aspirin and other NSAID-induced asthma (88,92), but this awaits confirmation. Aspirin withdrawal has been suggested as a possible cause of myocardial infarction (93).

Indomethacin has reduced cardiac output in patients with hyponaturemia (94), and this and other NSAIDs are well recognized to precipitate congestive cardiac failure in the elderly (95). Myocarditis and pericarditis have been reported to occur with the use of phenylbutazone, although these were part of hypersensitivity reactions, and did not occur as isolated events (96–98). There has been a case report of severe acral vasospasm in a patient who was given ibuprofen and tolmetin on two separate occasions (99).

There is an extensive literature concerning the effects of NSAIDs on hypertension and interaction with antihypertensive drugs (100). The NSAIDs appear to modestly increase blood pressure, on average 10 mmHg, and antagonize the effects of β-and α-adrenergic antihypertensive drugs (100). Nonprescription use of aspirin and ibuprofen has been noted to increase the blood pressure, but significantly only in patients who are hypertensive (101–103). On the whole, the effects of NSAIDs are mild, but rarely, a hypertensive crisis may occur, estimated at 1:100 a year, especially in the elderly and in patients with low-renin hypertension (100). NSAIDs also blunt the effect of thiazide and loop diuretics and of angiotensin-converting enzyme inhibitors (1,100).

Maternal treatment with indomethacin and other NSAIDs has been reported to cause persistent pulmonary hypertension in the newborn as a result of prostaglandin synthesis inhibition (104–107); however, the frequency of this complication is not known. Naproxen has been reported to cause hyponatremia and fluid retention in a neonate whose mother had received an overdose of naproxen (108).

V. KIDNEYS AND BLADDER

Salicyl edema was reported in patients receiving salicylate therapy by Hanzlick and colleagues in 1917 (109). Burns and colleagues identified that phenylbutazone could be associated with salt and water retention and possibly renal insufficientcy (119). Phenacetin was implicated as the principal cause of interstitial nephritis and papillary necrosis (111). It has since been identified that salicylates and other NSAIDs do not impair renal function in healthy adults, since prostaglandin production within the kidney is not necessary for the maintenance of renal blood flow in the healthy subject (112). However, if there is compromised renal function, such as occurs in altered volemic and osmolar states, there is increase in circulating norepinephrine, angiotensin II, and antidiuretic hormone, to support general homeostasis. The effects of these vasoconstrictors result in a potential decrease in renal perfusion, to which the kidney compensates by production of vasodilator prostaglandins (113). However, if NSAIDs are administered, there can be a rapid decrease in renal function, which is dose-dependent (114–116). The problem usually resolves on withdrawal of the NSAIDs, but rarely, ischemic tubular necrosis can occur, with associated acute irreversible renal failure and death (117–119). Elderly patients and patients with cardiovascular diseases, hepatic disease, and compromised renal function are at greatest risk of salt and water imbalance and for development of acute fluid retention and problems such as hyponatremia and hyperkalemia (29). Potassium supplements and potassium-sparing diuretics can result in hyperkalemia, with concomitant hyporeninemic hyperaldosteronism (114). Johnson reported that NSAIDs may be a risk factor for sudden death in marathon runners because of development of the hyperkalemia that is induced by strenuous exercise and dehydration (120).

Interstitial nephritis is an extremely rare complication of NSAID therapy (29). The complication usually commences after 6 months of therapy, with a range of 2 weeks to 18 months (121,122). Most patients have been elderly, and the most common offending drug has been fenoprofen (114,123), although it has also been reported with diclofenac, ibuprofen, and indomethacin (124). Oliguria is common, and proteinuria may be in the range associated with the nephrotic syndrome (123). The T lymphocytes of the cytotoxic suppressor subset and eosinophils are found in the interstitial tissues of the kidney, and eosinophiluria may be present (29). However, only a few patients have fever, rash, or eosinophilia (112). The complication is usually reversible. The use of high-dose corticosteroid therapy to assist recovery (29) requires further evaluation (124). Recurrence of acute interstitial nephritis has been reported after a second exposure to the same or to a different NSAID (125). In long-standing cases, glomerulosclerosis and interstitial fibrosis may develop (112).

Nephrotic syndrome is uncommon, and has been described in both children and adults. The condition usually resolves on withdrawal of the drug (126). The histological abnormality is that of a minimal-change glomerulopathy, with mild mesangial prominence, and glomerulosclerosis, with associated tubular damage, interstitial infiltration, and edema (112). Numerous T lymphocytes have been identified in the interstitial infiltrate, suggestive of a cytotoxic reaction (112). The development of a nephrotic syndrome has been identified with alclofenac, fenoprofen, ibuprofen, indomethacin, phenylbutazone, naproxen, sulindac, and tolmetin (112,127–129). A mild nephrotic syndrome has been reported with salsalate (130).

The clinical features of renal papillary necrosis, with chronic interstitial nephritis, are characterized by pain in the renal angle with associated hematuria. Sometimes there is interruption of urinary flow, and the patient passes a necrosed renal papilla. Pyelonephritis is common, as is hypertension and the development of renal failure owing to the production of a chronic interstitial nephritis, with fibrosis and end-stage renal disease (131,132). The mechanism of action of NSAID damage to the kidney is that of chronic tubular damage of the renal papilla and inner medulla, related to ischemia, resulting from prostaglandin synthesis inhibition (114). Volume depletion is probably also important in pathogenesis (133), and this may be why the complication has been frequently reported in Australia (134). Transitional cell carcinoma of the ureter and bladder are well-recognized complications of analgesic nephropathy (135). In a recent study, an increased incidence of kidney cancer was observed in elderly patients who took aspirin daily (136). Strictures of the ureters and retroperitoneal fibrosis are extremely rare complications of analgesic nephropathy (131).

Drug interactions, with resulting renal complications, are now well recognized (1), and can be broadly classified into pharmacokinetic and pharmacodynamic (137). Interactions between aspirin or other NSAIDs and methotrexate occur when high doses of the latter are prescribed, as in the treatment of malignancy. Interactions are uncommon in rheumatological practice in which low doses of methotrexate are used (138), but they have been described in children with arthritis (139) and in adult patients with renal dysfunction (140).

Hyperkalemia and renal insufficiency, secondary to cyclosporine, are thought to be potentiated with the use of the NSAIDs (112). Lithium toxicity is also enhanced, as is the toxicity of cisplatin, cadmium, acetylcholinesterase (ACE) inhibitors and digoxitin, and triamterene (112); (Table 1).

Phenylbutazone has been reported to cause uric acid precipitation in the tubule, with resultant hematuria, oliguria, and even anuria (141). A similar syndrome was reported with the use of the drug suprofen, which has since been withdrawn from the market (142).

Sulindac is a prodrug reputed to have a smaller effect on renal prostaglandins than other drugs. However, sulindac is converted in vivo to a biologically inactive sulfone and a biological active sulindac sulfide that is a potent prostaglandin inhibitor, and significant renal impairment has been reported (29). Hyponatremia has also been reported as has a drug interaction with furosemide and labetalol (1).

Ibuprofen has been reported to cause polyuria and nocturia (143), and naproxen has been reported to cause ejaculation dysfunction (144).

Finally, it should not be forgotten that aspirin increases the risk of postsurgical hemorrhage (145, 146).

VI. SYSTEMIC ANAPHYLACTOID REACTIONS

Several NSAIDs, including alclofenac, choline magnesium trisalcylate, diclofenac, ibuprofen, indoprofen, ketprofen, mefenamic acid, naproxen, phenylbutazone, sulindac, tolmetin, and zomepirac, and hypotension (147–160). These reactions have been fatal only with zomepirac, and were the reason for this drug's removal from the market (155). Anaphylactoid reactions appear to be more common with intermittent than with continuous use of an NSAID (155). According to O'Brien and Bagby, no anaphylactoid reactions

Table 1 Interactions With NSAIDs

Drug affected	NSAIDs implicated	Effect	Approach to management
Pharmacokinetic			
Antacids		The renal excretion of salicylates is extremely sensitive to changes in urinary pH and, as a consequence, there is an increased renal excretion of salicylates.	Monitor effect of antacid therapy on salicylate plasma levels, and adjust dose of salicylate accordingly.
Lithium	Probably all NSAIDs	Inhibition of renal excretion of lithium, increasing risk of toxicity.	Use sulindac, aspirin if NSAID unavoidable. Careful monitoring of lithium concentration and appropriate dose reduction.
Methotrexate (high-dose)	Probably all NSAIDs	Reduced clearance of methotrexate (mechanism unclear) increasing plasma concentration and risk of severe toxicity.	Simultaneous dosing is contraindicated. Use of NSAIDs between cycles of chemotherapy is probably safe.
Digoxin	All NSAIDs	Potential reduction in renal function (particularly in very young and very old), reducing digoxin clearance and increasing plasma concentration and risk of toxicity (no interaction if renal function normal).	Avoid NSAIDs if possible; if not, frequent checks of digoxin plasma concentration and plasma creatinine.

Aminoglycosides	All NSAIDs	Reduction in renal function in susceptible individuals, reducing aminoglycoside clearance and increasing plasma concentration.	Close plasma concentration monitoring and dose adjustment.
Probenecid	Probably all NSAIDs	Reduction in metabolism and renal clearance of NSAIDs.	May be used therapeutically to increase the response to given dose of NSAID.
Pharmacodynamic			
Antihypersensive agents: blockers, diuretics, ACE inhibitors, vasodilators	Indomethacin, other NSAIDs	Reduction in hypertensive effect, probably related to inhibition of renal prostaglandin synthesis (producing salt and water retention) and vascular prostaglandin synthesis (producing increased vasoconstriction).	Avoid all NSAIDs in treated hypertensive patients if possible; if not, use sulindac preferentially. May need additional antihypertensive therapy.
Diuretics	Indomethacin, other NSAIDs	Reduction in natriuretic and diuretic effects; may exacerbate congestive cardiac failure.	Avoid NSAIDs in patients with cardiac failure; use sulindac; monitor clinical signs of fluid retention.
Triamterene	Indomethacin	Potentiation of nephrotoxicity, including in subjects with normal renal function.	Combination contraindicated.
Potassium-sparing	All NSAIDs	Potassium retention and hyperkalemia.	Avoid combination; monitor K.

Source: Ref. 1.

have been reported with indomethacin (149), although this drug has been observed to cause the sudden onset of reproducible urticaria (161). Hypocomplementemia and antibodies to extractable nuclear antigens have been observed in several patients before the anaphylactoid reaction (149). Therefore, it is possible that certain patients may be inherently susceptible to reactions of this type (162).

Ibuprofen has been reported to cause fever, abdominal pain, nausea, vomiting, and elevated liver enzymes (149–151). It may seem strange, therefore, that this drug should have been licensed as an over-the-counter medication; but the reaction is extremely rare, and patients who have developed the syndrome have mostly suffered from systemic lupus erythematosus (SLE) or mixed connective tissue disease (149–151). Furthermore, only one patient has been reported to have died (163). Strangely, to date only ibuprofen has been reported to exacerbate systemic lupus erythematosus (164).

Lupuslike syndromes have been reported to occur with both ibuprofen (165) and phenylbutazone (166). These patients developed positive antinuclear factor tests (165, 166). Oxyphenbutazone was reported to cause thrombocytopenia associated with LE cells (167).

Alclofenac enjoyed a brief spell of popularity in the United Kingdom before being withdrawn from the market as a result of severe cutaneous vasculitis (168). Rare cases of vasculitis have been reported with the use of aspirin, diclofenac, fenbufen, flurbiprofen, ibuprofen, indomethacin, naproxen, and indomethacin (149,169–178). Most of these cases have involved the skin only (171,173,176,177), but others have involved the kidney in addition (169,170,172,174,178,179). Most of the patients with renal involvement recovered promptly on discontinuing treatment. However, a severe acute glomerulonephritis occurred in one patient after taking indomethacin (169), and Heaton and Bourke reported papillary necrosis, as a result of vasculitis, with ibuprofen (170).

Sudden death has been reported in children treated with indomethacin (179), and a fatal case of hemorrhagic chickenpox during treatment with indomethacin has been reported (180). The suggestion has been made that indomethacin and other NSAIDs may predispose to infection, but the case of fatal hemorrhagic chickenpox may have been incidental. The NSAIDs have been implicated in the reactivation of pulmonary tuberculosis by Canadian workers (181–183), but this has not been our experience. Indeed, low-dose oral corticosteroids are frequently prescribed to patients with healed pulmonary tuberculosis, without evidence of reactivation.

Sprung described a patient, with a hypersensitivity reaction to sulindac, who developed peripheral and mediastenal lymphadenopathy and erythema multiforme (184). There is no doubt, in this case, that sulindac was responsible because the illness improved when the drug was withdrawn, but recurred on rechallenge.

VII. DERMATOLOGICAL EFFECTS

The most common dermatological side effect of NSAIDs is a nonpruritic macular rash, which is rarely reported by clinicians except during clinical trials. The rare dermatological side effects of NSAIDs can usually be characterized as both unpleasant in appearance and in clinical symptoms. The most severe skin reactions to NSAIDs are erythema multiforme, Stevens–Johnson syndrome with involvement of the mouth and conjunctiva, and toxic epidermal necrolysis (Lyall's syndrome). Erythema multiforme has been reported caused by aspirin, diflunisal, sulindac, diclofenac, ibuprofen, fenbufen, naproxen, zomepirac, meclofenamic acid, phenylbutazone, oxyphenbutazone, and piroxicam (7). Stevens–Johnson syndrome has been reported with diflunisal, sulindac, diclofenac, ibuprofen, benoxaprofen, piroxicam, phenylbutazone, and oxyphenbutazone (7). Toxic epidermal necrolysis has been reported with indomethacin, sulindac, fenbufen, tolmetin, zomepirac, benoxaprofen, piroxicam, and phenylbutazone (7). It was the development of toxic epidermal necrolysis in patients receiving isoxicam that led to its withdrawal from the world markets (185,186). Pemphigus vulgaris has been reported secondary to piroxicam (187), and bullous pemphigus and Gougerot's syndrome have been reported with ibuprofen (188,189).

Photosensitivity has been identified with several nonsteroidal drugs including ketoprofen, naproxen, tiaprofenic acid, piroxicam, and carprofen (7,190–192). Benoxaprofen also caused a reaction in sun-exposed areas characteristic of bullous dermatitis (190,193), and similar reactions have been reported with piroxicam (194,195). Fixed drug eruptions, consisting of erythematous or brownish, eczemalike lesions, which recur when the drug is taken, have been reported with aspirin (196) and acetaminophen (197). However, the most common skin reaction to aspirin is urticaria (198). This occurs particularly in aspirin-sensitive patients. Aspirin also may cause an exacerbation in patients with chronic urticaria (199), which does not appear to be mediated by prostaglandin inhibition (200). Both indomethacin (201) and ibuprofen (202) have been reported to cause urticaria in aspirin-sensitive individuals. A single case of plasma cell granuloma was described in a patient with nonlipemic xanthomatosis who took indomethacin (203). Contact dermatitis has been reported with several proprionic acids, such as suprofen (204,205), and benoxaprofen has caused facial milia (206). Meclofenamic acid has exacerbated cutaneous features of psoriasis (207).

Hemorrhagic and bullous eruptions of the hand have been reported with phenylbutazone (7), and bullous eruptions, involving several parts of the body, have been reported with azapropazone (208). Phenylbutazone and oxyphenbutazone have also caused contact dermatitis and produced generalized pustular psoriasis (7). Also, phenylbutazone has caused acne necrotica (acne varioliformis) and localized ulcers of the lip (7). Ibuprofen has caused alopecia in patients using hair straighteners or dyes (209,210), and benoxaprofen has caused onycholysis and hypertrichosis (7).

The pathogenesis of dermatological reactions to NSAIDs has not been elucidated (211). In some instances it is not even certain whether the reaction is due to the drug or to an excipient (e.g., as in the case of aspirin urticaria, in which the offending allergen may be tartrazine; 198,212). An excipient might have been responsible for the severe dermatological complications of isoxicam, which occurred only with a Spanish-made product in France. Formulation factors need to be considered in further studies of dermatological reactions (213).

VIII. PULMONARY ADVERSE REACTIONS

Acute rhinitis, wheezing, and bronchospasm can occur in some 2–20% of asthmatic patients who take aspirin or other NSAIDs (7,214). Asthmatic patients with nasal polyps and hypersensitivity to aspirin are usually more severely affected (198). Adverse effects have been reported for indomethacin, ibuprofen, ketoprofen, fenoprofen, flurbiprofen, naproxen, zomepirac, and dipyrone, and fatal attacks have been identified (7). Aspirin-sensitive asthmatics can be desensitized by repeated challenges with low doses (215).

Cross-sensitivity has been observed with acetaminophen in aspirin-sensitive subjects with asthma (216), although acetaminophen can usually be safely given to aspirin-sensitive asthmatics (217). Fish oil has been reported to have a deleterious effect on patients with aspirin-intolerant asthma (218).

Acute pulmonary edema has been identified in patients suffering from salicylate intoxication (7). This has occurred in patients, with and without heart disease, and may occasionally be fatal (219). The management of the problem is immediate withdrawal of the drug, mechanical ventilation, and correction of any metabolic imbalance. Pulmonary edema can occur on the basis of acute salt and water retention and has been long recognized in elderly patients, with a history of cardiovascular disease, especially with phenylbutazone and oxyphenbutazone.

The NSAID-associated pneumonitis has been reported with fenbufen, ibuprofen, naproxen, phenybutazone, and sulindac (7,220,221). Patients have fever, cough, wheezing, and basal wet sounds. A chest x-ray film usually shows diffuse bilateral infiltrates. Eosinophilia is usually present, and eosinophils are usually abundant in the sputum. The illness subsides on stopping the NSAID and, if necessary, treatment with corticosteroids (7). A fatality has been reported with ibuprofen, as a result of this rare complication (222). A case of *Pneumocystis carinii* pneumonia complicating low-dose methotrexate treatment for psoriatic arthritis has been described (223).The authors suggested that this might have resulted from an interaction with NSAIDs, causing an increased plasma half-life of methotrexate. We would opine differently and consider it more likely to have been due to methotrexate.

IX. HEMATOLOGICAL ADVERSE REACTIONS

Aplastic anemia has been reported with aspirin and several other NSAIDs, including diclofenac, fenoprofen, ibuprofen, indomethacin, naproxen, piroxicam, and sulindac (149). The mortality rate in these iatrogenic cases was high, almost 70% (149). However, the NSAIDs that continue to be the leading cause of aplastic anemia in registries of drug adverse reactions are phenylbutazone and oxyphenbutazone (224–227) and, to a smaller extent, indomethacin (225–228). This is the reason that phenylbutazone and oxyphenbutazone have become obsolescent, if not obsolete, as antirheumatic agents (229). Aplastic anemia caused by NSAIDs is probably idiosyncratic (230), but phenylbutazone-induced aplastic anemia was noted to occur more frequently in women older than 50 years of age (224). O'Malley et al. reported that elderly people had a slower elimination rate of phenylbutazone (231); hence, it is possible that aplastic anemia in the elderly is related to higher blood drug concentrations. In support of this, patients who developed phenybutazone-induced aplastic anemia were noted by Cunningham et al. to have a slower elimination of acetanilide (232), which is biotransformed by the same liver enzymes as phenylbutazone.

Agranulocytosis induced by NSAIDs is extremely rare, being estimated as only 0.07 cases per million tablets for indomethacin (233). Again, phenylbutazone and oxyphenbutazone appear to be the main culprits (149), but the mortality is very much lower than for aplastic anemia (224). Neutropenia and agranulocytosis have been reported rarely with aspirin and the new NSAIDs, and fatalities even more rarely (149).

All NSAIDs inhibit platelet function by inhibition of cyclooxygenase. The effect of aspirin is due to acetylation of the cyclooxygenase; consequently, the effect is present for the life of the platelet. In contrast, the effort of other NSAIDs is present only for the life of the NSAID in plasma. Accordingly, aspirin is particularly likely to increase postoperative bleeding (234). Even topical application of aspirin has the potential to cause bleeding

(235). Other NSAIDs also have the potential to cause bleeding, but are much less likely to do so than aspirin. Indeed, ibuprofen can be used to treat hemophiliac arthritis (236).

Thrombocytopenia has very rarely been reported to occur with NSAIDs (149). However, again, phenylbutazone and oxyphenbutazone appear to be the main culprits (149).

Pure red cell anemia has been reported with fenoprofen, indomethacin, and phenylbutazone (149). In a patient with fenoprofen-induced red cell aplasia, reticulocytosis and an increase in hemoglobin concentration occurred immediately after the drug was discontinued (237). Pure red cell anemia, which responded to immunosuppressive therapy, has been reported in association with an IgG inhibitor in rheumatoid disease (238).

Autoimmune hemolytic anemia has been reported with several NSAIDs (239), but especially with mefenamic acid (149). This complication has been reported after less than 2 weeks of therapy in some cases, and after 1 year of treatment in others (149). In some reports, patients also had fever, thrombocytopenia, and hepatic and renal failure (149).

It has been suggested that phenylbutazone may be leukemogenic (149), and a controlled study in Australia certainly suggested that this might indeed be true (240). An American study of 409 patients with leukemia and lymphoma concluded that the use of phenylbutazone had been "somewhat more frequent" (241), but this may have been because musculoskeletal pain is a common feature in the early stages of these diseases and was the reason that phenylbutazone was prescribed (242,243). The jury will now probably require to remain out forever with the infrequent use of phenylbutazone.

Despite that most patients with glucose-6-phosphate dehydrogenase deficiency can safely be prescribed acetaminophen, aspirin, and phenylbutazone (244), there remains the possibility of inducing a hemolytic crisis (245). It must be remembered that some 150 mutant gene products have been identified (1); hence, care should be taken with the use of NSAIDs in patients known to have this enzymopathy.

X. MUSCULOSKELETAL ADVERSE REACTIONS

It has been suggested that potent prostaglandin inhibitors, such as indomethacin, might cause aseptic necrosis of the hip (246–248). A recent study by Rased et al. suggested a slower progression of hip osteoarthritis in patients receiving apazone (azapropazone; a weak prostaglandin inhibitor) (249). During inflammation of the hip, there is subchondral vasodilatation maintained by the local prostaglandin release. This blood supply is necessary for both subchrondral bone and cartilage. The use of a potent prostaglandin inhibitor will result in inhibition of cyclooxygenase, a reduction in vasodilator prostaglandin, and subsequent reduction in blood supply to subchondral bone and, hence, the development of aseptic necrosis. Interestingly, the clearance rate of intra-articularly injected radioactive xenon, ^{133}Xe, was reduced in rheumatoid arthritis by indomethacin, but not by sodium salicylate (250). Indomethacin may cause cartilage damage by inhibition of proteoglycan synthesis (251). On the other hand, Howell et al. have demonstrated biochemical and histological protection of cartilage by tiaprofenic acid in the Pond–Nuki canine model of experimental osteoarthritis (252). However, there remains considerable doubt about whether any of the NSAIDs cause acceleration of human osteoarthritis (253) and, also, for so-called chondroprotection (254).

There has been the suggestion that NSAIDs may increase the risk of hip fracture in the elderly (255), and that indomethacin may delay the healing of fractures (256). Aspirin may reduce heterotrophic ossification after hip arthroplasty for osteoarthritis, but this awaits confirmation by a controlled clinical trial. However, in a double-blind study, aspirin has been demonstrated to be an effective prophylactic of deep venous thrombosis after hip surgery (257).

Niflumic acid, a fluorinated NSAID, when given in high doses over long periods, may cause skeletal fluorosis (258) and osteomalacia (259). Preoperative administration of aspirin has been reported to reduce suxamethonium-induced myalgia (260).

Spanish workers have reported a 26-year-old male drug-user, who was human immunodeficiency virus (HIV)-positive and had Reiter's syndrome, who experienced worsening of his cutaneous lesions with indomethacin therapy (261). The skin lesions almost completely resolved after indomethacin was discontinued, but recurred when indomethacin therapy was reinstituted. This may be an example of an adverse virus–drug interaction, similar to that described with trimethoprim–sulfamethoxazole in acquired immunodeficiency syndrome (AIDS) patients treated for *Pneumocystis carinii* lung infection (262).

XI. CENTRAL NERVOUS SYSTEM

Aseptic meningitis has been reported as a result of treatment with ibuprofen, naproxen, sulindac, tolmetin, and trimethoprim–sulfamethoxazole (co-trimoxazole) (263,269). Symptoms are those of meningitis, with the cerebrospinal fluid showing an increase in polymorphonuclear leukocytes and a modest rise in protein concentration (270). The reaction has been reported most commonly with ibuprofen in patients with systemic lupus erythematosus and mixed connective tissue disease (270). One patient taking sulindac had an eosinophilic meningitis (267). The condition quickly settles on discontinuing the offending drug, and recovery is the rule (270). Even 1 tablet of ibuprofen has caused an exacerbation (270). Ibuprofen has been reported to cause an aseptic meningitis in New Zealand mice, which spontaneously develop systemic lupus erythematosis (271). Aseptic meningitis has been reported in patients with osteoarthritis and fractures (263,268). The reaction has also been reported as part of a generalized reaction, with pancreatitis, parotitis, pneumonitis, and acute renal failure (272,273).

Several ocular side effects have been reported with ibuprofen, including transient diplopia, color blindness, central field defects, and visual hallucinations (274–277). In one patient with decreased vision and color brightness, evoked visual potentials showed increased conduction times (278). These side effects all improved, albeit sometimes slowly, on stopping ibuprofen (270). One can only conclude that these ocular complications of ibuprofen are rare, since no ocular side effects have been reported in several large series of patients (270,279). Likewise, reports of corneal deposits and reduced retinal sensitivity with indomethacin therapy (280,281) are rare, as they have not been found in large series of patients who have been followed for several years (282). Transient myopia has been recorded with aspirin therapy (283), but must be extremely rare. The isolated report of ketoprofen-induced conjunctivitis (284) suggests *post hoc, ergo propter hoc* [after this, therefore an account of it; a fallacy of argument]. There is suggestive evidence that chronic aspirin therapy may protect against the development of cataracts (285–287), but there is no evidence, as had been suggested in the older literature, that aspirin treatment provides benefit in diabetic retinopathy (288).

Indomethacin is recognized as a common cause of severe depression and psychotic behavior in elderly patients (289–292). Rarely, however, these adverse rections have also been reported with other NSAIDs, including ibuprofen (293), sulindac (294), and tolectin

(295). A patient has been described who developed an encephalopathy while taking sulindac (296), and several cases of both grand mal and petit mal epilepsy have been reported with diclofenac, ibuprofen, and indomethacin (297–299). The patient who developed grand mal seizures with ibuprofen was, however, subsequently diagnosed as having systemic lupus erythematosis (299). These adverse reactions rapidly reversed on discontinuation of the drug. Cognitive function has been reported to be altered in elderly patients receiving ibuprofen and naproxen (300), although, on the other hand, there is evidence that daily aspirin therapy may improve or stabilize cognition in elderly patients with mutll-infarct dementia (301).

Salicylate therapy has long been recognized to cause tinnitus and deafness. What is perhaps less well recognized is that permanent deafness may result from habitual use of aspirin, although this must be rare (302,303). It is important to recognize that tinnitus and deafness can occur with plasma concentrations of salicylate less than 1.3 mmol/L (304,305). Day and his colleagues have demonstrated a linear relation between hearing loss and unbound salicylate concentrations (306).

Four patients have been described who developed peripheral neuropathy as a result of indomethacin therapy (307). Two further patients have been described with this complication while taking sulindac and dimethyl sulfoxide (308,309), but it is unclear which drug was responsible or whether the complication arose as a result of an interaction between the two drugs. Extrapyramidal symptoms and dyskinesia have been reported with mefenamic acid (310,311).

XII. PREGNANCY AND THE FETUS

There is no evidence that NSAIDs affect fertility (312). However, NSAIDs may increase the rate of fetal malformations (312), although several studies have failed to find any evidence of a causal association between NSAIDs and teratogenicity (313–315). The difficulties of interpretation of data on possible NSAID-induced fetal abnormalities have been recently reviewed by Bellamy et al. (106). Anti-inflammatory doses of aspirin have prolonged gestation and labor and have caused an increased blood loss at delivery (316). The effects of other NSAIDs on pregnancy and labor have not been studied, but similar to aspirin may infrequently be associated with neonatal bleeding and persistent pulmonary hypertension (317).

REFERENCES

1. Brooks PM, Buchanan WW. Prediction of the clinical efficacy of and intolerance to antirheumatic drug therapy. In: Bellamy N, ed. Prognosis in the rheumatic diseases. Lancaster, UK: Kluwer Academic Publishers, 1991:347–402.
2. Huskisson EC, Wojtulewski JA. Measurement of side effects of drugs. Br Med J 1974; 2:698–9.
3. Coles LS, Fries JF, Kraines RG, et al. From experience to experience: side effects of nonsteroidal anti-inflammatory drugs. Am J Med 1983; 74:820–8.
4. Steel K, Gertman PM, Crescenzi C, et al. Iatrogenic illness on a general medical service at a university hospital. N Engl J Med 1981; 304:638–42.
5. Naranjo LA, Busto U, Sellers EM, et al. A method for estimating the probability of adverse drug reactions. Clin Pharmacol Ther 1980; 30:239–45.
6. Girard M. Testing the methods of assessment for adverse drug reactions. Adverse Drug React Acute Poison Rev 1984; 4:237–44.
7. O'Brien WM, Bagby GF. Rare adverse reactions to nonsteroidal anti-inflammatory drugs. J Rheumatol 1985; 12:13–20.

8. Griffin JP, Weber JCP. Voluntary systems of adverse reactions reporting—Part II. Adverse Drug React Acute Poison Rev 1986; 6:23–55.
9. Rogers AS. Adverse drug events: identification and attribution. Drug Intell Clin Pharm 1987; 21:915–20.
10. Weber JCP. Epidemiology of adverse drug reactions to nonsteroidal anti-inflammatory drugs. Adv. Inflamm Res 1984; 6:1–7.
11. Gordon AJ, Sachs R. Potential biases influencing interpretation of data from worldwide spontaneous ADR reports. In: Rainsford KD, Velo GP, eds. Side-effects of anti-inflammatory drugs, part I. Clinical and epidemiological aspects. Lancaster, UK: MTP, 1987: 105–10.
12. Inman, WHW. Risks in medical intervention. PEM News 1984; 2:16–36.
13. Bell RL, Smith EO. Clinical trials in postmarketing surveillance of drugs. Control Clin Trials 1982; 3:61–8.
14. Porta MS, Hartzema AG. The contribution of epidemiology to the study of drugs. Drug Intell Clin Pharm 1987; 21:741–7.
15. Fries JF. Postmarketing drug surveillance: are our priorities right? J Rheumatol 1988; 15:389–90.
16. Inman WHW. Prescription event monitoring. Br Med J 1982; 285:809–10.
17. Lasagna L. Discovering adverse drug reactions. JAMA 1983; 249:2224–5.
18. Rossi AC, Knapp DE. Discovery of new adverse drug reactions—a review of the Food and Drug Administration's reporting system. JAMA 1984; 252:1030–3.
19. Fries JF, Williams CA, Bloch DA. The relative toxicity of nonsteroidal anti-inflammatory drugs. Arthritis Rheum 1991; 34:1353–60.
20. Sackett DL, Haynes RB, Tugwell P. Clinical epidemiology, a basic science for clinical medicine. Boston: Little, Brown & Co., 1985:226.
21. Strom BL. Overview of different logistical approaches to postmarketing surveillance. J Rhematol 1988; 15(suppl 17):9–13.
22. Tilson HH. Pharmacoepidemiology: the future. Drug Intell Clin Pharm 1988; 22:416–21.
23. Stergachis AS. Record linkage studies for post marketing drug surveillance: data quality and validity considerations. Drug Intell Clin Pharm 1988; 22:157–61.
24. Fox DA, Jick H. Nonsteroidal anti-inflammatory drugs and renal disease. JAMA 1984; 251:1299–1300.
25. Rossi AC, Knapp DE, Anello C, et al. Discovery of adverse drug reactions: a comparison of selected phase IV studies with spontaneous reporting methods. JAMA 1983; 249:2226–8.
26. Venning GR. Identification of adverse drug reactions to new drugs. IV—Verification of suspected adverse reactions. Br Med J 1983; 286:544–7.
27. Prescott LF. Liver damage with non-narcotic analgesics. Med Toxicol 1986; 1:44–56.
28. Prescott LF. The hepatotoxicity of non-steroidal anti-inflammatory drugs. In: Rainford KD, Velo GP, eds. Side effects of anti-inflammatory drugs. Dordrecht: Kluwer Academic Publishers, 1992:176–87.
29. Buchanan WW, Brooks PM. Prediction of organ system toxicity with antirheumatic drug therapy. In: Bellamy N, ed. Prognosis in the rheumatic diseases. Dordrecht: Kluwer Academic Publishers, 1991:403–50.
30. Gitlin N. Salicylate hepatotoxicity: the potential role of hypoalbuminemia. J. Clin Gastroenterol 1980; 2:281–5.
31. Zimmerman HJ. Effects of aspirin and acetaminophen on the liver. Arch Intern Med 1981; 141:333–42.
32. Tolman KG, Peterson P, Gray P, Hammar SP. Hepatotoxicity of salicylates in monolayer cell cultures. Gastroenterology 1978; 74:205–8.
33. Garber E, Craig RM, Bahu RM. Aspirin hepatitis. Ann Intern Med 1975; 82:592–3.
34. Paulus HE, Furst DE. Aspirin and other non-steroidal anti-inflammatory drugs. In: McCarty DJ, ed. Arthritis and allied conditions: a textbook of rheumatology. 11th ed. Philadelphia: Lea & Febiger, 1989:507–43.

35. Seaman WE, Plotz PH. Effect of aspirin on liver tests in patients with rheumatoid arthritis or SLE and in normal volunteers. Arthritis Rheum 1976; 19:155–60.
35. Seaman WE, Ishak KG, Plotz PH. Aspirin-induced hepatotoxicity in patients with systemic lupus erythematosus. Ann Intern Med 1974; 80:1–8.
36. Whaley K, Webb J. Liver and kidney disease in rheumatoid arthritis. Clin Rheum Dis 1977; 3:527–47.
37. Whaley K, Goudie RB, Williamson J, et al. Liver disease in Sjögren's syndrome and rheumatoid arthritis. Lancet 1970; 1:861–3.
38. Webb J, Whaley K, MacSween RNM, et al. Severe disease in rheumatoid arthritis and Sjögren's syndrome: prospective study using biochemical and serological markers of hepatic dysfunction. Ann Rheum Dis 1975; 34:70–80.
39. Starko KM, Mullick FG. Hepatic and cerebral pathology findings in children with fatal salicylate intoxication: further evidence for a causal relation between salicylate and Reye's syndrome. Lancet 1983; 1:326–9.
40. Everson GW, Krenzelok EP. Chronic salicylism in a patient with juvenile rheumatoid arthritis. Clin Pharm 1986; 5:334–41.
41. Trauner DA, Horvath E, Davis LE. Inhibition of fatty acid beta oxidations by influenza B virus and salicylic acid in mice: implications for Reye's syndrome. Neurology 1988; 38:239–41.
42. Tomasova H, Nevoral J, Pachl J, et al. Aspirin esterase activity and Reye's syndrome (letter). Lancet 1984; 2:43.
43. Stillman A, Gitter H, Shillignton D, et al. Reye's syndrome in the adult: case report and review of the literature. Am J Gastroenterol 1983; 78:365–8.
44. Tumiati B, Assalito C, Veneziani M. Reye's syndrome in an adult following therapy with salicylates in Still's disease. Medicina (Flor) 1989; 9:64–5.
45. Forsyth BW, Horwitz RI, Acampora D, et al. New epidemiologic evidence confirming that bias does not explain the aspirin/Reye's syndrome association. JAMA 1989; 261:2517–24.
46. Hurwitz ES. Reye's syndrome. Epidemiol Rev 1989; 2:249–53.
47. Strom BL. Aspirin and Reye's syndrome. In: Rainsford KD, Velo GP, eds. Side effects of anti-inflammatory drugs, 3. Dordrecht: Kluwer Academic Publishers, 1992:241–7.
48. Pinsky PF, Hurwitz ES, Schonberger LB, et al. Reye's syndrome and aspirin. Evidence for a dose–response effect. JAMA 1988; 260:657–61.
49. Orlowski JP, Campbell P, Goldstein S. Reye's syndrome: a case–control study of medication use and associated viruses in Australia. Cleve Clin J Med 1990; 57:323–9.
50. Editorial. A catch in the Reye is awry. Cleve Clin J Med 1990; 57:318–20.
51. Hansen JR, McCray PB, Bale JF Jr, et al. Reye syndrome associated with aspirin therapy for systemic lupus erythematosus. Pediatrics 1985; 76:202–5.
52. Rennebohm RM, Heubi JE, Daugherty CC, et al. Reye syndrome in children receiving salicylate therapy for connective tissue disease. J Pediatr 1985; 107:877–80.
53. Editorial. Reye's syndrome and aspirin: epidemiological associations and inborn errors of metabolism. Lancet 1987; 2:429–31.
54. Rowe PC, Valle D, Bruislow SW. Inborn errors of metabolism in children referred with Reye's syndrome: A changing pattern. JAMA 1988; 260:3169–71.
55. Ackerman Z, Flugelman Y, Wax Y, et al. Hepatitis during measles in young adults: possible role of antipyretic drugs. Hepatology 1989; 10:203–6.
56. Levy M, Ackerman Z. Liver toxicity of antipyretic drugs in conjunction with measles infections. In: Rainsford KD, Velo GP, eds. Side effects of anti-inflammatory drugs, 3. Dordrecht: Kluwer Academic Publishers, 1992:18–21.
57. Wolfe SM. Safety of piroxicam. Lancet 1986; 2:808–9.
58. O'Brien WM, Bagby GF. Rare adverse reactions to nonsteroidal anti-inflammatory drugs. J Rheumatol 1985; 12:562–7.
59. Hannequin JR, Doffoel M, Schmutz G. Les hepatites secondaires aux anti-inflammatoires non-steroidiens recents. Rev Rheum 1988; 55:983–8.

60. Katz LM, Love PY. NSAIDs and the liver. In: Famaey JP, Paulus HE, eds. Therapeutic applications of NSAIDs: Subpopulations and formulations. New York: Marcel Dekker, 1992:247–63.
61. Paulus HE. Government affairs: FDA arthritis advisory committee meeting. Arthritis Rheum 1982; 25:1124–5.
62. Zimmerman HJ, Lewis JH. Drug-induced cholestasis. Med Toxicol Adverse Drug Experience 1987; 2:112–60.
63. Benjamin SB, Ishak KG, Zimmerman HJ, et al. Phenylbutazone liver injury: a clinico-pathologic survey of 23 cases and review of the literature. Hepatology 1981; 225–263.
64. Lo TCN, Dymock IW. Azapropazone-induced hepatitis. Br Med J 1988; 297:1614.
65. Wouters JM, van Rijswijk MH, van de Putte LB. Adult onset Still's disease in the elderly: a report of two cases. J Rheumatol 1985; 12:791–3.
66. O'Brien WM. Adverse reactions to nonsteroidal anti-inflammatory drugs. Diclofenac compared with other nonsteroidal anti-inflammatory drugs. Am J Med 1986; 80:70–80.
67. Brooks PM. Side effects of nonsteroidal anti-inflammatory drugs. Bailliere's Clin Rheumatol 1988; 2:425–54.
68. Helfgott SM, Sandberg-Cook J, Zakim D, et al. Diclofenac-associated hepatotoxicity. JAMA 1990; 264:2660–2.
69. Ivenson TJ, Ryley NG, Kelley PMA, et al. Diclofenac associated hepatitis. J Hepatol 1990; 10:85–9.
70. Kromann-Anderson H, Pedersen A. Reported adverse reactions to and consumption of nonsteroidal anti-inflammatory drugs in Denmark over a 17 year period. Dan Med Bull 1988; 35:187–92.
71. Park GD, Spector R, Headstream T, et al. Serious adverse reactions associated with sulindac. Arch Intern Med 1982; 142:1292–4.
72. Llorca G, Larbe JP, Collet PH, et al. Changing the class of NSAID in cases of hepatotoxicity [letter]. Ann Rheum Dis 1988; 47:791.
73. Ferguson MM, Weistenfeld D, MacDonald DG. Oral mucosal lichenoid eruption due to fenclofenac. J Oral Med 1984; 39:39–40.
74. Speed BR, Spelman DW. Sialadenitis and systemic reaction associated with phenylbutazone. Aust NZ J Med 1982; 12:261–4.
75. Pearson DJ, Stones NA, Bentley SJ, et al. Proctocolitis induced by salicylate and associated with asthma and recurrent nasal polyps. Br Med J 1983; 287:1675.
76. Rutherford D, Stockdill G, Hamer-Hodges DW, et al. Proctocolitis induced by salicylate. Br Med J 1984; 288:794.
77. Baekelandt M, Vansteenberge R, van der Spek P, et al. Rectal stenosis following the use of suppositories containing paracetamol and acetylsalicylic acid. Gastrointest Radiol 1990; 15:171–3.
78. Lee P, Ahola SJ, Grennan D, et al. Observations on drug prescribing in rheumatoid arthritis. Br Med J 1974; 1:424–6.
79. Lee P, Anderson JA, Miller J, et al. Evaluation of analgesic action and efficacy of antirheumatic drugs. Study of 10 drugs in 684 patients with rheumatoid arthritis. J Rheumatol 1976; 3:283–95.
80. Benson GD. Acetaminophen in chronic liver disease. Clin Pharmacol Ther 1983; 33:95–101.
81. Black M. Acetaminophen hepatotoxicity. Annu Rev Med 1984; 35:577–93.
82. Kumar S, Rex DK. Failure of physicians to recognize acetaminophen hepatotoxicity in chronic alcoholics. Arch Intern Med 1991; 151:1189–91.
83. Lauterburg BH, Velez ME. Glutathione deficiency in alcoholics: risk factor for paracetamol hepatotoxicity. Gut 1988; 29:115–7.
84. Regal RE. Acetaminophen chronic toxicity [letter]. Drug Intell Clin Pharm 1986; 20:507.
85. Schlegel SI, Paulus HE. Non-steroidal and analgesic therapy in the elderly. Clin Rheum Dis 1986; 12:245–73.

86. Miwa K, Kambara H, Kawai C. Variant angina aggravated by aspirin [letter]. Lancet 1979; 2:1382.
87. Al-Abbasi AH. Salicylate-induced variant angina [letter]. Am Heart J 1983; 106:1450.
88. Ahmad S. Severe coronary spasm during zomepirac-induced allergic reaction [letter]. South Med J 1984; 77:938.
89. Wilkerson RD, Glenn TM. Influence of non-steroidal anti-inflammatory drugs on ouabain toxicity. Am Heart J 1977; 94:454–5.
90. Emmerson BT. Regimen of indomethacin in therapy in acute gouty arthritis. Br Med J 1967; 2:272–4.
91. McGregor M, Crelinsten GL. Possible interactions of indomethacin and nitrates in angina pectoris. Am J Cardiol 1984; 53:225–7.
92. Habbab MA, Szwed SA, Haft JI. Is coronary artery spasm, part of aspirin-induced asthma syndrome? Chest 1986; 90:141–3.
93. Louwerenburg JW, Suttorp MJ, Herie Kingma J. Aspirin withdrawal in a patient with essential thrombocytopenia: possible cause of myocardial infarction [letter]. Am J Med 1987; 83:1175.
94. Dzau VJ, Packer M, Lilly LS, et al. Prostaglandins in severe congestive heart failure: relation to activation of the renin–angiotensin system and hyponatremia. N Engl J Med 1984; 310:347–52.
95. van den Ouweland FA, Gribnau FW, Meyboom RH. Congestive heart failure due to nonsteroidal anti-inflammatory drugs in the elderly. Age Ageing 1988; 17:8–16.
96. Hodge PR, Lawrence JR. Two cases of myocarditis associated with phenylbutazone therapy. Med J Aust 1957; 1:640–1.
97. Shafar J. Phenylbutazone-induced pericarditis. Br Med J 1965; 2:797.
98. Ford MJ, Prescott LF. Phenylbutazone pericarditis. Scott Med J 1982; 27:252–3.
99. Siebold JR, Kim HC. Acral vasospasm complicating therapy with ibuprofen and tolmetin. J Rheumatol 1982; 9:647–8.
100. Houston MC. Nonsteroidal anti-inflammatory drugs and antihypertensives. Am J Med 1991; 90(suppl 5A):42–7.
101. Walter E, Kaufmann W, Oster P. Does chronic aspirin treatment increase blood pressure in man? Klin Worchenschr 1981; 59:297–9.
102. Waller PC, Ramsay LE. Arthritis and drug therapy in the hypertension clinic. Biomed Pharmacother 1988; 42:207–11.
103. Bradley JG. Nonprescription drugs and hypertension. Which ones affect blood pressure? Postgrad Med 1991; 89:195–7;201–2.
104. Dalens B, Dechelotte P, Gaulme J, et al. Maternal treatment with indomethacin and severe neonatal pulmonary hypertension. Arch Fr Pediatr 1981; 38:261–5.
105. Turner GR, Levin DL. Prostaglandin synthesis inhibition in persistent pulmonary hypertension of the newborn. Clin Perinatol 1984; 11:581–9.
106. Bellamy N, Grigor RR, Naden RP. Arthritis in pregnancy. In: Bellamy N, ed. Prognosis in the rheumatic diseases. Dordrecht: Kluwer Academic Publishers, 1991:279–319.
107. Besinger RE, Niebyl JR, Keyes WG, et al. Randomized comparative trial of indomethacin and ritodrine for the long-term treatment of preterm labour. Am J Obstet Gynecol 1991; 164:981–6.
108. Alun-Jones E, Williams J, Clwyd G. Hyponatremia and fluid retention in a neonate associated with maternal naproxen overdosage. Clin Toxicol 1986; 24:257–60.
109. Hanzlik PJ, Scott RW, Reycraft JL. The salicylates. VIII. Salicyl edema. Arch Intern Med 1917; 20:329–40.
110. Burns JJ, Rose RK, Chenkin T, et al. The physiological disposition of phenylbutazone in man and a method for its estimation in biological material. J Pharmacol Exp Ther 1953; 109:346–57.
111. Kincaid-Smith P. Analgesic nephropathy: a common form of renal disease in Australia. Med J Aust 1969; 2:1131–5.

112. Prescott LF, Martin U. Current status of nephrotoxicity by non-steroidal anti-inflammatory drugs. In: Rainsford KD, Velo GP, eds. Side effects of anti-inflammatory drugs, 3. Dordrecht: Kluwer Academic Publishers, 1992:223–35.
113. Clive DM, Stoff, JS. Renal syndromes associated with nonsteroidal anti-inflammatory drugs. N Engl J Med 1984; 310:563–72.
114. Blackshear JL, Napier JS, Davidman M, et al. Renal complications of nonsteroidal anti-inflammatory drugs: identification and monitoring of those at risk. Semin Arthritis Rheum 1985; 14:163–75.
115. Brater DC. Adverse effects of non-steroidal anti-inflammatory drugs on renal function. Ann Intern Med 1990; 112:559–60.
116. Gurwitz JH, Avorn J, Ross-Degnan O, et al. Nonsteroidal anti-inflammatory drug-associated azotemia in the very old. JAMA 1990; 264:471–5.
117. Boletis J, Williams RJ, Shortland JR, et al. Irreversible renal failure following mefenamic acid. Nephron 1989; 51:575–6.
118. Sarma PSA. Fatal acute renal failure after piroxicam. Clin Nephrol 1989; 31:54.
119. Itami N. Progressive renal failure despite discontinuation of mefanamic acid. Nephron 1990; 54:281–2.
120. Johnson RB. Use of NSAIDs in long distance runners: a risk factor for sudden death? South Med J 1989; 82:95.
121. Levin ML. Patterns of tubulo-interstitial damage associated with non-steroidal and anti-inflammatory drugs. Semin Nephrol 1988; 8:55–61.
122. Toto RD. Acute tubulointerstitial nephritis. Am J Med Sci 1990; 299:392–410.
123. Bender WL, Whelton A, Beschorner WE, et al. Interstitial nephritis, proteinuria and renal failure caused by nonsteroidal anti-inflammatory drugs. Am J. Med 1984; 76:1006–12.
124. Pierucci A, Patrano C. NSAIDs in renal impairment and dialysis. In: Famaey JP, Paulus HE, eds. Therapeutic applications of NSAIDs. subpopulations and new formulations. New York: Marcel Dekker, 1992:211–46.
125. Abraham PA, Keane WF. Glomerular and interstitial disease induced by nonsteroidal anti-inflammatory drugs. Am J Nephrol 1984; 4:1–6.
126. Tietjem DP. Recurrence and specificity of nephrotic syndrome due to tolmetin. Am J Med 1989; 87:354–5.
127. Chatterjee GP. Nephrotic syndrome due to tolmetin. JAMA 1981; 246:1589.
128. Lomvardias S, Pinn VW, Wadhwa ML, et al. Nephrotic syndrome associated with sulindac [letter]. N Engl J Med 1981; 304:424.
129. Kleinknecht D, Landais P, Goldfarb B. Analgesic and nonsteroidal anti-inflammatory drug-associated acute renal failure: a prospective collaborative study. Clin Nephrol 1986; 25:275.
130. Valles M, Tovar JL. Salsalate and minimal-change nephrotic syndrome [letter]. Ann Intern Med 1987; 107:116.
131. Prescott LF. Analgesic nephropathy: a reassessment of the role of phenacetin and other analgesics. Drugs 1982; 23:75–149.
132. Kincaid-Smith P. Renal toxicity of non-narcotic analgesics: at-risk patients and prescribing applications. Med Toxicol Adverse Drug Experience 1986; 1(suppl 1):14–22.
133. Robertson CE, Van Someren V, Ford MJ, et al. Mefenamic acid and nephropathy. Lancet 1980; 2:232–3.
134. Nanra RS, Stuart-Taylor J, de Leon AH, et al. Analgesic nephropathy: etiology, clinical syndrome and clinico-pathologic correlations in Australia. Kidney Int 1978; 13:79–92.
135. Taylor JS. Carcinoma of the urinary tract and analgesic abuse. Med J Aust 1972; 1:407–9.
136. Paganini-Hill A, Caao A, Ross RK, et al. Aspirin use and chronic diseases: a cohort study of the elderly. Br Med J 1989; 299:1247–50.
137. Tonkin AL, Wing LMH. Interactions of non-steroidal anti-inflammatory drugs. Bailliere's Clin Rheumatol 1988; 2:455–83.
138. Day RO, Furst DE, Graham GG, Champion GD. The clinical pharmacology of aspirin and

the salicylates. In: Paulus HE, Furst DE, Dromgoole SH, eds. Drugs for rheumatic disease. New York: Churchill-Livingstone, 1987: 227–63.
139. Dupius LL, Koren G, Shore A, et al. Methotrexate–nonsteroidal anti-inflammatory drug interaction in children with arthritis. J Rheumatol 1990; 17:1469–73.
140. Ahern M, Booth J, Loxton A, et al. Methotrexate kinetics in rheumatoid arthritis: is there an interaction with nonsteroidal anti-inflammatory drugs? J Rheumatol 1988; 15:1356–60.
141. Lipsett MB, Goldman R. Phenylbutazone toxicity: report of a case of acute renal failure. Ann Intern Med 1954; 41:1075–9.
142. Hart D, Ward M, Lifschitz MD. Suprofen-related nephrotoxicity: a distinct clinical syndrome. Ann Intern Med 1987; 106:235–8.
143. Novack SN. Side effect of ibuprofen therapy. Arthritis Rheum 1975; 18:628.
144. Wei N, Hood JC. Naproxen and ejaculatory dysfunction. Ann Intern Med 1980; 93:933.
145. Ruiz H, Saltzman B. Aspirin-induced bilateral renal hemorrhage after extracorporeal shock wave lithotripsy therapy: implications and conclusions. J Urol 1990; 143:791–2.
146. Watson CJ, Deane AM, Doyle PT, et al. Identifiable factors in post-prostatectomy haemorrhage: the role of aspirin. Br J Urol 1990; 66:85–7.
147. Smith FE, Lindberg PJ. Life-threatening hypersensitivity to sulindac. JAMA 1980; 244:269–70.
148. Rossi AC, Knapp DE. Tolmetin-induced anaphylactoid reactions. N Engl J Med 1982; 307:499–500.
149. O'Brien WM, Bagby GF. Rare adverse reactions to nonsteroidal anti-inflammatory drugs. J Rheumatol 1985; 12:347–53.
150. Sonnenblick M, Abraham AS. Ibuprofen hypersensitivity in systemic lupus erythematosus. B Med J 1978; 1:619–20.
151. Shoenfeld Y, Livni E, Shaklaim C, et al. Sensitization to ibuprofen in systemic lupus erythematosus [letter]. JAMA 1980; 244:547–8.
152. Stricker BH, Meyboom RH, Lindquist M. Acute hypersensitivity reactions to paracetamol. Br Med J 1985; 291:938–9.
153. Strom BL, Carson JL, Morse ML, et al. The effect of indication on hypersensitivity reactions associated with zomepirac sodium and other non-steroidal anti-inflammatory drugs. Arthritis Rheum 1987; 30:1142–8.
154. Nadkarmi MM, Peller CA, Retig J. Eosinophilic hepatitis after ingestion of choline magnesium trisalcylate. Am J Gastroenterol 1992; 87:151–3.
155. Strom BL, Carson JL, Schinnar R, Snyder ES, West S. Nonsteroidal anti-inflammatory drugs and hypersensitivity reactions. In: Rainsford KD, Velo GP, eds. Side effects of anti-inflammatory drugs, 3. Dordrecht: Kluwer Academic Publishers, 1992:22–6
156. Adverse drug reactions advisory committee. Phenylbutazone. Med J Aust 1979; 2:553.
157. Pavelka K, Schusta A. Behandlung der progredient chronischen polyarthritis mit einem nicht-steroidalen antirheumatikum mit langer halbwertszeit. Fortschr Med 1979; 97:965–7.
158. Dux Groslop I, Garty M, Rosenfeld JB. Anaphylactic shock induced by diclofenac. Br Med J 1983; 286:1861.
159. Fowler PD, Faragher EB. Drug and non-drug factors influencing adverse reactions to pyrazoles. J. Int Med Res 1977; 5(suppl 2):108–20.
160. Dromgoole SH, Furst DE. Naproxen. In: Paulus HE, Furst DE, and Dromgoole SH, eds. Drugs for rheumatic disease. New York: Churchill-Livingstone, 1987:347–64.
161. Katz AM, Pearson CM, Kennedy JM. A clinical trial of indomethacin in rheumatoid arthritis. Clin Pharmacol Ther 1965; 6:25–30.
162. Criep LH. Adverse drug reactions. Scope of the problem. Postgrad Med 1985; 78:208–9.
163. Lee RP, King EG, Russell AS. Ibruprofen: a severe systemic reaction. Can Med Assoc J 1983; 129:854–5.
164. Stratton MA. Drug-induced systemic lupus erythematosus. Clin Pharm 1985; 4:657–63.
165. Bar-sela S, Levo Y, Zeevi D, et al. A lupus-like syndrome due to ibuprofen hypersensitivity. J Rheumatol 1980; 1:379–80.

166. Farid N, Anderson J. SLE-like reaction after phenylbutazone. Lancet 1971; 1:1022–3.
167. Handley AJ. Thrombocytopenia and LE cells after oxyphenbutazone. Lancet 1971; 1:245–6.
168. Hort JF. Adverse reactions to alclofenac. Curr Med Res Opin 1975; 3:333–7.
169. Marsh FP, Almeyda JR, Levy IS. Non-thrombocytopenic purpura and acute glomerulonephritis after indomethacin therapy. Ann Rheum Dis 1971; 30:501–5.
170. Heaton JM, Bourke E. Papillary necrosis associated with calyceal arteritis. Nephron 1976; 16:57–63.
171. Grennan DM, Jolly J, Holloway LJ, et al. Vasculitis in a patient receiving naproxen. NZ Med J 1979; 89:48–9.
172. Plouvier B, Gosselin B, Hatron PY, et al. Vasculopathie allergique systemique induite par le naproxen. Ann Med Interne (Paris) 1979; 130:173–6.
173. Mordes JP, Johnson MW, Soter NA. Possible naproxen associated vasculitis. Arch Intern Med 1980; 140:985.
174. Leung AC, McLay A, Dobbie JW, Jones JM. Phenylbutazone-induced systemic vasculitis and crescentic glomerulonephritis. Arch Intern Med 1985; 145:685–7.
175. Stanziale P, Fuiano G, Balletta MM, et al. A case of relapsing renal micropolyarteritis: a possible association with assumption of non-steroidal anti-inflammatory drugs (NSAID). Adv Exp Med Biol 1989; 252:303–6.
176. Wei N. Flurbiprofen and cutaneous vasculitis [letter]. Ann Intern Med 1990; 112:550–1.
177. Gamboa PM, Tabar AI, Wong E. Indomethacin-induced vasculitis. Allergol Immunopathol 1988; 16:53–5.
178. Singhal PC, Faulkner M, Venkatesan J, Molho L. Hypersensitivity angiitis associated with naproxen. Ann Allergy 1989; 63:107–9.
179. Jacobs JC. Sudden death in arthritic children receiving large doses of indomethacin. JAMA 1967; 199:182–4.
180. Rodriguez RS, Barbabosa E. Hemorrhagic chickenpox after indomethacin. N Engl J Med 1971; 285:690.
181. Brennan M. Activation of latent tuberculosis by non-steroidal anti-inflammatory agents. Can Med Assoc J 1980; 122:400–2.
182. Brennan M. Latent tuberculosis and anti-inflammatory agents. Can Med Assoc J 1982; 126:21.
183. Tomasson HO, Brennan M, Bass MJ. Tuberculosis and nonsteroidal anti-inflammatory drugs. Can Med Assoc J 1984; 130:275–8.
184. Sprung DJ. Sulindac causing a hypersensitivity reaction with peripheral and mediastinal lymphadenopathy. Ann Intern Med 1982; 97:564.
185. Moore N, Paux G, Begaud B, et al. Adverse drug reaction monitoring: doing it the French way. Lancet 1985; 2:1056–8.
186. Albengres E. Features of the French postmarketing drug surveillance system. Application to cutaneous effects of nonsteroidal anti-inflammatory drugs. J Rheumatol 1988; 15(suppl 17):20–3.
187. Martin RL, McSweeney GW, Schneider J. Fatal pemphigus vulgaris in a patient taking piroxicam. N Engl J Med 1983; 309:795–6.
188. Pompeova L. Bulozni pemphigoid vyvolany uzivanim Brufenu. Cesk Dermatol 1981; 56:256–8.
189. Labbe A, Desvignes V, Souteyrand P. Tri-symptome de Gougerot induit par l'ibuprofene? Ann Dermatol Venerol 1982; 109:995.
190. Diffey BL, Daymond TJ, Fairgraves H. Phototoxic reactions to piroxicam, naproxen and tiaprofenic acid. Br J. Rheumatol 1984; 22:239–42.
191. Albengres E. Features of the French postmarketing drug surveillance system. Application to cutaneous effects of nonsteroidal anti-inflammatory drugs. J. Rheumatol 1988; 15(suppl 17):20–3.
192. Kantor TG. Ketoprofen: a review of its pharmacologic and clinical properties. Pharmacotherapy 1986; 6:93–102.

193. Du Vivier A. Bullous dermatitis with benoxaprofen. Lancet 1982; 1:47.
194. Stern RS. Phototoxic reactions to piroxicam and other nonsteroidal anti-inflammatory agents. N Engl J Med 1983; 309:186–7.
195. Stern RS, Bigby M. An expanded profile of cutaneous reactions to nonsteroidal anti-inflammatory drugs: reports to a specialty based system for spontaneous reporting of adverse reactions to drugs. JAMA 1984; 252:1433–7.
196. Shukla SR. Drugs causing fixed drug eruptions. Dermatologica 1981; 163:160–3.
197. Thomas RH, Munro DD. Fixed drug eruption due to paracetamol. Br J Dermatol 1986; 115:357–9.
198. Buchanan WW, Rooney PJ, Rennie JAN. Aspirin and the salicylates. Clin Rheum Dis 1979; 5:499–539.
199. Bailin PL, Matkaluk RM. Cutaneous reactions to rheumatological drugs. Clin Rheum Dis 1982; 8:493–516.
200. Settipaine GA. Adverse reactions to aspirin and related drugs. In: Side-effects of anti-inflammatory analgesic drugs. Adv Inflamm Res 1983; 6:189–201.
201. Matthews JI, Stage D. Indomethacin, aspirin, and urticaria. Ann Intern Med 1974; 80:771.
202. Gryglewski RJ, Szczeklik A, Czerniawska-Mysik G. Aspirin sensitivity: other drugs. Ann Intern Med 1975; 82:286–7.
203. Shelley WB, Rawnsley HM. Plasma cell granulomas in nonlipemic xanthomatosis: apparent induction by idomethacin. Acta Derm Venereol 1975; 55:489–92.
204. Dooms-Goossens A, Dooms M, Van Lint L, et al. Skin sensitizing properties of arylalcanoic acids and their analogues. Contact Dermatitis 1979; 5:324–8.
205. Valsecchi R, Falgheri G, Cainelli T. Contact dermatitis from ketoprofen. Contact Dermatitis 1983; 9:163–4.
206. Dawes PT, Raman D, Haslock I. Side effects of benoxaprofen. Br Med J 1982; 284:1631.
207. Meyerhoff JO. Exacerbation of psoriasis with meclofenamate. N Engl J Med 1983; 309:496.
208. Barker DJ, Cotterill JA. Azapropazone induced bullous drug eruptions. Acta Derm Venereol 1977; 57:461–2.
209. Meyer HC. Alopecia associated with ibuprofen. JAMA 1979; 242:142.
210. Herrick RT. Toxic alopecia associated with ibuprofen (Motrin) J Med Assoc Ala 1981; 51:16.
211. Rainsford KD. Mechanisms of rash formation and related skin conditions induced by non-steroidal anti-inflammatory drugs. In: Rainsford KD, Velo GP, eds. Side effects of anti-inflammatory drugs. Dordrecht: Kluwer Academic, 1992:287–301.
212. MacCara ME. Tartrazine: a potentially hazardous dye in Canadian drugs. Can Med Assoc J 1982; 126:910–4.
213. Florence AT, Salole EG, eds. Formulation factors in adverse reactions, London: Wright, 1990.
214. Aaron TH, Muttitt ELC. Reactions to acetylsalicylic acid. Can Med Assoc J 1982; 126:609–11.
215. Kowalski ML, Grzelewska-Rzymowska I, Rozniecki J, et al. Aspirin tolerance induced in aspirin-sensitive asthmatics. Allergy 1984; 39:171–8.
216. Settipane RA, Stevenson DD. Cross sensitivity with acetaminophen in aspirin-sensitive subjects with asthma. J Allergy Clin Immunol 1989; 84:26–33.
217. Falliers CJ. Acetaminophen and aspirin challenges in subgroups of asthmatics. J Asthma 1993; 20(suppl 1):39–49.
218. Picado C. Castillo JA, Schinca N, et al. Effects of a fish oil enriched diet on aspirin intolerant asthmatic patients: a pilot study. Thorax 1988; 43:93–7.
219. Davis PR, Burch RE. Pulmonary edema and salicylate intoxication. Ann Intern Med 1974; 80:553–4.
220. Adachi S, Nimura T, Monoe T, et al. A case of pneumonitis due to naproxen. Jpn J Thorac Dis 1986; 24:168–72.
221. Chuck AJ, Wilcox M, Bossingham DH. Fenbufen-associated pneumonites [letter]. Br J Rheumatol 1987; 26:475–6.

222. Bravo JF, Jacobson MP, Mertens BF. Fatty liver and pleural effusion with ibuprofen therapy. Ann Intern Med 1977; 87:200–1.
223. Wallis PJ, Ryatt KS, Constable TJ. *Pneumocystis carinii* pneumonia complicating low dose methotrexate treatment for psoriatic arthropathy. Ann Rheum Dis 1989; 48:247–9.
224. Inman WHW. Study of fatal bone marrow depression with special reference to phenylbutazone and oxyphenbutazone. Br Med J 1977; 1:1500–5.
225. Bottiger LE, Westerholm B. Drug-induced blood dyscrasias in Sweden. Br Med J 1973; 3:339–43.
226. Bottiger LE, Norlander M, Strandberg I. Deaths from drugs: an analysis of drug-induced deaths reported to the Swedish adverse drug reaction committee during a five year period (1966–1970). J Clin Pharmacol 1974; 14:401–7.
227. Bottiger LE. Phenylbutazone, oxyphenbutazone and aplastic anaemia. Br Med J 1977; 2:265.
228. Canada AT Jr, Burka ER. Aplastic anaemia after indomethacin. N Engl J Med 1968; 278:243–4.
229. The international agranulocytosis and aplastic anemia study. Risks of agranulocytosis and aplastic anemia. A first report of their relation to drug use with special reference to analgesics. JAMA 1986; 256:1749–57.
230. Vincent PC. Drug-induced aplastic anaemia and agranulocytosis. Incidence and mechanisms. Drugs 1986; 31:52–63.
231. O'Malley K, Crooks J, Duke E, Stevenson IH. Effect of age and sex on human drug metabolism. Br Med J 1971; 3:607–9.
232. Cunningham JL, Leyland MJ, Delamore IW, Price-Evans DA. Acetanilide oxidation in phenylbutazone-associated hypoplastic anaemia. Br Med J 1974; 3:313–7.
233. Arneborn P, Palmblad J. Drug-induced neutropenia—a survey for Stockholm 1973–1978. Acta Med Scand 1982; 212:289–92.
234. Carrick DG. Salicylates and post-tonsillectomy haemorrhage. J Larnyngol Otol 1984; 98:803–5.
235. Rose FA, Wiemer DR. Platelet coagulopathy secondary to topical salicylate use. Ann Plastic Surg 1983; 11:340–3.
236. McIntyre BA, Philp RB, Inwood MJ. Effect of ibuprofen on platelet function in normal subjects and hemophiliac patients. Clin Pharmacol Ther 1978; 24:616–21.
237. Weinberger KA. Fenoprofen and red cell aplasia. J Rheumatol 1979; 6:475.
238. Dessypris EN, Baer MR, Sergent JS, et al. Rheumatoid arthritis and pure red cell aplasia. Ann Intern Med 1984; 100:202–6.
239. Hughes JA, Sudell W. Haemolytic anaemia associated with naproxen. Arthritis Rheum 1983; 86:1054.
240. Leavesley GM, Stenhouse NS, Dougan L, et al. Phenylbutazone and leukaemia: is there a relationship? Med J Aust 1969; 2:963–5.
241. Fraumeni JF. Bone marrow depression induced by chloramphenicol or phenylbutazone: leukemia and other sequelae. JAMA 1967; 201:828–34.
242. Hart FD. Leukemia and phenylbutazone. Br Med J 1964; 2:569.
243. Friedman GD. Phenylbutazone, musculoskeletal disease, and leukemia. J Chron Dis 1982; 35:233–43.
244. Beutler E. Glucose-6-phosphate dehydrogenase deficiency. N Engl J Med 1991; 324:169–74.
245. Meloni T, Forteleoni G, Ogania A, et al. Aspirin-induced acute haemolytic anaemia in glucose-6-phosphate dehydrogenase-deficient children with systemic arthritis. Acta Haematol (Basel) 1989; 81:208–9.
246. Arora JS. Indomethacin arthropathy of hips. Proc R Soc Med 1968; 61:669.
247. Ronningen H, Langeland N. Indomethacin treatment in osteoarthritis of the hip joint: does the treatment interfere with the natural cause of the disease? Acta Orthop Scand 1979; 50:169–74.
248. Serup J, Ovensen JO. Salicylate-arthropathy. Accelerated coxarthrosis during long-term treatment with acetylsalicylic acid. Schweiz Rundschau Med Prax 1981; 70:359–61.

249. Rashed S, Revell P, Hemingway A, et al. Effect of nonsteroidal anti-inflammatory drugs on the course of osteoarthritis. Lancet 1989; 2:519–22.
250. Dick C, Dick PH, Nuki G, et al. Effect of anti-inflammatory drug therapy on clearance of ^{133}Xe from knee joints of patients with rheumatoid arthritis. Br Med J 1969; 3:278–80.
251. Dingle JT. NSAIDs and human cartilage metabolism. In: Rainsford KD, Velo GP, eds. Side-effects of anti-inflammatory drugs, 3. Dordrecht: Kluwer Academic Publishers 1992, 261–8.
252. Howell DS, Pita JC, Muller FJ, et al. Treatment of osteoarthritis with tiaprofenic acid: biochemical and histological protection against cartilage breakdown in the Pond–Nuki canine model. J Rheumatol 1981; 18(suppl 27):138–42.
253. Doherty M, Holt M, MacMillan P, et al. A reappraisal of "analgesic hip." Ann Rheum Dis 1986; 45:272–6.
254. Doherty M. "Chondroprotection" by non-steroidal anti-inflammatory drugs. Ann Rheum Dis 1989; 48:619–21.
255. Daly MP. Drugs and the risk of hip fracture [letter]. J Am Geriatr Soc 1990; 38:727–8.
256. Sudmann E. Indomethacin and fracture healing. Risk of delayed healing and development of pseudoarthrosis [letter]. Tidsskr Nor Laegeforen 1976; 96:52.
257. Putz P, Buyse H, Delvaux D, et al. Triflusal versus acetylsalicylic acid: a double-blind study for the prophylaxis of deep venous thrombosis after hip surgery. Acta Chir Belg 1991; 91:269–76.
258. Meunier PJ, Courpron P, Smoller JS. Niflumic acid-induced skeletal fluorosis: iatrogenic disease or therapeutic perspective for osteoporosis? Clin Orthop 1980; 148:304–9.
259. Bonvoisin B, Bouvier M, Meumier PJ, et al. Osteomalacie histologique induite par l'administration prolongee d'acide niflumique. Nour Presse Med 1982; 11:1636.
260. McLoughlin C, Nesbitt GA, Howe JP. Suxamethonium-induced myalgia and the effect of pre-operative administration of oral aspirin. A comparison with a standard treatment and an untreated group. Anaesthesia 1988; 43:565–7.
261. Allegue F, Boixeda P, Espana A, et al. Reiter's syndrome exacerbated by indomethacin. Med Cutan Ibero Lat Am 1989; 17:113–6.
262. Glatt AE, Chrigin K. *Pneumocystis carinii* pneumonia in human immunodeficiency virus-infected patients. Arch Intern Med 1990; 150:270–9.
263. Ruppert GB, Barth WF. Ibuprofen hypersensitivity in systemic lupus erythematosus. South Med J 1981; 74:241–3.
264. Ballas ZK, Donat ST. Sulindac-induced aseptic meningitis. Arch Intern Med 1982; 142:165–6.
265. Kremer I, Ritz R, Brummer F. Aseptic meningitis as an adverse effect of co-trimoxazole. N Engl J Med 1983; 308:1481.
267. Lorino GD, Hardin JG. Sulindac-induced meningitis in mixed connective tissue disease. South Med J 1983; 76:1185–7.
268. von Reyn CF. Recurrent aseptic meningitis due to sulindac. Ann Intern Med 1983; 99:343–4.
269. Perera DR, Seiffert AK, Greeley HM. Ibuprofen and meningoencephalitis. Ann Intern Med 1984; 100:619.
270. Sylvia LM, Forlenza SW, Brocavish JM. Aseptic meningitis associated with naproxen. Drug Intell Clin Pharm 1988; 22:399–401.
271. O'Brien WM, Bagby GF. Rare adverse reactions to nonsteroidal anti-inflammatory drugs. J. Rheumatol 1985; 12:785–90.
272. Berliner S, Weinberger A, Shoenfeld Y. Ibuprofen may induce meningitis in (NZB XNZW)F1 mice. Arthritis Rheum 1985; 28:104–7.
273. Ruppert GB, Barth WF. Tolmetin-induced aseptic meningitis. JAMA 1981; 245:67–8.
274. Treves R, Gastine H, Richard A, et al. Responsibilite de l'ibuprofen dans une meningite aseptique et une insuffisance renale aigue au cours d'un lupus erythemateux dissemine. Rev Rheum Mal Osteoartic 1983; 50:75–6.
275. Collum LM, Bowen DI. Ocular side effects of ibuprofen. Br J Ophthalmol 1971; 55:472–7.

276. Palmer CAL. Toxic amblyopia from ibuprofen. Br Med J 1972; 3:765.
276. Tullio CJ. Ibuprofen-induced visual disturbance. Am J Hosp Pharm 1981; 38:1362.
277. Asherov J, Schoenberg A, Weinberger A. Diplopia following ibuprofen administration. JAMA 1982; 248:649.
278. Hamberger HA, Beckman H, Thompson R. Visual evoked potentials and ibuprofen (Motrin) toxicity. Ann Ophthalmol 1984; 16:328–9.
279. Williamson J. Sturrock RD. An ophthalmic study of ibuprofen in rheumatoid conditions. Curr Med Res Opin 1976; 4:128–31.
280. Burns CA. Indomethacin, reduced retinal sensitivity, and corneal deposits. Am J Ophthalmol 1968; 66:825–35.
281. Palimeris G, Koliopoulos J, Velissaropoulos P. Ocular side effects of indomethacin. Ophthalmologica 1972; 164:339–53.
282. Carr RE, Siegel IM. Retinal function in patients treated with indomethacin. Am J Ophthalmol 1972; 75:302–6.
283. Sandford-Smith JH. Transient myopia after aspirin. Br J Ophthalmol 1974; 58:698–700.
284. Umez-Eronini EM. Conjunctivitis due to ketoprofen. Lancet 1978; 2:737.
285. Harding JJ, van Heyningen R. Drugs, including alcohol, that act as risk factors for cataract, and possible protection against cataract by aspirin-like analgesics and cyclopenthiazide. Br J Ophthalmol 1988; 72:809–14.
286. Sharma YR, Vajpayee RB, Bhatnagar R, et al. Systemic aspirin and systemic vitamin E in senile cataracts: cataract V. Indian J Ophthalmol 1989; 37:134–41.
287. Seddon JM, Christen WG, Manson JE, et al. Low-dose aspirin and risks of cataract in a randomized trial of US physicians. Arch Ophthalmol 1991; 109:252–5.
288. Early treatment diabetic retinopathy study research group. Effects of aspirin treatment on diabetic retinopathy. ETDRS report number 8. Ophthalmology 1991; 98(suppl 5):757–65.
289. Robinson R. Indomethacin in rheumatic disease: a clinical assessment. Med J Aust 1965; 1:266–9.
290. Carney MWP. Paranoid psychosis with indomethacin. Br Med J 1977; 2:994–5.
291. Gotz V. Paranoid psychosis with indomethacin. Br Med J 1978; 1:49.
292. Singh RPN, Sinha AKN. Organic psychosis with indomethacin. J Indian Med Assoc 1978; 71:210.
293. Griffith JD, Smith CH, Smith RC. Paranoid psychosis in a patient receiving ibuprofen, a prostaglandin synthesis inhibitor: case report. J Clin Psychiatry 1982; 43:499–500.
294. Kruis R, Barger R. Paranoid psychosis with sulindac. JAMA 1980; 243:1420.
295. Sotsky SM, Tossell JW. Tolmetin induction of mania. Psychosomatics 1984; 25:626–8.
296. Neufeld MY, Korczyn AD. Encephalopathy associated with sulindac. Hum Toxicol 1986; 5:55.
297. Heim M, Nadvorna H., Azaria M. Grand mal seizures following treatment with diclofenac and pentazocine. S Afr Med J 1990; 78:700–1.
298. Laan LA, de Weerd AW. Drug-induced absence status: the significance of EEG in diagnosis and treatment. EEG EMG 1990; 21:131–3.
299. Lortholary A, Varache N, Bouachour G, et al. Generalized status epilepticus after ingestion of ibuprofen (Brufen), disclosing systemic lupus erythematosus. Rev Med Interne 1990; 11:243–4.
300. Goodwin JS, Regan M. Cognitive dysfunction associated with naproxen and ibuprofen in the elderly. Arthritis Rheum 1982; 25:1013–15.
301. Meyer JS, Rogers RL, McClintic K, et al. Randomized clinical trial of daily aspirin therapy in multi-infarct dementia. A pilot study. J Am Geriatr Soc 1989; 37:549–55.
302. Myers EN, Bernstein JF, Fostiropolous G. Salicylate ototoxicity. N Engl J. Med 1965; 273:587–90.
303. Miller RR. Deafness due to plain and long-acting aspirin tablets. J Clin Pharmacol 1978; 18:468–71.

304. Halla JT, Hardin JG. Salicylate ototoxicity in patients with rheumatoid arthritis: a controlled study. Ann Rheum Dis 1988; 47:134–7.
305. Halla JT, Atchison SL, Hardin JG. Symptomatic salicylate ototoxicity: a useful indicator of serum salicylate concentration? Ann Rheum Dis 1991; 50:682–4.
306. Day RO, Graham GG, Bieri M, et al. Concentration–response relationships for salicylate-induced ototoxicity in normal volunteers. Br J Clin Pharmacol 1989; 28:695–702.
307. Eade OE, Acheson ED, Cuthbert MF, et al. Peripheral neuropathy and indomethacin. Br Med J 1975; 2:66–7.
308. Reinstein L, Mahon R, Russo GL. Peripheral neuropathy after concomitant dimethyl sulfoxide use and sulindac therapy. Arch Phys Med Rehabil 1982; 63:581–4.
309. Swanson BN, Ferguson RK, Raskin NH, et al. Peripheral neuropathy after concomitant administration of dimethyl sulfoxide and sulindac. Arthritic Rheum 1983; 26:791–3.
310. Remond AD. Dyskinesia induced by mefenamic acid? J R Soc Med 1981; 74:558–9.
311. Cremona -Barbaro A. Extrapyramidal symptoms following mefenamic acid. J R Soc Med 1983; 76:435
312. Roubenoff R, Hoyt J, Petri M, et al. Effects of anti-inflammatory and immunosuppressive drugs on pregnancy and fatality. Semin Arthritis Rheum 1988; 18:88–110.
313. Slone D, Heinonen OP, Kaufman DW, et al. Aspirin and congenital malformations. Lancet 1976; 1:1373–5.
314. Dudley DKL, Hardie MJ. Fetal and neonatal affects of indomethacin as a tocolytic agent. Am J Obstet Gynecol 1985; 15:181–4.
315. Miebyl JR, Witter FR. Neonatal outcome after indomethacin treatment for preterm labor. Am J Obstet Gynecol 1986; 155:747–9.
316. Ostensen M, Husby G. Anti-rheumatic drug treatment during pregnancy and lactation. Scand J Rheumatol 1985; 14:1–7.
317. Wilkinson AR, Aynsley-Green A, Mitchell MD. Persistent pulmonary hypertension and abnormal prostaglandin E levels in preterm infants after maternal treatment with naproxen. Arch Dis Child 1971; 54:942–5.

III

New Anti-Inflammatory Drugs and Analgesics

14

Ketorolac

JOHN M. YOUNG
Syntex Discovery Research
Palo Alto, California

JAMES P. YEE
Syntex Development Research
Palo Alto, California

I. INTRODUCTION

By the end of 1991, there were more than 15 nonsteroidal anti-inflammatory drugs (NSAIDs) approved for use in the United States. Ketorolac tromethamine is among the most recently approved drugs; the injectable form was approved at the end of 1989 and the oral tablet at the end of 1991. Ketorolac has the distinction of being the first NSAID approved in the United States for parenteral (intramuscular) administration as an analgesic.

Ketorolac was selected for development because of its especially potent analgesic activity in animal models at doses well separated from those causing gastrointestinal toxicity. The intrinsic high potency against arachidonic acid cyclooxygenase, together with excellent solubility characteristics and bioavailability, allowed development of a nonirritating, parenterally injectable form of the drug and a solution for topical ocular administration, as well as the more usual solid, tablet formulation for oral administration. The preclinical pharmacology studies predicted that ketorolac would be a potent analgesic agent, with relatively weaker anti-inflammatory and antipyretic activity (1,2).

II. PHYSICOCHEMICAL PROPERTIES OF KETOROLAC

Ketorolac tromethamine [(±)-5-benzoyl-2,3-dihydro-1H-pyrrolizine-1-carboxylic acid, 2-amino-2-(hydroxymethyl)-1,3-propanediol] (Fig. 1) has a molecular weight of 376.41 and is readily soluble in water with an *n*-octanol–water partition coefficient of 0.26. Similar to almost all NSAIDs, ketorolac is weakly acidic, with an ionization constant (pK_a) of 3.5. Ketorolac is structurally a pyrrolopyrrole and, thus, related to tolmetin. Ketorolac can be considered a cyclized propionic acid derivative, with a chiral center at the α-carbon (3). As with other NSAIDs, the biological activity of ketorolac appears to be associated primarily, perhaps exclusively, with the *S*-(–) enantiomer (4).

Most of the animal pharmacology studies were done with the free acid; however, the

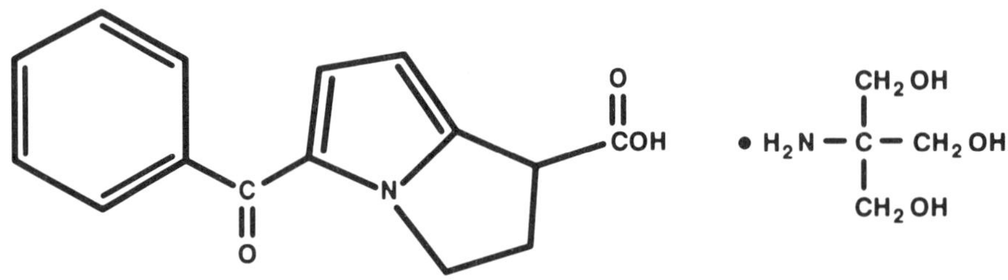

Figure 1 Chemical structure of ketorolac tromethamine.

tromethamine salt was eventually used for nearly all of the clinical development because of the enhanced aqueous solubility characteristics (> 30 mg/ml) of the tromethamine salt.

III. PRECLINICAL PHARMACOLOGY

A. Mechanism of Action Studies

In common with other NSAIDs, ketorolac was an effective inhibitor of arachidonic acid cyclooxygenase (Table 1). The selectivity for cyclooxygenase was evidenced by a lack of activity against human polymorphonuclear leukocyte 5-lipoxygenase, rabbit iris 5-lipoxygenase, washed human platelet 12-lipoxygenase, and rabbit reticulocyte 15-lipoxygenase, at concentrations up to 100 μM. When the purified enantiomers were examined in the sheep seminal vesicular microsome system, the *S*-(–)-enantiomer was active (median inhibitory concentration; IC_{50} = 3.3–5.0 μM), whereas the *R*-(+)-enantiomer was inactive at concentrations up to 100 μM. The enantioselectivity is consistent with the findings for other propionic acid derivatives, and the *S*-(–)-enantiomer possesses the typical NSAID activities in vivo, whereas the *R*-(+)-enantiomer is essentially inactive (4).

In view of the exceptional analgesic potency of ketorolac, considerable effort was spent to determine whether the compound possessed any additional mechanism of action other than cyclooxygenase inhibition (5). Ketorolac did not display significant binding to or interaction with μ-, κ-, or δ-opioid receptors. In other ligand-binding studies, ketorolac displayed weak affinity for both α_1- and α_2-adrenoceptors (pK_i = 4.2 and 4.0, respectively) of rat cerebral cortex, but significant occupancy of these receptors is unlikely to occur at pharmacologically relevant concentrations. There was no meaningful affinity for muscarinic receptors of rat cerebral cortex (M_1), heart (M_2), or submaxillary gland (M_3). Ketorolac did not display any inhibitory activity against either substance P- or

Table 1 Inhibitory Activity of Ketorolac Against Arachidonic Acid Cyclooxygenase

Test system	IC_{50} (μM)
Bovine seminal vesicular microsomes	0.26
Sheep seminal vesicular microsomes[a]	3.0–7.5
Rabbit renal medullary microsomes	0.4
Human platelet microsomes	0.19 ± 0.05
Collagen-induced human platelet aggregation	0.5
Arachidonic acid-induced human platelet aggregation	1.5

[a]Incubations in the presence of 1–100 μM arachidonic acid.

bradykinin-induced paw edema in the rat, nor against bradykinin-induced writhing in the mouse. In summary, ketorolac is a potent inhibitor of arachidonic acid cyclooxygenase and, at this writing, no other mechanism of action has been established.

B. Analgesic Activity

In an early series of tests using phenylquinone-induced writhing in the mouse and a 20-min oral predosing interval, ketorolac had approximately 350 times the potency of aspirin; it was considerably more potent than any other NSAID examined (1,3). In four of the assays listed in Table 2, ketorolac is active in the range of 0.13–0.3 mg/kg, orally (po). The lack of activity in the three tests indicated is consistent with ketorolac not possessing any opioid or morphinelike activity. The effective dose for the yeast-inflamed paw test was considerably higher than for other tests; nevertheless, ketorolac was more potent than other agents in our version of the test (1,2). In the mouse phenylquinone-induced writhing test, ketorolac possessed a long duration of action, lasting out to 6 h after dosing with 0.6 mg/kg. Ketorolac (as the acid and as the tromethamine salt) was compared with several standard agents in the mouse phenylquinone-induced writhing test (Table 3); the results are a combination of tests at 20 and at 60 min after oral drug administration.

Table 2 Analgesic Activity of Ketorolac in Animal Models

Test model	ED_{50}(mg/kg)
Mouse phenylquinone-induced writing	0.13
Mouse hot plate	No activity[a]
Rat phenylquinone-induce writhing	0.16
Rat adjuvant arthritis paw flexion	0.3
Rat adjuvant-inflamed tail pinch	0.15
Rat yeast-inflamed paw compression	1–3[b]
Rat electrically stimulated vocalization	No activity[c]
Mouse bradykinin-induced writhing	No activity[d]

[a]Tested at 1–49 mg/kg, ip.
[b]Minimum doses significantly elevating pain threshold in a series of tests.
[c]Tested at 3–30 mg/kg, ip.
[d]Tested at 0.5 and 1 mg/kg, po.

Table 3 Comparative Effective Doses of Ketorolac and Reference Agents in the Mouse Phenylquinone-Induced Writhing Test

Test material	ED_{50} (mg/kg) (95% confidence limits)	ED_{80}
Ibuprofen	13.7 (9–21)	22.1
Diclofenac	3.9 (3.0–5.0)	6.3
Indomethacin	2.3 (1.2–4.3)	3.7
Ketoprofen	0.8 (0.5–1.2)	1.3
Ketorolac	0.13[a] (0.09–0.19)	0.21
Ketorolac tromethamine	0.27[b] (0.16–0.44)	0.45

[a]Equivalent to 0.51 μmol/kg.
[b]Equivalent to 0.72 μmol/kg.

Ketorolac is equally potent when administered by either the oral or the subcutaneous route in rat and mouse analgesia tests. Also, when applied topically in ethanol solution, ketorolac was effective in the mouse phenylquinone-induced writhing test, although the median effective dose (ED_{50}) was about tenfold higher than that for the oral route of administration.

C. Anti-Inflammatory and Antipyretic Activity

Although ketorolac displayed anti-inflammatory activity, as would be expected for a typical NSAID, it was less potent than might have been anticipated on the basis of its analgesic activity (1,2). When ketorolac was compared with reference standards in the rat adjuvant-induced arthritis assay (prophylactic, bid dosing) as shown in Table 4, it was less active than diclofenac, indomethacin, and ketoprofen, which contrasted with the ranking of these drugs for analgesia (see Table 3). These results suggest that the analgesic effects of NSAIDs, and of ketorolac in particular, are separate from and do not depend on an anti-inflammatory action.

Ketorolac was tested for antipyretic activity using the model of yeast-induced pyresis in the rat. On the basis of reduction in body temperature 2 h after oral dosing, ketorolac was 20 times more potent than aspirin, with an ED_{50} of approximately 2.7 mg/kg (1). The potency of ketorolac here was again considerably less than might have been anticipated from its analgesic potency, but is consistent with its anti-inflammatory potency.

D. Gastrointestinal Irritancy

As with all drugs that inhibit cyclooxygenase, it was important to determine the potential of ketorolac to induce gastrointestinal irritation and toxicity. Ketorolac was evaluated for its gastric erosive properties 4 h after oral administration to 18-h–starved rats. When rats were maintained at normal room temperature, the ED_{50} for induction of visible erosions in the stomach and duodenum was 6.8 mg/kg; when the rats were additionally cold-stressed (3.3°C) during drug challenge, the ED_{50} was approximately 1.5 mg/kg. These doses were equal to or greater than those necessary to produce anti-inflammatory activity in rats, and at least tenfold greater than those necessary to achieve significant analgesia. In subchronic

Table 4 Comparative Effective Doses of Ketorolac and Reference Agents in the Prophylactic Adjuvant-Induced Arthritis Test in the Rat

Test material	ED_{50} (mg/kg per day) (95% confidence limits)
Ibuprofen	32 (3.6–302)
Diclofenac	0.60 (0.45–0.8)
Indomethacin	0.27 (0.16–0.42)
Ketoprofen	0.23 (0.09–0.61)
Ketorolac	1.40 (0.66–2.97)

bid dosing in rats, either 5 or 7 days, the minimum effective dose for induction of intestinal ulcers was ≥ 4.4 mg/kg. As indicated in Table 5, ketorolac possessed less ulcerogenic potency than the comparators, diclofenac, indomethacin, or ketoprofen, despite its increased analgesic potency.

The gastrointestinal-irritating property of ketorolac tromethamine was explored in rhesus monkeys by means of a gastroscope. With bid dosing for 3.5 days, 1.25 mg/kg ketorolac tromethamine caused no gastric lesions in four of four monkeys; 5 mg/kg produced lesions in only one of four monkeys; and 20 mg/kg produced lesions in two of four monkeys. Aspirin, at 5 mg/kg, produced lesions in two of two monkeys. In a second test, ketorolac tromethamine, at 5 mg/kg tid for 7.5 days, failed to cause lesions in three of three monkeys, although occult fecal blood loss occurred in one of three animals.

E. Ancillary Studies

Because of its high potency and good water solubility, it appeared that ketorolac tromethamine would be appropriate for routes of administration in addition to the oral. Both ketorolac and ketorolac tromethamine, at concentrations of 0.31–5.0% in sterile aqueous formulations, were administered intramuscularly to rabbits, 0.25 ml per injection. Histological evaluation of the sites 24-h postinjection showed that ketorolac tromethamine was no more irritating than the vehicle control, and ketorolac acid appeared to be less irritating than its vehicle control. In other studies, serum creatine phosphokinase was used as an indicator of tissue damage and, again, ketorolac and ketorolac tromethamine at 5.0%, injected intramuscularly, were no more irritating than the corresponding vehicles (2).

As a consequence of its high potency and low-irritation potential, ketorolac was examined for its topical anti-inflammatory activity in the eye (6). Isotonic solutions of up to 0.5% ketorolac tromethamine were nonirritating to the eyes of rats, rabbits, dogs, and rhesus monkeys, and no local anesthetic effect was manifest in the rabbit eye. Ketorolac tromethamine showed significant anti-inflammatory activity when applied locally in several models of ocular inflammation (Table 6). However, in contrast with corticosteroids, 0.5% ketorolac tromethamine solution did not enhance the spread of experimental ocular infections induced with *Candida albicans* or *Pseudomonas aeruginosa*.

Table 5 Comparative Intestinal Ulcerogenic Doses of Ketorolac and Reference Agents in a 5-Day–Dosing Study in the Rat

Test material	Minimum ulcerogenic dose[a] (mg/kg per day)	ED_{50} (mg/kg/day)[b] (95% confidence limits)
Ibuprofen	49	115 (97–135)
Diclofenac	3.6	8.3 (6.6–10)
Indomethacin	1.7	4.0 (2.9–5.5)
Ketoprofen	3.5	8.2 (6.2–11)
Ketorolac	4.4	10.2 (6.8–15)

[a]No-effect dose level calculated by extrapolation of a linear dose–response curve.
[b]Lesions were graded on a 0–5 scale with 5 indicating death caused by intestinal perforation before scheduled necropsy.

Table 6 Ophthalmic Pharmacology Studies with Ketorolac Tromethamine

Test system	Results summary
Silver nitrate corneal burn in the rat	Significant reduction of neovascularization with 0.25 and 0.5% KT,[a] 1 drop qid
Intravenous endotoxin-induced uveitis in the rabbit	Reduction of FITC[b]–dextran leakage with 0.5% KT
Arachidonic acid-induced increase in IOP[c] in the rabbit	0.5% KT blocked rise in intraocular pressure, did not change normal IOP
Arachidonic acid-induced vascular permeability and PMN[d] accumulation in the rabbit	0.5% KT blocked vascular leakage and PMN accumulation
Healing of surgical corneal wound in the rabbit	0.5% KT did not retard wound healing

[a]Ketorolac tromethamine.
[b]Fluorescein isothiocyanate.
[c]Intraocular pressure.
[d]Polymorphonuclear leukocyte.

IV. PHARMACOKINETICS AND METABOLISM

Preclinical animal pharmacology studies indicated that there was little or no difference in potency on a molar basis and time to onset for analgesia between ketorolac free acid and ketorolac tromethamine salt administered orally. Because ketorolac tromethamine was more soluble than the free acid and because a parenteral formulation was desired, development efforts proceeded with the tromethamine salt. The pharmacokinetics of ketorolac tromethamine (unlabeled and ^{14}C-labeled) have been explored in humans following administration intramuscularly (IM) and intravenously (IV) in solution, and orally in solution, capsules, and tablets (7–9). The [^{14}C]ketorolac tromethamine in solution was administered po and IV, and showed similar pharmacokinetics, metabolism, and excretion by each route. The main route of excretion was in the urine (91.4%), with low levels (6.1%) being recovered in the feces (Table 7). In plasma, 96% of the total radioactivity appeared as ketorolac, and minor amounts of radioactivity were identified as *p*-hydroxyketorolac; no conjugates were detected in plasma. In urine 58% of the total radioactivity appeared as ketorolac; 11% appeared as *p*-hydroxyketorolac; and 31% appeared as very polar metabolites, possibly conjugates.

The key pharmacokinetic characteristics of po and IV administered ketorolac are summarized in Tables 7 and 8. It may be noted that ketorolac is completely absorbed by either the intramuscular or oral administration routes in comparison with IV administration. Ketorolac has a plasma half-life of approximately 6 h, which is intermediate in comparison with other NSAIDs that tend to range from plasma half-lifes of 1 h to more than 24 h (10). There is little alteration of volume of distribution, clearance, and half-life in healthy elderly subjects in comparison with normal younger volunteers. Likewise, drug elimination was not altered in patients with hepatic impairment related to chronic alcoholic liver cirrhosis, indicating that only moderate or minimal residual hepatic function is necessary to achieve adequate metabolism of ketorolac to maintain its overall elimination from the body, which is preponderantly by renal clearance (8,11,12). As ketorolac is primarily eliminated by renal excretion, patients with renal impairment may have significantly decreased rates of drug clearance, roughly in proportion to the degree of renal impairment (11). Recent studies in anephric patients show that possibly adaptive

Table 7 Approximate Average Pharmacokinetic Parameters Following Intramuscular and Oral Doses of Ketorolac Tromethamine

Pharmacokinetic parameter (units)	Oral[a]	Intramuscular[b]		
	10 mg	15 mg	30 mg	60 mg
Bioavailability (extent)	100 %	100 %	100 %	100 %
T_{max}[d] (min)	20–60	30–60	30–60	30–60
C_{max}[e] (μg/ml; single dose)	0.7–1.1	1.0–1.4	2.2–3.0	4.0–4.5
C_{max} (μg/ml; steady-state qid)	0.7–1.2	1.1–1.7	2.3–3.5	N/A[c]
C_{min}[f] (μg/ml; steady-state qid)	0.2–0.3	0.2–0.3	0.3–0.7	N/A
C_{ave}[g] (μg/ml; steady state qid)	0.3–0.6	0.6–0.8	1.8–1.5	N/A
Vd(β)[h] (L/kg)	← 0.15–0.33 →			
% dose metabolized = <50				
% dose excreted in urine = 91				
% dose excreted in feces = 6				
% plasma protein binding = 99				

[a]Derived from po pharmacokinetic studies in 23 normal fasted volunteers.
[b]Derived from IM pharmacokinetic studies in 32 normal volunteers.
[c]Not applicable because 60 mg is recommended only as a loading dose.
[d]time-to-peak plasma concentration.
[e]Peak plasma concentration.
[f]Trough plasma concentration.
[g]Average plasma concentration.
[h]Volume of distribution (calculated from mean clearance and terminal half-life).

Table 8 The Influence of Age and Liver and Kidney Function on the Clearance and Terminal Half-Life of Intramuscular[a] and Oral[b] Ketorolac Tromethamine

Type of subjects	Total clearance (L/h per kg)		Terminal half-life (in h)	
	IM mean (range)	Oral mean (range)	IM mean (range)	Oral mean (range)
Normal subjects	0.023	0.025	5.3	5.3
IM (n=54), oral (n=77)	(0.010–0.046)	(0.013–0.050)	(3.5–9.2)	(2.4–9.0)
Healthy elderly subjects	0.019	0.024	7.0	6.1
IM (n=13), oral (n=12)	(0.013–0.034)	(0.018–0.034)	(4.7–8.6)	(4.3–7.6)
(mean age = 72, range = 65–78)				
Patients with hepatic dysfunction	0.029	0.033	5.4	4.5
IM and oral (n=9)	(0.013–0.066)	(0.019–0.051)	(2.2–6.9)	(1.6–7.6)
Patients with renal impairment	0.014	0.016	10.3	10.8
IM and oral (n=9)	(0.007–0.043)	(0.007–0.052)	(8.1–15.7)	(3.4–18.9)
(serum creatinine 1.9–5.0 mg/dl)				
Renal dialysis patients	0.016		13.6	
IM (n=9)	(0.003–0.036)		(8.0–39.1)	

[a]Estimated from 30-mg single IM doses of ketorolac tromethamine.
[b]Estimated from 10-mg single oral doses of ketorolac tromethamine.

mechanisms of elimination may occur in such severely renally impaired patients. Renal dialysis patients had ketorolac clearance that was approximately 58% that of healthy volunteers. Dialysis had minimal effects on elimination of ketorolac.

The pharmacokinetics of ketorolac tromethamine following single or multiple po or IM doses, are linear (e.g., plasma levels are approximately proportional to dosage).

Steady-state plasma levels are achieved after dosing every 6 h for 1 day. No changes in clearance occur with chronic dosing. To minimize the time delay in achieving adequate analgesic effect from the initial dose of a given regimen, it has been recommended that a loading dose equal to twice the maintenance dose be given. This recommendation is based on the pharmacokinetic principle (13) that when the dosing interval is near the drug's half-life, the target steady-state plasma level is achieved faster if the first dose is twice the maintenance dose (Fig. 2). This principle is true whether the drug is administered by the oral or IM route; the levels achieved depend on the amount of administered dose, not the route. Although steady-state plasma concentrations are achieved after a period of dosing equivalent to three to five half-lives without use of a loading dose (13), use of a loading dose can be useful in acute pain situations when maximal, early relief of pain is the goal.

Ketorolac does not readily penetrate the blood–brain barrier (14). A study has shown that levels of ketorolac in the cerebral spinal fluid (median 2.1 ng/ml, range 0.4–5.7 ng/ml between 62 and 277 min after dosing) are remarkably lower than those found in plasma (median 5.3 μg/ml, range 2.1–8.4 μg/ml) after IM administration. This feature of distribution of ketorolac may indicate a relatively minor role of central nervous system (CNS) activity of the drug and possibly reduce the likelihood of adverse events from CNS penetration by the drug (14).

Concurrent use of probenecid with ketorolac will reduce the elimination of ketorolac. This interaction of probenecid on the urinary excretion of ketorolac is commonly seen with other NSAIDs. Use of ketorolac in patients concurrently receiving furosemide may decrease the diuretic effect of furosemide. Again, this drug interaction is known to occur with other NSAIDs.

V. CLINICAL EFFICACY

A. Perspectives on Clinical Studies Evaluating the Analgesic Effect of Ketorolac

Ketorolac tromethamine has been available for study in a variety of formulations suitable for oral (tablets, capsules), IM or IV (1 or 3% w/v aqueous solution), rectal suppository,

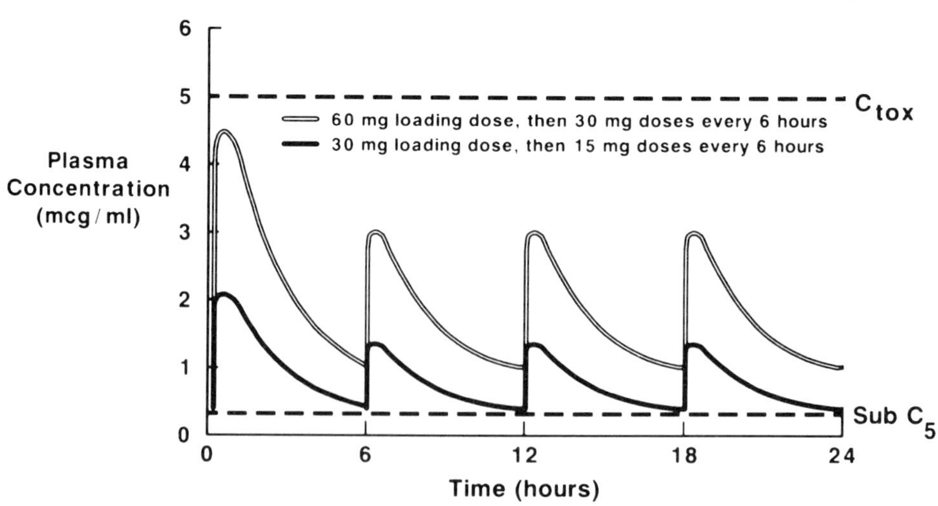

Figure 2 Plasma levels of ketorolac after recommended dosing schedules of ketoralac tromethamine.

topical dermal (1% gel), and topical ophthalmic (0.5% drops) application. The po and Intramuscular routes of administration, as described in the foregoing, give rapid and complete absorption in healthy volunteers. However, in some clinical settings, oral administration of analgesic medication may be an impractical (e.g., immediate postoperative period) or a less reliable route of administration. The parenteral route of administration of ketorolac provided a new opportunity for use of an analgesic from the NSAID pharmacological class in the United States. Ketorolac tromethamine is very well suited for parenteral use because of its high aqueous solubility, high milligram potency, and relatively nonirritating chemical characteristics. In contrast with IM administered diclofenac, ketorolac IM injection does not cause significant release of creatine phosphokinase into the bloodstream, reflecting the relative absence of muscle irritation or damage (15). The IM route of delivery permitted administration of ketorolac earlier in postoperative pain than is generally feasible with oral drug administration. Morphine and meperidine were the most commonly used IM analgesic comparators for study of the efficacy of ketorolac in acute postoperative pain. In contrast, in analgesic trials comparing orally administered analgesics, aspirin, acetaminophen, or acetaminophen plus codeine were considered the best-established active standards. It should be noted in studies of either the po or IM routes of drug administration, conventional study designs have called for restriction of use of other analgesics for 4 or 6 h before the study test drug administration to minimize or eliminate carryover effects of prior analgesics or other potentially confounding medications. In routine clinical settings, little or no washout period from prior anesthetic or analgesic use is imposed before initiating postoperative analgesic administration. To the contrary, preoperative and intraoperative analgesics or analgesia-potentiating drugs are often given to enhance the management of pain and reduce the degree of initial postoperative pain. The experimentally measured apparent onset, peak, and duration of effect of any analgesic is also influenced by the underlying etiology of pain (e.g., upper abdominal and thoracic surgical procedures tend to be associated more often with very severe pain that requires a longer duration of analgesic administration and more frequent repeat doses of opiate than does pain management following superficial procedures performed on the extremities). The apparent duration of analgesic effect of a drug will tend to be greater on the day after surgery than in the immediate hours after completion of surgery. Patients experience their most severe pain in immediate post-anesthesia period. The IV route of delivery is the most rapid and convenient method to administer analgesia in this immediate postoperative period. However, as will be described in greater detail later, the duration of effect is shorter and peak effect of ketorolac is less, as with other drugs, in this very acute, severe pain setting (16).

The most practical and sensitive analgesic efficacy studies to define the specific relative efficacy of a new analgesic, such as ketorolac, have been acute pain conditions, such postoperative pain, especially the pain from extraction of bony impaction of mandibular third molars. This pain model can sensitively distinguish the relative efficacy of test and standard analgesics (both parenteral and oral standards). Chronic pain conditions, such as cancer pain, low-back pain, or from osteoarthritis, give a much cruder assessments of relative efficacy of analgesics.

B. Dose Definition in Human Analgesic Trials

Over the span of clinical development, a wide range of doses have been tested in a variety of clinical pain models. Single or multiple doses of ketorolac 2.5, 5, 10, 12.5, 20, 30,

90, 100, and 200 mg have been tested using IM, po, or IV routes of administration (17,18). In particular, for the pivotal efficacy studies of IM ketorolac, single doses of 10, 30, or 90 mg were included in five individual trials. To enhance the power of detecting statistically significant differences in degree of efficacy associated with this range of doses of IM ketorolac, a pooled study analysis has been performed. Individual studies usually have sample sizes of n = 30–40 patients per treatment group. The results from five postoperative pain studies have been pooled in which single doses of ketorolac IM, 10, 30, and 90 mg, were compared to IM opiate doses of either morphine 12 mg and morphine 6 mg or meperidine 100 mg and meperidine 50 mg. In these double-blind studies of parallel, randomized design, patients had moderate or severe pain at baseline and were reevaluated at 0.5, 1, 2, 3, 4, 5, and 6 h following IM analgesic administration (19–23). When the results are looked at in their entirety (Table 9), it may be concluded that ketorolac (KT) doses of 30 and 90 mg are more effective, mainly in duration of activity, than KT 10 mg for all the subtypes of postoperative pain studied. Ketorolac doses of 30 and 90 mg are superior to meperidine (MEP) 50 mg or morphine (MS) 6 mg both at early time points as well as with summed pain intensity difference scores or total pain relief score for the first 3 and 6 h in all the subgroups. Ketorolac doses of 90 and 30 mg are comparable with MS, 12 mg, and MEP, 100 mg, at the early time points, 0.5 and 1.0 h, and equal to or superior to these doses of the opiates when assessed over the summed 3- and 6-h scores. From this series of study results, it may be concluded that with ketorolac doses of 10, 30, or 90 mg, the main advantage of using the high doses in this range is to achieve a somewhat more rapid onset of action and, perhaps more importantly, gain a longer duration of action than achieved by the 10-mg dose. [*Note*: In another study,

Table 9 Pooled Results from Five Studies

Treatment comparison	SPID[a]		TOTPAR[b]		%	PID[d]		PAR[e]	
	3 h[f]	6 h	3 h	6 h	TIA[c]	0.5 h	1.0 h	0.5 h	1.0 h
HO > LO	+		+	+		+		+	+
KT10 > LO	+	+	+	+	+				+
KT30 > LO	+	+	+	+	+	+	+	+	+
KT90 > LO	+	+	+	+	+	+	+	+	+
KT10 > HO	+	+		+	+			–	
KT30 > HO	+	+	+	+	+				
KT90 > HO	+	+	+	+	+				
KT90 > KT10	+	+	+	+	+	+	+	+	+
KT30 > KT10	+	+	+	+	+		+	+	+
KT90 > KT30					+				

Key: HO, high-dose opiate (morphine 12 mg or meperidine 100 mg); LO, low-dose opiate (morphine 6 mg or meperidine 50 mg); KT, ketorolac tromethamine 10, 30, or 90 mg; +, statistically significant difference between the treatments in relative efficacy as indicated by ">" (greater than) sign; –, reverse statistically significant relative efficacy.

[a]Summed pain intensity difference: area under the PID-by-time curve.

[b]Total pain relief: area under the pain relief-time curve.

[c]Percentage of patients terminating because of inadequate efficacy within 6 h of dosing.

[d]Pain intensity difference from baseline.

[e]Average pain relief from last baseline.

[f]Time from dosing.

multiple doses of KT, 90 mg (given four times a day or 360 mg/day for 5 days), caused peptic ulcers, so the KT 90-mg dose was not further pursued as a suitable clinical dose for repeated use.] In subset analyses, patients with pain from major surgeries are more likely to benefit from a greater degree of efficacy from initial doses of ketorolac that are higher than 10 mg (e.g., 30- or 60-mg initial-loading dose) than patients with more moderate pain from minor surgery. Doses higher than 30 mg four times following a 60-mg initial-loading dose are not recommended because of the greater risk of gastrointestinal intolerance, including peptic ulceration, that may be associated with regular daily dosages of more than 120 mg/day (see Sect. VI.A). For use in pain conditions requiring more than 5 days of therapy, maximum daily dosages of 10 mg qid probably give the optimal therapeutic index for ketorolac.

C. Studies of the Efficacy of Intramuscular Ketorolac

Ketorolac IM has been studied in a variety of postoperative pain situations, including orthopedic, gynecological, abdominal, and dental surgery (extraction of bony impactions of third molars) procedures. In comparison with IM meperidine or morphine, ketorolac, 30 mg IM, is approximately equal to 100 mg of meperidine or 10–12 mg of morphine on a single-dose basis (19–23). On a repeated-dose basis, a higher cumulative maximal analgesic effect of ketorolac probably is not accrued by increasing the dosage or dosage frequency beyond a total of about 120 mg/day (24–26). This maximal analgesic effect of ketorolac, in part, may be related to saturation of its probable primary mechanism of action (i.e., suppression of prostaglandin synthesis). In this situation, for severe pain states, supplemental use of an analgesic with a different mechanism of action (i.e., an opiate) has increased the overall degree of pain control with a suitable absence of significant drug interactions (27,28). Patients with pain from surgical procedures involving the abdomen (e.g., abdominal hysterectomy, cholecystectomy) may benefit from some supplemental use of opiates for maximal pain control in the immediate postoperative period, when analgesic demands are the greatest. Clinicians should adjust the analgesic dosage regimen in accordance with the pattern of diminishing pain intensity with time elapsed following surgery; the apparent duration of efficacy of a dose of ketorolac will, as with other analgesics, effectively increase with greater elapsed time from the initial surgical trauma.

In addition to postsurgical pain, IM ketorolac has been evaluated for pain from renal colic (29) and cancer pain (30). Ketorolac, 10 mg IM, was as effective as, and ketorolac, 90 mg IM, was longer-acting than, meperidine, 100 mg IM, in renal colic. Ketorolac doses of 10, 30, and 90 mg IM were more effective than placebo in the cancer pain study.

D. Studies of Efficacy of Intravenous Ketorolac

The same formulation of ketorolac used for intramuscular injection has been studied intravenously. The efficacy and safety of IV ketorolac has been primarily evaluated in patients with acute postoperative pain. Intravenous ketorolac has been routinely administered much earlier in the postoperative recovery course than feasible with po or IM ketorolac. In this setting, ketorolac 20–60 mg (given as two 10-mg or two 30-mg boluses) IV is comparable with 4–8 mg (given as two 2-mg or 4-mg boluses) morphine IV (16,18). In clinical settings where repeated doses of IV morphine in amounts greater than a total of 8 mg within 2 h are required to gain adequate pain control, two doses of ketorolac IV, 10 or 30 mg (20 or 60 mg total), may not be an adequate, sole analgesic agent for such patients. A higher maximum analgesic effect is not achievable with larger doses of IV ketorolac, but can be achieved with cumulative, repeated doses of IV morphine. However, such maximally effective, large doses of opiates are often avoided for fear of respiratory depression, excessive sedation, or drug addiction. Therefore, giving supplemental doses of opiates (in the limited range of doses commonly accepted as safe) in addition to giving the recommended doses of ketorolac may be a suitable method to achieve maximal control of very severe pain, while reducing use of high doses of opiates and the associated undesirable opiate-related side effects (27). Studies are currently underway using IV ketorolac in association with patient-controlled morphine and also using ketorolac in a patient-controlled analgesic administration device.

E. Studies of the Efficacy of Oral Ketorolac

Ketorolac administered in the form of capsules or tablets has been studied in orthopedic (31–34), dental (35,36), and abdominal (37) postoperative pain settings, as well as in postpartum uterine-cramping pain (38), and cancer pain (39,40). The clearest definition of the relative efficacy of ketorolac, compared with established standards, is derived from the dental surgery studies (extraction of third molars; 35,36). In these studies, ketorolac, 10 mg, has been more effective than acetaminophen, 600 mg plus codeine 60 mg, or aspirin, 650 mg, or plain acetaminophen, 600 mg. These active comparators were more effective than placebo. Ketorolac, 10 mg po, has also been comparable with naproxen sodium 550 mg and ibuprofen 400 mg (one study of each comparator). Other comparators that have been evaluated in single-dose efficacy studies of ketorolac, 10 mg, include diflunisal, 500 mg; glafenine, 400 mg; propoxyphene, 200 mg with aspirin; pentazocine, 100 mg; morphine, 10 mg IM, and ketobemidone, 10 mg. Ketorolac was usually equal to or, in some instances, more effective than these comparators.

F. Clinical Experience with Ketorolac Gel Applied Topically

Ketorolac gel when applied to the skin is slowly absorbed (in comparison with po or IM route of drug administration), with a maximum plasma concentration achieved 12–23 h after initial administration. A relatively small amount of ketorolac is absorbed if applied in a nonoccluded fashion (3–5% bioavailability). However, occlusion significantly increases the amount of absorption, although variability still occurs (16–59% absorption).

Ketorolac administration topically to the skin covering painful joints or injured soft tissues has been studied (41). A major objective of drug administration by the topical route of delivery is to increase the therapeutic index of the drug. Acute soft-tissue injuries, such as sprains and strains of the ankle from sports or work injuries, that cause pain have been considered suitable models for testing. Some study designs have been aimed at establishing a local effect of drug administration. Proof of such local action has been difficult because, for most of the pain conditions under study, placebo response rates are much higher than ordinarily observed with systemic administration of analgesic medications. As many as 40–60% of patients have been reported to respond to placebo topical agents in trials of acute sprains and strains (42). This high placebo rate may be related to the therapeutic benefit of local massage during drug application and the tendency for spontaneous improvement of these injuries. In a double-blind study comparing topical ketorolac, 2% gel, with etofenamate, 5% gel, and placebo in the treatment of ankle sprains, both active agents were superior to placebo in reducing swelling. Ketorolac was equal or superior to etofenamate in reduction of pain scores at various time points of assessment on days 2 through 8 of treatment (41).

G. Clinical Experience with Ketorolac Ophthalmic Solution

A 0.5% ophthalmic solution of ketorolac has been studied in a variety of potential indications, including seasonal allergic conjunctivitis, postophthalmic surgical inflammation, acute ocular pain from trauma, chronic cystoid macular edema, prevention of cystoid macular edema, treatment of acute cystoid macular edema, and maintenance of intraoperative mydriasis. Reduction of ocular itching and conjunctival injection has been demonstrated in allergic conjunctivitis related to ragweed and other seasonal allergens. In studies where 1 or 2 drops were applied to the affected eyes for 7 days consecutively, clinical signs and symptoms were assessed on days 3 and 4 and 7 and 8 by the investigator and patient. Significant reductions in conjunctival inflammation scores and in eye-itching scores have been reported.

Ketorolac ophthalmic drops have also been demonstrated to reduce postoperative (removal of lens for cataracts) inflammation by measuring fluorescein leakage into the posterior chamber (43–45). In a placebo-controlled, double-blind, randomized trial, significant improvement of visual acuity in patients with chronic cystoid macular edema was found with ketorolac ophthalmic 0.5% drop treatment (46). The prophylactic administration of ketorolac, 0.5% eye drops, reduced the incidence of postcataract surgery-associated aphakic cystoid macular edema in comparison with a control group randomized to receive placebo (vehicle) drops (47).

VI. CLINICAL SAFETY

A. Adverse Events Observed with Limited Duration Use of Intramuscular Ketorolac

Most clinical situations in which IM analgesic administration is suitable involve a limited duration of use (e.g., most postoperative pain requires no more than 2–5 days of parenteral analgesic administration). Adverse reaction rates from the short-term use of NSAIDs are generally low, and this has been observed with the use of IM ketorolac. Short-term use of ketorolac permits higher daily doses (120 mg/day) to be employed than total daily doses found suitable for longer-term, but limited duration, use (40 mg/day). The overall incidence of adverse events associated with ketorolac IM use in lower than seen with meperidine or morphine use (Table 10), particularly with a lower incidence of drowsiness, nausea, or vomiting, with ketorolac than with morphine, 12 mg (16,18–20,24,25).

The initial use of ketorolac, IM 30 mg prn (120 mg maximum per day), followed by ketorolac oral, 10 mg prn (10 mg qid prn), was compared with meperidine, 100 mg IM prn, followed by acetaminophen, 600 mg plus codeine 60 mg, in a study of pain following major abdominal or gynecological surgery. The efficacy of ketorolac was comparable with the meperidine–acetaminophen–codeine regimen. Patients received 1–2 days of IM analgesia (mean number of doses 4.3 ketorolac, 5.4 doses of meperidine) and 10 days of oral medication (mean 26 doses ketorolac, 28 doses of acetaminophen plus codeine). The adverse events are summarized in Table 11. (*Note*: Some of the events in both groups may be attributable to surgery, the anesthetic, or other peri- or postoperative medications given to the patients).

Ketorolac is contraindicated for use in patients with a previous history of allergic or

Table 10 Unabridged Incidence of Adverse Events

Adverse events	Ketorolac 30 mg (n = 509)	Morphine 10–12 mg (n = 151)
Nervous system		
Somnolence	15%	34%
Headache	5%	9%
Dizziness	3%	6%
Digestive system		
Nausea	16%	28%
Vomiting	6%	11%
Skin and appendages		
Pruritus	1%	13%
Injection site		
Injection site pain	4%	7%
Body as a whole	3%	7%
Urogenital	1%	6%

Table 11 Incidence of Adverse Events Following IM to Oral Transition in Dosing in Patients with Postoperative Pain

Body system and term	Meperidine 100 mg IM followed by acetominophen 600 mg + codeine 60 mg n = 104	Ketorolac 30 mg IM followed by ketorolac 10 mg oral n = 106
Gastrointestinal		
Nausea	66%	39%
Constipation	24%	8%
Diarrhea	3%	9%
Nervous system		
Dizziness	28%	8%
Somnolence	28%	8%
Dry mouth	20%	9%
Insomnia	9%	14%
Nervousness	2%	6%
Tremor	5%	0%
Skin		
Pruritus	10%	4%
Rash	6%	3%
Urogenital		
Urinary retention	8%	0%

hypersensitivity reactions to aspirin or other NSAIDs. Prescribing physicians have reported patients' experiencing cross-sensitivity to this class of drugs (48,49), but cases of anaphylaxis also have been reported, even though no previous history of allergic disposition was identified. On the other hand, one of the specific benefits of ketorolac is the absence of respiratory depression that is a feared adverse event associated with employing fully optimal analgesic doses of opiates (50,51). Ketorolac also has minimal effects on psychomotor function, compared with opiates such as buprenorphine (15).

Ketorolac may, even in limited-duration use, be occasionally associated with peptic ulceration or upper gastrointestinal bleeding in high-risk patients (52,53). However, such gastrointestinal adverse events are rare in comparison with the rates typically observed with long-term use of ketorolac, as is true with other NSAIDs (see Sect. VI.B). Opiates have a strong tendency to cause constipation and reduced gastrointestinal motility; ketorolac use, compared with opiate analgesia, has been associated with earlier return of bowel function in patients following major abdominal surgery (54–56). Impairment of renal function, including acute renal failure, may occur with ketorolac use, as with other NSAIDs, particularly if there is a significant reduction in blood volume related to intravascular volume depletion from surgery or underlying renal compromise with discontinuation of ketorolac use.

Similar to other drugs that inhibit cyclooxygenase activity, ketorolac inhibits platelet aggregation and may prolong bleeding time (57,58). There have been postmarketing reports of postoperative wound hematomas, particularly noted in patients undergoing cosmetic plastic surgery procedures who received the drug intraoperatively. Thus, in surgical settings for which strict hemostasis is required and in any patient who has an underlying coagulation disorder or is receiving drug therapy that interferes with hemostasis (therapeutic doses of heparin or warfarin), caution should be used if ketorolac is administered (57). Ketorolac should also be avoided in settings for which other NSAIDs are routinely avoided because of effects on platelets (e.g., before renal lithotripsy). The effect of ketorolac on platelet function is reversed within approximately 24 h of drug administration, as the drug is eliminated from the body.

B. Adverse Events Observed with Use of Oral Ketorolac

Ketorolac has been approved in the United States for limited-duration use for the management of pain. This limited duration of use is, in part, based on observations from a long-term (1-year) safety and efficacy study, comparing ketorolac with aspirin, involving 823 patients with chronic pain (59). The overall therapeutic effect of ketorolac, administered 10 mg po, qid, as needed, for pain (with an average daily dosage of about 30 mg/day), was superior to aspirin (650 mg, qid as needed for pain; average daily dosage 1950 mg/day), as measured by the lower frequency of patients discontinuing treatment owing to lack of adequate efficacy (20% for ketorolac compared with 32% for aspirin; $p < 0.001$). The rate of terminations before 1 year for safety-related reasons (adverse events, clinical laboratory abnormalities, intercurrent disease, or multiple termination reasons that included one of these) was 27% for ketorolac and 30% for aspirin ($p = 0.31$). The cumulative symptoms reported by patients are summarized in Table 12 (59). This study showed that the most important serious risk from long-term use of ketorolac, as with other NSAIDs, was the development of peptic ulcers or upper gastrointestinal tract bleeding.

The time-adjusted percentages of patients who developed peptic ulcers or upper gastrointestinal bleeding are as follows:

Interval of use (mo)	Ketorolac (average daily dose 30 mg/day)	Aspirin (average daily dose 1950 mg/day)
≤ 3	0.69%	0%
≤ 6	1.59%	0.73%
≤ 12	3.09%	2.44%

Table 12 Incidence of Adverse Events During Long-Term Treatment with Oral Ketorolac

Adverse effect	Percentage of patients: Ketorolac 10 mg (*n*=553)	Percentage of patients: Aspirin 650 mg (*n*=270)
Gastrointestinal events		
Gastrointestinal pain	24	21
Dyspepsia	22	30
Nausea	18	19
Diarrhea	14	9
Constipation	8	10
Central nervous system events		
Headache	30	24
Dizziness	14	12
Somnolence	8	6
Other adverse events		
Body as a whole	27	27
Respiratory (sinusitis, rhinitis, cough, dyspnea)	23	19
Musculoskeletal (arthralgias, myalgias)	17	17
Special senses (tinnitis)	13	13
Cardiovascular (chest pain, hypertension, migraine)	12	9
Skin and appendages	11	9
Metabolic/nutritional disorders	10	7
Urogenital	9	4
Hematological and lymphatic	3	4

Ketorolac administered orally is bioequivalent to ketorolac given IM. The principal reason for recommending lower dosages of ketorolac for oral use (i.e., 10 mg qid) compared with IM use (i.e., 60-mg loading dose followed by 30 mg q6h or qid prn) is that in most clinical settings requiring parenteral analgesic, the duration of use of ketorolac will be very short. In short-term use, the gain in efficacy with the higher dosage regimen (120 mg/day) is achieved without a significant increase in adverse events, compared with the lower dosage regimen (40 mg/day). This advantage may not be maintained in use beyond 5 days (i.e., the efficacy difference of ketorolac, 30 mg qid, compared with 10 mg qid is not sufficiently great to offset the difference in tolerance between the dosage regimens if given for more than 5 days). Oral ketorolac is not recommended for long-term use.

VII. SUMMARY

Ketorolac is in the pharmacological class of nonsteroidal anti-inflammatory analgesic drugs. It has the attributes of high potency, low chemical irritancy to body tissues, and high aqueous solubility, which have given it a unique and favorable therapeutic profile for use as a parenterally administered analgesic. Because ketorolac is an NSAID, rather than an opioid category agent, use of ketorolac avoids the adverse events associated with opiate pharmacological activities. Prescribers must balance these advantages with the risks that are associated with use of an NSAID: the most serious potential adverse events are gastrointestinal bleeding, with or without peptic ulcers, renal failure, and allergic reactions. The gastrointestinal and renal risks can be minimized by limited duration use of appropriate doses of ketorolac. The incidence of allergic reactions can perhaps be reduced by carefully screening patients for a prior history of NSAID allergy or a strong history of atopy or asthma. Ketorolac also is available as an orally administered, solid-dose formulation and has efficacy that has compared favorably with available oral analgesics. Ketorolac oral is recommended for limited duration use to manage pain. Ketorolac topical gel is undergoing further clinical evaluation and may have the advantage of local efficacy with minimal or no systemic side effects. Ketorolac ophthalmic drops have been used clinically and have shown promising efficacy in a variety of inflammatory eye conditions.

REFERENCES

1. Rooks WR II, Tomolonis AJ, Maloney PJ, Wallach MB, Schuler ME. The analgesic and anti-inflammatory profile of (±)-5-benzoyl-1,2-dihydro-3*H*-pyrrolo[1,2*a*]pyrrole-1-carboxylic acid (RS-37619). Agents Actions 1982; 12:684–90.
2. Rooks WH II, Maloney JP, Shott LD, Schuler ME, Sevelius H, Strosberg AM, Tanenbaum L, Tomolonis AJ, Wallach MB, Waterbury D, Yee JP. The analgesic and anti-inflammatory profile of ketorolac and its tromethamine salt. Drugs Exp Clin Res 1985; 11:479–92.
3. Muchowski JM, Unger SH, Ackrell J, Cheung P, Cooper GF, Cook J, Gallegra P, Halpern O, Koehler R, Kluge AF, Van Horn AR, Antonio Y, Carpio H, Franco F, Galeazzi E, Garcia I, Greenhouse R, Guzman A, Iriarte J, Leon A, Pena A, Perez V, Valdez D, Ackerman N, Ballaron SA, Krishna Murthy DV, Rovito JR, Tomolonis AJ, Young JM, Rooks WR. Synthesis and antiinflammatory and analgesic activity of 5-aroyl-1,2-dihydro-3*H*-pyrrolo [1,2*a*-]pyrrole-1-carboxylic acids and related compounds. J Med Chem 1985; 28:1037–49.
4. Guzman A, Yuste F, Toscano RA, Young JM, Van Horn AR, Muchowski JM. Absolute configuration of (–)-5-benzoyl-1,2-dihydro-3*H*-pyrrolo[1,2*a*]pyrrole-1-carboxylic acid, the active enantiomer of ketorolac. J Med Chem 1986; 29:589–91.
5. Lopez M, Waterbury LD, Michel A, Seavey W, Yee J. Lack of addictive potential of ketorolac tromethamine. Pharmacologist 1987; 29:136.
6. Waterbury L, Kunysz E, Beuerman R. Effects of steroidal and non-steroidal anti-inflammatory agents on corneal wound healing. J Ocul Pharmacol 1987; 3:43–54.
7. Mroszczak EJ, Lee FW, Combs D, Sarnquist FH, Huang BL, Wu AT, Tokes LG, Maddox ML, Cho DK. Ketorolac tromethamine absorption, distribution, metabolism, excretion and pharmacokinetics in animals and humans. Drug Metab Dispos 1987; 15:618–26.
8. Jung D, Mroszczak E, Bynum L. Pharmacokinetics of ketorolac tromethamine in humans after intravenous, intramuscular and oral administration. Eur J Clin Pharmacol 1988; 35:423.
9. Jung D, Mroszczak EJ, Wu A, Ling TL, Sevelius H, Bynum L. Pharmacokinetics of ketorolac and *p*-hydroxyketorolac following oral and intramuscular administration of ketorolac tromethamine. Pharm Res 1989; 6:62–5.
10. Brooks PM, Day RO. Nonsteroidal antiinflammatory drugs—differences and similarities. N Engl J Med 1991; 324:1716–25.
11. Martinez JJ, Garg DC, Pages LJ, Jallad NS, Yee JP, Mroszczak ES, Renneke GA, Weidler DJ. Single dose pharmacokinetics of ketorolac in healthy young and renal impaired subjects. J Clin Pharmacol 1987; 27:722.
12. Pages LJ, Martinez JJ, Garg DC, Yee JP, Mroszczak ES, Renneke GA, Weidler DJ. Pharmacokinetics of ketorolac tromethamine in hepatically impaired vs young healthy subjects. J Clin Pharmacol 1987; 27:724.
13. Peck CC, Conner DP, Murphy MG. Bedside clinical pharmacokinetics. Vancouver, Wash: Applied Therapeutics, 1989; 27, 31, 39, 40.
14. O'Sullivan CM, Rice ASC, Miller C, Lloyd J, Bullingham RES. Ketorolac transfer (KT) into CSF. Eur J Clin Pharmacol 1989; 36(suppl):A316.

15. MacDonald FC, Gough KJ, Nicoll RAG, Dow RJ. Psychomotor effects of ketorolac in comparison with buprenorphine and diclofenac. Br J Clin Pharmacol 1989; 27:453–9.
16. Peirce RJ, Fragen RJ, Pemberton DM. Intravenous ketorolac tromethamine versus morphine sulfate in the treatment of immediate postoperative pain. Pharmacotherapy 1990; 10(suppl): 111S–5.
17. Brown CR, Moodie JE, Dickie G, Wild VM, Smith BA, Clarke PJ, Evans SA, Bynum LJ. Analgesic efficacy and safety of single-dose oral and intramuscular ketorolac tromethamine for postoperative pain. Pharmacotherapy 1990; 10(suppl):59S–70.
18. Brown CR, Moodie JE, Wild VM, Bynum LJ. Comparison of intravenous ketorolac tromethamine and morphine sulfate in the treatment of postoperative pain. Pharmacotherapy 1990; 10(suppl):116S–21.
19. Yee JP, Koshiver JE, Allbon C, Brown CR. Comparison of intramuscular ketorolac tromethamine and morphine sulfate for analgesia of pain after major surgery. Pharmacotherapy 1986; 6:253–61.
20. O'Hara DA, Fragen R, Kinzer M, Pemberton D. Ketorolac tromethamine as compared with morphine sulfate for treatment of postoperative pain. Clin Pharmacol Ther 1987; 41:556–61.
21. Stanski DR, Cherry C, Bradley R, Sarnquist FH, Yee JP. Efficacy and safety of single doses of intramuscular ketorolac tromethamine compared with meperidine for postoperative pain. Pharmacotherapy 1990; 10(suppl):40S–4.
22. Fricke J, Angelocci D. The analgesic efficacy of IM ketorolac and meperidine for the control of postoperative dental pain. Clin Pharmacol Ther 1987; 41:181.
23. Brown CR, Moodie JE, Phillips E. Different responses to postoperative analgesics by inpatients and outpatients. Clin Pharmacol Ther 1991; 49:183.
24. Brown CR, Mazzulla JP, Mok MS, Nussdorf RT, Rubin PD, Schwesinger WH. Comparison of repeat doses of intramuscular ketorolac tromethamine and morphine sulfate for analgesia after major surgery. Pharmacotherapy 1990; 10(suppl):45S–50.
25. Spindler JS, Mehlisch D, Brown CR. Intramuscular ketorolac and morphine in the treatment of moderate to severe pain after major surgery. Pharmacotherapy 1990; 10(suppl):51S–8.
26. Black AMS, Goodman NW, Bullingham RES, Lloyd J. Intramuscular ketorolac and morphine during patient-controlled analgesia (PCA) after hysterectomy: does PCA lock-out time reveal an efficacy limitation of ketorolac? Eur J Anaesthesiol 1990; 7:9–17.
27. Baumann TJ. Place of ketorolac in pain management [editorial]. Clin Pharm 1990; 9:938.
28. Power I, Noble DW, Douglas E, Spence AA. Comparison of IM ketorolac trometamol and morphine sulfate for pain relief after cholecystectomy. Br J Anaesth 1990; 65:448–55.
29. Oosterlink W, Philp NH, Charig C, Gillies G, Hetherington JW, Lloyd J. A double-blind single dose comparison of intramuscular ketorolac tromethamine and pethidine in the treatment of renal colic. J Clin Pharmacol 1990; 30:336–41.
30. Staquet MJ. A double-blind study with placebo control of intramuscular ketorolac tromethamine in the treatment of cancer pain. J Clin Pharmacol 1989; 29:1031–6.
31. McQuay HJ, Poppleton P, Carroll D, Summerfield RJ, Bullingham RES, Moore RA. Ketorolac and acetaminophen for orthopedic postoperative pain. Clin Pharmacol Ther 1986; 39:89–93.
32. Honig WJ, Van Ochten J. A multiple-dose comparison of ketorolac tromethamine with diflunisal and placebo in postmeniscectomy pain. J Clin Pharmacol 1986; 26:700–5.
33. Galasko CSB, Russel S, Lloyd J. Double-blind investigation of the efficacy of multiple oral doses of ketorolac tromethamine compared with dihydrocodeine and placebo. Curr Ther Res 1989; 45:844–52.
34. Johansson S, Josefsson G, Malstam J, Lindstrand A, Stenstroem A. Analgesic efficacy and safety comparison of ketorolac tromethamine and doleron for the alleviation of orthopaedic postoperative pain. J Int Med Res 1989; 17:324–32.
35. Forbes JA, Butterworth GA, Burchfield WH, Beaver WT. Evaluation of ketorolac, aspirin, and an acetaminophen–codeine combination in postoperative oral surgery pain. Pharmacotherapy 1990; 10(suppl):77S–93.

36. Forbes JA, Kehm CJ, Grodin CD, Beaver WT. Evaluation of ketorolac, ibuprofen, acetaminophen, and acetaminophen–codeine combination in postoperative oral surgery pain. Pharmacotherapy 1990; 10(suppl):94S–105.
37. Kagi P. A multiple-dose comparison of oral ketorolac and pentazocine in the treatment of postoperative pain. Curr Ther Res 1989; 45:1049–59.
38. Bloomfield SS, Cissell G, Peters N, Nelson E, Hopson CN, Frieberg RA, Barden TP, Ketorolac analgesia for postoperative pain. Clin Pharmacol Ther 1988; 43:160.
39. Carlson RW, Borrison RA, Sher HB, Eisenberg PD, Mowry PA, Wolin EM. A multi-institutional evaluation of the analgesic efficacy and safety of ketorolac tromethamine, acetaminophen plus codeine, and placebo in cancer pain. Pharmacotherapy 1990; 10:211–6.
40. Estape J, Vinolas N, Gonzalez B, Ingles F, Bofill T, Guzman MC, Tarrago E. Ketorolac, a new non-opioid analgesic: a double-blind trial versus pentazocine in cancer pain. J Int Med Res 1990; 18:298–34.
41. Diebschlag W, Nocker W, Bullingham R. A double-blind study of efficacy of topical ketorolac tromethamine gel in the treatment of ankle sprain, in comparison to placebo and etofenamate. J Clin Pharmacol 1990; 30:82–9.
42. Editorial. Topical NSAIDs: a gimmick or a godsend? Lancet 1989; 2:779–80.
43. Flach AJ, Jaffe NS, Akers WA. The effect of ketorolac tromethamine in reducing postoperative inflammation: double-mask parallel comparison with dexamethasone. Ann Ophthalmol 1989; 21:407–11.
44. Flach AJ, Lavelle CJ, Olander KWE, Retzlaff JA, Sorenson LW. The effect of ketorolac tromethamine solution 0.5% in reducing postoperative inflammation after cataract extraction and intraocular lens implantation. Ophthalmology 1988; 95:1279–84.
45. Flach AJ, Graham J, Kruger LP, Stegman RC, Tanenbaum L. Quantitative assessment of postsurgical breakdown of the blood–aqueous barrier following administration of 0.5% ketorolac tromethamine solution. A double-masked, paired comparison with vehicle–placebo solution study. Arch Ophthalmol 1988; 106:344–7.
46. Flach AJ, Dolan BJ, Irvine AR. Effectiveness of ketorolac tromethamine 0.5% ophthalmic solution for chronic aphakic and pseudophakic cystoid macular edema. Am J Ophthalmol 1987; 103:479–86.
47. Flach AJ, Stegman RC, Graham J, Kruger LP. Prophylaxis of aphakic cystoid macular edema without corticosteroids. A paired-comparison, placebo-controlled double-masked study. Ophthalmology 1990; 97:1253–8.
48. Fournier DC, Linehan AT, Hilman BC. A case of ketorolac induced asthma in an adult with aspirin sensitivity. J Allergy Clin Immunol 1991; 87(suppl):275.
49. Vicks SD, Dean RJ, Tenholder MF. Ketorolac induced respiratory failure in an aspirin sensitive asthmatic. Immunol Allergy Pract 1991; 13:23–5.
50. Brandon Bravo LJC, Mattie H, Spierdijk J, Bovill JG, Burm AGL. The effects on ventilation of ketorolac in comparison with morphine. Eur J Clin Pharmacol 1988; 35:491–4.
51. Kenney GNC, McArdle CS, Aitken HH. Parenteral ketorolac: opiate-sparing effect and lack of cardiorespiratory depression in the perioperative patient. Pharmacotherapy 1990; 10(suppl): 127S–31.
52. Fleming BM, Coombs DW. Bleeding diathesis after perioperative ketorolac. Anesth Analog 1991; 73:235.
53. Lanza FL, Karlin DA, Yee JP. A double-blind placebo-controlled endoscopic study comparing the mucosal injury seen with an orally and parenterally administered new nonsteroidal analgesic ketorolac tromethamine at therapeutic and supratherapeutic doses. Am J Gastroenterol 1987; 82:939.
54. Rubin P, Yee JP, Murthy VS, Seavey W. Ketorolac tromethamine (KT) analgesia: no postoperative respiratory depression and less constipation. Clin Pharmacol Ther 1987; 41:182.
55. Yee MK, Evans WD, Facey PE, Hayward MWJ, Rosen M. Gastric emptying and small bowel transit in male volunteers after IM ketorolac and morphine. Br J Anaesth 1991; 67:426–31.

56. Goodman E. Use of ketorolac in sickle-cell disease and vaso-occlusive crisis. Lancet 1991; 338:641–2.
57. Spowart K, Greer IA, McLaren M, Lloyd J, Bullingham RES, Forbes CD. Haemostatic effects of ketorolac with and without concomitant heparin in normal volunteers. Thromb Haemost 1988; 60:382–6.
58. Conrad KA, Fagan TC, Mackie MJ, Mayshar PV. Effects of ketorolac tromethamine on hemostasis in volunteers. Clin Pharmacol Ther 1988; 43:542–6.
59. Rubin P, Yee JP, Ruoff G. Comparison of long-term safety of ketorolac tromethamine and aspirin in the treatment of chronic pain. Pharmacotherapy 1990; 10:106S–110.

15

Bromfenac

JOSEPH S. WAJDULA, IVAN VAVRA, DIANE SULLIVAN, and JAMES ERMER
Wyeth–Ayerst Research
Philadelphia, Pennsylvania

MOHAMED OSMAN
Wyeth–Ayerst Research
Princeton, New Jersey

I. INTRODUCTION

Bromfenac sodium, a phenylacetic acid derivative, exhibits pronounced analgesic and anti-inflammatory activity. Its actions appear to be primarily related to the inhibition of prostaglandin synthesis. Its pharmacological profile is marked by a demonstrable dose–response curve, an acceptable therapeutic window, a fast onset of action, and a long duration of analgesic activity, despite rapid excretion.

II. CHEMISTRY

Bromfenac sodium, or 2-amino-3-(4-bromobenzyl)phenylacetic acid sodium salt sesquihydrate (Fig. 1), is structurally related to diclofenac and to ketoprofen. The insertion of a bromine substituent in the 4-position of the benzoyl ring was determined to increase the duration of analgesic activity and to increase anti-inflammatory potency (1). Bromfenac is fully ionized at physiological pH (pK_a 4.29) and exhibits limited lipophilicity, as indicated by a partition coefficient of 3.22 at pH 7.41. The compound is not optically active. Bromfenac is an orange-yellow crystalline powder that has a slight odor; it is soluble in water, methanol, and dilute base, but insoluble in chloroform and in dilute acid. Acidic conditions favor the degradation of bromfenac to a heterocyclic inactive product.

III. PRECLINICAL PHARMACODYNAMIC PROPERTIES

A. Receptor-Binding and Enzymatic Studies

Bromfenac has undergone extensive in vitro pharmacological screening to determine its effect on various receptors and enzyme systems. No significant interaction was detected on

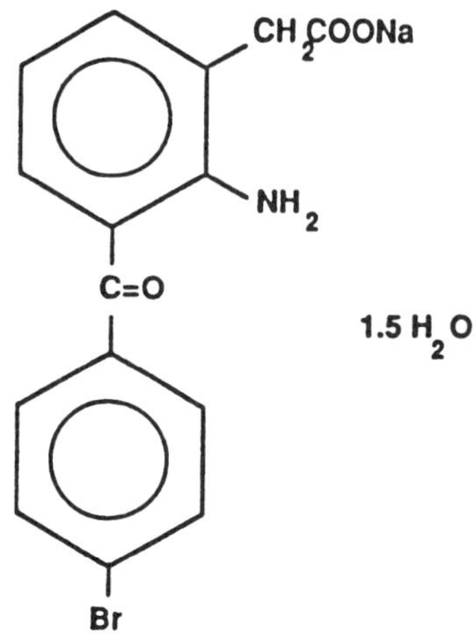

Figure 1 Structure of bromfenac sodium.

the adrenergic-, serotoninergic-, excitatory amino acids-, γ-aminobutyric acid (GABA)-, adenosine-, opioid-, bradykinin-, or substance P-binding sites. The compound is a highly potent inhibitor of cyclooxygenase; the 50% inhibitory concentration (IC_{50}) of bromfenac was 11 ± 1 μM, whereas the standards, indomethacin and aspirin, yielded IC_{50} values of 25 and 1000 μM, respectively. Complementary biochemical studies have indicated that bromfenac competes with arachidonic acid for binding to cyclooxygenase, resulting in decreased formation of prostaglandins. No significant effects have been observed on the synthesis of other eicosanoids (e.g., leukotrienes). However, bromfenac differs from indomethacin and flurbiprofen in that its competitive-binding constant is not affected by lipid hydroperoxide, an inflammatory peroxide responsible for the priming of cellular prostaglandin H (PGH) synthase and for oxygenation of unesterified arachidonic acid. The high potency and the limited effect of hydroperoxide differentiate the biochemical activity of bromfenac from other nonsteroidal anti-inflammatory drugs (NSAIDs).

B. Effects on Prostaglandin Synthesis

Data from comparative pharmacological studies show that bromfenac is 6–32 times more potent than indomethacin and 70–300 times more potent than ibuprofen in inhibiting the formation of PGE_2 and $PGF_{2\alpha}$ in microsomes of bovine seminal vesicle, rabbit uterus, and rabbit renal medulla. Studies examining the in vitro inhibitory effect of bromfenac on arachidonic acid-induced platelet aggregation have also demonstrated that bromfenac interferes with prostaglandin biosynthesis; the IC_{50} for bromfenac was 0.39 μM. Presumably, bromfenac reduced the fraction of arachidonic acid available for subsequent transformation to thromboxane A_2 (TXA_2), a potent platelet aggregator.

Local reduction in the tissue concentrations of prostaglandins is generally believed to account for many of the pharmacological actions of NSAIDs. A multitude of physiological and pathophysiological effects have been linked to prostaglandins, including the transduction of painful stimuli at nociceptors and the augmentation of the inflammatory response. Thus, a bromfenac-induced reduction in the local concentration of prostaglandins theoretically translates to reduced transduction of painful stimuli (i.e., analgesia).

However, no experiments have as yet correlated the prostaglandin-inhibiting capacity of bromfenac to its analgesic and anti-inflammatory activity.

C. Antinociceptive Studies

Classic analgesic models have been employed to investigate the antinociceptive activity of bromfenac in animals (1). Specifically, the acetylcholine- and phenylbenzoquinone (PBQ)-induced writhing tests and the tail pinch test in mice have been used. Bromfenac was a more potent inhibitor of the mouse writhing response to acetylcholine than zomepirac, piroxicam, suprofen, or pemedolac, and was equipotent to ketorolac. The 50% effective dose (ED_{50}) of bromfenac was approximately 0.08 mg/kg of body weight when administered orally 60 min before acetylcholine. The writhing-inhibiting effects of bromfenac were remarkably stable over 300 min. In contrast, the suppression of the writhing response by suprofen and piroxicam decreased during this time. Additionally, bromfenac was about six times more potent than zomepirac in blocking the nociceptive response to bradykinin in dogs; however, it has no specific affinity for the bradykinin receptor. The antibradykinin activity of bromfenac was probably due to the inhibitory effect of the compound on other mediators of pain and inflammation (i.e., prostaglandins).

Bromfenac, similar to other NSAIDs, is characterized by its nonnarcotic mode of action (1). Tolerance to the analgesic effect of bromfenac did not appear following 13 consecutive doses of 0.316 mg/kg, given to mice over 5 days. Under the same conditions, tolerance developed to the analgesic activity of meperidine, given at a comparable analgesic dose (31.6 mg/kg). Moreover, 5 mg of naloxone administered subcutaneously (sc) antagonized the analgesic activity of meperidine, but did not block the activity of bromfenac. Bromfenac, 3.16 mg/kg by mouth (po), was inactive in blocking the nociceptive response to an artery clip placed at the base of the tail of mice, whereas meperidine (100 mg/kg, po) did block this response.

The duration of analgesic action of bromfenac (Fig. 2) has been examined in the PBQ-induced writhing assay. Significant antinociceptive activity was seen in mice within 30 min of administration of 1 mg/kg po; the activity persisted at 1, 2, 4, and 8 h. Inhibition of the writhing response was not significant at 16 and 24 h after bromfenac administration. Maximal writhing inhibition (83–94%) occurred within the first 2 h, and declined to 55% at 8 h, and to 28% at 24 h. Plasma concentrations of bromfenac were highest 0.5 h after dose administration, indicating rapid absorption, and fell below the level of detection (30 ng/ml) 16 h after the dose. Application of an E_{max} model (Fig. 3) showed an apparent positive relation between plasma concentration and analgesia. However, some pharmacological activity persisted 16 h after dose administration, despite almost complete disappearance of bromfenac from plasma. The basis for this persistent antinociceptive activity is unclear.

D. Anti-Inflammatory Studies

The anti-inflammatory activity of bromfenac has been explored using the Evans blue–carrageenan pleural effusion assay, the carrageenan foot edema assay, and the adjuvant-induced arthritis model (1). In the carrageenan foot edema assay, rats were given doses of bromfenac, ranging from 0.01 to 3.16 mg/kg po, 1 h before carrageenan challenge. The anti-inflammatory activity of bromfenac was optimal at doses between 0.10 and 3.16 mg/kg. The ED_{50} value for the anti-inflammatory activity of bromfenac was calculated to be 0.05 mg/kg. Blood samples taken at the time of anti-inflammatory activity

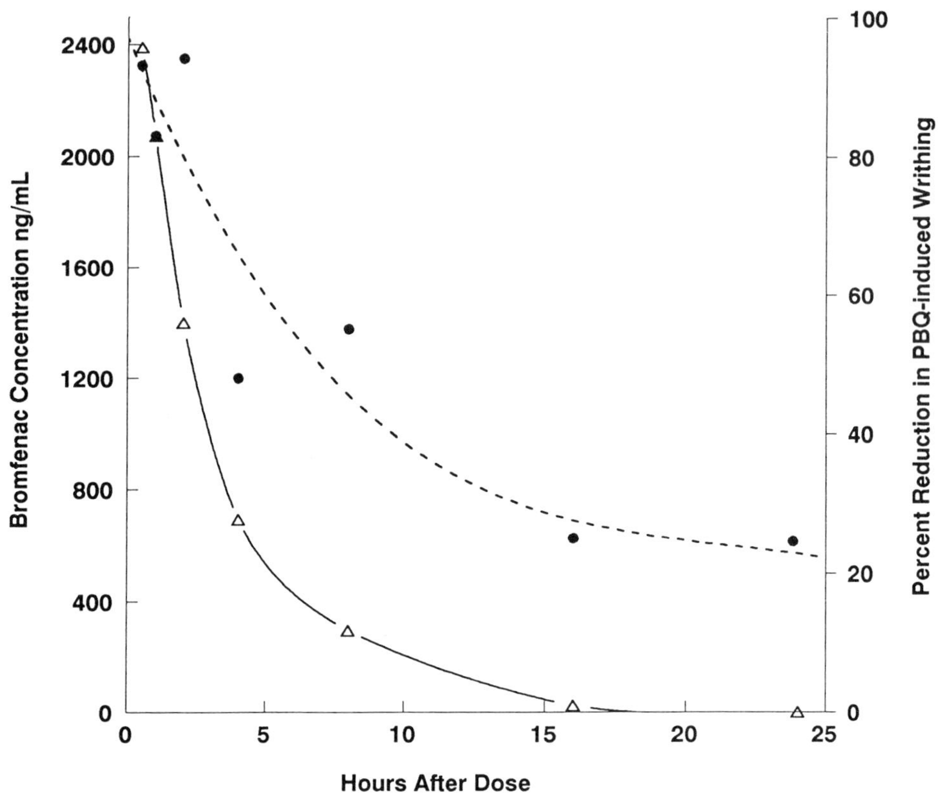

Figure 2 Bromfenac plasma levels (△) and antinociceptive activity (●) following a single oral dose (1 mg/kg) in mice.

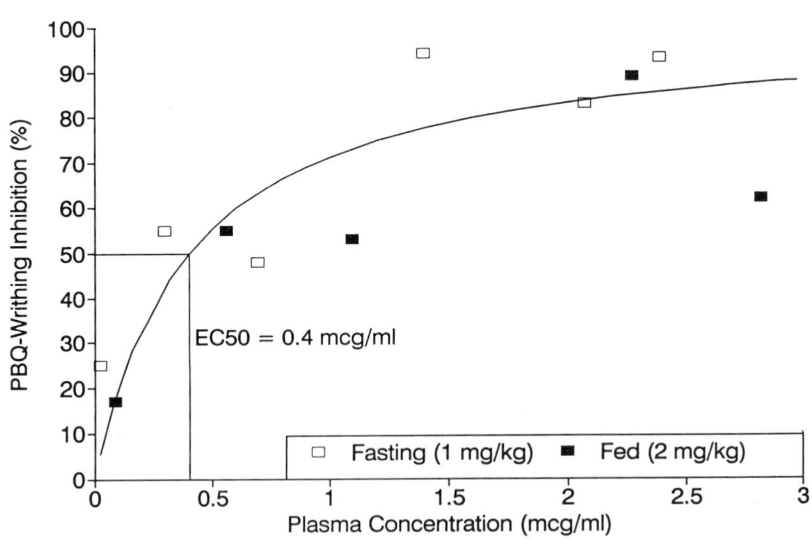

Figure 3 Effect–concentration (PK/PD) relation generated with an E_{max} model for bromfenac-treated mice.

measurements revealed that bromfenac concentrations greater than 0.25 μg/ml were generally needed to produce maximal activity. Blood levels increased beyond this point produced no significant increase in anti-inflammatory activity, indicating a ceiling to the pharmacological effect.

In the Evans blue–carrageenan pleural assay in rats, bromfenac (0.8 and 4.0 mg/kg, po) significantly reduced the exudate production 5 and 17 h after the dose (1). Bromfenac was 7.5 times more potent than indomethacin in suppressing the 5-h pleural response and 20 times more potent than indomethacin in suppressing the 17-h pleural response. The maximal effects of bromfenac and indomethacin were similar in magnitude.

Bromfenac and indomethacin were therapeutically administered to rats following the induction of Freund's adjuvant arthritis. Bromfenac was 3.7 times more potent than indomethacin in this test. Both compounds significantly increased the gain in body weight, reflecting an improvement in the general condition (i.e., an increased appetite) of the animals.

The duration of anti-inflammatory response was assessed in the carrageenan-induced edema assay (2). Bromfenac was administered orally at 0.316 mg/kg to fasted male Sprague-Dawley rats at various times (0.5–48 h) before the carrageenan injection. Significant inhibition of the inflammatory response was noted when bromfenac was given 0.5–24 h before carrageenan challenge. Concentrations of bromfenac in the plasma were detectable for 24 h after administration; highest plasma concentrations (1.61 μg/ml) were measured at 0.5 h and fell to 0.04 μg/ml 24 h after the dose.

E. Antipyretic Activity

Oral doses of bromfenac were effective in lowering the rectal temperature of hyperthermic rats, without affecting the rectal temperature of normothermic rats (1). The onset of the antipyretic action of bromfenac occurred within 30 min and persisted longer than 3 h following oral administration.

F. Gastrointestinal Toxicity

The liability of bromfenac to induce gastric and intestinal injury was shown to be similar to that of indomethacin (1). Oral administration of bromfenac to rats produced gastric damage in a dose-dependent manner; gastric lesions were seen in 29% of the animals after doses of 1 mg/kg and in 100% of the rats after 9 mg/kg. No intestinal lesions were present at the 0.75 mg/kg dose level, whereas 100% of the animals displayed mucosal damage in the gut after the 3.0 and 6.0 mg/kg doses. The relative acute therapeutic index of bromfenac (the ratio of its anti-inflammatory activity to its gastric toxicity) was 5.4, compared with an index of 1.0 for indomethacin.

IV. PRECLINICAL PHARMACOKINETIC PROPERTIES

The pharmacokinetic profile of bromfenac was evaluated in mice, rats, and monkeys (Table 1). After rapid absorption, bromfenac is widely distributed, with highest tissue concentrations in the organs of elimination. The plasma metabolic profile of bromfenac has not been completely characterized, but studies with radiolabeled bromfenac have detected a substantial fraction of radioactivity that is not reflective of parent compound. The elimination of bromfenac occurs rapidly, by renal and biliary excretion routes.

Table 1 Summary of Pharmacokinetic Parameters in Various Species

Species	Dose (mg/kg)	Route	n	C_{max} (μg/ml)		t_{max} (h)		$AUC_{0\text{-}48}$ (μg/ml)		$t_{1/2}$ (h)		Absolute bioavailability (%)
				^{14}C	BRO	^{14}C	BRO	^{14}C	BRO	^{14}C	BRO	
Mouse	1.0	po	64	—[a]	2.4	—	0.5	—	8.9[c]	—	2.4	—
Rat	0.6	po	3	2.8	2.8	0.25	0.25	26.8	18.0	7.9	3.5	68.7
	6.0	po	3	23.8	23.5	0.25	0.25	266.9	167.7	8.6	4.8	50.0
	0.3	iv	3	NA[b]	NA	NA	NA	17.7	13.1	7.4	4.4	100
	3.0	iv	3	NA	NA	NA	NA	198.5	168.8	7.0	4.7	100
Monkey												
Rhesus	15	po	2	42.7	33.3	0.33	0.33	97.3	58.7	5.9	4.3	74.1
	45	po	2	170	150	0.67	0.67	362.5	247.1	5.2	NA	64.6
	15	iv	2	NA	NA	NA	NA	130.9	79.2	7.5	4.9	100
	45	iv	2	NA	NA	NA	NA	764.8	382.4	12.4	6.4	100
Cynomolgus	3.0	po	2	5.6	5.3	0.92	0.92	16.9	10.5	—	—	49
	30	po	2	37.2	36.8	2.8	2.8	183.4	132.9	—	—	28
	3.0	iv	2	NA	NA	NA	NA	28.6	21.4	—	—	100
	30	iv	2	NA	NA	NA	NA	573.2	472.3	—	—	100
Cynomolgus												
Fed	15	po	4	—	29	—	0.21	—	53.7[c]	—	—	NA
Fasted	15	po	4	—	85.1	—	0.42	—	100.6[c]	—	—	NA

BRO, bromfenac (unchanged compound);
[a] indicates data not available;
[b] NA indicates data not applicable;
[c] $AUC_{0\text{-}24}$.

A. Absorption

1. Rat

The time course of plasma radioactivity was investigated in male and female rats following single oral or intravenous doses of [^{14}C]bromfenac. After oral doses of 0.6 and 6.0 mg/kg of [^{14}C]bromfenac, the respective peak plasma concentrations (C_{max}) of radioactivity were equivalent to 2.8 and 23.8 μg/ml at 0.25 h. The average terminal elimination half-life of [^{14}C] after the oral and intravenous doses was 7.7 ± 0.7 hr. After both oral doses, all of the plasma radioactivity at the C_{max} was due to the unchanged drug. The absolute bioavailabilities following single doses of 0.6 and 6 mg/kg were 68.7 and 50.0%, respectively. The average terminal elimination half-life for unchanged bromfenac after the oral and intravenous doses was 4.4 ± 0.6 h.

2. Monkeys

The time course of plasma radioactivity was investigated in male and female rhesus and cynomolgus monkeys following single oral and intravenous doses of [^{14}C]bromfenac (see Table 1). Oral doses of 15 and 45 mg/kg of [^{14}C]bromfenac were given to rhesus monkeys, and doses of 3.0 and 30.0 mg/kg were administered to cynomolgus monkeys. The C_{max} values when normalized for dosage were higher in rhesus monkeys than in cynomolgus monkeys. Measurement of plasma radioactivity at the C_{max} revealed a larger fraction represented by parent drug in cynomolgus monkeys (97%) than in rhesus monkeys (83%). In addition, the absolute bioavailability of bromfenac appeared to be less in cynomolgus monkeys than in rhesus monkeys.

3. Effects of Food on Absorption

The relative availability of bromfenac was evaluated after administration of 15 mg/kg in male and female cynomolgus monkeys under fed and fasted conditions (see Table 1). The C_{max} was 29.0 and 85.1 μg/ml at 0.21 and 0.42 h after the dose in fed and fasted monkeys, respectively. Data from this study indicate that the relative bioavailability of bromfenac is approximately 50% less in fed cynomolgus monkeys than in monkeys that have received the drug following an overnight fast. A similar profile of reduced bioavailability was observed in rats after the postprandial administration of bromfenac.

The mechanisms underlying the apparent food-induced reduction in the bioavailability are uncertain. Preliminary data indicate that exposure of the compound for extended periods to an acid environment similar to the in vivo postprandial gastric conditions may enhance the degradation of bromfenac. In vitro experiments showed that hydrochloric acid concentrations of pH 4 or less are associated with the spontaneous degradation of bromfenac to an inactive heterocyclic product. Inasmuch as the bioavailability of the parent compound is reduced when administered concurrently with food, radiolabeled bromfenac given to fed and fasted cynomolgus monkeys displayed an interesting excretion pattern (Table 2). The net amount of radioactive recovery in the urine and feces was essentially identical for fed and fasted conditions. Thus, both the parent compound and the gastric degradation products appear to be absorbed across the gastrointestinal mucosa.

B. Distribution

Binding of bromfenac to red blood cells in dogs and humans is minimal. The erythrocyte/plasma ratio of bound bromfenac was about 0.10. The in vitro plasma protein-binding of bromfenac in dogs and humans was greater than 99%. The fraction of

Table 2 Recovery of Radioactivity in the Excreta of Cynomolgus Monkeys Given a Single 1 mg/kg oral dose of [^{14}C] bromfenac

	Collection interval (h)	% of dose		
		Urine	Feces	Total
Fasted	0–24	62.2 ± 35.2	7.1 ± 6.6	
	0–168	69.9 ± 1.7	22.1 ± 7.6	92.0
Fed	0–24	54.9 ± 14.9	7.2 ± 7.3	
	0–168	64.6 ± 15.2	30.3 ± 8.6	94.9

unbound bromfenac measured in in vitro tests is species-dependent and concentration-independent (Table 3). Reflective of the high degree of protein binding, the volume of distribution (V_d) is correspondingly low; V_d was 0.15 L/kg in rats and 0.87 L/kg in cynomolgus monkeys.

The distribution of radioactivity in pigmented rats was studied by whole-body autoradiography after 7 daily consecutive oral (1.5 mg/kg per day) and intravenous (1.0 mg/kg per day) doses of [^{14}C]bromfenac. Radioactivity, measured 15 min after the last intravenous dose, was widely distributed throughout the tissues. Distribution was generally similar in male and female rats and was qualitatively similar after oral and intravenous doses. Much of the radioactivity was associated with the gastrointestinal (hepatic) and renal tracts, as expected for systems of biotransformation and excretion. Radioactivity was still associated with the harderian glands, walls of the great arteries, salivary glands, and livers of the rats 48 h after the last dose.

Solutions containing [^{14}C]bromfenac were administered orally to male and female cynomolgus monkeys. Doses of 3 or 30 mg/kg were used. The presence of radioactivity in blood and nearly all tissues at 0.5 h after dose administration indicated rapid absorption and distribution of [^{14}C]bromfenac. The distribution of radioactivity in tissues showed no appreciable tendency for accumulation in any tissues other than the organs of elimination and excretion (liver, kidneys, gallbladder, and lower gastrointestinal tract). Radioactivity was undetectable in many of the tissues by 36 h after the dose.

C. Metabolism

Preliminary metabolic profiles for bromfenac have been determined in plasma, urine, and bile. In plasma samples obtained from the lactating rat, the only metabolites detected

Table 3 In Vitro Protein-Binding of Bromfenac

	% unbound bromfenac		
Species	2 μg/ml	10 μg/ml	50 μg/ml
Mouse	2.5	2.7	3.3
Rat	0.5	0.5	0.5
Dog	0.2	0.2	0.2
Cynomolgus monkey	0.4	0.4	0.5
Rhesus monkey	0.3	0.3	0.4
Human	0.2	0.2	0.2

were bromfenac and AHR-11665 (a benzoic acid derivative), indicating that the parent compound is not extensively metabolized. Hepatic biotransformation during the 4-h period after dosing accounted for the detection of five major biliary metabolites in the rat; these included free and conjugated bromfenac and AHR-11655, and AHR-10240, the cyclic amide of bromfenac. The percentage of excreted radioactivity of conjugated bromfenac and AHR-11665, and free bromfenac and AHR-11655, and AHR-10240 were 28.7, 4.3, 11.1, 16.8, and 18.6%, respectively. In contrast with rats, the plasma compartment of cynomolgus monkeys revealed only the parent compound. Metabolites detected in urine included four glucuronide conjugates of unknown aglycones and the cyclic amide. Figure 4 depicts the structure of bromfenac and its known metabolites.

D. Elimination

Oral administration of radiolabeled bromfenac to rats resulted in an apparent plasma elimination half-life of about 7–9 h for total radioactivity and about 3–5 h for unchanged drug. An average of 78% of the total radioactivity was recovered in the excreta after either intravenous or oral administration; approximately 27% of the radioactivity was eliminated in the urine. The excretion pattern (see Table 2) in cynomolgus monkeys shows that both total recovery and the percentage excreted in urine were higher than those in the rats. Additionally, clearance of intravenously administered bromfenac was shown to be high (140 ml h^{-1} kg^{-1}) in cynomolgus monkeys.

V. HUMAN PHARMACOKINETICS

The pharmacokinetics of bromfenac has been studied in young and elderly subjects. Additionally, the effect of food on the absorption of bromfenac and the metabolic disposition of bromfenac have been investigated. These studies examined the pharmacokinetic characteristics of bromfenac over the dose range of 25–200 mg.

The first study was conducted to assess dose proportionality. Twelve young male subjects were given single 25-, 50-, 100-, and 200-mg oral doses of bromfenac as a solution. As shown in Figure 5, bromfenac plasma concentrations reached a maximum

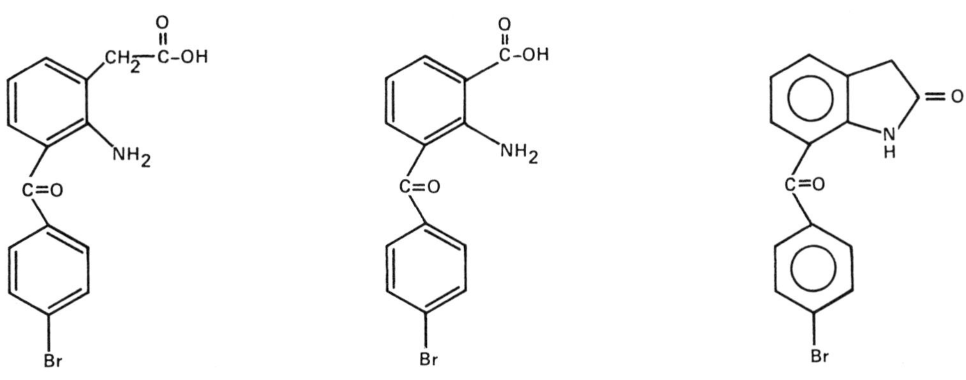

(AHR-10282)
Bromfenac

AHR-11665

AHR-10240

Figure 4 Structures for bromfenac and known metabolites.

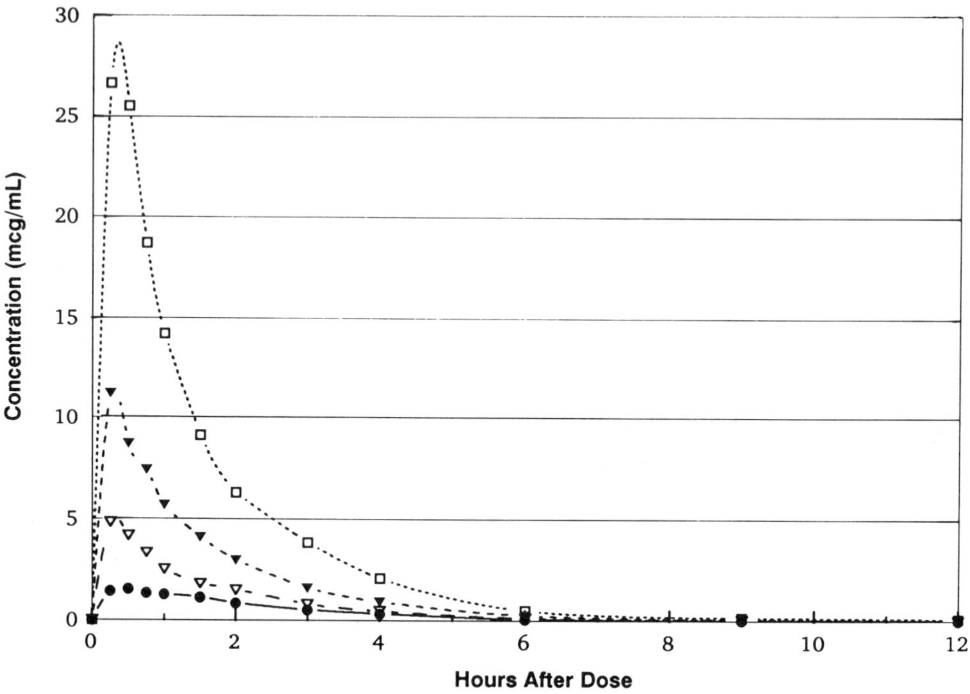

Figure 5 Mean plasma levels obtained from male subjects after a single dose of bromfenac 25 mg (●), 50 mg (▽), 100 mg (▼), or 200 mg (□).

level within 20–40 min and declined rapidly, with a half-life of approximately 1 h. Total plasma clearance was approximately 90 ml/ h^{-1} kg^{-1}, and protein-binding of bromfenac was greater than 99.8%. Both C_{max} and area under the plasma concentration–time curve (AUC) were linearly proportional within the projected therapeutic range of 10–100 mg; at 200 mg there was a 35% deviation from linearity.

The effects of age and sex on bromfenac pharmacokinetics were studied in a preliminary study. Twenty subjects, ten men and ten women, mean age of 69 years (range, 65–84 years), received single 50-mg oral doses of bromfenac. The pharmacokinetic profile was similar to that attained in young subjects given the same dose in a different study (Table 4). Notably, excretion rates for bromfenac did not appear to be age-related, as the mean elimination half-lives were constant, and only small plasma clearance variations were measured in young and elderly subjects.

The metabolic disposition of bromfenac was investigated in six male volunteers following oral administration of 50 mg of [^{14}C]bromfenac sodium as a single dose. Consistent with studies using unlabeled bromfenac, absorption of radiolabeled drug was rapid; a mean C_{max} equivalent to 4.87 ± 1.78 μg/ml was reached at 1.0 ± 0.5 h after dosing. Similar to the cynomolgus monkey, virtually all of the radioactivity in plasma within 2 h of dosing was attributed to the parent compound; a minor unidentified metabolite was detected at later time points. The drug was primarily eliminated by the urine (82.4%) as four glucuronide conjugates of unidentified aglycones and the cyclic amide. None of the urinary metabolites were detected in the plasma.

Another study assessed the absorption of bromfenac when administered with food.

Table 4 Comparison of Mean (SD) Pharmacokinetic Parameters in Young and Elderly Volunteers Receiving a Single 50-mg Oral Dose of Bromfenac

	Young subjects	Elderly subjects	
Parameter[a]	Male (n=7)	Male (n=10)	Female (n=10)
AUC (mg/L h)	10.3 ± 3.2	9.6 ± 2.7	13.7 ± 3.4
C_{max} (mg/L)	7.0 ± 2.4	5.2 ± 1.5	8.1 ± 1.7
t_{max} (h)	0.6 ± 0.1	0.8 ± 0.4	0.7 ± 0.2
$t_{1/2}$ (h)	1.3 ± 0.15	1.3 ± 0.3	1.3 ± 0.2
CL/F(ml h^{-1} kg^{-1})	79 ± 23	72 ± 27	60 ± 14
V_d/F(L/kg)	0.15 ± 0.04	0.13 ± 0.02	0.11 ± 0.02

[a]AUC, area under the plasma concentration–time curve; C_{max}, maximum plasma concentration; t_{max}, time to C_{max}; $t_{1/2}$, terminal elimination half-life; CL/F, oral clearance; V_d/F, apparent volume of distribution.

Seven subjects completed the crossover study. After the subjects had eaten a standard breakfast, bromfenac C_{max} and AUC were significantly lower than the values measured under fasting conditions. Specifically, the mean values for C_{max} and AUC were 7.0 μg/ml and 10.3 μg h/ml, respectively, when bromfenac was administered after a fast, compared with 1.5 μg/ml and 3.7 μg h/ml, respectively, after a meal. Mean time to C_{max} (t_{max}) was 2.6 times longer in fed subjects than in those who had fasted. The influence of gastric acid secretion on the bioavailability of bromfenac was also examined in this study, since in vitro experiments indicated that the drug was acid-labile. Accordingly, the study was repeated in the same subjects, who this time received cimetidine, 300 mg every 6 h for 24 h, before the administration of bromfenac. Cimetidine caused a small increase in bromfenac AUC values, but had no substantial effect on the difference in bromfenac bioavailability between fed and fasted subjects. Further investigation is planned to elucidate the mechanism by which food affects the absorption characteristics of bromfenac.

VI. THERAPEUTIC EFFICACY AND HUMAN PHARMACODYNAMICS

A. Analgesic Studies

Bromfenac has been clinically tested in standard analgesic models (3–6). From these studies, a single-dose data base has been generated for the analgesic efficacy of bromfenac compared with that of other NSAIDs (Table 5). In every comparison between bromfenac and an NSAID of established analgesic activity, the activity of bromfenac has either equaled or surpassed the activity of the standards. The salient features of bromfenac shown in these studies include high potency, a demonstrable dose–response curve, and an acceptable efficacy–tolerability profile.

1. *Oral Surgery Studies*

In each of the three oral surgery studies described in Table 5, standard analgesic methods were employed. Single oral doses of bromfenac at multiple strengths were compared with positive control drugs and placebo under double-blind conditions. Pain relief and pain intensity were measured at regular intervals with standard analgesic scales. Derived measures of efficacy were also computed from the pain relief and pain intensity data;

Table 5 Summary of Single-Dose Analgesic Studies with Bromfenac

Model (Ref)	Bromfenac dose (mg)	Comparators	Duration of assessment (h)	Results
Oral surgery (unpublished)	5, 25, 50	Aspirin, 650 mg; placebo	6	Bromfenac, 25 mg and 50 mg, superior to aspirin, 650 mg
Oral surgery (3)	5, 10, 25	Aspirin, 650 mg; ibuprofen, 400 mg; placebo	8	Bromfenac, 25 mg, superior to aspirin and at least as effective as ibuprofen, 400 mg
Oral surgery (4)	10, 25, 50, 100	Aspirin, 650 mg; ibuprofen, 400 mg, placebo	8	Bromfenac, 100 mg, superior to ibuprofen, 400 mg
Orthopedic surgery (5)	5, 10, 25	Acetaminophen, 1000 mg; placebo	6	Bromfenac, 25 mg, was at least as effective as acetaminophen
Orthopedic surgery (6)	25, 50, 100	Ibuprofen, 200 mg; ibuprofen, 400 mg	8	Bromfenac, 100 mg, superior to ibuprofen, 200 mg; all bromfenac doses equivalent to ibuprofen, 400 mg

these measures included pain intensity difference (PID), summed pain intensity difference (SPID), summed analogue pain intensity difference (SPAID), and total pain relief (TOPAR).

In a double-blind, randomized, placebo-controlled trial, 202 men and women received single oral doses of either bromfenac (5, 25, or 50 mg), aspirin (650 mg), or placebo for moderate or severe pain secondary to erupted or impacted tooth extraction. Results showed that all active treatments were significantly ($p < 0.05$) more efficacious than placebo according to SPID, SPAID, and TOPAR scores and remedication rates at 4 and 6 h. The 25- and 50-mg doses of bromfenac produced significantly better scores than aspirin for SPID, SPAID, and TOPAR. In addition, a significantly larger portion of patients in each of the bromfenac treatment groups than in the placebo group made a "good" or "excellent" global evaluation, and the two higher-dose groups were significantly superior to aspirin according to this variable.

In another study (3) involving pain after oral surgery, the relative safety and efficacy of bromfenac (5, 10, and 25 mg), aspirin (650 mg), ibuprofen (400 mg), and placebo were compared. This was a single-dose, double-blind, randomized, parallel trial in which 269 patients took study medication. All three doses of bromfenac and ibuprofen (400 mg) were significantly superior to placebo for every measure of total and peak analgesia. The mean pain relief results over the course of the assessment period are illustrated in Figure 6. Bromfenac (10 and 25 mg) and ibuprofen (400 mg) had manifested an analgesic effect by hour 1. The effect was significant for bromfenac (5 mg) and aspirin (650 mg) by hour 2, but persisted only until hour 3. The effect of bromfenac (10 mg) persisted until hour 5; that of bromfenac (25 mg) and ibuprofen persisted for 8 h. Overall, the results of this

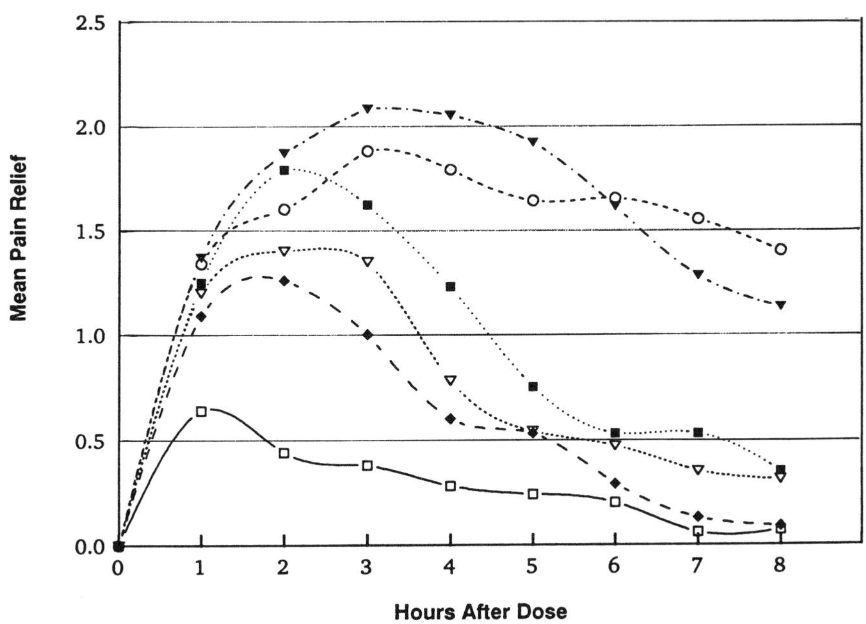

Figure 6 Mean pain relief registered in patients following oral surgery after a single oral dose of placebo (□), ibuprofen (○); aspirin, 650 mg (◆); bromfenac, 5 mg (▽); 10 mg (■); or 25 mg (▼). (From Ref. 3)

study indicated that the analgesic efficacy of bromfenac (25 mg) was similar to that of ibuprofen (400 mg).

Another single-dose oral surgery study (4) was performed with higher doses of bromfenac to more fully characterize the dose–response relation. In this study, 317 oral surgery patients were randomly assigned to receive one of seven treatments: bromfenac (10, 25, 50, or 100 mg), aspirin (650 mg), ibuprofen (400 mg), or placebo. All doses of bromfenac and ibuprofen were significantly superior to placebo for most measures of analgesia. Aspirin was significantly superior to placebo for 3-h TOPAR and 3-h SPID scores. Bromfenac (10 mg) was significantly superior to aspirin for TOPAR at 3 and 8 h and for SPID at 8 h. Bromfenac doses of 100, 50, and 25 mg were superior to aspirin for TOPAR and SPID at both 3 and 8 h. Figure 7 depicts the pain relief time curves for each treatment. The data show that peak analgesic activity is achieved with bromfenac, 25 mg; higher doses do not produce increased levels of analgesia, but provide a longer duration of analgesia. Comparison of 8-h SPID and TOPAR scores for each treatment (Fig. 8) show that the maximal response was associated with bromfenac, 50 and 100 mg. Statistical analysis indicated that the 8-h mean TOPAR value was significantly higher ($p < 0.01$) for bromfenac (100 mg) than for ibuprofen (400 mg).

In an effort to estimate a potential therapeutic dose range in humans, a pharmacodynamic (E_{max}) model was applied to the data obtained from two clinical pain studies in patients who had undergone surgical extraction of impacted third molars (3,4). The PID data from these two analgesia studies, which encompassed the dose range of 5–100 mg, were pooled and combined with predicted plasma concentration profiles based on the

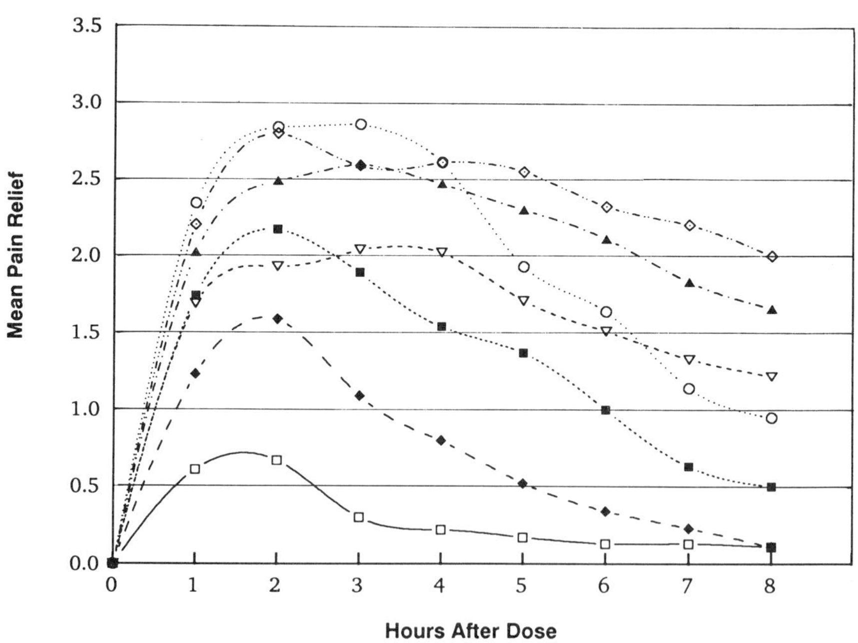

Figure 7 Mean pain relief registered in patients following oral surgey after a single oral dose of placebo (□); aspirin, 650 mg (◆); ibuprofen, 400 mg (▽); bromfenac, 10 mg (■); 25 mg (○); 50 mg (▲); or 100 mg (◇). (From Ref. 4)

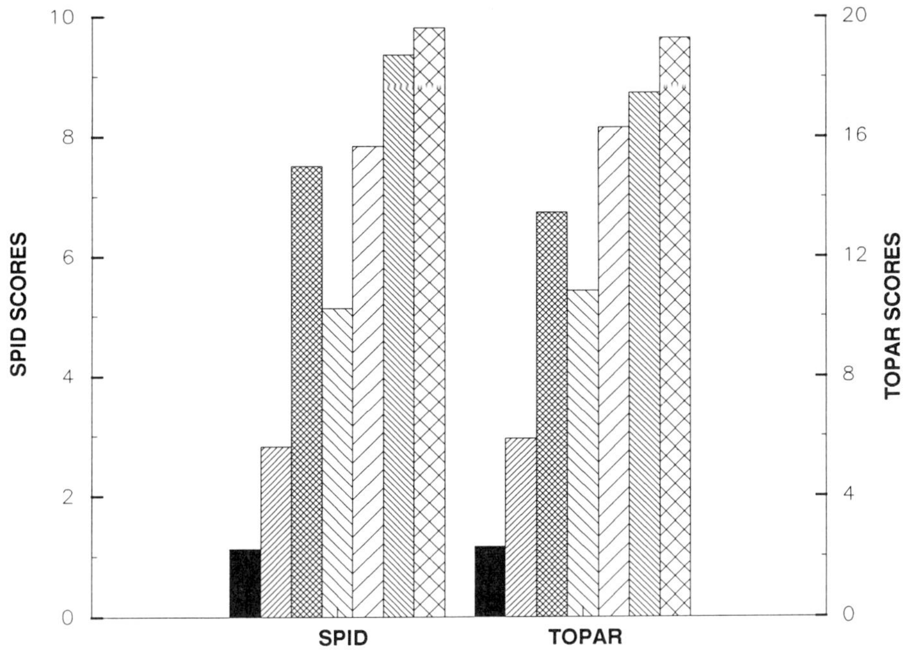

Figure 8 Mean sum of pain intensity difference (SPID) and total pain relief (TOPAR) scores from patients following oral surgery after a single oral dose of placebo (■); aspirin, 650 mg (▨); ibuprofen 400 mg (▩); bromfenac, 10 mg (⧅); 25 mg (▨); 50 mg (▧); 100 mg (⊠). (From Ref 4)

pharmacokinetic studies. The data were analyzed using the Verotta–Sheiner semiparametric procedure; the resulting model is shown in Figure 9. The effective concentration at the effect site that produced 50% of the maximal pain relief (EC_{50}) was approximately 0.4 μg/ml. The equilibrium half-life between the plasma and effect site was approximately 3 h. Thus, despite a rapid decline in bromfenac plasma concentrations, the concentrations at the site of action may be sustained long enough to produce a therapeutic effect for more than 8 h after a 50-mg dose (Fig. 10). Of interest is that the same EC_{50} (0.4 μg/ml) was obtained from animal pharmacokinetic and pharmacodynamic (PBQ writhing) data; this coincidence suggests that this animal test may be relevant in predicting the therapeutic dose in humans.

2. *Orthopedic Pain Studies*

A single-dose, double-blind, randomized study was conducted to compare the efficacy of three oral doses of bromfenac (5,10, and 25 mg), acetaminophen (1000 mg), and placebo in relieving pain after orthopedic surgery. The results from 159 patients revealed an apparent dose response for bromfenac (5). In contrast to oral surgery studies, the 5-mg dose did not produce significant analgesia, as compared with placebo. However, higher doses of bromfenac (10 and 25 mg) and acetaminophen were clearly separated from the negative control, as indicated by the 6-h SPID and TOPAR scores. Summary analgesic indexes also indicated that bromfenac (25 mg) provided significantly greater analgesia than bromfenac (5 mg). Inspection of the pain relief data (Fig. 11) for the 6-h evaluation shows that the high dose of bromfenac provided the longest duration of action, compared

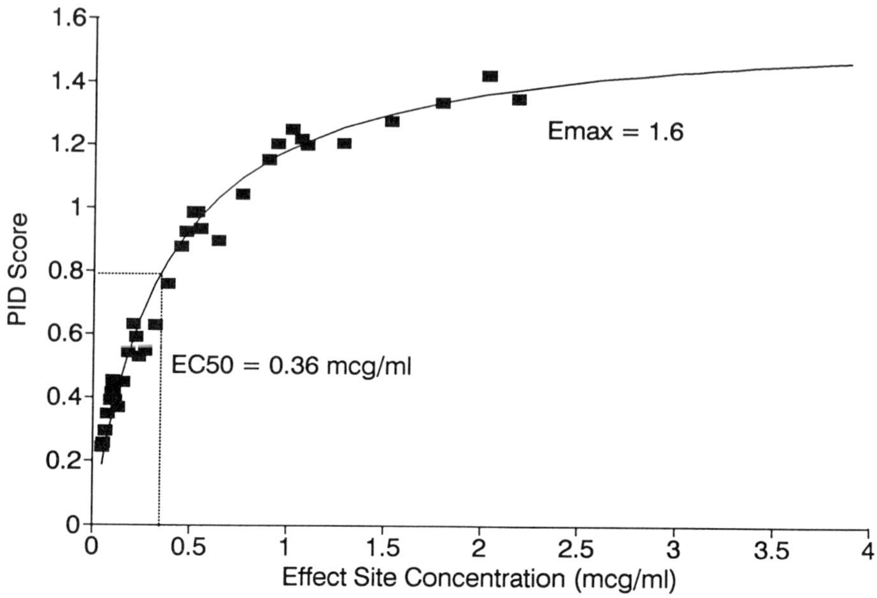

Figure 9 Relation between pain intensity difference (PID) scores and effect site concentrations using an E_{max} model. Bromfenac PK/PD response in humans.

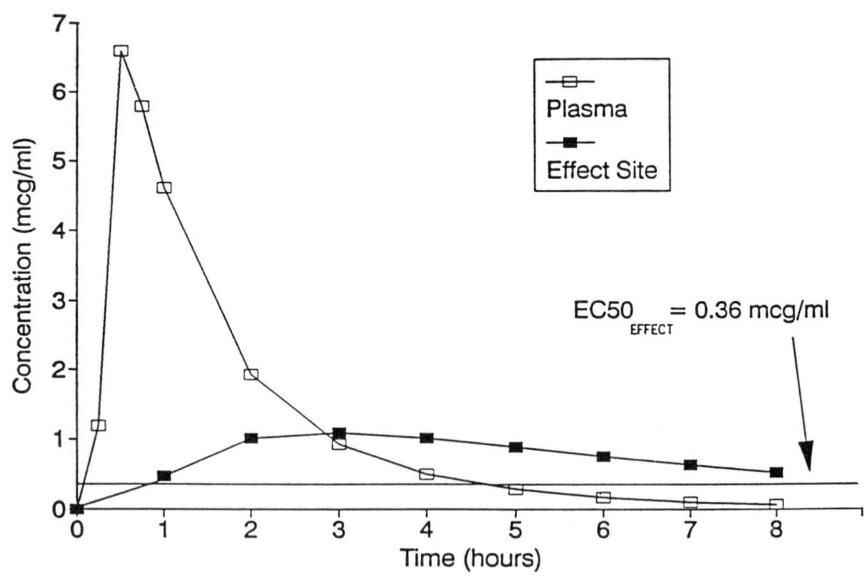

Figure 10 Plasma and effect site concentrations as a function of time in fasting subjects receiving a single 50-mg dose of bromfenac.

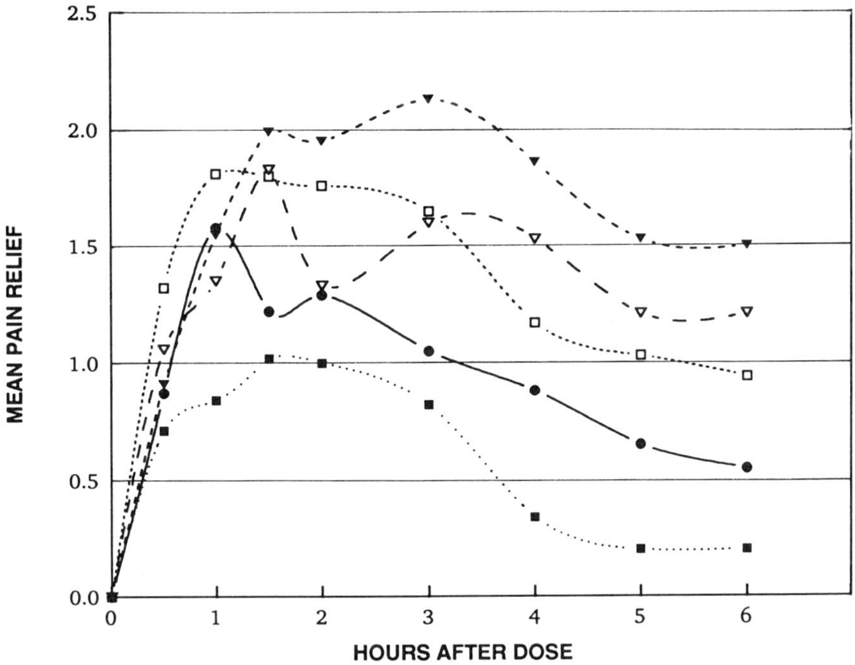

Figure 11 Mean pain relief scores in patients treated with bromfenac, acetaminophen (APAP), or placebo for postoperative orthopedic pain: placebo (■); APAP, 1000 mg (□); bromfenac, 5 mg (●); 10 mg (▽); 25 mg (▼).

with the other doses of bromfenac and acetaminophen (1000 mg). Overall, these data indicate that acetaminophen (1000 mg) provides a degree of analgesia similar to that produced by bromfenac (10 or 25 mg) in the orthopedic pain model.

The efficacy of bromfenac was examined in another single-dose study with 200 patients experiencing pain secondary to orthopedic surgery (6). The efficacy of bromfenac (25, 50, and 100 mg) and ibuprofen (200 and 400 mg) were compared under double-blind conditions. Even though a placebo control was not used, the trial was validated by a statistical separation between the low and high doses of ibuprofen. The three doses of bromfenac did not produce a dose-related response; bromfenac (25 mg) could not be separated from the two higher doses of bromfenac for any measure of analgesia. All doses of bromfenac appeared to produce analgesia equivalent to that produced by ibuprofen (400 mg), whereas bromfenac (25 and 100 mg) produced significantly higher levels of analgesia than ibuprofen (200 mg). These results indicate that bromfenac provides therapeutic levels of analgesia comparable with that obtained with ibuprofen (400 mg) in postoperative orthopedic pain.

B. Studies in Arthritis

Multicenter long-term studies of bromfenac in osteoarthritis and rheumatoid arthritis are in progress, One Phase II study comparing the efficacy of three dosages of bromfenac (20, 40, and 100 mg daily), aspirin (2600 and 4000 mg daily), and placebo has been completed. A total of 144 patients received one of the treatments for up to 6 weeks. The doses were taken four times a day with meals. End-points of efficacy included weight-bearing pain, the physician's global assessments, and the patient's global assessments. A preliminary analysis indicated that all doses of bromfenac were equally effective and, on the average, as active as the high dose of aspirin (4000 mg daily). All bromfenac treatments and the higher dose of aspirin were superior to placebo in all three variables. A small pilot dose–range study with 40, 100, and 200 mg of bromfenac per day was also completed in patients with rheumatoid arthritis.

VII. SAFETY PROFILE

The safety profile of bromfenac is based on limited experience, as Phase III studies have just recently been initiated. As with other NSAIDs, adverse events related to central nervous and gastrointestinal systems are preponderant in the safety profile obtained in the single-dose analgesic studies; the frequency of these effects was comparable with those observed with ibuprofen and aspirin. The most common complaints were dizziness, nausea, headache, vomiting, somnolence, abdominal pain, dyspepsia, and flatulence. No relation was detected between the dose and rates of adverse events.

The safety profile observed in the long-term studies is also characteristic of the NSAID class. Minor gastrointestinal complaints, headache, somnolence, and dizziness were most frequent. Among the laboratory signs, small and transient elevations in blood urea nitrogen and creatinine levels, as well as elevated transaminase activity have been observed.

VIII. PLACE OF BROMFENAC IN THERAPY

Bromfenac is a promising investigational agent for the treatment of acute and chronic pain. With its potent and long-lasting analgesic properties, bromfenac may provide an alternative to other analgesics. Remarkably, bromfenac (25–100 mg) appears to provide at least the same pain relief as ibuprofen (400 mg), a recognized benchmark in analgesic research. At this developmental stage, additional clinical research is required relative to the analgesic activity of bromfenac compared with other analgesics, including opioids, to define the usefulness of this compound in the treatment of pain. Additionally, the short- and long-term safety profile of bromfenac requires further quantification, a task presently being undertaken in Phase III trials.

REFERENCES

1. Sancilio LF, Nolan JC, Wagner LE, Ward JW. The analgesic and anti-inflammatory activity and pharmacologic properties of bromfenac. Drug Res 1987; 37:513–9.
2. Nolan HC, Osman MA, Cheng LK, Sancilio LF. Bromfenac, a new nonsteroidal anti-inflammatory drug: relationship between the anti-inflammatory and analgesic activity and plasma drug levels in rodents. J Pharmacol Exp Ther 1990; 254:104–8.
3. Forbes JA, Edquist IA, Smith FG, Schwartz MK, Beaver WT. Evaluation of bromfenac, aspirin, and ibuprofen in postoperative oral surgery pain. Pharmacotherapy 1991; 11:64–70.
4. Forbes JA, Beaver WT, Jones KF, Edquist IA, Gongloff CM, Smith WK, Smith FG, Schwartz MK. Analgesic efficacy of bromfenac, ibuprofen, and aspirin in postoperative oral surgery pain. Clin Pharmacol Ther 1992; 51:343–52.
5. McQuay HJ, Carroll D, Frankland T, Harvey M, Moore A. Bromfenac, acetaminophen, and placebo in orthopedic postoperative pain. Clin Pharmacol Ther 1990; 47:760–6.
6. Bostrom AS, Forbes JA, Adolfsson C, Beaver WT, Vavra I, Bell WE. An evaluation of bromfenac and ibuprofen in postoperative pain following orthopedic surgery. Pharmacotherapy 1993; (in press).

16

Pemedolac

THUY T. CHAU and BARRY M. WEICHMAN
Wyeth–Ayerst Research
Princeton, New Jersey

MARIE SANDA
Wyeth–Ayerst Research
Radnor, Pennsylvania

I. INTRODUCTION

Analgesics are broadly divided into two categories: the centrally acting and the peripherally acting analgesics. In the first category, strong narcotic analgesics, such as morphine, have been used for centuries to alleviate moderate to severe pain. Weaker narcotics, such as codeine or *d*-propoxyphene, are appropriate for the relief of mild pain. The clinical efficacies of these analgesics are, however, clouded by their side effects, which include tolerance after repeated administration, dependence liability, decreased intestinal motility, and most importantly, respiratory depression. Other centrally acting analgesics, such as antidepressants, cannabinoids, or neuropeptides, have shown promise in animal models, but their efficacies and side effect liabilities in clinical pain states remain uncertain.

The second category of analgesics, which also possess anti-inflammatory and antipyretic properties, belong to the broad class of nonsteroidal anti-inflammatory drugs (NSAIDs). These analgesics are widely prescribed, with two members, aspirin and ibuprofen, available over-the-counter (OTC). Inhibition of the cyclooxygenase pathway of arachidonic acid metabolism, resulting in inhibition of prostaglandin (PG) biosynthesis has been postulated as the major mechanism of action of NSAIDs (1). The inhibition of PG biosynthesis may occur at sites along the pain pathway during transmission of pain signals, or at an anti-inflammatory site, with the locations of such inhibition not only in the periphery, but also in the brain (2–7). The concomitant inhibition of PG biosynthesis in the gastronintestinal (GI) mucosa, where PGE_2 and PGI_2 exert cytoprotective actions, may result in the GI side effects commonly exhibited by the NSAIDs (8–10). This can lead to severe bleeding and, therefore, curtail their prolonged use in chronic pain.

Efforts in many laboratories have focused on identifying more efficacious and safer analgesics, which can be taken over a long period for the relief of moderate to severe pain. As a result, recently marketed NSAIDs have been developed that have effectiveness in cancer pain (ketorolac; 11) and may have a wider safety margin (etodolac; 12–14). A compound that is efficacious, safe, and at the same time demonstrates analgesic selectivity is even more desirable in conditions when pain is not accompanied by inflammation. The search in our laboratories has led to the identification of pemedolac, *cis*-1-ethyl-1,3,4,9-tetrahydro-4-(phenylmethyl)pyrano-[3,4,*b*]indole-1-acetic acid (Fig. 1), which is structurally related to etodolac (15). It is a white solid, with a molecular weight of 349.43, a p*K*a= 5.0, and is freely soluble in ethanol, chloroform, and dimethyl sulfoxide. However, despite inhibiting PG biosynthesis as an activity that pemedolac shares with NSAIDs, the compound offers a unique pharmacological profile distinct from the NSAIDs.

II. PRECLINICAL PHARMACOLOGICAL PROFILE

A. Analgesic Effects

The analgesic potency of pemedolac has been demonstrated in various animal models, using either chemical or mechanical stimuli (16,17). In the commonly employed writhing assays, the compound efficiently inhibited the abdominal contractions induced by *p*-phenylbenzoquinone (PBQ), acetic acid, or acetylcholine, either in mice or in rats, with a median effective dose (ED_{50}) values ranging from 0.3 to 2 mg/kg po. The potency of pemedolac in these tests was similar to that of the more potent NSAIDs, such as indomethacin, piroxicam, zomepirac, or ketoprofen, as well as to that of morphine. However, pemedolac was 16–80 times more potent than ibuprofen, aspirin, and etodolac against PBQ writhing in mice (Table 1), and 15–150 times more potent in other writhing models.

The analgesic effects of pemedolac were also demonstrated in the paw pressure model of hyperalgesia in rats (16). Injections of brewer's yeast, Freund's complete adjuvant (FCA), or PGE_2 into rat paws produced an acute inflammatory effect and lowered the pain threshold in response to the application of pressure to the edematous paws, as evidenced by paw withdrawal or a vocalization response of the animals. In contrast to opiates, which raise the pain threshold of both normal and inflamed paws, peripheral analgesics act on the injected paw only. In these tests, the oral ED_{50} of pemedolac was estimated to be 0.02 mg/kg (see Table 1). The dose–response curve however, was typified by a flat slope, which made the determination of an accurate ED_{50} difficult. Nevertheless, in these models of hyperalgesia, the potency of pemedolac was minimally equal to that of morphine, indomethacin, piroxicam, and ketoprofen, all of which exhibited dose–response curves steeper than that of pemedolac. The reason for the flat dose–response curve

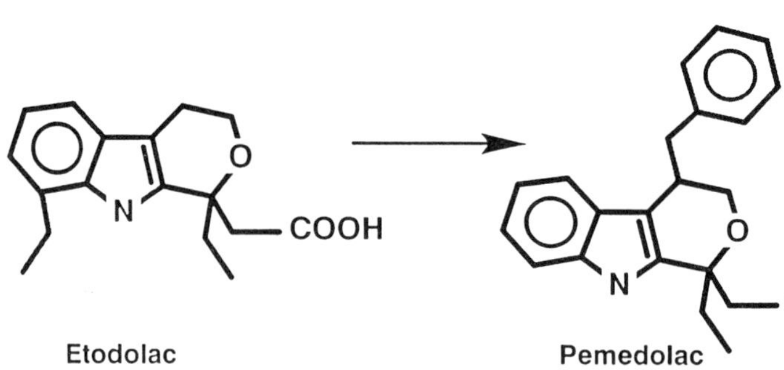

Figure 1 Pemedolac, *cis*-1-ethyl-1,3,4,9-tetrahydro-4-(phenylmethyl)pyrano[3,4-*b*]indole-1-acetic acid, a structural analogue of the NSAID, etodolac.

Table 1 Comparative Effects of Pemedolac and Reference Analgesics in Animal Models of Pain

	Oral ED_{50} (mg/kg)			
Drug	Mouse PBQ writhing[a]	Rat acetic acid writhing[a]	Rat paw pressure[b]	Dog urate synovitis[c]
Pemedolac	1.0	2.0	≤ 0.02	0.17
Indomethacin	1.5	3.6	0.4	0.2
Ketaprofen	2.3	11.0	2.0	
Piroxicam	3.4	7.0	0.35	
Naproxen	57.3	4.5	13.6	
Aspirin	89.0	81.3	28.4	23.0
Ibuprofen	32.4	54.8	64.5	1.6
Etodolac	168.0		4.5	

[a]The writhing response was induced by ip injections of a 0.02% solution of PBQ (0.15 ml/10 g body weight) to male CD mice (20–28 g) or 1% acetic acid (0.5 ml/100 g body weight) to male Sprague-Dawley rats (140–190 g). Drugs were administered by gavage 1 h before the noxious challenge. The number of writhes was determined for 15 min following PBQ or 20 min following acetic acid. The ED_{50} was the dose that decreased the number of writhes by 50% (26,27).

[b]Rats were injected with 0.1 ml FCA (5 mg/ml dead *Mycobacterioum butyricum*) into the hind paw. At 24 h drugs or vehicle were administered orally. Determination of the pain threshold (paw withdrawal) was performed 1 h later. A 50% increase in the pain threshold was considered a positive response. The ED_{50} was the dose that produced positive response in 50% of the animals (28).

[c]Synovitis was induced by the injection of 5 mg sodium urate crystal in the right knee joint of mongrel dogs (15–20 kg). Paw pressure was determined by an automated measuring platform at regular intervals, for 2 h before oral administration of drugs, and thereafter, for another 3 h. The ED_{50} was the dose that reestablished the injected paw pain threshold to 50% of the normal threshold (29).

remains to be determined, but it is unlikely that it is due to an unusual effect of pemedolac in the rat, inasmuch as the drug's inhibition of acetic acid writhing in rats is described by a steeper dose–response curve that is similar to that of other analgesics.

The analgesic potency of pemedolac was also observed in the dog, in which it inhibited the hyperalgesia associated with urate synovitis (ED_{50} = 0.17 mg/kg po). In this model, pemedolac was equipotent with indomethacin. Thus, pemedolac exhibited analgesic activity against experimental pain in three species; mice, rats, and dogs.

In the writhing assay in mice and paw pressure assay in rats, pemedolac exhibited a long duration of action. At a dose that produced approximately 80% analgesic effect, substantial antinociception was still maintained 10–12 h after administration. This duration of action suggests that, in clinical situations, the compound may not require frequent administration, thereby minimizing the possibility for the development of tolerance. In animal studies, no tolerance to the analgesic effects of pemedolac was observed after repeated administration in the mouse PBQ writhing or rat paw pressure assays (16).

Pemedolac does not appear to exert its analgesic effects by either a central or peripheral opiate mechanism (16). Because tolerance is a well-known characteristic drawback of opiates, its absence implies that pemedolac differs from the opiates. Further evidence is provided by the failure of naloxone to antagonize pemedolac's analgesic effects, either in the mouse writhing or in the rat paw pressure tests. Under the same experimental conditions, the antinociceptive effects of morphine were completely abolished by naloxone. Furthermore, high doses of pemedolac were inactive in the mouse hot plate and tail-flick tests, which are analgesic models more sensitive and specific for opiates. The possibility that pemedolac may be an opiate agonist–antagonist, being inactive against heat-induced nociception, was ruled out by pemedolac's lack of effect on the potency of morphine in the mouse tail-flick test. Also, unlike morphine, pemedolac did not elicit the jumping response in mice when challenged with naloxone after acute or repeated administrations. Because the jumping response is one of the characteristics of the withdrawal syndrome in mice and is indicative of dependence liability, the data strongly suggest that pemedolac will not produce physical dependence in humans by an opiate mechanism.

B. Separation of Analgesic from Anti-Inflammatory and Ulcerogenic Effects

Unlike other NSAIDs, pemedolac presents a unique analgesic-selective profile. When assessed for its anti-inflammatory activity against rat carrageenan paw edema, a model of acute inflammation, pemedolac inhibited the edema by 50% or less at doses from 100 to 200 mg/kg po (16). Likewise, the primary inflammatory response induced in the rat paw 3 days after the injection of FCA was inhibited by 37% by pemedolac at a daily dose of 25 mg/kg po for 3 days. Similarly, in another model of acute inflammation, reverse passive Arthus pleurisy in rats, pemedolac showed a weak inhibitory effect on fluid accumulation with an ED_{30} of 46 mg/kg po (17). The weak anti-inflammatory effects of pemedolac were observed at doses that were higher than the analgesic doses in rats. In contrast, reference NSAIDs, such as indomethacin, naproxen, piroxicam, and ibuprofen, displayed similar analgesic and anti-inflammatory potencies in these animal models (Table 2).

Table 2 Effects of Pemedolac and Reference NSAIDs in Models of Acute Inflammation in Rats

	Oral ED_{50} (mg/kg)	
Drug	Carrageenan paw edema[a]	Preventive adjuvant edema[b]
Pemedolac	48% inhib. at 100 mg/kg	37% inhib. at 25 mg/kg
Indomethacin	2.9	1.0
Piroxicam	1.3	3.2
Naproxen	2.9	31.5
Phenylbutazone	20.4	95.0
Etodolac	23.0	11.2
Ibuprofen	20.7	51.0
Aspirin	124.5	309.0

[a]Edema was induced by 0.1 ml carrageenan (2% suspension in saline) injected into the left hind paws of CD rats. Paw volumes were measured 3 h postcarrageenan application. Drugs or vehicle were administered by gavage 1 h before the phlogistic agent. The ED_{50} was the dose that decreased the edema volume by 50% (30).

[b]CA (0.1 ml of 5 mg *Mycobacterium butyricum* per milliliter of mineral oil) was injected into the left hind paws of CD rats on day 0. Drugs or vehicle were administered by gavage on days 0, 1, and 2. Paw volumes were measured on day 3. The ED_{50} was the dose that decreased the edema volume by 50% (31).

Pemedolac displayed antipyretic activity at doses intermediate to the analgesic and anti-inflammatory doses. Although the body temperature of normal rats was not affected, pemedolac reduced elevated body temperature in rats rendered hyperthermic by subcutaneous injections of brewer's yeast in a dose-related manner over the 5- to 20-mg/kg–po dose range, with the effect lasting for 6 h. Typical NSAIDs, such as ibuprofen, naproxen, and indomethacin, reduced the fever at doses identical with or lower than the analgesic doses. For instance, naproxen at 3 mg/kg po or ibuprofen at 10 mg/kg po was found to inhibit hyperthermia almost completely in rats.

In situations when immediate relief of pain is necessary, a parenterally administered analgesic would be more advantageous. The availability of a soluble sodium salt formulation of pemedolac offers the potential use of the compound as an injectable analgesic. In the rodent writhing assays, the potency of pemedolac sodium was similar whether it was given orally, intramuscularly, or intravenously, indicating that the compound was readily bioavailable. This observation was confirmed in hyperalgesia models. The duraction of analgesic action (time at which the compound lost 50% of its original analgesic activity) was longest when the intramuscular route of administration was employed (about 12 h in rats, or 16 h in mice, for an ED_{80} dose). As expected, the intravenous route of administration offered the shortest duration of action (5 h). Again, as noted previously for orally administered pemedolac, repeated parenteral administrations did not result in either accumulated effects or in tolerance (18).

Besides its selective analgesic properties, pemedolac presents a unique safety profile. Reference NSAIDs produced gastric irritation in rats at doses similar to those at which analgesic and anti-inflammatory actions were noted (16). In rats, pemedolac given orally, either in one single dose to fasted rats, or once daily for 4 days to fed rats, showed UD_{50} values (dose at which 50% of the animals have a GI effect ranging from mild irritation to ulcers) of 107 mg/kg and 140 mg/kg per day, respectively. Therefore, the safety index, calculated as the ratio between the analgesic ED_{50} in rats (2 mg/kg in the acetic acid-induced writhing or 0.02 mg/kg in the paw pressure assay) and the UD_{50}, is at least 50, which implies that pemedolac has a large safety index. Interestingly, the gastric effects of pemedolac occur at doses associated with the drug's anti-inflammatory activity.

In several pharmacological safety studies, pemedolac showed unremarkable activity at doses that were several times the analgesic doses. In the charcoal meal test in mice, pemedolac had no constipating effects at 100 mg/kg po, nor antidiarrheal activity at the same dose in the castor oil test in rats. The compound did not affect experimental cardiovascular variables in spontaneously hypertensive rats at doses up to 30 mg/kg po. It did not significantly affect urine output nor sodium excretion of saline-loaded rats. Likewise, it did not exhibit central nervous system (CNS) effects, as indicated by its inactivity in locomotor tests in mice and rats. Pemedolac appeared devoid of metabolic effects, for it did not alter food intake; plasma glucose, serum cholesterol, or triglyceride levels; or liver weight in rats.

Recently, much attention has been focused on the chirality of therapeutic agents, with the goal of minimizing clinical variability and toxicity (19). Several known NSAIDs are mixtures of two optical isomers, with the pharmacological activities usually residing in the (+)-isomer (20). The ratio between the activities of the two isomers, however, varies with the compound used, the animals tested and, most importantly, the rate of interconversion of the isomers. Pemedolac has the 4-(phenylmethyl) group and the 1-acetic acid group on the same side of a plane containing the flat indole moiety. The molecule is asymmetric and exists as a mixture of two optical isomers, (1*S*, 4*R*)-(+)-pemedolac and (1*R*, 4*S*)-(–)-pemedolac, from here on referred to as (+)-pemedolac and (–)-pemadolac, respectively. Thus, it was important to evaluate the biological properties of the isomers to determine which possessed the analgesic activity.

In the analgesic models employed, the activity of pemedolac appeared exclusively in the (+)-isomer. In the PBQ, acetic acid, or acetylcholine writhing assays in rodents, the potency of the (+)-isomer equaled that of the racemic compound, whereas the (–)-isomer was inactive at doses 10- to 50-fold higher than the ED_{50} of either pemedolac or the eutomer. Similar results were also obtained in the rat paw pressure models. It is not yet known why the potency of the (+)-isomer was not twice that of the racemate, because there is a 1:1 ratio of the two isomers in the racemic mixture. It is likely that the inherent variabilities of the in vivo models do not allow the consistent detection of a twofold difference in potency. However, pharmacokinetics and tissue distribution may be other factors contributing to the observed similar potency of the racemic pemedolac and its enantiomer. As expected, (+)-pemedolac was devoid of effects in the hot plate and tail-flick tests, and its analgesic activity in the writhing assays was not affected by naloxone. Again, as seen with the racemic compound, repeated administrations of the active enantiomer did not result in tolerance or dependence.

In acute or chronic models of inflammation, similar to the racemate, the (+)-enantiomer exhibited anti-inflammatory activity, but it was weaker, relative to the analgesic potencies. The anti-inflammatory activity of (+)-pemedolac was at least 30 times weaker than that of indomethacin. For instance, in the carrageenan paw edema model of acute inflammation, (+)-pemedolac inhibited the edema in a non–dose-related manner from 60 to 240 mg/kg po, with 56% inhibition at the highest dose. Indomethacin, in this assay, showed an ED_{50} of 3 mg/kg po. In the adjuvant arthritis model of chronic inflammation, the ED_{50} values of (+)-pemedolac and indomethacin were 4–8 mg/kg po and 0.1–0.3 mg/kg po, respectively. The (–)-isomer also showed some weak anti-inflammatory effects in the carrageenan paw edema model (minimum effective dose = 90 mg/kg), but was inactive in the chronic model of adjuvant arthritis at doses up to 36 mg/kg per day. All animals treated with high doses of pemedolac or its isomers appeared to tolerate the compounds and gained weight steadily, as exemplified by the 9-day treatment period in rats with established adjuvant arthritis. This may reflect the weak gastroirritant effects of pemedolac. In acute studies, the separation between the dose of (+)-pemedolac that caused gastric lesions (72 mg/kg) and that that produced analgesia in the rat paw pressure test (0.07 mg/kg) was large. The (–)-enantiomer also exhibited gastroirritant effects at a very high dose (200 mg/kg). Thus, the analgesic activities of pemedolac are due to the (+)-isomer, wheras preliminary results suggest that high doses of (–)-pemedolac may have weak anti-inflammatory and gastroirritant effects. Studies are now underway to fully define the pharmacokinetics of the isomers and the racemate.

III. MECHANISM AND SITE OF ACTION

Inasmuch as pemedolac is a member of the pyranocarboxylic acid drug class and, therefore, structurally related to the NSAID etodolac, it is not surprising that pemedolac inhibits prostaglandin biosynthesis. However, pemedolac's profile of relative analgesic selectivity and its wide safety margin in animals distinguishes it from some other NSAIDs and implies that pemedolac may possess an additional mechanism or site of action different from the NSAIDs.

Whereas pemedolac inhibited the cyclooxygenase pathway of arachidonic acid metabolism, it did not affect the 5-lipoxygenase pathway. For example, in rat peritoneal exudate cells, A23187-induced thromboxane B_2 and PGE_2 biosyntheses were inhibited with IC_{50} values of 2×10^{-8} M and 3×10^{-8} M, respectively, whereas 5-hydroxyeicosatetraenoic acid (5-HETE), and leukotriene (LT)B_4 biosyntheses were not inhibited by pemedolac at concentrations as high as 1×10^{-5} M. Similarly, pemedolac inhibited PGE_2 biosynthesis in isolated bovine articular chondrocytes, with an IC_{50} of 1×10^{-8} M. Thus, as an inhibitor of PG biosynthesis, pemedolac possessed a potency similar to its structural analogue, etodolac. Interestingly, pemedolac inhibited acetic acid-induced 6-keto-$PGF_{1\alpha}$ production in the mouse peritoneal cavity, with an ID_{50} of 0.44 mg/kg po, an effect that correlated with its ability to inhibit the acetic acid writhing response (21). Despite being similar to etodolac in potency in vitro, pemedolac appeared approximately 100-fold more potent in this pain model in vivo. This observation suggests that pharmacokinetic considerations may help explain the difference between these two analogues. Inasmuch as the volume of distribution was greater for pemedolac, it may have the capability of distributing to a greater part of the body. The calculated log P for pemedolac is 4.4, indicating that it is approximately tenfold more lipophilic than etodolac (log P = 3.5) (22). Despite these theoretical considerations, drug distribution studies using [^{14}C] pemedolac did not uncover any unusual site of drug accumulation.

Noxious stimuli induce pain either by acting directly at the nociceptive neurons or by releasing endogenous mediators, such as prostaglandins, that sensitize the neurons to the actions of other pain mediators (2,3,23,24). Inhibition of the formation of prostaglandins at the periphery is believed to be a primary mechanism of action of NSAIDs. This, however, does not exclude a central mechanism, either by inhibition of prostaglandin synthesis or by another mechanism. Several NSAIDs that exhibit analgesic and antipyretic properties without having significant anti-inflammatory activity (e.g., acetaminophen) have inhibited the cyclooxygenase enzyme in nervous tissues (25).

The fact that [^{14}C]pemedolac was not detected in significant amounts in brain tissue of rats following parenteral administration implied that the major site of drug action is peripheral. Furthermore, studies were performed with pemedolac sodium administered intracerebroventricularly (icv) in the mouse PBQ writhing assay. Pemedolac sodium, given icv, produced a dose-dependent antinociceptive response in the mice challenged with PBQ, with an ED_{50} of 40 μg per mouse. However, if one considers the iv potency (4 mg/kg or 80 μg per mouse), the iv/icv ratio is only 2, whereas with a typical centrally acting analgesic, the ratio of parenteral/central doses is much higher (e.g., 80 for morphine). This observation implies that the central component, if it exists, is not likely the main mechanism of action of pemedolac. It also suggests that the analgesic effect in these icv studies is due to a leakage of the compound into the peripheral circulation. This suggestion was supported by the ability of icv pemedolac to inhibit acetic acid-induced 6-keto-$PGF_{1\alpha}$ biosynthesis in the peritoneal cavity. Furthermore, it is unlikely that pemedolac is an opiate, since the icv effects in the mouse writhing assay were not sensitive to naloxone. Pemedolac sodium was not active either in the tail-flick or hot plate tests when administered icv to the mouse. Indeed, the significance of these observations depends on the ability of the compound to cross the blood–brain barrier.

The ability of pemedolac to interfere with the actions of other pain mediators was investigated in several in vitro and in vivo models. Using radioligand-binding techniques in vitro, pemedolac did not compete for the receptor-binding sites for bradykinin (BK), substance P, opiates, and serotonin, nor those of 33 other binding sites. In vivo, pain responses elicited by bradykinin were not blocked by pemedolac, but were antagonized by the bradykinin receptor BK_2 antagonist, NPC567. Finally, as before, the analgesic actions of pemedolac in rat and mouse models were not affected by the opiate antagonist, naloxone.

Because pemedolac is a racemate, studies were undertaken to ascertain if one of the enantiomers affected the biological activity of the other as an explanation for pemedolac's profile. However, analgesic activity resided exclusively in the (+)-enantiomer, and was not affected by coadministration of the (–)-enantiomer in the PBQ writhing assay. The profile of the (+)-enantiomer was indistinguishable from that of the racemate, implying that interactions between the enantiomers do not account for pemedolac's unique profile.

Thus, the present understanding of pemedolac's mechanism of action is that, similar to the NSAIDs, it is capable of inhibiting prostaglandin biosynthesis. Unlike the NSAIDs, it has weak anti-inflammatory and gastroirritant effects, actions that are noted at doses higher than those at which analgesia occurs. The reason for this preclinical profile remains to be elucidated and confirmed by clinical trials.

IV. TOXICOLOGY STUDIES

The results of 1-month and 6-month toxicology studies in rats and dogs confirmed the wide safety margin projected in the preclinical pharmacology studies. In acute toxicity studies, the LD_{50} of pemedolac in male and female mice ranged from 853 to 994 mg/kg po and in male and female rats from 317 to 334 mg/kg po. Therefore, the therapeutic index of pemedolac was minimally 425 in mice and 160 in rats.

In the 1-month toxicology study in rats, the major limiting effect was gastrointestinal lesions noted in a few animals receiving the high dosage of 180 mg/kg per day. These gastrointestinal effects were not noted in rats receiving 10, 20, or 50 mg/kg per day. In dogs receiving pemedolac daily for 1 month, no drug-related effects were noted on gross or microscopic observations at doses of drug up to 50 mg/kg per day.

In the 6-month study in rats, a dosage of 10 mg/kg per day was without biological effect, whereas a dosage of 50 mg/kg per day produced some renal papillary necrosis and interstitial nephritis and alterations in clinical chemistry values. The effects noted in rats at the 100-mg/kg per day dosage were more pronounced. In dogs, remarkable effects were not noted at 5, 10, or 40 mg/kg per day, but a dosage of 80 mg/kg per day was associated with gastrointestinal ulceration and secondary tubular nephrosis, secondary hematological changes, and changes in clinical chemistry values.

Pemedolac was not mutagenic in the Ames test, the in vitro Chinese hamster ovary chromosomal aberration test, the in vitro unscheduled DNA synthesis rat hepatocyte assay, or the in vivo micronucleus assay in mice.

V. CLINICAL PHARMACOLOGY

The tolerability of orally administered pemedolac has been investigated in two studies with healthy volunteers. Forty-two men participated in the first study, which had a double-blind, placebo-controlled, ascending single-dose design. There were six dose level groups, with the pemedolac dose ranging from 5 to 160 mg. At each dose level, five subjects received active drug and two subjects received placebo. Pemedolac was well tolerated after single doses. Subsequently, the tolerability of multiple daily dosages of pemedolac was studied in healthy men. Again, a double-blind, placebo-controlled, ascending-dose design was used. Dosages of 5–80 mg bid or matching placebo were given to 22 healthy male subjects for 2 weeks. Pemedolac was generally well tolerated. No significant differences in safety evaluation between pemedolac treatment and placebo were observed.

A preliminary pharmacokinetic evaluation was performed in conjunction with the tolerability studies. The results indicate that pemedolac was rapidly absorbed following oral administration, with peak serum concentrations occurring within 1–2 h. Mean oral dose clearance was high (1.5 L h^{-1} kg^{-1} after single doses, 1.8 L h^{-1} kg^{-1} at steady state) and was consistent among the dose levels. The mean apparent oral dose steady-state volume of distribution was large (3–7 L/kg) and variable, and the mean $t_{1/2}$ was approximately 7 h. The results after the single doses and at a steady state suggested that the serum concentration of pemedolac was in linear proportion to the dose administered.

VI. SUMMARY

In conclusion, pemedolac is a potent, long-acting, nonopiate analgesic, with an apparent peripheral mechanism of action. Although it structurally derives from the NSAID etodolac and shares one mechanism of action in common with classic NSAIDs, the compound distinguishes itself by its analgesic selectivity and gastrointestinal safety. The mechanism underlying this difference, as well as a demonstration of clinical efficacy remain to be established for pemedolac. Inital Phase I studies suggested that this drug was well tolerated by healthy volunteers. At this stage, other possible mechanisms of action have been discounted, since pemedolac does not interact with a series of receptor-binding sites or other enzyme systems. Preliminary studies have indicated that the analgesic activity of the compound resides in the (+)-isomer, and that high doses of the (–)-isomer have gastroirritant effects. The availability of a soluble sodium salt makes parenteral formulation of pemedolac possible for use as an injectable in the immediate relief of pain. As clinical trials progress, it will be interesting to ascertain if the profile exhibited by pemedolac in animals is borne out in humans.

REFERENCES

1. Vane JR. Inhibition of prostaglandin synthesis as a mechanism of action for aspirin-like drugs. Nature 1971; 231:232–5.
2. Ferreira SH, Vane JR. New aspects of the mode of action of non-steroid antiinflammatory drugs. Annu Rev Pharmacol 1974; 14:57–73.
3. Ferreira SH, Lorenzetti BB, Correa FMA. Central and peripheral antialgesic action of aspirin-like drugs. Eur J Pharmacol 1978; 53:39–48.
4. Okuyama S, Aihara H. The mode of action of analgesic drugs in adjuvant arthritic rats as an experimental model of chronic inflammatory pain: possible central analgesic action of acidic non-steroidal antiinflammatory drugs. Jpn J Pharmacol 1984; 35:95–103.
5. Okuyama S, Aihara H. Hyperalgesic action in rats of intracerebroventricularly administered arachidonic acid, PGE_2, and $PGF_{2\alpha}$: effect of analgesic drugs on hyperalgesia. Arch Int Pharmacodyn 1985; 278:13–22.
6. Nakamura H, Shimoda A, Ishii K, Kadokawa T. Central and peripheral analgesic action of non-acidic non-steroidal antiinflammatory drugs in rats and mice. Arch Int Pharmacodyn 1986; 282:16–25.
7. Taiwo YO, Levine JD. Indomethacin blocks central nociceptive effects of $PGF_{2\alpha}$. Brain Res 1986; 373:81–4.
8. Whittle BJR. Relationship between the prevention of rat gastric erosions and the inhibition of acid secretion by prostaglandins. Eur J Pharmacol 1976; 40:233–9.
9. Whittle BJR. Temporal relationship between cyclooxygenase inhibition, as measured by

prostacyclin biosynthesis, and the gastrointestinal damage induced by indomethacin in the rat. Gastroenenterology 1981; 80:94–8.
10. Main IHM, Whittle BJR. Investigation of the vasodilator and antisecretory role of prostaglandins in the rat gastric mucosa by use of non-steroidal antiinflammatory drugs. Br J Pharmacol 1975; 53:217–24.
11. Buckley MM-T, Brogden RN. Ketorolac. A review of its pharmacodynamic and pharmacokinetic properties, and therapeutic potential. Drugs 1990; 39:86–109.
12. Humber LG. Etodolac: the chemistry, pharmacology, metabolic disposition, and clinical profile of a novel antiinflammatory pyranocarboxylic acid. Med Res Rev 1987; 7:1–28.
13. Karbowski A. A global safety evaluation of etodolac. Clin Rheum 1989; 8:73–9.
14. Zvaifler N. A review of the antiarthritic efficacy and safety of etodolac. Clin Rheum 1989; 8:43 53.
15. Katz AH, Demerson CA, Shaw C-C, Asselin AA, Humber LG, Conway KM, Gavin G, Guinosso C, Jensen NP, Mobilio D, Noureldin R, Schmid J, Shah U, Van Engen D, Chau TT, Weichman BM. Synthesis and analgesic activity of pemedolac (*cis*-1-ethyl-1,3,4,9-tetrahydro-4-(phenylmethyl)pyrano[3,4-*b*] indole-1-acetic acid). J Med Chem 1988; 31:1244–50.
16. Chau TT, Weichman BM. Pemedolac: a novel and long acting non-narcotic analgesic. J Pharmacol Exp Ther 1989; 248:907–15.
17. Weichman BM, Chau TT. Pemedolac: a novel nonopiate analgesic. In: Zor U, Naor Z, Danon A, eds. Leukotrienes and prostanoids in health and disease. New trends in lipid mediators research. vol. 3. Basel: S Karger, 1989:124–9.
18. Chau TT, Weichman BM. Analgesic profile of the sodium salt of pemedolac. Pharmacologist 1988; 30:103.
19. Lee EJD, Williams KM. Chirality: clinical pharmacokinetic and pharmacodynamic considerations. Clin Pharmacokinet 1990; 18:339–45.
20. Bellamy N, Cox S, Campbell J. Relationship between enantiomer levels of flurbiprofen and clinical response in rheumatoid arthritis. Inflammopharmacology 1991; 1:37–47.
21. Berkenkopf JW, Weichman BM. Production of prostacyclin in mice following intraperitoneal injection of acetic acid, phenylbenzoquinone, and zymosan: its role in the writhing response. Prostaglandins 1988; 36:693–709.
22. Mobilio D, Humber LG, Katz AH, Demerson CA, Hughes P, Brigance R, Conway K, Shah U, Williams G, Labbadia F, DeLange B, Asselin A, Schmid J, Newburger J, Jensen NP, Weichman BM, Chau T, Newman G, Wood DD, Van Engen D, Taylor N. Structure–activity relationships among analogues of pemedolac, *cis*-1-ethyl-1,3,4,9-tetrahydro-4-(phenylmethyl)pyranol[3,4-]*b*]-indole-1-acetic acid, a potent analgesic agent. J Med Chem 1988; 31:2211–7.
23. Ferreira SH, Nakamura M, Castro NS. The hyperalgesic effect of prostacyclin and prostaglandin E_2. Prostaglandins 1978; 16:31–7.
24. Willis AL. Parallel assay of prostaglandin-like activity in rat inflammatory exudate by means of cascade perfusion. J Pharm Pharmacol 1969; 21:126–8.
25. Flower RJ, Vane JR. Inhibition of prostaglandin synthesis in brain explains the antipyretic activity of paracetamol (4-acetamidophenol). Nature 1972; 240:410–1.
26. Siegmund E, Cadmus R, Lu G. A method for evaluating both non-narcotic and narcotic analgesics. Proc Soc Exp Biol Med 1957; 95:729–31.
27. Niemegeers CJE, VanBruggen JAA, Janssen PAJ. Suprofen, a potent antagonist of acetic acid-induced writhing in rats. Arzneimittelforschung 1975; 25:1505–9.
28. Randall LD, Selitto JJ. A method for measurement of analgesic activity on inflamed tissue. Arch Int Pharmacodyn Ther 1957; 111:409–19.
29. Carlson RP, Dakto LJ, Welch TM, Parvis WF, Shaw GW, Thompson JL, Brunner TR. An automated microcomputer-based system for determining canine paw pressure quantitatively in the dog synovitis model. J Pharmacol Methods 1986; 15:95–104.

30. Winter CA, Risley EA, Nuss GW. Carrageenan-induced edema in hindpaw of the rat as an assay for antiinflammatory drugs. Proc Soc Exp Biol Med 1962; 3:544–7.
31. Wax J, Tessman DK, Winder CV, Stephens MD. A sensitive method for the comparative bioassay of non-steroidal antiinflammatory compounds in adjuvant-induced primary inflammation in the rat. J Pharmacol Exp Ther 1975; 192:166–71.

17

Pravadoline

A Dual-Mechanism Aminoalkylindole Analgesic

SUSAN J. WARD
Sterling Winthrop Pharmaceutical Research Division
Rensselaer, New York

I. INTRODUCTION

Pravadoline (Fig. 1), the maleate salt of WIN 48098, was originally synthesized as a putative cyclooxygenase inhibitor in which the inclusion of a basic amine was designed to limit gastric irritancy relative to typical acidic nonsteroidal anti-inflammatory drugs (NSAIDs). Pravadoline indeed proved to be a cyclooxygenase-inhibiting antinociceptive agent, devoid of gastrointestinal toxicity. Unexpectedly, however, pravadoline was found to possess several additional properties uncharacteristic of cyclooxygenase inhibitors. Most importantly, pravadoline was effective against a greater range of nociceptive stimuli than are NSAIDs and, against some inflammatory stimuli, was also more efficacious.

The clinical attractiveness suggested by pravadoline's superior preclinical profile prompted both an intensive investigation to identify its underlying molecular mechanism, and clinical assessment of pravadoline's analgesic actions. A series of studies revealed that pravadoline, in common with related aminoalkylindoles, has agonist activity at the cannabinoid receptor that may contribute to pravadoline's analgesic and behavioral profile. Clinical evaluation revealed pravadoline to be effective against moderate and moderately severe postoperative pain in humans.

Pravadoline was discontinued from further clinical development when evidence of nephrotoxicity was observed following multiple administrations in humans. A nephrotoxic potential was also observed in dogs. However, subsequent studies in dogs also revealed that this toxicity is associated with the maleate salt in pravadoline, and *not* with the WIN 48098 molecule per se. Thus, an alternative, nonnephrotoxic salt form of WIN 48098 may yet become of clinical use.

II. BIOCHEMICAL PROPERTIES

Pravadoline is a member of a series of aminoalkylindoles in which molecules possess varying degrees of two distinct biochemical properties: inhibition of cyclooxygenase (1),

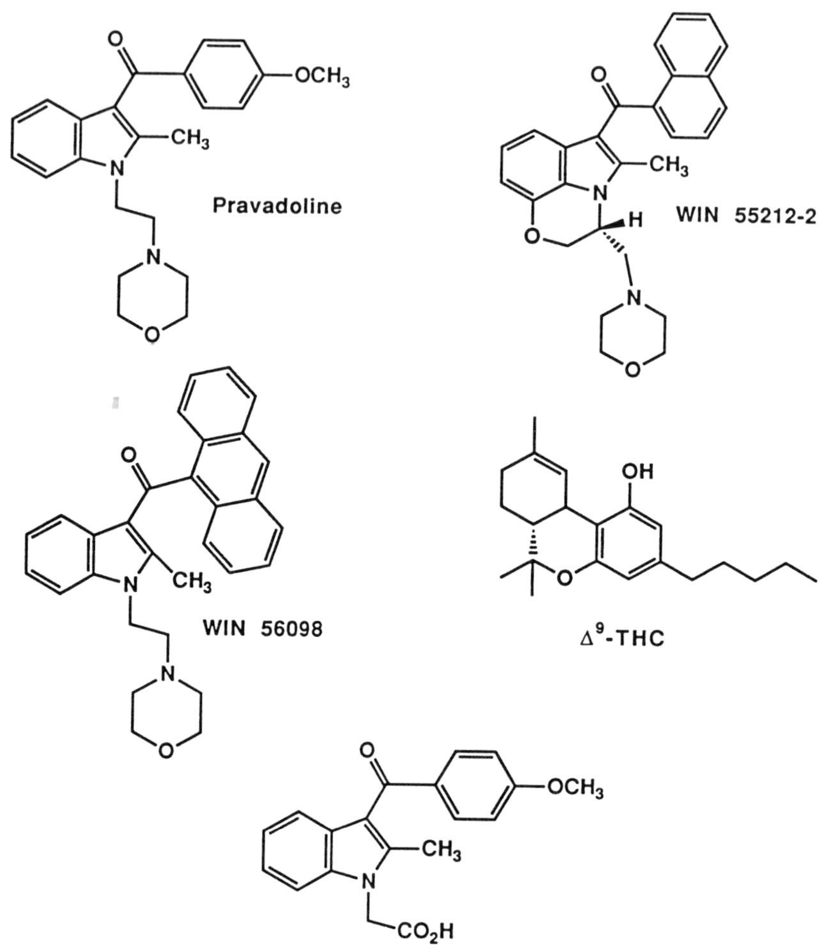

WIN 31041

Figure 1 The structures of the base forms of pravadoline; WIN 55212-2, an aminoalkylindole cannabinoid receptor agonist; WIN 56098, a cannabinoid receptor antagonist; Δ^9-tetrahydrocannabinol (THC); and WIN 31041, a major metabolite of pravadoline.

and agonist activity at cannabinoid receptors (2). Although some molecules in the series possess only one activity or the other (1), pravadoline possesses both properties (3–5).

A. Inhibition of Cyclooxygenase

Pravadoline inhibits prostaglandin formation in mouse brain microsomes in vitro, and attenuates ex vivo the 2-min postmortem rise in prostaglandin E_2 (PGE_2) formation that occurs in the brain (6) (Fig. 2). It is probable that the mechanism by which pravadoline inhibits formation of prostaglandins is by inhibition of cyclooxygenase, since, in the same concentration range, pravadoline also inhibits arachidonic acid-induced oxygen consumption (a more direct measure of cyclooxygenase activity; 7) (see Fig. 2). Pravadoline is

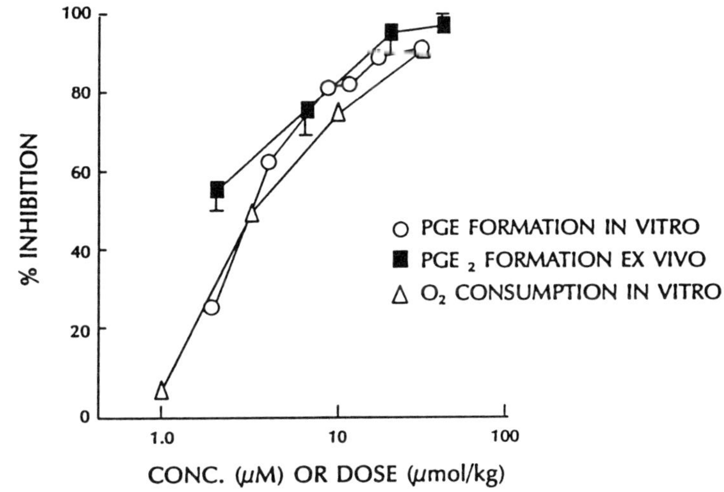

Figure 2 Inhibition of cyclooxygenase by pravadoline: inhibition of prostaglandin formation from [^{3}H]arachidonic acid by the microsomal fraction of mouse brain in vitro (○), inhibition of O_2 consumption by cyclooxygenase in homogenates of bovine seminal vesicles in vitro (△), and inhibition ex vivo of the postmortem rise in PGE_2 in mouse brain 2 min following sacrifice (■). Values are the mean ± SEM of three separate determinations in vitro, and of at least five determinations ex vivo. (From Ref. 3 and Miller M, unpublished observations; △).

more potent as a cyclooxygenase inhibitor than acetaminophen and ibuprofen, has similar potency to naproxen, and is less potent than zomepirac and indomethacin (Table 1).

B. Agonist at Cannabinoid Receptors

Unexpectedly, pravadoline and a subseries of related aminoalkylindoles possessed an agonist action at cannabinoid receptors. This cannabinoid property was discovered by elucidating the mechanism underlying initial observations suggesting that pravadoline possesses a distinct additional, non–cyclooxygenase-related mechanism (2–5). The cannabinoid actions of pravadoline are illustrated in Figure 3. Pravadoline binds to cannabinoid receptor-binding sites (2,8–10) labeled by either the classic cannabinomimetric [^{3}H]CP-55940 (11,12) or by the aminoalkylindole [^{3}H]WIN 55212-2 (13) (see Fig. 1) (8–10). Although the affinity of pravadoline for the cannabinoid receptor is low compared with classic cannabinoids and some aminoalkylindole analogues (Table 2), the interaction appears competitive, since the Hill coefficient approximates –1 (9).

The binding affinity of pravadoline for cannabinoid receptors is reflected in an agonist action. Thus, in a manner similar to cannabinoids (14,15), pravadoline inhibits adenylate cyclase activity in rat cerebellar membranes, and inhibits electrically stimulated contractions of the mouse isolated vas deferens (see Table 2) (4). These actions are mediated by the cannabinoid receptor, since pravadoline's actions (a) are antagonized by the selective cannabinoid receptor antagonist WIN 56098 (see Figs. 1 and 4) (2,4,16), and (b) are not antagonized by other G-protein-coupled receptor antagonists (2,4). Moreover, pravadoline falls on the line of correlation between binding affinity and functional activity for other cannabinoid receptor agonists (Fig. 5).

Table 1 Effects of Pravadoline and Reference Cyclooxygenase Inhibitors on Prostaglandin Synthesis in Mouse Brain

Compounds	IC_{50} In vitro (μM) PG formation[a]	O_2 consumption[b]	ED_{50} Ex vivo[c] (mg/kg po)
Pravadoline	4.9 (3.6–6.8)	3.4 (2.8–4.2)	20 (9–38)
Ibuprofen	12.5 (7.8–20)		2.3 (0.8–5.7)
Indomethacin	0.5 (0.47–0.76)	0.7 (0.2–.1)	0.1 (0.04–0.3)
Naproxen	6.7 (1.5–30)	9.9 (4.6–21.2)	1.7 (0.8–3.0)
Zomepirac	0.4 (0.23–0.83)	2.2 (0.3–16.8)	0.3 (0.2–0.6)
Acetaminophen	362 (231–569)	~ 2500	113 (61–290)

IC_{50} and ED_{50} values with 95% CL were calculated from a graded dose–response analysis of the concentration–effect curve (56).
[a]Cyclooxygenase activity was measured in vitro in the microsomal fraction of mouse brain in the presence of 13 μM [^{14}C]arachidonic acid; the four radiolabeled products were isolated by thin-layer chromatography.
[b]Cyclooxygenase activity was measured directly by inhibition of 0_2 consumption in the conversion of μM arachidonic acid by homogenates of bovine seminal vesicles.
[c]PGE_2 formation was measured ex vivo by assessing accumulation of PGE_2 over a 2-min period after decapitation. PGE_2 concentration was assessed by radioimmunoassay.
Sources: Data adapted from [a]Ref. 3; [b]Miller M, unpublished observations; [c]Ref. 6.

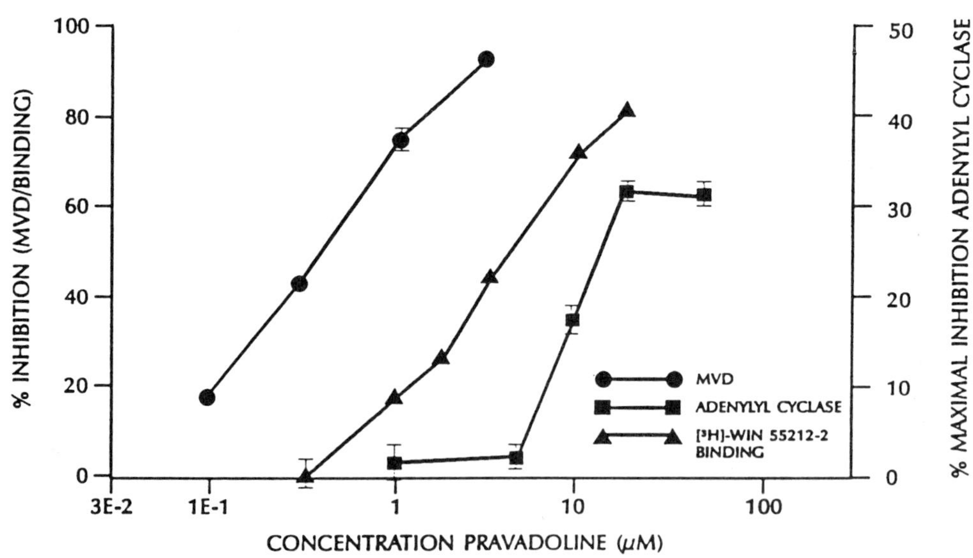

Figure 3 Cannabinoid properties of pravadoline (i.e., effect of pravadoline at the cannabinoid receptor): inhibition of specific binding of [^{3}H]WIN 55212-2 to rat cerebellar homogenates (▲), inhibition of basal adenylate cyclase activity in rat cerebellar homogenates (■), and inhibition of electrically stimulated contractions of the mouse isolated vas deferens preparation (●). Values are the mean ± SEM of three or more separate determinations. (Data from Refs. 4,5,8–10).

Table 2 Effects of Pravadoline, AAI Analogues, and Cannabinoids at Cannabinoid Receptors in Vitro

	K_i (nM)		IC_{50}	
Compound	[^{3}H]WIN 55212-2[a]	[^{3}H]CP55940[b]	Adenylate cyclase (μ)M[c]	Mouse vas deferens (nM)[d]
Pravadoline	2511 ± 177	12% at 1 μM	3.6 ± 1.4	319 ± 63
WIN 55212-2	2.2 ± 0.26	1.1	0.32 ± 0.08	0.4 ± 0.1
Δ^9-THC	10.2 ± 0.78	1.6 ± 0.56		4.0 ± 0.49
CP-55940	0.35 ± 0.044	0.07 ± 0.007	0.15 ± 0.03	0.3 ± 0.03
Levonantradol			0.12 ± 0.04	0.93 ± 0.28
Cannabidiol	2420 ± 323	>500		>10,000

[a]Specific inhibition of [^{3}H]WIN 55212-2 binding to rat cerebellar membranes. Values are mean of at least three determinations. Hill coefficients do not deviate significantly from 1.
[b]Specific inhibition of [^{3}H]CP 55940 binding to P_2 homogenates of rat brain. Values are the mean of three determinations.
[c]Inhibition of [^{3}H]cAMP production in low pH-treated rat cerebellar membranes. Values are mean of at least three determinations.
[d]Inhibition of electrically stimulated contractions of the mouse isolated vas deferens preparation. Values are the mean of at least three determinations.
Source: [a]Refs. 8–10; [b]Refs. 8–12; [c]Refs. 4,57; [d]Ref. 8.

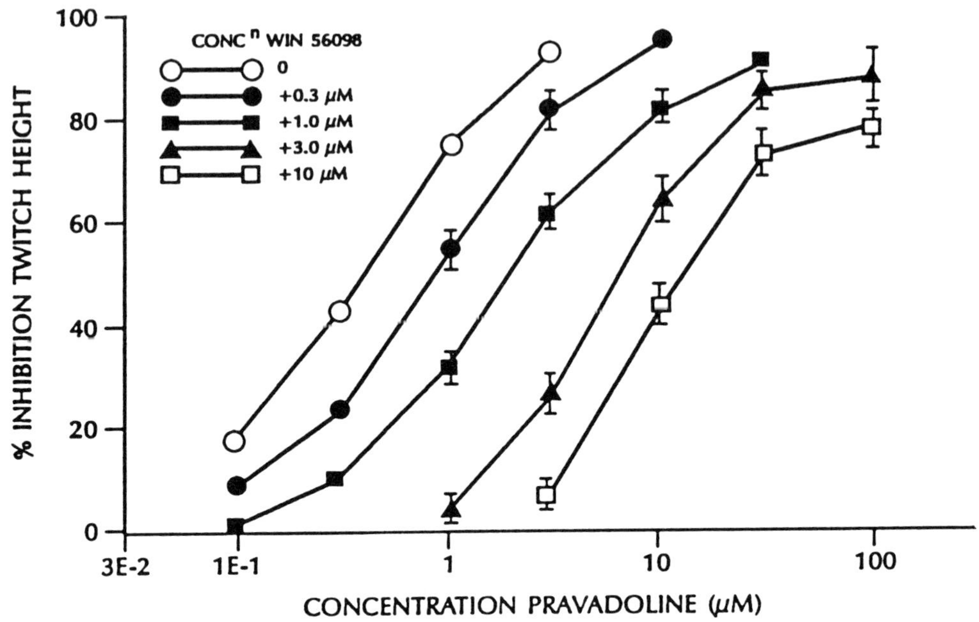

Figure 4 Antagonism of cannabinoid agonist actions of pravadoline by the cannabinoid antagonist WIN 56098: Inhibition of electrically stimulated contractions of the mouse isolated vas deferens preparation by pravadoline in the absence (○) and in the presence of 0.3 μM (●), 1 μM (■), 3 μM (▲), and 10 μM (□) WIN 56098. Values are the mean ± SEM of three to five separate determinations. (Data from Ref. 4)

III. PRECLINICAL THERAPEUTIC PROFILE

A. Antinociceptive Profile

Assessment in a range of nociceptive assays that incorporate chemical, thermal, and inflammatory stimuli, demonstrates that pravadoline has greater antinociceptive efficacy than do classic NSAIDs. This enhanced efficacy is manifest in two ways:

First, in many nociceptive assays, classic NSAIDs have a "ceiling" to their antinociceptive action, such that higher doses do not produce a greater antinociceptive effect. The actions of zomepirac in three chemical nociceptive assays and in the adjuvant arthritis rat model illustrate this point (Fig. 6). In contrast with zomepirac, and in a manner more similar to morphine, pravadoline produces steep dose–response curves in these assays and a high maximal effect (see Fig. 6).

Second, pravadoline is effective against a greater range of nociceptive stimuli than are classic NSAIDs and other cyclooxygenase inhibitors (Table 3) (3). In common with most cyclooxygenase inhibitors, pravadoline is antinociceptive against intraperitoneal acetylcholine, intraperitoneal acetic acid, and intra-arterial bradykinin (see Table 3). Also, in common with most cyclooxygenase inhibitors, pravadoline is effective against brewer's yeast-induced hyperalgesia, although pravadoline's potency in this assay is higher (relative to potency in other assays in the same species) than one would predict for a typical cyclooxygenase inhibitor (see Table 3). Moreover, whereas other cyclooxygenase inhibitors are essentially ineffective (maximal effect $\leq$ 30%) against intraperitoneal prostaglandin E_2 (PGE_2), high-dose (3 mg/kg) intraperitoneal p-phenylbenzoquinone

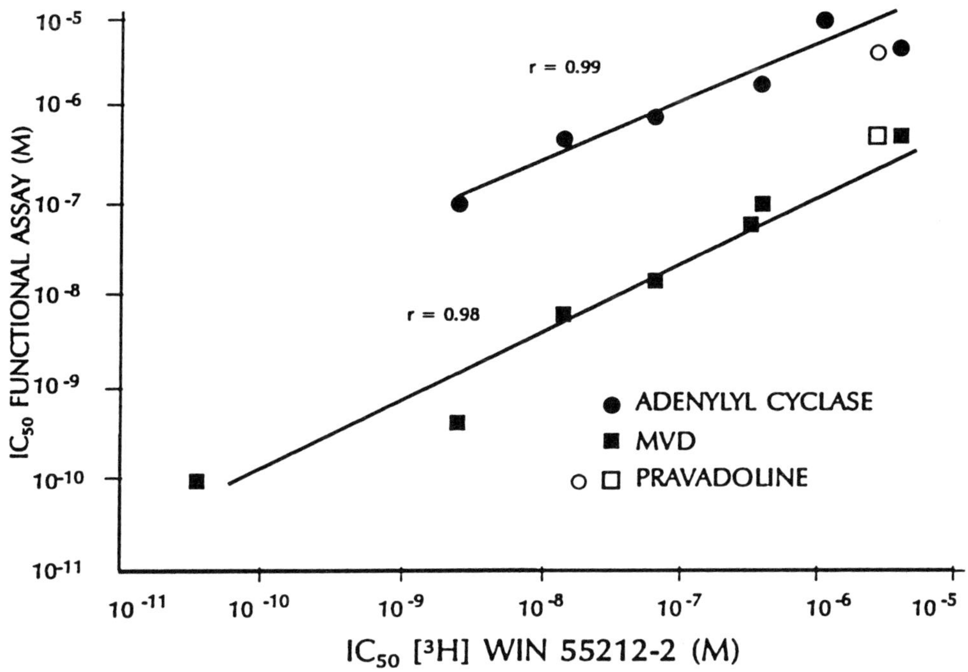

Figure 5 Correlation of binding affinity and agonist actions of pravadoline and cannabinoids: binding affinity of aminoalkylindole (AAI) and classic cannabinoids is shown as a function of agonist potency to inhibit basal adenylate cyclase activity in rat cerebellar homogenates (●) ($r = 0.93$), and to inhibit electrically stimulated contractions of the mouse isolated vas deferens preparation (■) ($r = 0.97$). Values for pravadoline in each paradigm are also shown (○,□) and lie within the 95% confidence limits for the correlations of affinity versus function. (Data from Ref. 2, 4, and 9).

(PBQ), or a 55°C thermal nociceptive stimulus, pravadoline is antinociceptive in all of these assays (see Table 3).

B. Mechanism of Antinociception

The mechanism by which pravadoline displays greater antinociceptive range and efficacy than other cyclooxygenase inhibitors is likely a consequence of its dual molecular mechanism. In a manner similar to pravadoline and morphine, cannabinoid receptor agonists, such as Δ^9-tetrahydrocannabinol (THC; see Fig. 1) and levonantradol, are effective against a 55°C thermal stimulus (17–19) and against both high-dose intraperitoneal PBQ (3 mg/kg) and intraperitoneal PGE_2 (20). Similarly, cannabinoid receptor agonists, such as pravadoline, and in contrast with cyclooxygenase inhibitors, demonstrate a high maximal effect in assays, such as the acetic acid-induced writhing model (Table 4). Thus, in these assays, pravadoline's antinociceptive activity may be mediated by cannabinoid agonist action. The relative contribution of pravadoline's two molecular mechanisms is less clear in assays, such as the acetylcholine-induced writhing assay, in which classic NSAIDs are active. Thus, as illustrated in Figure 7, in the acetylcholine-induced writhing assay, pravadoline falls on the line of the correlation between antinociceptive activity and molecular mechanism for *both* cyclooxygenase inhibitors and cannabinoid receptor agonists.

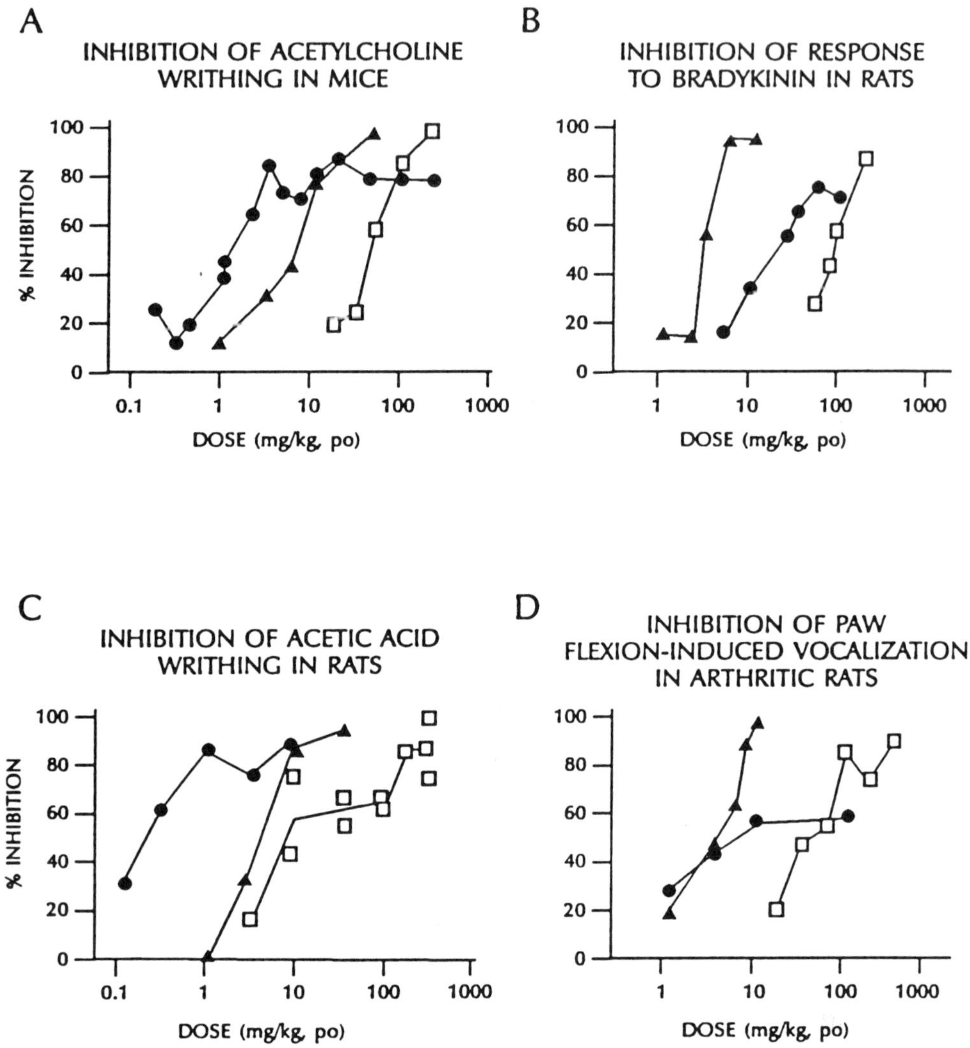

Figure 6 Antinociceptive profile of pravadoline (□) compared with morphine (▲) and zomepirac (●) following oral administration in rodents: inhibition of nociceptive responding to (A) intraperitoneal acetylcholine (3.2 mg/kg) in mice, (B) intra-arterial bradykinin (0.1–0.5 μg) in rats, (C) intraperitoneal acetic acid (0.5 ml of 9%), and (D) flexion of the hind paw in rats administered a subplantar injection of Freund's adjuvant 14 days previously. In panel (D), morphine was administered subcutaneously. (Data from Ref. 3).

The locus of antinociceptive action of pravadoline has not been established. The NSAIDs are traditionally thought to produce antinociception by an action in the periphery (21); however, a central site of action should not be discounted (22,23). It may be pertinent that pravadoline is effective in the acetylcholine-induced writhing assay following intracerebroventricular administration (ED_{50} = 124 nmol per mouse) (24) and after intrathecal administration (ED_{50} = 11 nmol per mouse; Ward SJ, unpublished observations); pravadoline potency after intravenous administration is 4 mg/kg, or approximately 230 nmol per mouse. Analysis of the distribution of cannabinoid receptor-binding sites has as

Table 3 Antinociceptive Potency of Pravadoline and Reference Analgesic Drugs

Compound	Acetylcholine writhing[a] (mouse)	Acid writhing[b] (rat)	IA bradykinin[c] (rat)	Randall–Selitto[d] (rat)	PGE_2 writing[e] (mouse)	PBQ writhing[f] (mouse)	Tail immersion[g] (55°C) (mouse)
Pravadoline	41 (26–61)	14.6 (13.9–15.5)	78 (72–84)	1	24 (18–31)	44 (17–114)	100
Aspirin	88 (37–209)	25.3 (18.1–35.3)	121 (46–455)	100		>300	>300
Ibuprofen	9.2 (4.6–18)	43.5 (15.3–124)	70 (43–114)	3	178 (126–252)	>300	>300
Indomethacin	3.2 (2.4–4.3)	2.4 (1.4–4.2)	18.2 (7.5–44)	10		>30	>100
Naproxen	10.9 (4.2–29)	1.1 (0.57–2.0)	4.6 (2.5–8.6)	100	>550[h]	>30	300
Zomepirac	0.8 (0.3–2.3)	0.34 (0.11–1.0)	3.1 (2.1–4.7)	17.3	>300[h]	>100	>1000
Acetaminophen	139 (85–229)	143 (73–280)	126 (85–188)	300	173 (123–245)	>300	>300
Timegadine	71 (38–127)	4.2 (2.3–7.6)		3	682 (132–3528)		
Morphine	6.2 (4.6–8.3)	5.2 (3.4–7.7)	~30[i]	3	0.7 (0.4–1.3)	8 (5–16)	3

[a]Values are ED_{50} (mg/kg, po) (95% confidence limits; *CL*) to inhibit the percentage of mice demonstrating nociceptive response to ACh bromide (3.2 mg/kg, ip).
[b]Values are ED_{50} (mg/kg, po) (95% CL) to inhibit the nociceptive response of rats given 0.5 ml of 9% acetic acid ip
[c]Values are ED_{50} (mg/kg, po) (95% CL) to inhibit the nociceptive response of rats given an intracartotid threshold dose of bradykinin (0.1–0.5 μg/0.2 ml injection) (58).
[d]Values are MED (mg/kg, po) to attenuate the mechanical hyperalgesia induced by 0.1 ml subplantar injection of a 20% suspension of brewer's yeast into rat hind paw.
[e]Values are ED_{50} (mg/kg, po) (95% CL) to inhibit the percentage of mice demonstrating a nociceptive response to PGE_2 (0.3 mg/kg, ip).
[f]Values are ED_{50} (mg/kg, po) (95% CL) to inhibit the percentage of mice demonstrating a nociceptive response to PBQ (3 mg/kg, ip).
[g]Values are MED (mg/kg, sc) to increase latency of mice to withdraw their tail from emersion into 55°C water (59).
[h]Less than 30% effect at maximally tested dose.
[i]An accurate ED_{50} could not be determined because of the steepness of the dose–response curve.
Sources: Data from [a–e,g] Ref. 3; [f]Ref. 60.

Table 4 Antinociceptive[a] Effects of Pravadoline, AAI Analogues and Cannabinoids

Compound	ED_{50} (mg/kg, po) ACh	ED_{50} (mg/kg, po) PBQ	Acetic acid ED_{50} (CL) (mg/kg po)	Acetic acid E_{max} (%)
Pravadoline	41 (26–61)	388[b]	14–6 (13.9–15.5)	>95
WIN 55212-2	33 (20–56)	30[b]	7.5	>95
Δ^9-THC	32	106 (55–205)	~ 5[b]	>95
Levonantradol	0.7	2.6 (1.3–5.3)		

[a]Assay systems described in Table 2.
[b]Confidence limits could not be calculated owing to inadequate number of data points between 16 and 84%.
Source: Data from Ref. 20.

yet failed to reveal any specific sites in peripheral tissue. Within the central nervous system (CNS), the concentration of cannabinoid receptors in laminar II of the dorsal horn of the spinal cord (25), and the ability of cannabinoids to produce antinociception after intrathecal administration (26–28), suggests the spinal cord as one potential locus of action.

C. Predicted Clinical Analgesic Profile

Collectively, the data suggest that pravadoline may be effective against more diverse, and possibly more severe, pain than are NSAIDs. Although some preclinical antinociceptive models can distinguish relative efficacy between NSAIDs and opioids, generally these assays are not designed to distinguish among the more efficacious drugs (e.g., between pentazocinelike and morphinelike compounds). Thus, even though the antinociceptive profile of pravadoline in preclinical assays is similar to that of morphine, one cannot conclude that pravadoline's efficacy in humans will fully mimic that of morphine. Cannabinoid agonists, including THC, levonantradol, and nabilone, are analgesic in humans against postoperative and cancer pain (11,29–32). Thus, one might predict that both of pravadoline's molecular properties could mediate analgesia in humans. The absence of direct comparisons of maximal efficacy of cannabinoids and NSAIDs in humans leaves open the question of whether pravadoline could possess analgesic activity against more severe pain as a consequence of its cannabinoid receptor agonist property.

IV. BIODISPOSITION

Pravadoline is well absorbed from the gastrointestinal tract in mice, rats, dogs, monkeys, and humans (33–35). It is cleared preponderantly by metabolism in all species, and the indole acetic acid analogue of pravadoline, WIN 31041 (1) (see Fig. 1), is always a major metabolite. Key biodispositional parameters of pravadoline in humans, estimated from studies with radiolabeled pravadoline, are summarized in Table 5; biodisposition is similar to that seen preclinically. The t_{max} and $t_{1/2}$ values do not differ for pravadoline and its major

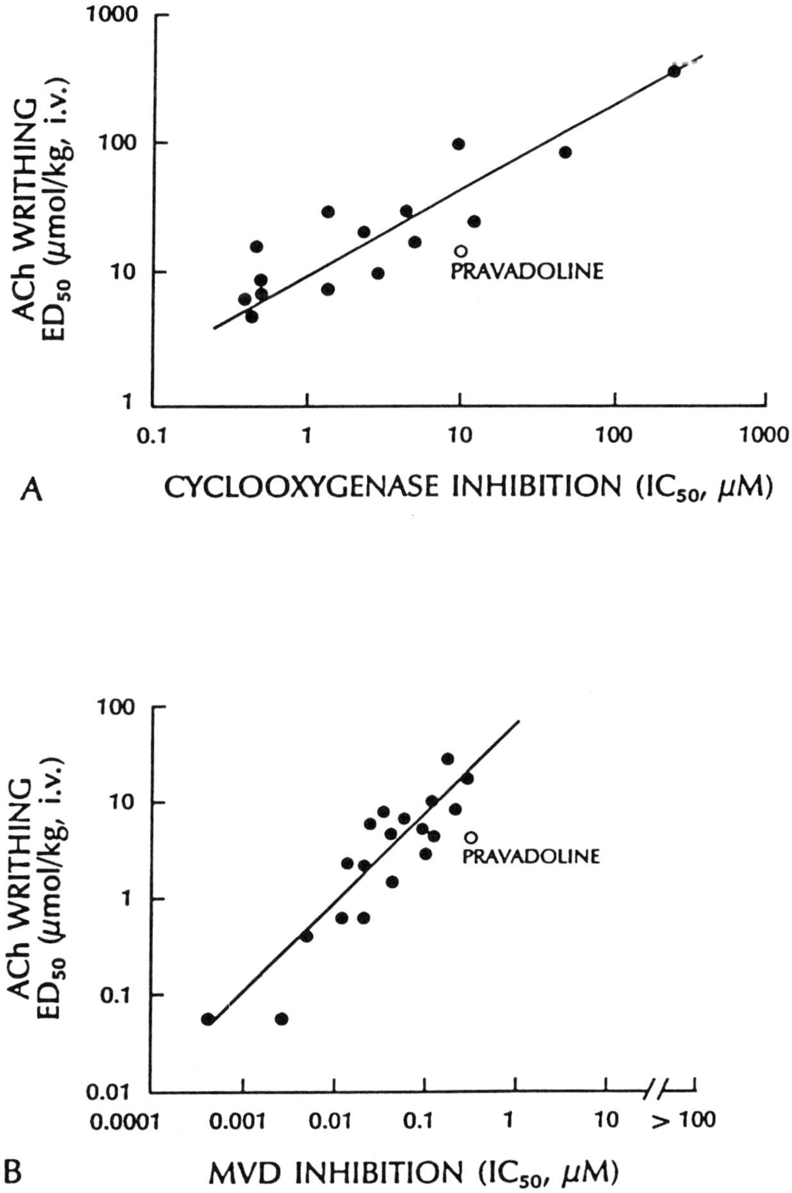

Figure 7 Molecular mechanism of pravadoline-induced antinociception: Antinociceptive potency of (A) cyclooxygenase inhibitors, and (B) cannabinoid agonists to attenuate the acetylcholine-induced nociceptive response in mice is shown as a function of affinity for molecular target in vitro (r = 0.82 and 0.87, respectively). Values for pravadoline are also shown (○) and lie within the 95% confidence limits for the correlations of affinity versus antinociceptive potency. (Data from Refs. 2, 3, and 20).

metabolite; C_{max} and the area under the concentration–time curve (AUC) are approximately two times higher for pravadoline (see Table 5). Consistently, at peak plasma levels, pravadoline and WIN 31041 represent approximately 20–35% and 10–15% of total radioactivity in plasma. In a comparison of biodisposition in fed and fasted states in humans (34), the t_{max} of pravadoline was 1.4 h in both instances, and the $t_{1/2}$ in plasma ranged from 6.9 to 7.6 h. Appurtenant to a possible central site of action of pravadoline (see foregoing), studies in mice indicate that brain levels of pravadoline are approximately three times higher than those seen in plasma, and that levels of WIN 31041 in brain are below detection limits (Rosi D, Miller MS, Ward SJ, unpublished observations). The pK_a of pravadoline is 4.3. The degree to which pravadoline is protein-bound in plasma has not been determined.

V. ANCILLARY PHARMACOLOGY AND TOXICOLOGY

A. Lack of Gastrointestinal Irritancy

Pravadoline does not produce gastric lesions following either single-dose or multiple-dosing regimens to rats, mice, or dogs, even at lethal doses (3). Table 6 compares pravadoline with

Table 5 Biodisposition of [^{14}C]Pravadoline in Normal Male Volunteers. Values Are Mean ± Standard Deviation Derived from Plasma Measurements in $N = 5$ Subjects

	t_{max} (h)	C_{max} (mg/ml)	$t_{1/2}$ (h)	AUC (mg h/ml)
Pravadoline	1.6 ± 0.2	3.52 ± 0.71	5.7 ± 1.4	12.2 ± 2.9
WIN 31041	1.6 ± 0.2	1.43 ± 0.39	8.3 ± 6.8	5.80 ± 2.03

The dose of pravadoline maleate was equivalent to 600 mg base, and contained approximately 92 μCi of ^{14}C (in the aroyl ring of pravadoline).
Source: Baker JF, unpublished observations.

Table 6 Comparative Effects of Pravadoline and Reference Compounds on Gastric Lesion Scores in Rodents After Acute po Dosing

	Single-dose studies MED (mg/kg po)				Two-dose studies ED_{50} (mg/kg po × 2) (95% confidence limits)
Compound	Mouse	Therapeutic ratio[c]	Rat	Therapeutic ratio[d]	Mouse
Pravadoline	>1000[a]	>24	>1000[a]	>68	>1730[a,b]
Aspirin	30	0.3	30	1.2	>1000[a]
Ibuprofen	10	1	30	0.7	199 (136–291)
Indomethacin	3	1	10	4	16 (11–23)
Naproxen (Na)	100	9	3	3	220 (130–308)
Zomepirac (Na)	0.55	0.6	10	29	41 (14–120)
Acetaminophen	>1000[a]	>7	>1000[a]	>7	
Carprofen	>1000[a]	>12	100	>17	

[a]Compound did not significantly increase lesion scores at the highest dose tested.
[b]Two of eight mice died at this dose; stomachs of the mice that died were not examined.
[c]Ratio relative to ED_{50} in ACh-induced writhing assay.
[d]Ratio relative to ED_{50} in acetic acid-induced writhing assay.
Source: Ref. 3.

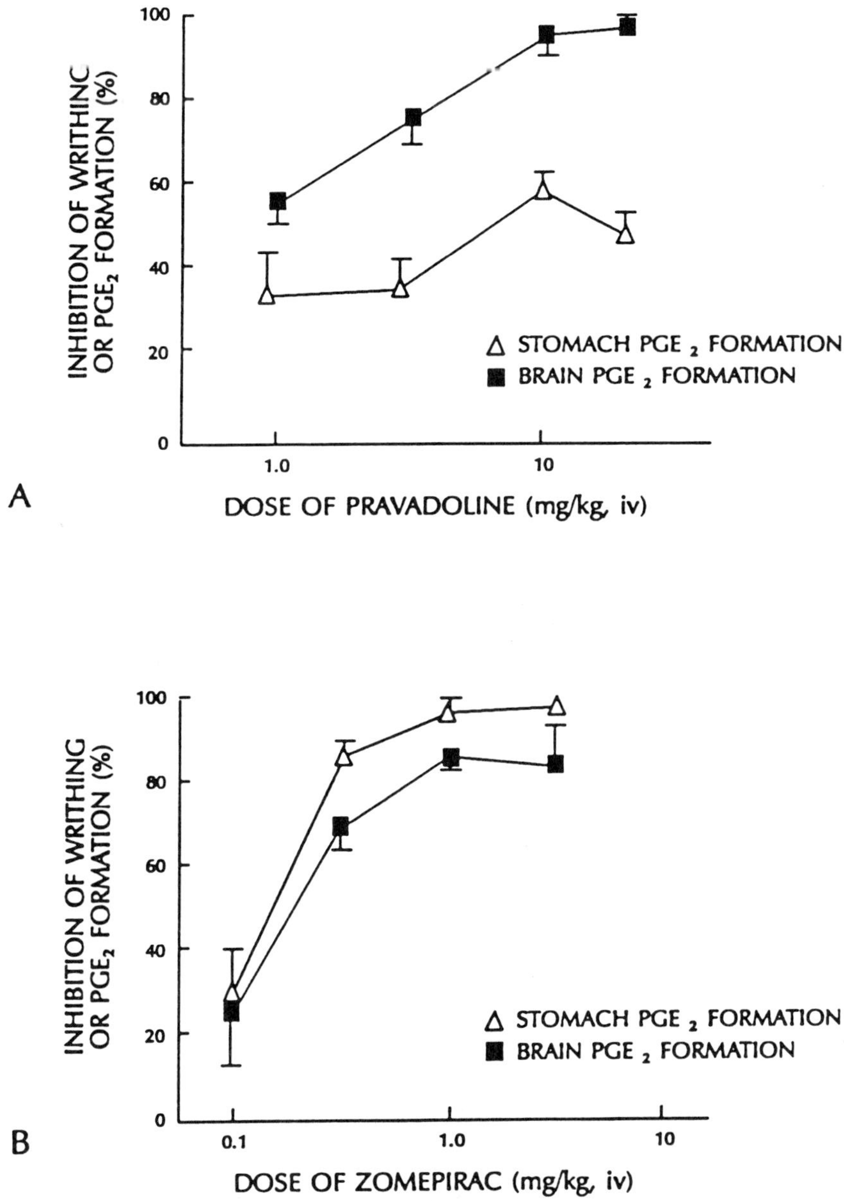

Figure 8 Selective inhibition of ex vivo PGE_2 formation in brain by pravadoline: Inhibition of the postmortem rise in PGE_2 2 min following sacrifice in brain (□) and in stomach (△) by (A) pravadoline and (B) zomepirac. Values are the mean ± SEM of at least five separate determinations. (Data from Ref. 3).

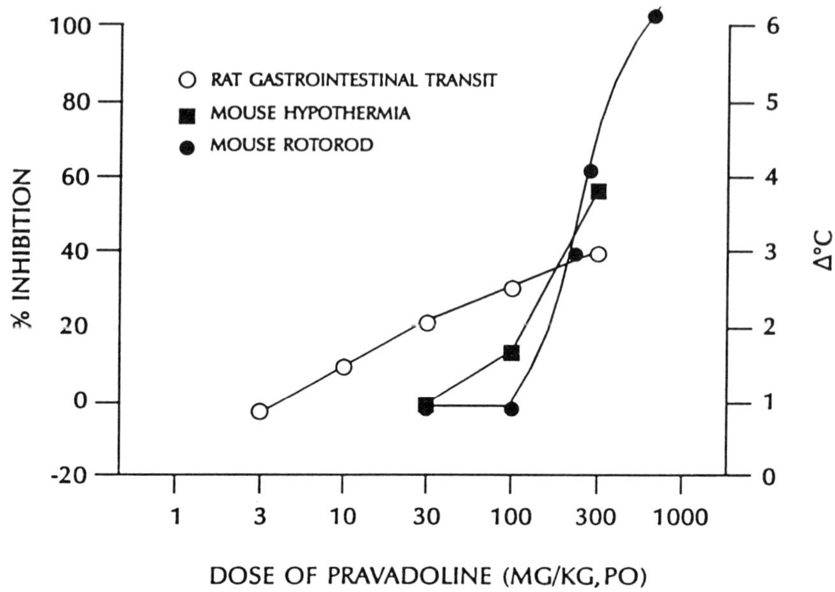

Figure 9 Ancillary pharmacology of pravadoline: The inhibitory effects of pravadoline on transit of a gum tragacanth charcoal meal in rats (○), on body temperature in mice (■), and on performance on a rotating rod in mice (●). (Data from Refs. 3 and 20).

other cyclooxygenase inhibitors on measures of gastrointestinal lesion production in rodents. Whereas most acidic NSAIDs produce gastric lesions at antinociceptive doses, the therapeutic ratio for pravadoline, as with acetaminophen and carprofen, is not limited by gastric irritancy.

The mechanism underlying pravadoline's lack of gastric irritancy has not been clearly elucidated. Although it is generally accepted that the mechanism of NSAID-induced gastric irritancy is related, at least in part, to these agents' inhibition of prostaglandin formation (36–38), the mechanism underlying the lower propensity for gastric irritation by some cyclooxygenase inhibitors (e.g., acetaminophen and carprofen) is not resolved. Several possibilities for pravadoline's lack of gastric irritancy may be considered. First, the obvious consideration that pravadoline may act as a prodrug for its acid metabolite is improbable. Although the acid metabolite has some cyclooxygenase inhibitory activity (IC_{50} = 5.4 μM), this molecule itself, like pravadoline, does not cause gastric irritancy (orally or intravenously), nor does it demonstrate the superior preclinical antinociceptive profile of pravadoline (Baizman DA, Miller MS, Ward SJ, unpublished observations). The possibility that the cannabinoid agonist property of pravadoline could ameliorate gastric irritancy driven by cyclooxygenase inhibition is also unlikely, because cannabinoid receptor agonists when coadministered with NSAIDs do not attenuate the latter's induction of gastric irritancy (Baizman DA, Ward SJ, unpublished observations).

A third possibility is that at nociceptive doses, pravadoline inhibits prostaglandin formation in the gut to a smaller extent than do NSAIDs. In support of this hypothesis, antinociceptive doses of pravadoline inhibit the ex vivo postmortem rise in PGE_2 levels in mouse brain; higher doses are required to inhibit ex vivo postmortem PGE_2 formation in the stomach (Fig. 8A). The converse is true for zomepirac (see Fig. 8B) and other

NSAIDs (24). Whether this "brain-selectivity" may reflect differences in drug distribution, or a differential ability to inhibit cyclooxygenase that is activated postmortem from different tissues, is unclear. It will be interesting to determine if differential affinity for the recently discovered constitutive and inducible forms of cyclooxygenase (39) may underlie the range of gastrointestinal liability displayed by NSAIDs.

Finally, it may be that the original premise for the design of pravadoline (1), does indeed underlie its lack of gastric irritancy—namely, that by virtue of its weakly basic pK_a and moderate lipophilicity, pravadoline may be poorly absorbed in the stomach and, as such, may not accumulate in a manner postulated to predispose cyclooxygenase inhibitors toward gastric irritancy (40–42).

B. Cannabinoid Receptor Pharmacology

Pravadoline produces hypothermia and ataxia (as defined by impairment of rotorod performance) in rodents in doses at and above the ED_{70} for antinociception (Fig. 9). Such effects are consistent with an agonist action at cannabinoid receptors (19,43–44), which are densely located in rodent hypothalamus and cerebellum (25,45). Although cannabinoids can have effects on motor behaviors in humans (30,46), this effect is less pronounced at psychoactive doses than might be anticipated from data in rodents. Interestingly, the rat cerebellum demonstrates a strikingly higher density of cannabinoid receptors than does human cerebellum (25,47).

Also, in a manner similar to cannabinoids (48), pravadoline produces a modest inhibition of gastrointestinal transit of a charcoal meal in mice (see Fig. 9) (3).

In animals and humans, cannabinoids also produce ocular hypotension (49) and are antiemetic (50) and anticonvulsant (46,51). Pravadoline has not been evaluated for any of these potential actions.

C. Renal Effects

Although pravadoline does not cause nephrotoxicity in mice, rats, or monkeys (at doses of 650, 400, or 100 mg/kg po, respectively) (52), studies in dogs revealed that pravadoline produces evidence of acute tubular nephrotoxicity following single oral doses of 40, 60, or 100 mg/kg (35). Nephrotoxicity in the dog was evident from histomorphological assessments and from increases in serum creatinine and urea nitrogen, with or without glucosuria. Nephrotoxic potential was confirmed in humans in a multiple dose Phase I study in which pravadoline, at doses of 400 and 600 mg, elicited a uricosuria suggestive of renal toxicity (53). Recent studies designed to elucidate the nephrotoxic moiety of pravadoline maleate revealed that nephrotoxicity in the dog is elicited by equimolar doses of the maleate salt, but not by equimolar doses of an alternative salt form of pravadoline, the ethanesulfonate (35). Pertinently, neither cyclooxygenase-inhibiting nor cannabinoid classes of drugs are known to produce uricosuria in humans. Thus, the possibility is raised that other salt forms of pravadoline may not produce in humans the suggestion of nephrotoxicity seen with pravadoline maleate.

VI. PHASE II CLINICAL STUDIES

A. Analgesic Actions

Pravadoline produced dose-related analgesia against postoperative pain in oral doses, ranging from 200 to 800 mg, in an eight-center, 458-patient, double-blind study using

Table 7 Analgesic Efficacy of Pravadoline Against Postoperative Gynecological and Orthopedic Pain

Parameter	Placebo	Acetaminophen (650 mg)	Acetaminophen (650 mg) + codeine (30 mg)	Pravadoline 200 mg	Pravadoline 400 mg	Pravadoline 800 mg
N	79	77	73	76	76	77
Mean 6 H. Totpar[a]	5.9	10.7	12.2	9.2	10.9	11.8
Median 6 H. Totpar	2.0	11.5	13.0	9.0	10.5	14.8
% of patients remedicated within 12 h	80	75	77	81	74	57
Median time to remedication (h)	3.3	5.8	6.3	5.5	6.1	9.0
Patient global (% good or better)	38	62	77	57	59	71

[a]Total pain relief scores.
Source: Data from Ref. 54.

acetaminophen and acetaminophen plus codeine as comparator agents (Table 7) (54,55). Time to onset and global pain relief were significantly different from placebo for all drug groups. Total pain relief scores for pravadoline (800 mg) and acetaminophen plus codeine were almost identical (12 and 12.2, respectively), although neither group differed significantly from total pain relief scores from lower doses of pravadoline or from acetaminophen alone. Of all treatment groups, pravadoline (800 mg), consistent with its plasma half-life, had the longest duration of action (8.3 h).

B. Adverse Events

No serious adverse events were observed in the foregoing analgesic study, but pravadoline (800 mg) tended to have higher incidences of adverse events than other treatment groups, notably of sedation, dizziness or lightheadedness, and nausea. It may be pertinent that the principal effects of classic cannabinoids at analgesic doses are drowsiness and dizziness (27,43,51). In a multiple-dose study (40 mg/kg per dose), two male subjects developed "cell-urea," proteinuria, and gluosuria (53). These effects, which were rapidly reversed after cessation of treatment, are consistent with observations in dogs (52), in which the maleic acid in the pravadoline formulation induced similar evidence of nephrotoxicity.

VII. SUMMARY

Pravadoline is a novel analgesic with demonstrated efficacy in humans. The duality of its mechanism of action—inhibition of cyclooxygenase and agonist activity at cannabinoid receptors—could confer advantages relative to each constituent mechanism alone. Thus, the cannabinoid agonist component of pravadoline clearly confers greater antinociceptive efficacy relative to NSAIDs in preclinical paradigms. Conversely, the potential disadvantages of a cannabinoid action may be offset by a concomitant second analgesic mechanism (inhibition of cyclooxygenase). Nevertheless, it remains unclear whether the current regulatory climate in which potent cannabinoids (such as nabilone and THC) are scheduled drugs would impinge on pravadoline. Importantly, although pravadoline is a cannabinoid receptor agonist, its potency at this site is modest, and frank THC-like "highs" have not been observed in the clinic.

Pravadoline's complete lack of gastrointestinal irritancy is important, not only clinically, but also mechanistically. Thus, elucidation of the mechanism by which pravadoline and structurally related cyclooxygenase inhibitors obviate the gastrointestinal liabilities of many NSAIDs could lead to important new therapeutic agents.

ACKNOWLEDGMENTS

The author wishes to thank Drs. D. Luttinger, D. Haycock, M. Eissenstat, R. Everett, and J. Baker for their review and suggestions on the manuscript, and is indebted to Ms Y. Micheli and Mr. E. Gower for typing and graphics assistance.

REFERENCES

1. Bell MR, D'Ambra TE, Kumar V, Eissenstat MA, Herrmann JL Jr, Wetzel JR, Rosi D, Philion RE, Daum SJ, Hlasta DJ, Kullnig RK, Ackerman JH, Haubrich DR, Luttinger DA,

Baizman ER, Miller MS, Ward SJ. Antinociceptive aminoalkylindoles. J Med Chem 1991; 34:1099–110.

2. Ward SJ, Baizman ER, Bell M, Childers S, D'Ambra T, Eissenstat M, Estep K, Haycock D, Howlett A, Luttinger D, Miller M, Pacheco M. Aminoalkylindoles (AAIs): a new route to the cannabinoid receptor? Natl Inst Drug Abuse Monogr 1990; 105:304–5.
3. Haubrich DR, Ward SJ, Baizman E, Bell MR, Bradford J, Ferrari R, Miller M, Perrone M, Pierson AK, Saelens JK, Luttinger D. Pharmacology of pravadoline: a new analgesic agent. J Pharmacol Exp Ther 1990; 255:511–22.
4. Pacheco M, Childers SR, Arnold R, Casiano F, Ward SJ. Aminoalkylindoles: actions on specific G-protein-linked receptors. J Pharmacol Exp Ther 1991; 257:170–83.
5. Ward SJ, Mastriani D, Casiano F, Arnold R. Pravadoline: profile in isolated tissue preparations. J Pharmacol Exp Ther 1990; 255:1230–39.
6. Ferrari RA, Ward SJ, Zobre CM, Van Liew DK, Perrone MH, Connell MJ, Haubrich DR. Estimation of the in vivo effect of cyclooxygenase inhibitors on prostaglandin E_2 levels in mouse brain. Eur J Pharmacol 1990; 179:25–34.
7. Van Der Ouderaa FJ, Buytenhek M, Nugteren DH, Van Dorp DA. Purification and characterization of prostaglandin endoperoxide synthetase from sheep vesicular glands. Biochim Biophys Acta 1976; 487:315–31.
8. Kuster JE, Haycock DA, Howlett AC, Subramanian B, Ward SJ. Aminoalkylindole binding data suggests a new approach for studying cannabinoid activity. Neurosci Abstr 1990; 16:697.
9. Kuster JE, Stevenson JI, Ward SJ, D'Ambra TE, Haycock DA. Aminoalkylindole binding in rat cerebellum: selective displacement by natural and synthetic cannabinoids. J Pharmacol Exp Ther 1992; (in press).
10. Haycock DA, Kuster JE, Stevenson JI, Ward SJ, D'Ambra T. Characterization of aminoalkylindole binding: selective displacement by cannabinoids. Proc Comm Probl Drug Depend 1990; 105:304–5.
11. Johnson MR, Melvin LS. The discovery of nonclassical cannabinoid analgetics. In Mechoulam R, ed. Cannabinoids as therapeutic agents. Boca Raton: CRC Press, 1986:121–45.
12. Devane WA, Dysarz FA III, Johnson MR, Melvin LS, Howlett AC. Determination and characterization of a cannabinoid receptor in rat brain. Mol Pharmacol 1988; 34:605–13.
13. D'Ambra TE, Estep KG, Bell MR, Eissenstat MA, Josef KA, Ward SJ, Haycock DA, Baizman ER, Casiano FM, Beglin NC, Chippari SM, Grego JD, Kullnig RK, Daley GT. Conformationally restrained analogues of pravadoline: nanomolar potent, enantioselective, (aminoalkyl) indole agonists of the cannabinoid receptor. J Med Chem 1992; 35:124–35.
14. Howlett AC. Cannabinoid inhibition of adenylate cyclase: biochemistry of the response in neuroblastoma cell membranes. Mol Pharmacol 1985; 27:429–36.
15. Howlett AC, Johnson MR, Melvin LS, Milne GM. Nonclassical cannabinoid analgetics inhibit adenylate cyclase: development of a cannabinoid receptor model. Mol Pharmacol 1988; 33:297–302.
16. Casiano F, Arnold R, Haycock D, Kuster J, Ward SJ. Putative aminoalkylindoles (AAI) antagonists. Natl Inst Drug Abuse Res Monogr 1990; 105:427–8.
17. Melvin LS, Johnson MR, Harbart CA, Milne GM, Weissman A. A cannabinoid derived prototype analgesic. J Med Chem 1984; 27:67–71.
18. Little PJ, Compton DR, Johnson R, Melvin LS, Martin BR. Pharmacology and stereoselectivity of structurally novel cannabinoids in mice. J Pharmacol Exp Ther 1988; 247:1046–51.
19. Martin BR, Compton DR, Thomas BF, Prescott WR, Little MD, Razdan RK, Johnson MR, Melvin LS, Mechoulam R, Ward SJ. Behavioral, biochemical, and molecular modeling evaluations of cannabinoid analogs. Pharmacol Biochem Behav 1991; 40:471–8.
20. Luttinger D, Baizman ER, Miller MS, Ward SJ. The in vivo effects of aminoalkylindoles, a new class of compounds which interact with a cannabinoid binding site. Comm Probl Drug Depend Abstr 1990.
21. Lim RKS. Pain. Annu Rev Physiol 1970; 32:269–88.

22. Ferreira SH, Lorenzetti BB, Correa FMA. Central and peripheral antianalgesic action of aspirin-like drugs. Eur J Pharmacol 1978; 53:39–48.
23. Malmberg AB, Yaksh TL. Hyperalgesia mediated by spinal glutamate or substance P blocked by spinal cyclooxygenase inhibition. Science 1992; 257:1276–8.
24. Miller MS, Zobre C, Kiefer D, Ferrari R, Ward SJ. WIN 48098-induced antinociception: a central component. Pharmacologist 1986; 28:140.
25. Herkenham M, Lynn AB, Johnson MR, Melvin LS, de Costa BR, Rice KC. Characterization and localization of cannabinoid receptors in rat brain: a quantitative in vitro autoradiographic study. J Neurosci 1991; 11:563–83.
26. Yaksh TL. The antinociceptive effects of intrathecally administered levonantradol and desacetyllevonantradol in the rat. J Clin Pharmacol 1981; 21:334S–40S.
27. Segal M. Cannabinoids and analgesia. In: Mechoulam R, ed. Cannabinoids as therapeutic agents. Roca Raton: CRC Press, 1986:105–20.
28. Welch SP, Stevens DL. Antinociceptive activity of intrathecally administered cannabinoids alone, and in combination with morphine, in mice. J Pharmacol Exp Ther 1992; 262:10–7.
29. Noyes R Jr, Brunk SF, Avery DH, Canter A. The analgesic properties of delta-9-tetrahydrocannabinol and codeine. Clin Pharmacol Ther 1975; 18:84–9.
30. Razdan RK, Howes JF. Drugs related to tetrahydrocannabinol. Med Res Rev 1983; 3:119–46.
31. Smith PB, Martin BR. delta-9-Tetrahydrocannabinol biodisposition and effects following intrathecal administration. Brain Res 1992; (in press).
32. Archer RA, Stark P, Lemberger L. Nabilone. In: Mechoulam R, ed. Cannabinoids as therapeutic agents. Boca Raton: CRC Press, 1986:85–103.
33. Johnson JA, Gonyea GJ, Baker JF. Investigation of pravadoline metabolites by thermospray mass spectrometry [abstract]. Presented at 37th ASMS Conf Mass Spectrometry Allied Topics, 1989:959–60.
34. Cook JA, Crawmer BP, O'Neil A, Boddy W, Dorflinger EE, Stroshane RM. The effects of food, milk and antacid on the bioavailability of pravadoline. Pharm Res 1989; 6:S231.
35. Everett RM, Descotes G, Rollin M, Greener Y, Bradford JC, Benziger DP, Ward SJ. Nephrotoxicity of pravadoline maleate (WIN 48098-6) in dogs: evidence of maleic acid-induced acute tubular necrosis. Fundam Appl Toxicol 1992; (in press).
36. Miller TA. Protective effects of prostaglandins against gastric mucosal damage: current knowledge and proposed mechanisms. Am J Physiol 1983; 245:G601–G623.
37. Fromm D. Mechanisms involved in gastric mucosal resistance to injury. Annu Rev Med 1987; 38:119–28.
38. Shorrock CJ, Reese WDW. Overview of gastroduodenal mucosal protection. Am J Med 1988; 84(suppl 2A):25–34.
39. O'Banion MK, Winn VD, Young DA. cDNA cloning and functional activity of a glucocorticoid-regulated inflammatory cyclooxygenase. Proc Natl Acad Sci, USA 1992; 89:4888–92.
40. McCormack K, Brune K. Classical absorption theory and the development of gastric mucosal damage associated with the non-steroidal antiinflammatory drugs. Arch Toxicol 1987; 60:261–9.
41. Rainsford KD, Fox SA, Osborne DJ. Comparative effects of some non-steroidal anti-inflammatory drugs on the ultrastructural integrity and prostaglandin levels in the rat gastric mucosa: relationship to drug uptake. Scand J Gastroenterol [Suppl] 1984; 101:55–68.
42. Deardon JC, Nicholson RM. Antiinflammatory drug design: correlation of gastric irritancy with hydrophobicity in a heterogeneous group of drugs. J Pharm Pharmacol 1987; 39(suppl): 101P.
43. Razdan RK. Structure–activity relationships in cannabinoids. Pharmacol Rev 1986; 38:75–149.
44. Consroe P, Snider SR. Therapeutic potential of cannabinoids in neurological disorders. In: Mechoulam R, ed. Cannabinoids as therapeutic agents. Boca Raton: CRC Press, 1986:21–49.

45. Jansen EM, Haycock DA, Ward SJ, Seybold VS. Distribution of cannabinoid receptors in rat brain determined with aminoalkylindoles. Brain Res 1992; 575:93–102.
46. Dewey WL, Harris LS, Howes JF, Kennedy JS, Anderson RN. A pharmacological investigation of some of the peripheral effects of the constituents of marijuana. Comm Probl Drug Depend 1970; pp 6883–9.
47. Herkenham M, Lynn AB, Little MD, Johnson MR, Melvin LS, DeCosta BR, Rice KC. Cannabinoid receptor localization in brain. Proc Natl Acad Sci USA 1990; 87:1932–6.
48. Dewey WL. Cannabinoid pharmacology. Pharmacol Rev 1986; 38:151–78.
49. Adler MW, Geller EB. Ocular effects of cannabinoids. In: Mechoulam R, ed. Cannabinoids as therapeutic agents, Boca Raton: CRC Press, 1986:51–70.
50. Levitt M. Cannabinoids as antiemetics in cancer chemotherapy. In: Mechoulam R, ed. Cannabinoids as therapeutic agents. Boca Raton: CRC Press, 1986:71–83.
51. Consroe P, Sandyk R. Potential role of cannabinoids for therapy of neurological disorders. In: Murphy L, Bartke A, eds. Marijuana/cannabinoids neurobiology and neurophysiology. Boca Raton: CRC Press, 1992:459–524.
52. Greener Y, Mayes BA, Everett RM, Dean JH. Assessment of the acute oral toxicity of Win 48098-6 in beagle dogs. Toxicologist 1990; 10:269.
53. Shapiro BE, Halstenson CE, Abraham PA, Dorflinger E, Fritz AK, Keane WF. Nonsteroidal anti-inflammatory agents (NSAID) and uric acid excretion. Clin Pharmacol Ther 1990; 47:193.
54. Grieco G, Deandrade J, Dorflinger E, Kantor T, Saelens J, Sunshine A, Wang R, Wideman G, Zelman V. Pravadoline maleate, a new non-opioid oral analgesic, in the treatment of post-operative pain. Clin Pharmacol Ther 1989; 45:123.
55. Minehart IM, Steen SN, Zelman V, Matta J, Mok MS. A comparative clinical study of pravadoline maleate for post-operative analgesia. Acta Anaesthesiol Scand [Suppl] 1989; 91:124.
56. Tallarida RJ, Murray RB. Manual of pharmacological calculations with computer programs. New York: Springer-Verlag, 1981.
57. Childers SR, Pacheco MA, Ward SJ. Cannabinoids and aminoalkylindoles bind to common receptors to inhibit adenylyl cyclase in brain. Neurosci Abstr 1990; 16:1302.
58. Berkowitz BA, Way EL. Analgesic activity and central nervous system distribution of the optical isomers of pentazocine in the rat. J Pharmacol Exp Ther 1971; 177:500–8.
59. Luttinger D. Determination of drug efficacy in mice by use of different water temperatures in a tail-immersion test. J Pharmacol Methods 1985; 12:351–7.
60. Luttinger D, Koonz D, Chippari S. Phenyl-*p*-quinone writhing in mice: can it predict analgesic efficacy? Pharmacologist 1988; 30:A155.

18

Romazarit

DAVID BRADSHAW and PETER E. O. WILLIAMS
Roche Products Ltd.
Welwyn Garden City, Hertsfordshire, England

I. INTRODUCTION

Currently available disease-modifying antirheumatic drugs (DMARDs) are of limited use owing to their poor therapeutic margins, the severity of their side effects, and concern over their effectiveness (1). A new generation of DMARDs is required the activity and safety of which will permit their use as first-line agents, thereby enabling more widespread benefit.

One of the few compounds to have shown some promise of fulfilling these requirements was clobuzarit (Clozic), a compound originally developed by ICI as an antihyperlipidemic agent. The rationale for assessing the efficacy of clobuzarit as an antirheumatic agent came from the observation that, in patients with atherosclerosis, the compound reduced levels of the acute-phase protein, fibrinogen (2). This coincided with the suggestion that an important difference between the symptomatic therapies and the remission-inducing drugs used in arthritis was the ability of the latter to lower the elevated levels of acute-phase reactants such as C-reactive protein (CRP), haptoglobin, and fibrinogen (3). In patients with rheumatoid arthritis (RA), the beneficial clinical response produced by clobuzarit could be clearly differentiated from that of nonsteroidal anti-inflammatory drugs (NSAIDs) in that it was associated with a reduction in various clinical variables, including erythrocyte sedimentation rate (ESR), acute-phase proteins, and immune complexes. In addition, there was a trend toward reducing radiological progression (2). Although clobuzarit was generally well tolerated in humans, its development was terminated following four cases of Stevens–Johnson syndrome and adverse findings in animal toxicology studies, such as the occurrence of hepatomas in male mice. This latter finding may have been associated with another property of clobuzarit, namely, its ability to induce a marked proliferation of liver peroxisomes in rodents.

Because of the interesting clinical profile of clobuzarit, plus an ability to distinguish clobuzarit from NSAIDs in experimental animal models, we embarked on a program to

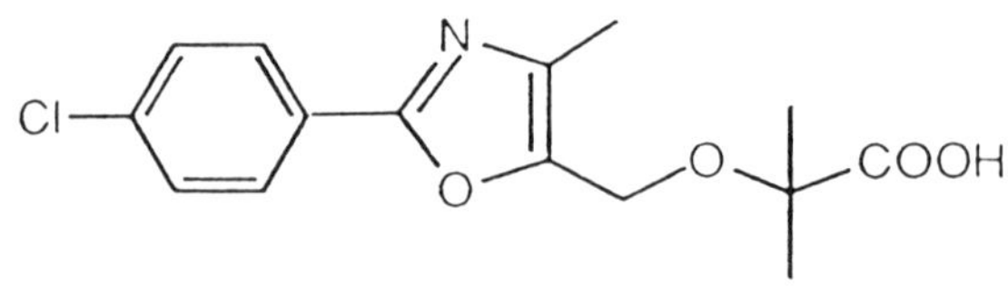

Romazarit (Ro 31-3948) (Mol wt 331.73; solubility in water > 100 g/100 ml)

synthesize and evaluate a series of analogues of this molecule. Our aim was to identify a new clinical candidate that showed similar or superior efficacy to clobuzarit, but with a reduced potential to produce adverse effects, particularly the induction of hepatic peroxisomal proliferation. Detailed in the following are the biological properties of romazarit (see structure), which led to its selection (as its sodium salt) for clinical evaluation, followed by a review of the clinical studies undertaken with this compound.

II. PRECLINICAL STUDIES

A. Adjuvant Arthritis

Induction of arthritis in rats by the injection of *Mycobacterium tuberculosis* in mineral oil permits the evaluation of antiarthritic compounds using a variety of different protocols. In one protocol, compounds are administered from the day of sensitization of the animals, and the arthritis is allowed to develop for 5 days. A distinction between cyclooxygenase-inhibiting NSAIDs and potential DMARDs can then be made by measuring their effects on the edematous component of the arthritis, in comparison with their ability to modify the acute-phase protein response (3). In this type of experiment, romazarit inhibited paw inflammation, with a minimum effective dose (MED) of 30 mg/kg and reduced the plasma levels of the acute-phase reactants, seromucoid and haptoglobin (4). This latter property distinguishes the activity of romazarit from that of NSAIDs (3). Similar activity was found in adrenalectomized animals, indicating that the therapeutic activity of romazarit is not attributable to stimulation of the pituitary–adrenal axis.

When romazarit was tested using a protocol in which the arthritis was allowed to develop for 15 days, a dose-related improvement of all the clinical signs of the disease was observed, with a minimum effective dose of 25 mg/kg. This was accompanied by a more extensive restoration of acute-phase reactant levels toward normal values than was seen at the 5-day time point (4).

In a test in which romazarit was administered to animals with an established disease, the increase in paw volume that occurred between days 21 and 28 after adjuvant injection was reduced from 1.45 ml in untreated rats to 0.59 ml in the group treated with romazarit (30 mk/kg), and this difference was statistically significant.

B. Collagen Arthritis

Intradermal injection of type II collagen emulsified with Freund's incomplete adjuvant was used to sensitize rats, which went on to develop hind-paw arthritis about 15 days later. Romazarit, at doses of 20 mk/kg or above, when administered using a therapeutic-dosing schedule on days 15–29 after sensitization, reduced paw volume and decreased the radiographic changes occurring in the hind paws of the rats (4). The median effective dose (EC_{50}) for these effects was approximately 50 mg/kg. Romazarit had no effect on levels of circulating anticollagen antibody.

Romazarit was also effective when employed using a prophylactic-dosing schedule (i.e., when compound administration was started at sensitization and thus preceding arthritis development). Dose-dependent inhibition of paw inflammation (Fig. 1) was accompanied by a reduction in the bony changes in the talus and tarsus regions of the hind paws assessed radiologically, these changes being statistically significant at doses of 10 mg/kg and higher.

In one experiment, romazarit was administered therapeutically for 1 week and then withdrawn. Hind-paw volumes increased following withdrawal and eventually paralleled those of an untreated arthritic control group. By contrast, a group of animals treated continuously with romazarit continued to show improvement up to termination of the experiment 36 days after the start of dosing (Fig. 2).

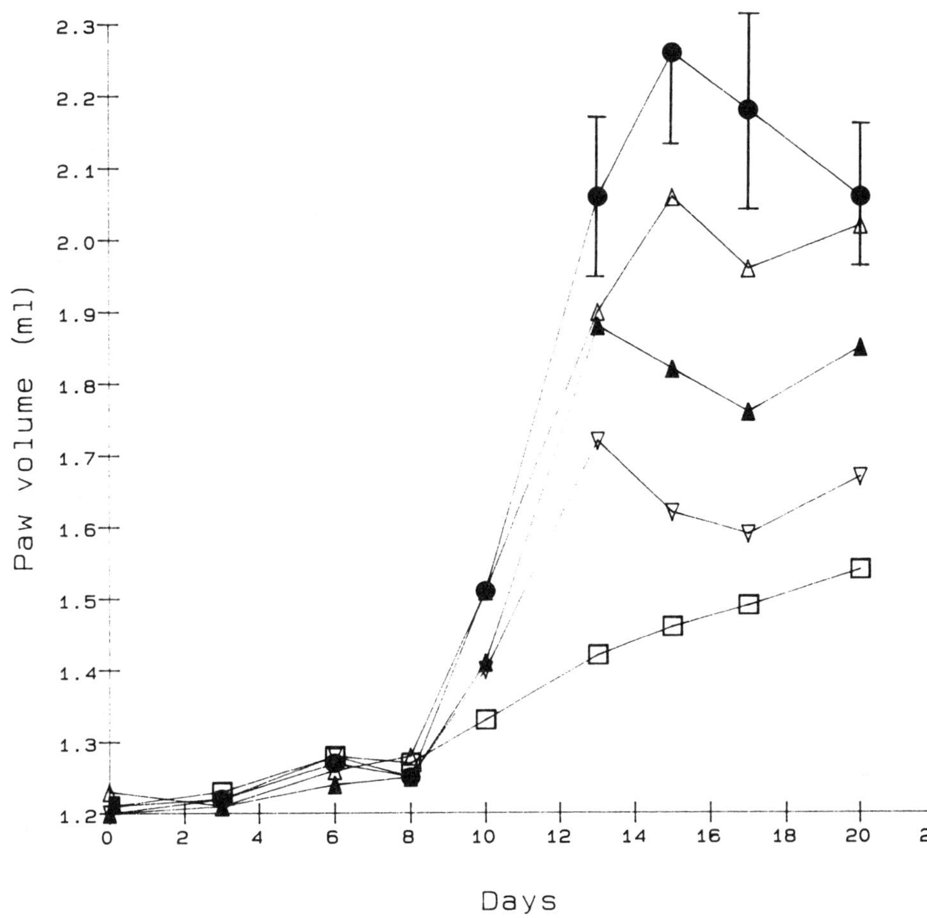

Figure 1 Effect of prophylactic administration of romazarit on collagen arthritis in rats. Groups of eight animals received romazarit orally, 1 day before sensitization with collagen (sensitization on day 1) and then once daily throughout the experiment. The increase in paw volumes of nonarthritic rats is due to normal growth. Control (●); romazarit: 15 mg/kg (△); 40 mg/kg (▲); 60 mg/kg (▽); nonarthritic (□).

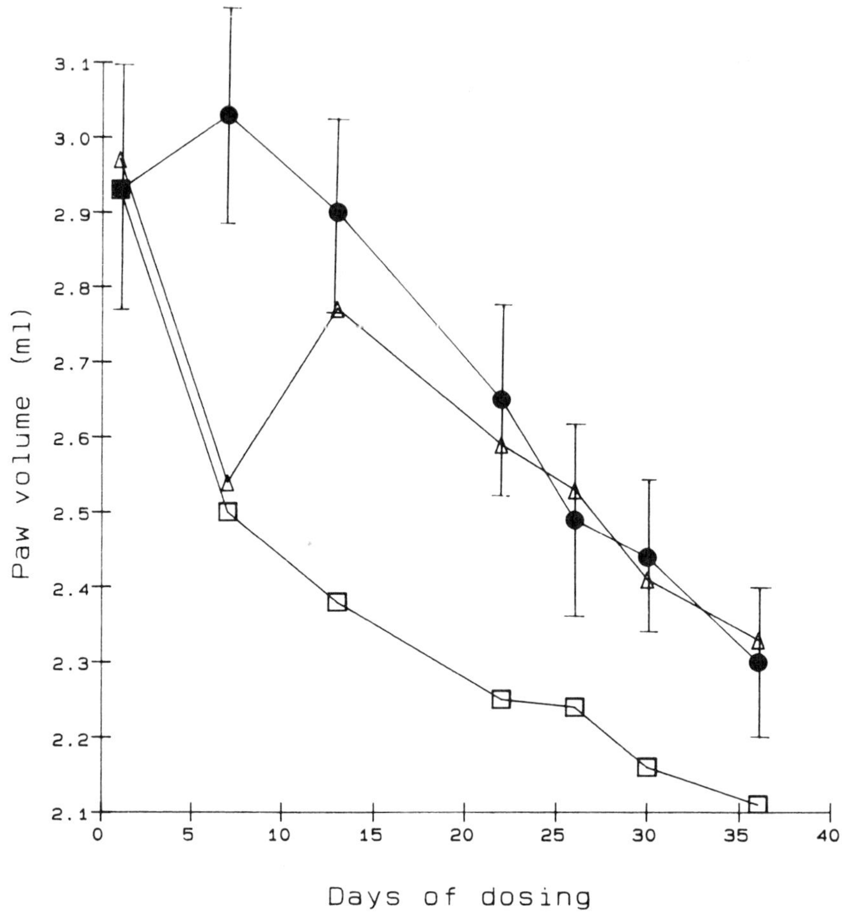

Figure 2 Effect of withdrawal of romazarit from rats with collagen arthritis. Romazarit was administered orally, once daily, to animals with an established arthritis. In one group, romazarit was withdrawn after 7 days, whereas in another group, compound administration was continued throughout the experiment. Control (●); romazarit, 50 mg/kg (□); romazarit withdrawn (△).

The results in adjuvant and collagen arthritis indicate, therefore, that romazarit is effective whether given prophylactically or therapeutically, and some distinction from the effects of NSAID can be made. Withdrawal of romazarit leads to a reversal of the antiarthritic effect, but not a rebound above control levels, whereas continuous administration of romazarit remains beneficial.

C. MRL/lpr Mouse

The MRL/lpr mouse carries an autosomal recessive gene that is responsible for the development of a lupuslike syndrome and an arthritis that is serologically and histologically similar to rheumatoid arthritis. The daily, oral administration of romazarit at 100 or 200 mg/kg per day to MRL/lpr mice from the age of 8 weeks, for a period of 12 weeks, significantly reduced the development of arthritis (Fig. 3). The compound also reduced

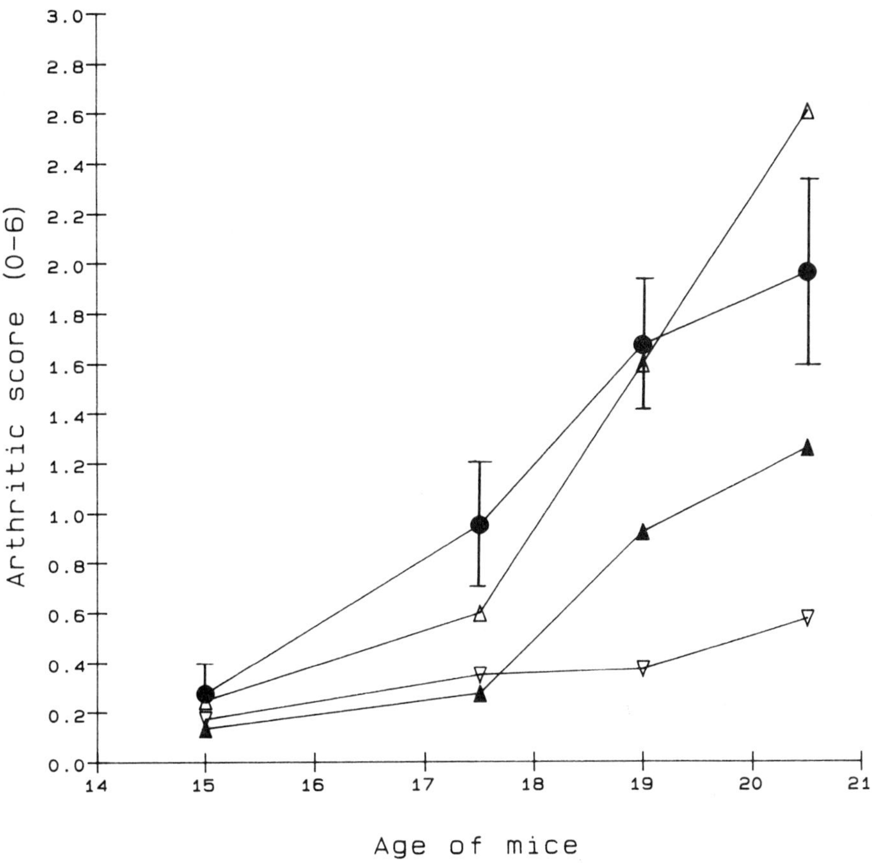

Figure 3 Effect of romazarit on spontaneous arthritis in MRL/lpr mice. Romazarit was administered orally, once daily, to MRL/lpr mice from the age of 8 weeks, for a period of 12 weeks. Arthritis was assessed using a visual scoring system. Control (●); romazarit: 30 mg/kg (△); 100 mg/kg (▲); 200 mg/kg (▽).

immune complex formation, the development of anti-DNA autoantibody, lymphoid hyperplasia, the increase in serum IgG levels, and the development of proteinurea. Romazarit, therefore, was active in reducing both the arthritis and the lupuslike syndrome in this model (data on file, Hoffmann–La Roche).

D. Humoral and Cell-Mediated Immunity

Romazarit had no effect on the production of antibodies to sheep red blood cells in mice, suggesting that the mode of action of romazarit does not involve modification of humoral immunity.

Induction of paw edema by a delayed hypersensitivity response to methylated bovine serum albumin (mBSA) has previously been shown to be inhibited by immunosuppressive agents when administered at the time of sensitization and by NSAIDs when given at the time of antigen challenge (5). Romazarit had no effect when administered during the sensitization phase in an experiment in which azathioprine reduced the response by 43%.

The compound was also ineffective when given during the elicitation period in an experiment in which indomethacin caused a 38% inhibition. Romazarit thus showed no indication of either an acute anti-inflammatory effect or an inhibition of cell-mediated immunity.

E. Arachidonate Metabolism

Romazarit, at concentrations up to 300 μM, had no significant effect on the production of prostaglandin E_2 (PGE_2) by human peripheral blood mononuclear cells exposed to phytohemagglutinin. In rat adherent peritoneal cells, romazarit (100 μM) had no effect on ionophore-induced arachidonic acid release, leukotriene-B_4 (LTB_4) production or 6-keto-PGF_1 production.

Romazarit showed extremely weak inhibition of PG synthetase activity in both sheep seminal vesicle and rat renal medulla cell-free preparations, with a median inhibiting concentration (IC_{50}) against the sheep enzyme of 6500 μM, showing the compound to be at least 4000-fold less potent than indomethacin. These results suggest that it is unlikely that direct inhibition of phospholipase A_2, lipoxygenase, or cyclooxygenase represents the mechanism of the anti-inflammatory action of romazarit. Metabolic conversion to an inhibitor of arachidonic acid metabolism is also unlikely, since administration of the compound to rats for 1 week at 100 mg/kg per day had no effect on urinary PGE_2 production.

As might be expected from this lack of effect on prostaglandin production, romazarit had no ulcerogenic effect at 100 mg/kg in a stressed rat model, whereas indomethacin was ulcerogenic with an ED_{50} value of 2.9 mg/kg.

F. Models of Acute Inflammation

The lack of effect of romazarit on the enzymes involved in arachidonic acid metabolism was reflected in models of acute inflammation. Thus, romazarit had no effect on the inflammatory response induced in rabbit skin by the injection of a mixture of bradykinin and arachidonic acid and had only a slight effect on UV-induced erythema in guinea pig skin and, then, only when a multiple dose schedule was used.

In a carrageenan-induced pleurisy model in the rat, romazarit had no effect on exudate volume or polymorphonuclear leukocyte accumulation in experiments employing either a single dose of five daily doses of 100 mg/kg. However, the infiltration of mononuclear cells was reduced by romazarit, and it is possible that this is of relevance to the mode of action of the compound as an antiarthritic agent (4).

G. Interleukin-1-Induced Responses

1. Mediator Synthesis by Human Fibroblasts

Receptor studies indicated that romazarit did not affect either binding of interleukin-1 (IL-1) to cells or the internalization of the IL-1 receptor–ligand complex. However, romazarit does show inhibition of IL-1-stimulated cellular events in vitro, and this may have some relevance to its mode of action. In particular, the release of PGE_2 from human rheumatoid synovial fibroblasts stimulated with recombinant human IL-1α was inhibited by romazarit, with an IC_{50} of 150 μM (Table 1). Romazarit also inhibited the release of collagenase from IL-1-stimulated human dermal fibroblasts with an IC_{50} of 200 μM (see Table 1). In these experiments, indomethacin (0.1 μM) prevented prostaglandin release

Table 1 Effect of Romazarit on IL-1-Induced PGE_2 and Collagenase Release by Human Fibroblasts

	% Inhibition	
Concentration of romazarit (μM)	PGE_2 synthesis (mean ± SEM)[a]	Collagenase synthesis[b]
25	6.8 ± 7.9	–13
50	22 ± 8	39
100	41 ± 2	39
200	58 ± 7	46
400	74 ± 4	74
IC_{50}	150 μM	200 μM

[a]Six experiments on rheumatoid synovial cells.
[b]Dermal fibroblast cell line CCD-43.

by its inhibition of PG synthetase, but it had no effect on the release of the degradative enzyme collagenase (data on file, Hoffmann–La Roche).

2. *Interleukin-1-Induced Serum Amyloid P in Mice*

Interleukin-1 administered subcutaneously to mice induces an elevation in circulating levels of the acute-phase protein, serum amyloid P (SAP), over the subsequent 24 h. Administration of romazarit 1 day and then again 1 h before injection of IL-1 resulted in a reduction in the SAP response (Table 2).

H. Hepatic Effects

1. *Peroxisomal Proliferation*

Clobuzarit is a powerful inducer of hepatic peroxisomal proliferation in rodents, and this type of effect has been associated with the production of hepatomas in rodent toxicological studies (6). Romazarit was compared with clobuzarit for its ability to induce peroxisomal proliferation by measuring the effect of the compounds on liver catalase and PPA80 (6) following administration to rats for 15 days. These studies showed romazarit to be approximately 15-fold less potent than clobuzarit as an inducer of peroxisomal proliferation (4).

2. *Acute-Phase Proteins*

Romazarit had a significant effect on the levels of only one acute-phase protein, haptoglobin, following administration for 15 days to animals in which no experimental

Table 2 Effect of Romazarit on IL-1-Induced Elevation of Serum Amyloid P Levels in Mice

	Plasma SAP concentration (mg/L)			
Treatment	0 h	6 h	18 h	24 h
IL-1 (2000 U)	23 ± 0.8	47 ± 6.6	122 ± 11	90 ± 3.0
IL-1 (2000 U) + 100 mg/kg romazarit	21 ± 2.5	38 ± 7.7	93 ± 7.3	64 ± 9.2[a]

[a]Figure underlined represents statistically significant ($p < 0.05$) difference in response from control IL-1-treated group.

inflammatory or arthritic response had been induced (designated normals). By contrast, clobuzarit caused significant decreases in the plasma levels of ceruloplasmin, iron, and seromucoid, and a significant increase in the level of fibrinogen. Clobuzarit also caused significant increases in liver weight and catalase activity, whereas romazarit had no effect on these measurements (Table 3). These findings may indicate a direct effect of clobuzarit on hepatic protein synthesis and suggest that the effects of clobuzarit on acute-phase reactants in arthritic models are not exclusively related to an effect on the inflammatory response.

I. Concluding Comments on the Preclinical Studies

Romazarit is clearly distinguishable from conventional NSAIDs in that its marked beneficial effects in chronic models of arthritis are not accompanied by an acute anti-inflammatory effect. Its similarities to clobuzarit, a compound for which clinical benefit in rheumatoid arthritis has been demonstrated, suggested that romazarit was potentially a new disease-modifying antirheumatic drug. Coupled with its markedly fewer hepatic effects, compared with clobuzarit, this led to the decision to progress this compound into clinical trials.

III. CLINICAL STUDIES

After some comments on the preclinical pharmacokinetic data that contributed to the choice of dosages in the clinical studies, two tolerability–pharmacokinetic studies in humans will be described, and this section will end with some results from the efficacy study of romazarit in patients with rheumatoid arthritis.

A. Background Information

Romazarit is a fairly small hydrophilic drug, with good UV-absorbance and a pK_a of 4.5 for the carboxyl group in the propionic acid moiety. These properties imply that the measurement of drug concentrations in biological fluids by high-performance liquid chromatography (HPLC) is not complex. After protein precipitation with acetonitrile, reverse-phase HPLC has been used to quantify romazarit concentrations in plasma samples (200 μl). For urine, each sample was analyzed before and after hydrolysis for 60 mins with 2 M sodium hydroxide solution. The assays were sensitive, with quantification limits of 0.01 or 0.10 mg/L, accurate, and precise; coefficients of variation for the quality control samples were 8% or less (further details are given in Ref. 7).

Blood samples were taken for drug analysis from rats at the end of a pharmacological study of the efficacy of romazarit against arthritis induced by type II collagen. After 15 daily oral doses of 20 mg/kg, plasma concentrations of romazarit averaged 64 mg/L, with a standard deviation of 27 mg/L. This finding suggested that a reasonable target concentration range in patients with rheumatoid arthritis was 50–100 mg/L, if the studies in animals predicted therapeutic response in humans. Such predictions were true for clobuzarit, which appeared to be about half as potent as romazarit throughout the preclinical pharmacology. Clobuzarit was more effective in those patients whose plasma concentrations exceeded 150 mg/L (2), substantiating the suggested target range for romazarit.

Blood samples were also taken from rats and marmosets at the end of the 26-week toxicity studies of romazarit. At dosages of 50 mg/kg per day in rats and 60 mg/kg per

Table 3 Effect of Romazarit on Liver Weight and Acute-Phase Proteins in Normal Animals

Treatment group	Liver weight (g/100 g BW)	Acute-phase reactants							
		Catalase (ksec-1 g^{-1})	Cer (mg L^{-1})	Fib (g L^{-1})	Alb (g L^{-1})	Iron (μg/100 ml)	Sero (g L^{-1})	Hapto (g L^{-1})	Chol (mg/100 ml)
Control (0.1 M $NaHCO_3$)	5.3 ± 0.2 (n = 7)	158 ± 12	679 ± 27	1.03 ± 0.18	32.5 ± 0.5	374 ± 22	3.79 ± 0.23	0.36 ± 0.04	58.4 ± 4.8
Ro 31-3948/000 (100 mg kg^{-1})	5.6 ± 0.2	144 ± 5	756 ± 44	1.51 ± 0.17	33.4 ± 0.4	348 ± 25	3.82 ± 0.47	0.25* ± 0.01	59.0 ± 5.5
Clobuzarit (100 mg kg^{-1})	6.7*** ± 0.2	256*** ± 12	539** ± 25	1.83** ± 0.10	31.9 ± 0.70	168*** ± 16	2.05** ± 0.08	0.24 ± 0.06	42.7* ± 2.3

Compounds were administered orally once daily for 15 days. Results represent mean ± SEM.
Number of animals (n) = 8 unless otherwise stated.
BW, body weight; Cer, ceruloplasmin; Fib, fibrinogen; Alb, albumin; Sero, seromucoid; Hapto, haptoglobin, Chol, cholesterol.

day in marmosets, both of which lacked significant toxicity, mean plasma drug concentrations were 363 mg/L at 5 h and 307 mg/L at 2 h, respectively. Therefore, safety margins in excess of threefold could be derived in comparison with the upper limit of the target therapeutic range in patients.

B. Human Studies

Apart from investigating the tolerability of romazarit in humans, the first two clinical studies had an objective of estimating the oral dosage required to achieve the target plasma concentration range at steady state.

For the first administration of romazarit to humans, a double-blind, placebo-controlled study of tolerability and pharmacokinetics was performed (7). Groups of nine healthy male volunteers received single oral doses of placebo (n = 3) or romazarit (40, 100, 200, 300, 450, 700, 1000, 1200, 1500 mg). No subject received more than three of these doses, which were always separated by at least 2 weeks. Volunteers fasted overnight before and for 3 h after dosing. Vital signs were recorded for 12 h after each dose. Blood and urine samples were collected for laboratory safety tests immediately before, 2 days and 5 days after each dose. Venous blood samples for the measurement of romazarit concentrations were obtained at intervals up to 120 h after dosing. Timed collections of all urine were made over the same period.

The volunteers averaged 26 years of age and 73 kg bodyweight. A total of 57 single oral doses of romazarit were administered during the study and 27 placebo doses. There were nine adverse events reported by four different volunteers; headaches (four reports) and gastrointestinal discomfort (two reports) were the most common events. None of the subjects required treatment or withdrew from the study because of the adverse events. The minor changes in vital signs were of equal magnitude and incidence after romazarit and after placebo, suggesting effects of the study, rather than the drug. Elevations in liver enzyme activities led to the withdrawal of two volunteers, possibly rather than probably related to the drug. The mean pharmacokinetic parameters of romazarit are shown in Table 4.

The mean peak concentrations were directly proportional to dose, and there was a slight tendency for the times to peak concentrations to increase with dose. The mean apparent plasma clearance decreased from 9.7 L/h after the 40-mg dose to 1.7 L/h after the 700-mg dose, but did not decrease with further increases in dose. The urinary recovery of drug-related material averaged 70% across all doses. More than 90% of the material was present in the form of labile metabolites, probably ester glucuronides. The rate of appearance of these glucuronides in urine was correlated with the concurrent area under the concentration–time curve (AUC), for example, the AUC to 8 h was 98% of the total area after 100-mg doses and the urinary recovery in the first 8 h was 94% of the total recovery.

The results of this study indicated that single oral doses of romazarit, up to 1500 mg, were well tolerated by young male volunteers. The pharmacokinetic data suggested that romazarit was rapidly and extensively absorbed. Renal clearance of glucuronide conjugates seemed to account for the decline in romazarit concentrations in plasma (i.e., the conjugation of romazarit with glucuronic acid followed by the renal excretion of the conjugates appeared to be the primary elimination mechanism of the drug). The secretion of the glucuronides by the kidney tubules may be saturable. If romazarit glucuronides are retained in the plasma for a relatively longer time after higher doses, they could be

Table 4 Pharmacokinetic Parameters of Romazarit After Single Oral Doses in Healthy Volunteers

Dose (mg) (No. of evaluable volunteers)	Mean (%CV) parameter value (units)				
	C_{max} (mg/L)	t_{max} (h)	AUC_t (mg h/L)	Cl/F (L/h)	UR (% dose)
40	2.95	0.542	4.43	9.66	79.2
(n = 6)	(76)	(90)	(36)	(28)	(33)
100	11.1	0.833	22.1	4.56	71.9
(n = 6)	(26)	(75)	(14)	(14)	(31)
200	21.2	1.46	63.3	3.48	61.3
(n = 6)	(32)	(91)	(37)	(32)	(20)
300	25.6	0.850	60.0	5.13	81.7
(n = 5)	(14)	(49)	(17)	(20)	(11)
450	40.6	0.950	152	3.16	60.9
(n = 5)	(40)	(54)	(29)	(29)	(14)
700	79.8	1.25	439	1.74	66.9
(n = 6)	(17)	(49)	(35)	(31)	(21)
1000	104	1.83	691	1.60	76.1
(n = 6)	(22)	(54)	(38)	(32)	(5.4)
1200	118	1.62	787	1.69	68.8
(n = 6)	(13)	(76)	(43)	(28)	(19)
1500	144	1.42	958	1.73	68.1
(n = 6)	(34)	(40)	(36)	(33)	(22)

hydrolyzed back to romazarit, which would be seen as reduced clearance of the parent drug. This reversible glucuronidation has been described for ketoprofen (8) and clofibrate (9), which are both structurally similar small acidic drugs. At doses higher than 700 mg, the romazarit plasma clearance did not decrease further, suggesting that an alternative nonsaturable (or unsaturated) clearance mechanism, such as renal filtration or biliary excretion of the conjugates, was also present. From this study, it seemed that there would be little accumulation during multiple dosing, despite the partially saturable clearance of romazarit. An oral dosage regimen of 700 mg tid was predicted to give steady-state plasma concentrations in the target range, between 50 and 100 mg/L.

Because of the possibility that the pharmacokinetics of romazarit could be different in patients with RA from those in healthy volunteers, a second study was undertaken to provide a better estimate of the appropriate dosing regimen. A total of 24 patients, with definite rheumatoid arthritis according to ARA criteria, were recruited to the study (10) in three sequential groups of eight. Within each group, six patients received romazarit and two received placebo. The first group of patients received a single dose of 100-mg romazarit, followed by 100 mg tid for 19 doses. The second group received 350-mg romazarit as a single dose, followed by 350 mg tid for 19 doses. Concurrent drug analyses in plasma suggested that the proposed regimen of 700 mg tid was too high a dosage rate, and so the third group received 350-mg romazarit as a single dose followed by 350 mg bid for 13 doses. Blood and urine samples were collected over a 49-hr period after the first dose and the last of the multiple doses. An interval of 5 days between the single dose and the start of the multiple dosing allowed interim analysis of the drug concentrations in each patient before proceeding. Tolerability was assessed by daily observation of vital signs and by laboratory safety tests on days 0, 7, 9, 13, and 15. Romazarit concentrations were measured in plasma and urine by HPLC methods (see Sect. III.A).

The 7 male and 17 female patients had a mean age of 61 years, a mean height of 173 cm, and a mean weight of 61 kg. By using the equation of Cockcroft and Gault (11), a mean creatinine clearance of 59.4 ml/min was derived. Adverse events (80 reports in 19 patients) were mainly minor complaints of drowsiness, headache, tingling of the lips, nausea, and rash. These events were evenly distributed across the three dosage groups and the amalgamated placebo group, and did not increase in incidence with increasing dose. One patient in each dose group experienced vomiting, which was thought to be possibly drug-related, and one of these patients withdrew from the study. There were no changes in the vital signs or laboratory safety tests that were thought to be clinically significant.

Mean plasma concentrations of romazarit are illustrated in Figures 4 and 5, and pharmacokinetic parameters are shown in Table 5. After the single 100- and 350-mg doses, the plasma levels of romazarit rose to peaks of 8.1 and 42 mg/L, respectively. The AUC to the last point with detectable drug concentration, AUC_t, seemed to be a reasonable estimate of the infinite area in each patient, because the concentration at the t time point was so much lower than the peak. There was a tenfold increase in AUC_t for a 3.5-fold increase in the single dose from 100 to 350 mg, indicating the nonlinearity of romazarit kinetics and, hence, the inappropriateness of calculating elimination half-lives from these data. The mean urinary recovery of drug-related material was 71%, suggesting extensive romazarit absorption.

After the last of the multiple doses, considerable drug accumulation occurred, especially in the group who received 350 mg tid. Plasma romazarit concentrations rose

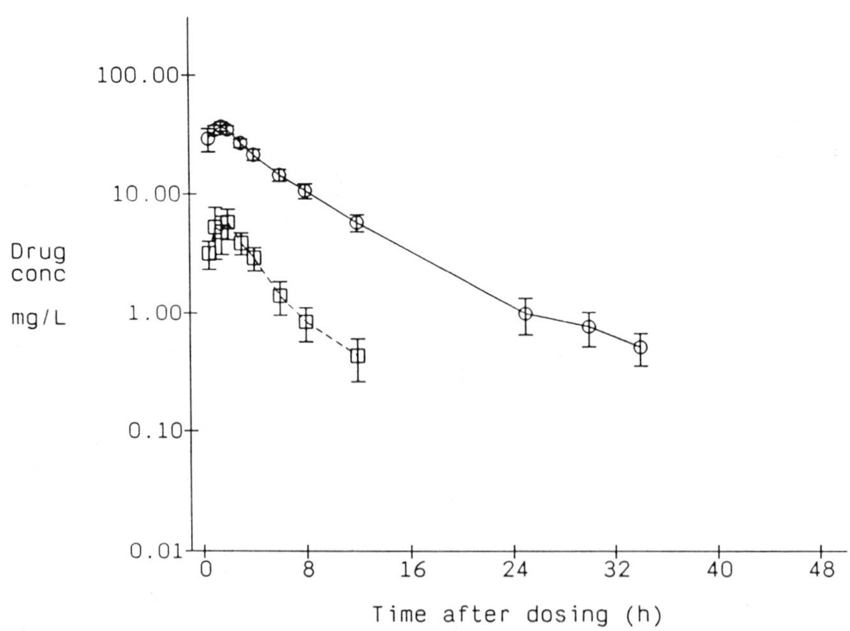

Figure 4 Mean plasma concentrations after single oral doses of romazarit in patients with rheumatoid arthritis. Bars indicate standard error. (-○-) 350 mg, n = 12; (—□—) 100 mg, n = 5.

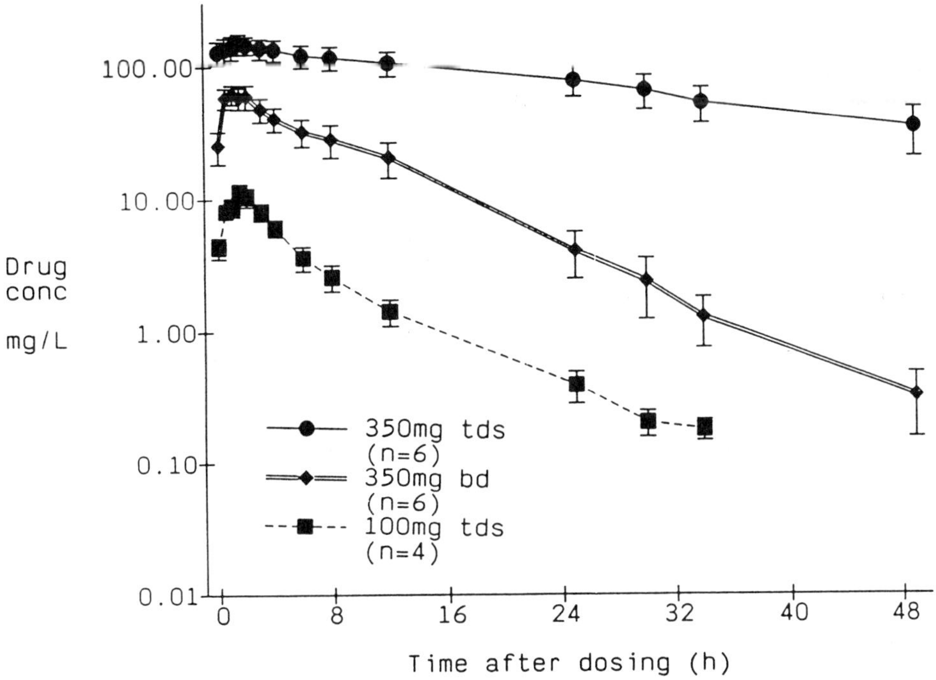

Figure 5 Mean plasma concentrations after multiple oral doses of romazarit in patients with rheumatoid arthritis. Bars indicate standard error.

Table 5 Pharmacokinetic Parameters of Romazarit

Dosage (No. of evaluable patients)	Mean (%CV) parameter values [Units]					
	C_{max} (mg/L)	t_{max} (h)	AUC_d (mg h/L)	AUC_t (mg h/L)	CL/F (L/h)	Ae(49) (% dose)
100-mg single dose	8.1	2.00	22	25	4.93	73
(n = 5)	(58)	(61)	(40)	(40)	(67)	(39)
350-mg single dose before	45.5	1.00	190	216	1.79	76
bid dosing (n = 6)	(37)	(45)	(33)	(32)	(36)	(14)
350-mg single dose before	38.7	2.00	179	281	1.57	64
tds dosing (n = 6)	(16)	(27)	(33)	(35)	(72)	(26)
100 mg tds	11.8	1.38	50	NC	2.11	
last dose (n = 4)	(26)	(18)	(28)		(24)	
350 mg bid last	66.7	1.00	436	NC	1.05	
dose (n = 6)	(40)	(55)	(54)		(57)	
350 mg tds last dose (n = 6)	159	1.33	1050	NC	0.745	
	(37)	(39)	(45)		(150)	

Key: C_{max}, peak plasma concentration; t_{max}, time to peak; AUC, area under the plasma concentration versus time curve (d = during the dosing interval, t to the last time-point with detectable drug); CL/F, apparent plasma clearance, calculated from dose/AUC_t after the first doses and dose/AUC_d after the last doses of each regimen Ae(49), total urinary recovery of drug-related material; NC, implies not calculated.

to mean peaks of 11.8, 159, and 66.7 mg/L after 100 mg tid, 350 mg tid, and 350 mg bid, respectively. A steady state was reached in each patient by the day of the last dose. Then the mean apparent plasma clearances were 2.11, 0.745, and 1.05 L/h from the three regimens. Five of the six patients who received 350 mg tid had plasma clearance below 0.32 L/h. A regression of plasma clearance at steady state on creatinine clearance was significant ($p < 0.01$), but explained only 50% of the variation in the drug clearance values. As the data from the second group became available, it was clear that accumulation in RA patients was greater than that predicted from single doses in healthy volunteers, and so the planned third regimen of 700 mg tid was replaced by 350 mg bid.

Romazarit elimination appeared to be a nonlinear process that was slower in RA patients than in healthy volunteers because of greater dependence on one or more saturable processes, such as tubular secretion of the glucuronide conjugates. In turn, this greater dependence may have arisen because the patients were

1. Suffering from rheumatoid arthritis, which can reduce body weight and renal tubular secretion (11)
2. Older than the healthy volunteers (range 42–73 years vs 20–35 years)
3. More often women, all the volunteers were men
4. Receiving concomitant medication, such as NSAIDs

This second study did not define the pharmacokinetics of romazarit in patients with RA because of the marked nonlinearity. However, simple interpolation between the dosage regimens tested in this study suggested that 450 mg bid should achieve plasma concentrations within the estimated therapeutic range of 50–100 mg/L.

The efficacy study of romazarit was designed to provide statistically significant evidence of the effects of the drug on various markers of disease activity, including Ritchie Articular Index (RI) and C-reactive protein (CRP). Patients, with an RI higher than 12 and other signs of rheumatoid arthritis, were randomly assigned to receive either 200 mg romazarit or 450 mg romazarit, or placebo every 12 h by mouth for 6 months. Efficacy and safety (laboratory tests including drug assay, vital signs, and adverse events) were assessed at baseline and after 2, 4, 8, 12, 16, 20, 24, and 28 weeks. A blood sample, for drug analysis, was taken 50–70 min after dosing at each of these clinic visits. The investigator was to be informed within a week of sampling if any of these analyses detected a plasma romazarit concentration in excess of 200 mg/L.

A total of 224 patients were recruited to the study by 11 investigational centers. There were 59 men and 165 women. They had a mean age of 55 years and a mean weight of 67 kg. At baseline, the mean RI value was 22 in each dose group, but there were significant differences in mean RI between the investigational centers. The adverse events were neither more common nor more severe in the patients given romazarit, compared with those who received placebo, except for a slight trend toward a smaller incidence of blood pressure changes, diarrhea, and abdominal pain in the latter. The biochemical and hematological tests did not reveal any drug-related trends that reached statistical significance.

Plasma concentrations of romazarit varied widely within and between patients in the 200-mg and especially the 450-mg dose groups. The mean ($\pm$CV%) concentrations within dosage groups remained fairly constant throughout the 24 weeks of dosing at 17 (60) mg/L in the 200-mg group and 56 (90) mg/L in the 450-mg group. Thus, the mean concentrations after the higher dose were close to the lower limit of the target therapeutic range. The lower dosage of 200 mg bid was chosen to give plasma concentrations threefold lower than the higher dosage, and this choice was successful. Only three patients had a plasma romazarit concentration greater than 200 mg/L after 2 weeks of dosing; two of these patients were withdrawn from the study, because of gastrointestinal discomfort and elevated serum creatinine, respectively, and one continued to receive romazarit. There did not appear to be a common characteristic of these three that would have predicted their substantial accumulation of the drug.

The mean RI decreased in all groups during the study. By 12 weeks, but not at later time points, there were sufficient patients remaining for an analysis-of-variance of the RI values as changes from baseline. The mean RI in the 200-mg group was 3 units lower than placebo ($p = 0.07$), and the mean RI in the 450-mg group was 4.5 units lower than placebo ($p = 0.01$). The two romazarit groups did not differ significantly from each other. None of the biochemical markers of anti-inflammatory activity such as C-reactive protein or plasma viscosity changed in a significant way during the course of the study.

The statistical analysis of this study was extended by applying the NONMEM suite of programs for mixed effects modeling. Rather than analysis-of-variance at a fixed time point, a multiple linear regression model was tested, which allowed all the RI values from each patient to depend on treatment duration and dosage simultaneously. This regression analysis allowed the construction of a dose–response relationship after 24 weeks of treatment. From a baseline mean RI of 22, placebo gave a decrease of 2.5 units, 200 mg bid gave a decrease of 4.9 units, and 450 mg gave a decrease of 7.8 units. This alternative statistical approach reached the same conclusions as the standard approach, but also incorporated results from patients who completed fewer than 12 weeks treatment and those who completed the full 24 weeks of the study.

Detailed analysis of all of the preclinical and clinical data on romazarit led to the conclusion that the therapeutic margin was not sufficiently favorable to justify progression of the compound to the marketplace, and thus clinical development was discontinued in late 1990.

ACKNOWLEDGMENT

We would like to thank all of our Roche colleagues, too numerous to mention individually, who contributed to the identification and development of romazarit, and we acknowledge that a short review such as this does not do justice to their tremendous efforts.

REFERENCES

1. Goddard D, Butler R, eds. Rheumatoid arthritis: the treatment controversy. London: Macmillan Press, 1984.
2. Billingham MEJ, Rushton AR. Clozic. In: Rainsford K, ed. Anti-inflammatory and anti-rheumatic drugs. vol 3. Boca Raton: CRC Press, 1985:31–63.
3. Lewis EJ, Bishop J, Cashin CH. Automated quantification of rat plasma acute phase reactants in experimental inflammation. J Pharmacol Methods 1989:183–94.
4. Bloxham DP, Bradshaw D, Cashin CH, Dodge BB, Lewis EJ, Westmacott D, Self CR. Biologic properties of romazarit (Ro 31-3948), a potential disease-modifying antirheumatic drug. J Pharmacol Exp Ther 1990; 252:1331–40.
5. Cashin CH, Gill J, Jones SA, Kennedy AJ. An assessment of the delayed hypersensitivity reaction to methylated serum albumin in the mouse and its use in the evaluation of drug effects on cell mediated immune reactions. Agents Actions 1979; 9:553–9.

6. Reddy JK, Lalwani ND. Carcinogenesis by hepatic peroxisomal proliferators: evaluation of the risk of hypolipidemic drugs and industrial plasticizers to humans. CRC Crit Rev Toxicol 1983; 12:1–58.
7. Williams PEO, Muirhead GJ, Worth E, Zimmer R, Lücker P. Pharmacokinetics and tolerance of romazarit after oral administration of ascending single doses to healthy human volunteers. Eur J Drug Metab Pharmacokinet 1990; 15:317–22.
8. Verbeeck RK, Wallace SM, Loewen GR. Reduced elimination of ketoprofen in the elderly is not necessarily due to impaired glucuronidation. Br J Clin Pharmacol 1984; 17:783–4.
9. Meffin PJ, Zilm DM, Veenendaal JR. Reduced clofibric acid clearance in renal dysfunction is due to a futile cycle. J Pharmacol Exp Ther 1983; 22:732–8.
10. Williams PEO, Bird HA, Minty S, Helliwell PS, Muirhead GJ, Bentley J, York A. A pharmacokinetic and tolerance study of romazarit in patients with rheumatoid arthritis. Biopharm Drug Dispos 1992; 13:119–129.
11. Cockcroft DW, Gault MH. Prediction of creatinine clearance from serum creatinine. Nephron 1976; 16:31–41.

19

Tilomisole

RICHARD P. CARLSON,
FRANCIS J. GREGORY,*
and RICHARD L. FENICHEL
Wyeth–Ayerst Research
Princeton, New Jersey

STEVEN C. GILMAN
Sterling Winthrop, Inc.
Collegeville, Pennsylvania

W. CRAIG DANIEL
Wyeth-Ayerst Research
Radnor, Pennsylvania

I. INTRODUCTION

Experiments conducted by Renoux and Renoux (1) using levamisole in Lewis lung tumor-bearing mice established the concept that modulation of the cellular immune system can inhibit the growth and spread of malignant tumors. Similarly, clinical trials with this agent showed efficacy in rheumatoid arthritis patients, although toxicity (manifested by agranulocytosis) has limited its use (2). At Wyeth–Ayerst laboratories, we have developed tilomisole, an anti-inflammatory agent with immunomodulating activities, for the treatment of rheumatoid arthritis and perhaps other diseases involving the immune system (3). In this chapter we will review the immunopharmacology, anti-inflammatory, and antiarthritic activities of tilomisole (Fig. 1) and summarize the current clinical results obtained with this compound.

II. EFFECT ON CELLULAR IMMUNITY

A. T-Cell Proliferation

Stimulation of resting T cells by antigens or mitogens induces activation and proliferation of the cells. Cellular proliferation is a critical means by which sufficient numbers of T cells can be generated to protect the host from microbial, cellular, or viral invasion and, in addition, T cells play a major role in the induction and development of autoimmune diseases such as rheumatoid arthritis and lupus. This response can be conveniently measured in vitro by the uptake of [^{3}H]thymidine into DNA in lymphocytes exposed to mitogenic or antigenic stimuli. As illustrated in Table 1, the antigen-induced proliferative response of splenic T cells from ovalbumin-immunized rats was augmented in the presence of tilomisole (4). Tilomisole also enhanced the proliferative response of human lympho-

*Retired.

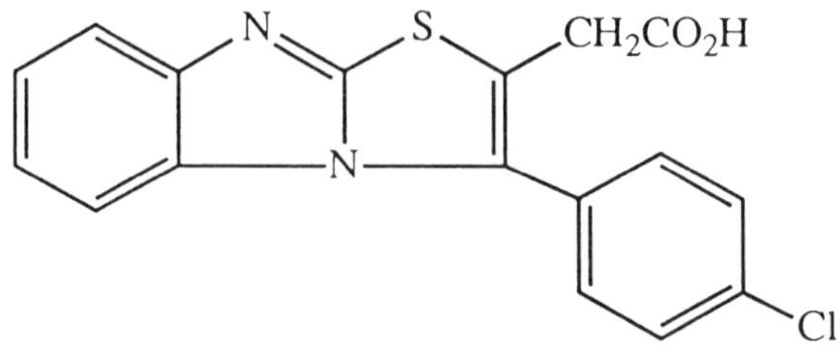

Figure 1 Tilomisole: 3-(*p*-chlorophenyl)thiazolo[3,2-*a*]benzimidazole-2-acetic acid.

cytes to the T-cell mitogen, phytohemmagglutinin (PHA) (5). However, in studies using mouse spleen cells, a mixed pattern of stimulation and inhibition of concanavalin A (Con A)-induced proliferation was observed (stimulation at 0.05 and 0.1 μg per culture) (6,7). In all of these studies, tilomisole was not directly stimulatory to T cells, but instead, increased the reponse of the cells to another stimulus.

Tilomisole has also demonstrated T-cell stimulatory properties in vivo. Administration of 1–10 mg/kg po to rats augmented the ex vivo proliferative response of their spleen cells to the T-cell mitogens Con A and PHA and to ovalbumin antigen (Fig. 2). The ability of tilomisole in vitro (1–10μM) to enhance interleukin-2 (IL-2) production, an important T-cell proliferation factor (8), from rat spleen cells was first demonstrated using (CTLL-2 cells), a murine T-cell line that is absolutely dependent on IL-2 for growth (4). However, this stimulation of IL-2 was seen only when using suboptimal Con A concentrations (O.1 μg/ml). In studies employing peripheral blood leukocytes (PBL) from normal human donors, tilomisole (1–50 μg/ml) also significantly augmented IL-2 production in vitro (3). When developing adjuvant-arthritic rats (see Sect. IV.D), with depressed spleen cell proliferative responses, were treated with tilomisole, 100 mg/kg per day po, for 16 days, IL-2 synthesis was enhanced and the arthritic spleen cells were restored to near-normal proliferative responses (when cultured in vitro with Con A; 9) (Fig. 3). The increase in IL-2 production induced by tilomisole may explain the ability of this compound to augment T-cell proliferation.

B. Interferon gamma

When activated in autologous mixed leukocyte reactions (auto-MLR) in vitro, T cells from normal individuals produce interferon gamma (INF-γ), which can be assessed by the ability of culture supernatant fluids to suppress Epstein–Barr virus-induced prolifera-

Table 1 Effects of Tilomisole on In Vitro Antigen-Specific Proliferative Responses of Spleen Cells from Ovalbumin-Immunized Rats[a]

Tilomisole concentration (μM)	Proliferative response (mean dpm [^{3}H]thymidine uptake $\times 10^{-3} \pm$ SD)
0	16.7 ± 2.9
1	14.3 ± 2.9
10	38.9 ± 5.9*

[a]Spleen cells from ovalbumin-immunized rats were cultured in vitro for 4 days with 100 μg/ml ovalbumin (antigen) in the presence or absence of tilomisole. Uptake of [^{3}H]thymidine in cultures without OA was less than 2000 disintigrations per minute (dpm) and was not changed by drug treatment.

*Statistically significant compared with cultures without tilomisole ($p \leq 0.05$, Dunnett's *t*-test).

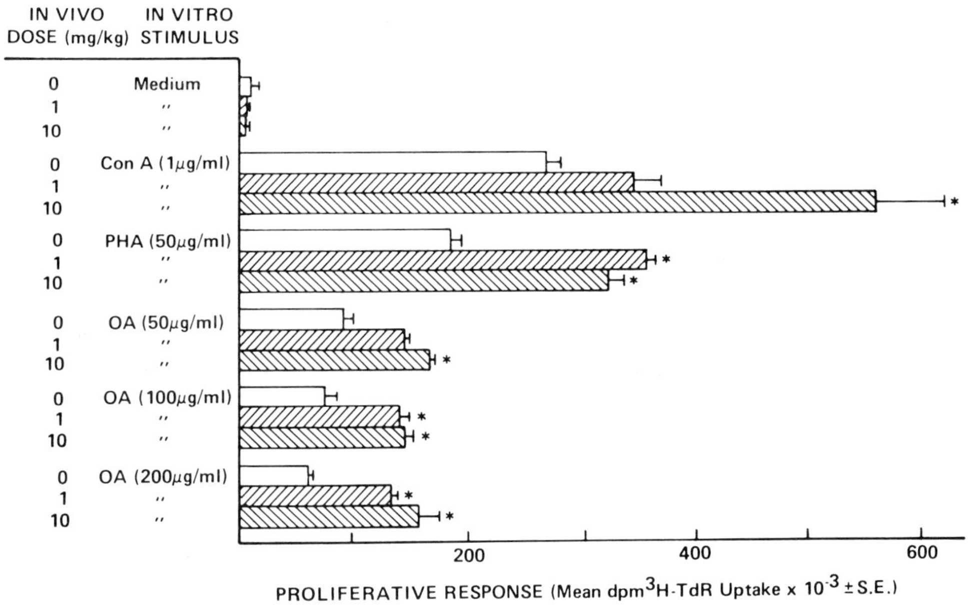

Figure 2 In vivo effects of tilomisole on subsequent in vitro proliferative responses of rat spleen cells. Groups of OA-immunized rats ($N=3$) were given two daily oral doses of vehicle, 1 mg/kg or 10 mg/kg of tilomisole; 24 h after the last dose their spleens were removed, and in vitro spleen cell proliferative responses were assessed. $^*p \leq 0.05$ vs vehicle-treated group (Dunnett's test).

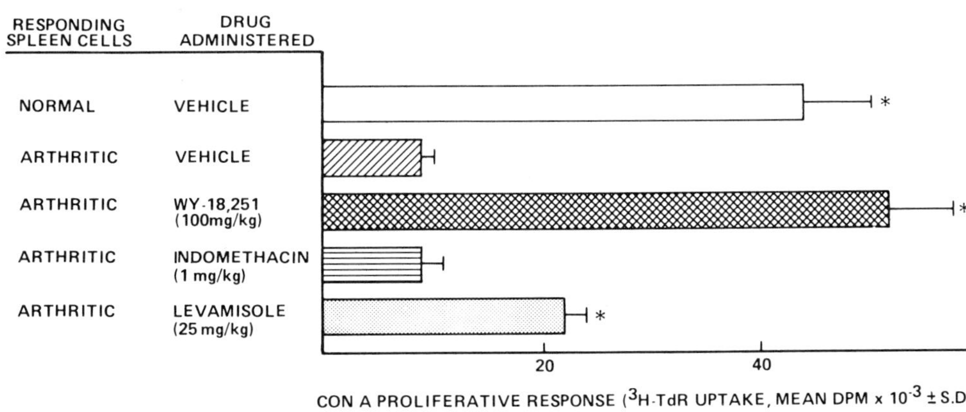

Figure 3 Effects of drug therapy on splenic immune function in rat developing adjuvant-induced arthritis: *M. butyricum*-injected rats were treated daily for 16 days with 100 mg/kg tilomisole (WY-18,251), 25 mg/kg levamisole, or 1 mg/kg indomethacin (po). In vitro spleen cell proliferative responses to T-cell mitogen Con A were then assessed. $^*p<0.05$ compared with vehicle-treated arthritic animals.

tion of normal B cells (10). In contrast, T cells from patients with rheumatoid arthritis (RA) are deficient in their ability to generate INF-γ in auto-MLR. Addition of tilomisole (0.1–100 μg/ml) to the auto-MLR did not affect the production of INF-γ by normal T cells, but 100 μg/ml of tilomisole restored to normal the defective INF-γ synthesis by RA T cells (Fig. 4). Indomethacin (1 μg/ml), but not levamisole (0.1–100 μg/ml), had a similar effect (11).

C. Suppressor T Cells

The effects of tilomisole on the generation of T-suppressor cells was also examined. In vitro culture of normal BALB/c spleen cells with staphylococcal enterotoxin B (SEB) activates antigen nonspecific suppressor T cells (Ts), which can be assayed by their ability to suppress antibody production by B cells in a plaque assay. Tilomisole augmented the generation of Ts cells in this system. Thus, addition of 10–100 μM tilomisole to cultures of spleen cells plus SEB significantly increased Ts activity relative to cultures without the drug (12) (Fig. 5). Similar results were obtained with levamisole, but, in contrast, indomethacin (1–10 μM) inhibited SEB-induced Ts activity (12). That tilomisole may activate Ts cells was further suggested by studies that showed that the drug inhibited

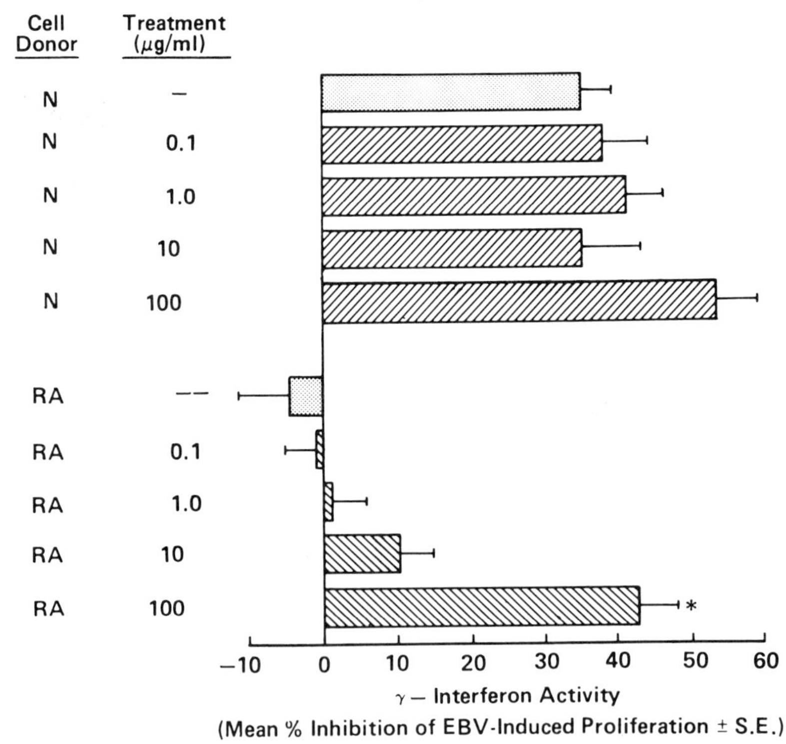

Figure 4 Effects of tilomisole on interferon-γ production by normal and RA lymphocytes. Normal (n=6) and RA (n=8) lymphocytes were cultured for 24 h, with or without 0.1–100 μg/ml tilomisole, in autologous mixed lymphocyte cultures. Supernatant fluids from these cultures were assayed for IFN-γ activity by their ability to suppress EBV-induced B-cell proliferation. *$p \leq 0.05$ vs drug-free control.

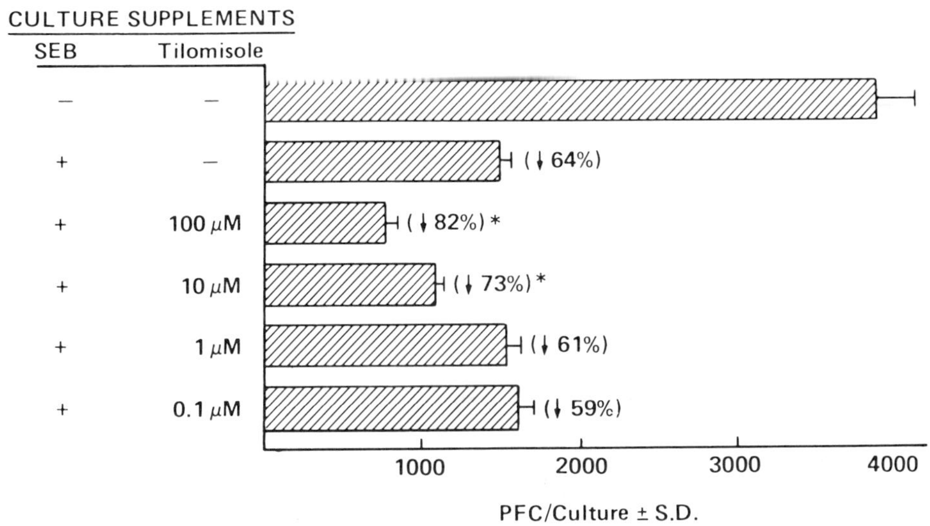

Figure 5 Effects of tilomisole on the SEB-induced production of suppressor T cells (Ts) in vitro. Normal spleen cells were cultured for 48 h at 37°C with 10 μg/ml SEB plus the indicated concentration of tilomisole. The cells were then collected, washed and assayed for Ts activity in a secondary Mishell–Dutton culture system. Note that SEB stimulation induces Ts activity and that tilomisole (10 and 100 μM) increase this Ts activity: ( ) =% suppression relative to no SEB, no drug; $p \leq 0.05$ vs SEB, no drug.

immunoglobulin secretion by methylprednisone-treated pokeweed mitogen-stimulated human peripheral blood leukocytes (13).

D. Natural Killer Cell Activity

Natural killer (NK) cells, leukocytes that have the capacity to lyse a variety of tumor or virus-infected cells, are believed to perform an important protective function against tumor growth and metastasis and to have protective effects against certain viral and bacterial infections (14). The NK cells can directly destroy target cells, but can also lyse cells coated with antibody in a process termed antibody-dependent cellular cytotoxicity (ADCC).

Tilomisole (0.1–10 μM) did not affect the in vitro NK activity of spleen cells from normal rats (4). In addition, when tilomisole was given to mice (1 or 10 mg/kg, ip), either as a single dose or on two occasions 1 week apart, it did not alter the ADCC activity of splenocytes harvested 1 week after drug administration.

E. Effect on Phagocytosis

Clearance of intravenously administered carbon from the blood by the reticuloendothelial system (liver and spleen) provides one measure of phagocytic capacity in mice. Carbon clearance was not enhanced in mice given tilomisole intravenously at doses of 1.25, 5, and 10 mg/kg (15). In contrast, levamisole, at an intravenous dose of 4 mg/kg, did enhance carbon clearance. However, neither tilomisole (1–100 mg/kg) nor levamisole (3–30 mg/kg) was effective when administered orally 24 h before carbon injection (15). These results show that tilomisole does not effect phagocytic activity in the reticuloendothelial system.

F. Delayed-Type Hypersensitivity

The effect of tilomisole on delayed hypersensitivity was measured in both cyclophosphamide-immunosuppressed guinea pigs using dinitrochlorobenzene (DNCB) as an antigen (3) and normal mice sensitized to suboptimal doses of methylated bovine serum albumin (mBSA) (16). Tilomisole, at oral doses of 50–150 mg/kg significantly enhanced the delayed-type hypersensitivity reaction in the guinea pigs, indicative of its capacity to enhance cellular immunity (Table 2).

III. EFFECT ON HUMORAL IMMUNITY

Tilomisole demonstrated condition-dependent effects on immunoglobulin production. oral doses of 10 and 100 mg/kg reduced plaque-forming cell (PFC) formation in the spleens of normal mice (4) and in vitro PFC formation by enhancing the generation of suppressor T cells which, in turn, down-regulated antibody production (see Sect. II.C).

In contrast to these murine studies, tilomisole had little effect on immunoglobulin secretion by human B cells. Thus, concentrations of 0.1–10 μM did not significantly affect the pokeweed mitogen-induced secretion of immunoglobulins by cultured human peripheral blood mononuclear (PBM) cells (17). As mentioned earlier (see Sect. II.C), tilomisole produced a small, but statistically significant, reduction of IgM and IgG secretion by pokeweed mitogen-stimulated methylprednisolone-treated human PBM. This effect was most dramatic when the cells were preincubated with tilomisole and then washed before addition of pokeweed mitogen and methylprednisolone (13). Collectively, these data indicate that tilomisole treatment results in a diminution of immunoglobulin synthesis by B cells, but that this effect is mediated by indirect mechanisms such as T-suppressor cells.

IV. EFFECTS ON INFLAMMATION: ARTHRITIC IMMUNOINFLAMMATORY STUDIES IN RATS

Antiinflammatory activity is not a characteristic of most immunomodulating agents, such as *d*-penicillamine, levamisole, and gold. Although considerable interest has centered on the use of immunomodulators in the treatment of rheumatoid arthritis and other

Table 2 Effect of Tilomosile on the Delayed-Type Hypersensitivity Reaction to DNCB in Immunosuppressed Guinea Pigs

Oral dose (mg/kg)	No. guinea pigs	Area of erythema (mm^2 ± SE)
0	16	671 ± 40
50	10	860 ± 46*
100	10	888 ± 42*
150	7	913 ± 41*

$^*p < 0.01$, Student's *t*-test.

autoimmune diseases, it is assumed that these agents act by restoring toward normal the derangements in immune function that are believed to play a role in the pathophysiology of these diseases. Data presented in the following sections indicate that tilomisole possesses aspirinlike anti-inflammatory activity, similar to other nonsteroidal anti-inflammatory drugs, with resultant inhibition of prostaglandin synthesis. Also, the possession of immunomodulating activities makes tilomisole a more suitable drug to treat rheumatoid arthritis and other autoimmune diseases.

A. Carrageenan-Induced Paw Edema

In this standard model of inflammation, carrageenan is injected into the subplantar region of the hind paw of rats, and paw volume is measured at zero time and at 3 h. Oral administration of 50–100 mg/kg tilomisole 1 h before injection of carrageenan into the footpad significantly reduced the resultant inflammatory response at 3 h (ED_{50} = 200 mg/kg; 15). In comparison, aspirin and indomethacin produced ED_{50} of 130 and 7.5 mg/kg, respectively. Levamisole also showed some minor effects (about 40% at 30 mg/kg) in this model, but failed to inhibit the response in a dose-related fashion. Moreover, the anti-inflammatory action of levamisole was abolished by prior adrenalectomy of the rats, whereas the response to tilomisole remained intact (15). In acute combination studies in the rat carrageenan edema model using naproxen and aspirin, only the tilomisole–aspirin mixture (60:40) showed a less than addictive effect (17).

B. Gastric Tolerance in Rats

Gastric tolerance of tilomisole was assessed in rats fasted for 16 h before oral drug administration. Gastric irritancy was measured in terms of the number of rats with ulcers and the increase in gastric fluid contents (gastric swelling) 4 h after drug administration (15). Tilomisole and aspirin produced gastric swelling at doses of 120 mg/kg and higher, but no gastric ulcers. Indomethacin produced gastric ulcers at doses of 5 mg/kg and higher, but no gastric swelling.

C. Rat Hyperesthesia and Yeast-Induced Fever

Tilomisole demonstrated significant analgesic activity as assessed by the Randall–Selitto yeast-induced hyperalgesia test, but only at a very high dose (300 mg/kg) (15). Its activity was not as great as that of aspirin in this model. Tilomisole was not antipyretic; oral administration of doses of 25, 50, and 100 mg/kg did not prevent the development of fever in rats injected subcutaneously with brewer's yeast (15).

D. Rat Adjuvant-Induced Arthritis

The adjuvant arthritis model is an experimental arthritic disease model that shares some features in common with rheumatoid arthritis in human (18). Dessicated *Mycobacterium butyricum*, suspended in mineral oil, is injected into the paw of a rat, and 16 days later the immunologically induced inflammatory response ("secondary edema") in the uninjected paw is measured. In this developing model, tilomisole demonstrated anti-inflammatory activity, depending on the dosing schedule employed (15).

For example, different oral dosing schedules for tilomisole produced different effects on paw edema at day 16 [i.e., days 2, 3, 4 regimen at 50 and 100 mg/kg near the time of antigen presentation augmented the paw edema; 90 mg/kg on a daily schedule (0–15) inhibited paw edema; and a regimen on days 16, 17, 18, at 50 and 100 mg/kg inhibited established paw edema].

Rats undergoing developing adjuvant arthritis, demonstrate markedly reduced spleen cell proliferative responses to Con A, PHA, and pokeweed mitogen (PWM) by day 16, which correlates with the development of inflammation (paw edema) and bone damage (erosions) (9,19,20). This reduction in arthritic spleen cell proliferation is probably due to a reduction in IL-2 synthesis from these cells (see Sect. II.A). However, this reduction in spleen cell proliferative response may have no part in the pathogenesis of T-cell-mediated adjuvant arthritis. Treatment of arthritic rats with 100 mg/kg po of tilomisole restored to normal the reduced spleen cell proliferative response (see Fig. 3) and inhibited paw edema by approximately 37%. Indomethacin, 1 mg/kg, inhibited only paw edema (about 44%). Levamisole (25 mg/kg) partially restored spleen cell proliferation without affecting the paw edema.

Daily administration of 50–200 mg/kg po of tilomisole in the rat established adjuvant arthritic model from day 16 to 29 following *M. butyricum* injection on day 0, significantly inhibited paw edema in a dose-related manner (Table 3) and bone lesions at 200 mg/kg (ie., erosions, osteoporosis, periosteal reaction, increase in soft tissue, and calcification) in the uninjected paw (Table 4) (9). In this model, tilomisole (ED_{50} = 200 mg/kg) was two to three times more potent than aspirin, but 125 times less potent than indomethacin. In a second study using the rat established adjuvant model, a tilomisole–naproxen mixture (80:20) produced greater than additive anti-inflammatory effects (reduction in paw edema and bone erosion) at low-dose combinations (i.e., tilomisole, 1 mg/kg, and naproxen, 4 mg/kg), and no gastroirritation was observed at these doses (17). The immunomodulatory activity of tilomisole may play a role in this synergistic action, although tilomisole has a very high-binding affinity to plasma albumin (>99%), which may make the more potent naproxen available to reduce inflammation at the sites of inflammation at lower doses.

Table 3 Effect of Tilomisole, Aspirin, and Indomethacin on Paw Edema in Rats with Established Adjuvant-Induced Arthritis[a]

Treatment group	Oral dose (mg/kg)	Left paw edema (mean ml ± SEM)	% change
Arthritic control		1.64 ± 0.10	
Tilomisole	50	1.18 ± 0.15	–28
	100	1.11 ± 0.10	–33*
	200	0.78 ± 0.06	–53*
Aspirin	75	1.46 ± 0.11	–11
	150	1.35 ± 0.08	–18
	300	1.07 ± 0.06	–38*
Indomethacin	0.4	1.16 ± 0.10	–29*
	0.8	0.97 ± 0.06	–41*
	1.6	0.73 ± 0.05	–55*

[a]Lewis rats were injected on day 0 with 0.5 mg *M. butyricum* emulsion in the right hind paw. Sixteen days later groups of 8–10 animals were given the indicated drugs daily *po* for 14 days. Edema in the uninjected paw was then measured using a mercury plethysmograph.

*Significantly different from athritic control group ($p < 0.05$, Dunnett's *t*-test).

Table 4 Effect of Tilomisole, Aspirin, and Indomethacin on Radiographic Assessment of Bony Changes in Rats with Established Adjuvant Arthritis[a]

Drug	Oral Dose (mg/kg)	Osteoporosis		Erosion		Periosteal reraction		Increase in soft tissue		Calcification	
		Mean ±SE	% Change	Mean ±SE	% Change	Mean ±SE	% Change	Mean ±SE	% Change	Mean ±SE	% Change
Arthritic control		2.45 ± 0.1		2.50 ± 0.2		2.45 ± 0.1		2.50 ± 0.2		2.30 ± 0.3	
Tilomisole	50	1.85 ± 0.2	–24*	1.65 ± 0.2	–34*	1.85 ± 0.2	–24*	2.10 ± 0.1	–16	1.45 ± 0.2	–37
	100	2.21 ± 0.1	–10	2.07 ± 0.2	–17	2.36 ± 0.1	–4	2.29 ± 0.1	–8	1.86 ± 0.2	–19
	200	1.19 ± 0.1	–51*	0.94 ± 0.2	–62*	1.13 ± 0.2	–54*	1.75 ± 0.3	–30*	1.00 ± 0.2	–57*
Aspirin	75	2.29 ± 0.1	–7	2.36 ± 0.1	–6	2.14 ± 0.1	–13	2.43 ± 0.1	–3	1.93 ± 0.2	–16
	150	2.31 ± 0.2	–6	2.31 ± 0.3	–8	2.38 ± 0.2	–3	2.50 ± 0.1	0	1.94 ± 0.3	–16
	300	1.30 ± 0.2	–47*	1.40 ± 0.2	–44*	1.15 ± 0.2	–53*	1.85 ± 0.1	–26*	1.15 ± 0.3	–50*
Indomethacain	0.4	2.00 ± 0.2	–18	2.07 ± 0.3	–17	2.00 ± 0.2	–18	2.00 ± 0.2	–20	1.36 ± 0.5	–41
	0.8	2.30 ± 1.3	–6	1.80 ± 0.2	–28	2.25 ± 0.1	–8	2.10 ± 0.2	–16	1.45 ± 0.3	–37
	1.6	1.05 ± 0.1	–57*	0.75 ± 0.2	–70*	0.80 ± 0.1	–67*	1.20 ± 0.1	–52*	0.40 ± 0.2	–83*

[a]Lewis rats were injected on day 0 with 0.5 *M butyricum* emulsion in the right hind paw. Sixteen days later, groups of 8–10 rats were treated daily for 14 days with the indicated drug (*po*). X-rays of the uninjected paws were taken using a General Electric 1000 dental x-ray machine (0.5 sec, 52 kV). Radiographs were examined under code for severity of pathological changes (erosion, osteoporosis, periosteal reaction, increase in soft tissue, and calcification) using the following rating system: 0, none; 1, mild; 2, moderate; 3, severe.

*Significantly different from arthritic control group ($p \leq 0.05$) Dunnett's *t*-test.

E. Rat Type II Collagen-Induced Arthritis

Subcutaneous injection of type II collagen (bovine articular cartilage) in incomplete Freund's adjuvant in the paw and 7 days later in the tail produces a polyarthritic disease similar to adjuvant arthritis, but less severe. This model was boosted with muramyl dipeptide to increase incidence and severity. Oral administration of tilomisole at 10 mg/kg daily for 14 days (starting at day 21) significantly reduced paw edema by about −26% (15).

F. Mouse (MRL/l) Lupus Model

MRL/l mice spontaneously develop an autoimmune disease similar to systemic lupus erythematosus in humans. However, MRL/l mice have a severe lymphoadenopathy intertwined with the lupus manifestations. Tilomisole (1–100 mg/kg, po) and levamisole (0.3–30 mg/kg, po) were not effective in preventing or reducing the lupuslike disease in MRL/l mice. Thus, 78 consecutive days of drug administration did not alter any clinical parameters of the disease including glomerular nephritis, autoimmune antibodies, peripheral blood lymphocytosis, lymphadenopathy, or mortality (3).

V. EFFECTS ON ENZYME SYSTEMS

A. Arachidonic Acid Cascade

Arachidonic acid, liberated from phospholipid pools during cellular activation processes, can be metabolized into a number of inflammatory lipid mediators. Products of the cyclooxygenase pathway, particularly prostaglandin E_2 (PGE_2), play an important role in many inflammatory and immune reactions (21).

Inhibition of prostaglandin synthesis is believed to be responsible for much of the anti-inflammatory activity of nonsteroidal anti-inflammatory drugs. More recently, it has become evident that products of the lipoxygenase enzyme pathway of arachidonic acid metabolism, leukotrienes and hydroxyeicosatetraenoic acids (HETEs), are also potent immunoinflammatory mediators (22).

1. Prostaglandin Synthetase

Tilomisole inhibited prostaglandin synthetase activity in a cell-free preparation from sheep seminal vesicles (IC_{50} = 4.7 μM) and was more potent than aspirin (IC_{50} = 190 μM) in this (15). In addition, tilomisole produced a dose-dependent inhibition of PGE_2 formation by zymosan-stimulated mouse peritoneal macrophages (Fig. 6). Again, tilomisole (IC_{50} = 2 μM) was more potent than aspirin (IC_{50} = 10 μM), but less potent than indomethacin (IC_{50} = 0.003 μM); levamisole was inactive (≤20% inhibition at 100 μM) (15). Similar results were obtained when the prostacyclin metabolite, 6-keto-$PGF_{1\alpha}$, biosynthesis was measured. None of the drugs directly influenced marcrophage phagocytosis or cell viability.

2. Lipoxygenase Enzymes

Although tilomisole inhibited prostaglandin synthetase, it did not inhibit lipoxygenase enzymes. Although the synthesis of 5-HETE by rat neutrophils was inhibited by nordihydroguaiaretic acid (IC_{50} = 1 μM), concentrations as high as 100 μM of tilomisole or indomethacin did not reduce 5-HETE synthesis by more than 30%. Similarly, the synthesis of 15-HETE by a cell-free preparation of soybean 15-lipoxygenase was unaffected by tilomisole (15).

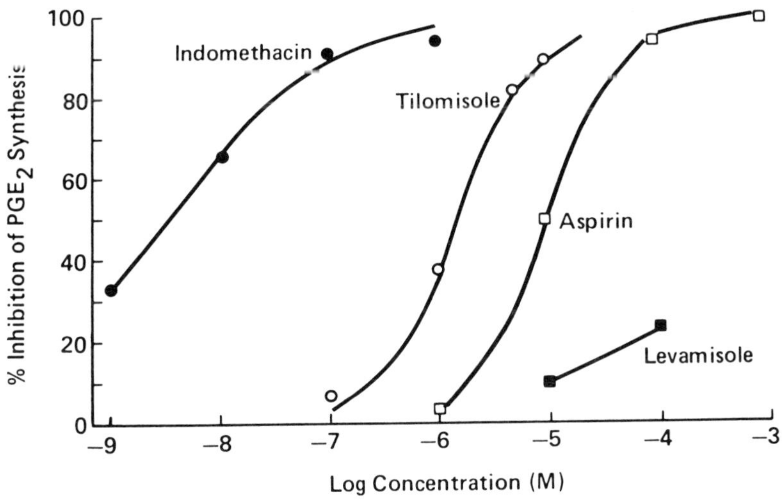

Figure 6 Effect of tilomisole (○——○), indomethacin (●——●), aspirin (□——□), and levamisole (■——■) on in vitro PGE_2 biosynthesis in zymosan-stimulated mouse peritoneal macrophages.

B. Collagenase

The action of collagenase may be involved both in the mediation of joint damage in rheumatoid arthritis and in the spread of metastatic tumor cells. Both of these processes involve the breakdown or penetration of connective tissues. Collagenase is formed excessively in rheumatoid lesions and has been identified at the cartilage–pannus junction (23). Thus, the capacity of a drug to inhibit collagenolysis may contribute to its antirheumatic activity.

When tested at Wyeth–Ayerst against two different concentrations of collagenase obtained from human skin fibroblasts, tilomisole displayed weak inhibitory activity (near 80% at 1 mM; unpublished data). In comparison, indomethacin showed little activity (near 14% at 1 mM).

VI. ANCILLARY PHARMACOLOGY AND TOXICOLOGY

Tilomisole is well tolerated by a variety of experimental animals. For example, assessment of the oral acute toxicity of tilomisole gave an LD_{50} of 969 mg/kg for male mice and 1033 mg/kg for male rats (24,25). In subacute toxicity studies, lasting 3 months, dogs receiving an oral dose of 54 mg/kg once weekly exhibited emesis on the day of dosing, but other adverse drug-related effects were small, inconsistent, or absent (26,27). Following oral administration, bioavailability of tilomisole is 75–85% in dogs and rhesus monkeys, and peak plasma concentrations of 79–100 μgEq/ml can be reached. The plasma half-lives of tilomisole, measured by radiolabeled drug, were about 8 and 15 h in the dog and monkey, respectively (28,29). Tilomisole is metabolized primarily by glucuronidation and fecal excretion (greater than 80%) is the preponderant route of elimination in dogs, and rhesus monkeys (30). Moreover, tilomisole is not teratogenic and is Ames test-negative.

Tilomisole did not demonstrate clinically significant pharmacological effects in variety of cardiovascular, central nervous system, endocrine, or metabolic tests.

VII. CLINICAL TRIAL WITH TILOMISOLE

A. Pharmacokinetics

An initial pilot study was performed to determine the pharmacokinetics of a single oral dose of 250 mg of tilomisole (free acid) in four healthy men between 30 and 44 years of age (31). Anticoagulated venous blood samples for plasma determinations were collected at 0 time and 1, 2, 4, 6, 8, 12, 24, and 48 hours after drug administration. Complete 48-h urine specimens were also obtained. Peak plasma concentrations of 21–25 μg/ml were achieved 2–4 h after dose administration. The plasma half-life was 6.1–14.4 h, with clearances ranging from 20.2 to 34.9 ml/min; volumes of distribution were 18.6–33 L (31). Urinary excretion of the drug over 48 h evidenced a mean of 24 ± 9% (SD). No adverse effects were reported in this study.

An open-label dose proportionality study (six subjects) was performed to determine the pharmacokinetics of single oral doses of tilomisole (2, 10, and 25 mg/kg) in healthy normal subjects. A three-period crossover design was used that included 1 week washout intervals between doses. Plasma was separated from heparinized blood samples before each dose, at 30-min intervals through 4 h, and after 5, 6, 9, 12, 18, 24, 48, and 96 h. Plasma concentrations of tilomisole were detected 30 min to 48 h after ingestion. Table 5 summarizes the pharmacokinetic values obtained from the plasma concentration–time data for each dose of tilomisole.

The mean lag time (t_{lag}) before the start of absorption was 20–30 min after each dose of tilomisole; average total absorption time was about 90 min. The mean time for peak concentration (t_{max}) ranged from 1.9 to 2.5 h for the three doses; the peak concentrations (C_{max}) were not linearly proportional to dose. The mean terminal dispositions half life ($t_{1/2}$) and the mean apparent volume of distribution at steady state (V_{ss}/F) were dose-dependent. The total areas under the plasma concentration–time curve (AUC) were dose-proportional, with mean ratios of 1:15:12. In this study, 16–26% of each dose of tilomisole, was recovered in the urine within 24 h after drug administration.

One subject withdrew from the study after his first dose of tilomisole (25 mg/kg)

Table 5 Pharmacokinetic Parameters of Oral Tilomisole in Healthy Volunteers

Parameters	Dose: 2 mg/kg	Dose: 10 mg/kg	Dose: 25 mg/kg
C_{max} (μg/ml)	16 (10–22)[a]	54 (28–84)	96 (49–168)
t_{max} (h)	1.9 (1.4–2.7)	2.2 (2.0–2.6)	2.5 (1.6–3.0)
t_{lag} (min)	26 (12–40)	23 (15–40)	34 (7–56)
t_{abs} (h)	1.5 (0.9–2.6)	1.6 (1.2–2.2)	1.5 (0.7–2.5)
AUC [(μg/ml)hr]	84 (54–121)	449 (255–706)	988 (417–1631)
C1/F (m/h^{-1} kg^{-1})	29 (18–43)	26 (11–36)	28 (15–47)
$t_{1/2}$ (h)	7 (2–10)	10 (8–12)	13 (8–19)
V_{ss}/F (ml/kg)	114 (64–177)	193 (126–326)	304 (145–501)

[a]Numbers represent the mean values with the range in parentheses.

because of mild nausea and dizziness that began 130 min after drug administration and persisted for 3 h before disappearing spontaneously. There were no other clinically significant adverse effects.

B. Efficacy

An early Phase II, open-label clinical trial was initiated in patients with severe rheumatoid arthritis who had not been adequately controlled by conventional NSAID therapy; most had also not responded to remission-inducing agents, such as gold or penicillamine.

Twenty-four patients, 24–46 years of age, with active rheumatoid arthritis participated in this study. Active disease was defined as the presence of six or more swollen joints, and at least two of the following criteria (1) six or more tender joints on pressure, (2) sedimentation rate of at least 25 mm/h, or (3) morning stiffness of at least 45-min duration. Patients were permitted to take aspirin or NSAIDs during the study. Prednisone (or its equivalent), up to 10 mg po daily, was also allowed.

Tilomisole was given orally on a twice-a-day schedule for 24 weeks; the morning dose was administered 1 h after breakfast and the evening dose 12 h later. Patients received 250 mg of tilomisole bid the first week, 500 mg bid during week 2, and 1000 mg bid during weeks 3–24. Evaluations performed every 4 weeks included joint counts for tenderness and swelling, as well as physician and patient global assessment.

The results of this study are shown in Table 6. At 3 months, most of patients showed at least 30% improvement from baseline in the primary efficacy measures. At 6 months, more than half of the patients demonstrated at least 50% improvement in key efficacy

Table 6 Mean Decreases From Pretherapy Baseline During Initial 24 Weeks of Tilomisole Therapy

Efficacy assessment	Study week	n	Baseline mean	Therapy mean	Mean decrease
Number of tender joints	4	23	32.9	29.3	−3.5*
	12	22	32.3	22.5	−9.7*
	24	12	28.8	18.3	−10.5*
	Final	23	32.9	21.0	−11.9*
Number of swollen joints	4	23	25.4	22.6	−22.8[b]
	12	22	24.8	15.4	−9.4*
	24	12	22.5	7.8	−14.7*
	Final	23	25.4	13.9	−11.6*
Physician's[a] assessment	4	23	55.2	47.8	−7.3*
	12	22	55.6	37.5	−18.1*
	24	12	53.8	25.6	−28.2*
	Final	23	55.2	36.1	−19.1*
Patient's[a] assessment	4	23	62.3	55.7	−6.6[b]
	12	22	61.7	42.6	−19.1*
	24	12	63.0	30.7	−32.3*
	Final	23	62.3	41.0	−21.2*

[a]Assessment was made using a 100-mm visual analog scale with 0 representing feeling perfectly well and 100 representing feeling as bad as possible.

[b]$0.05 < p < 0.06$.

*Statistically significant at the 0.05 level.

variables (32); none of the patients had a 10% or greater worsening relative to baseline in any primary efficacy measure. At 6 months, significant ($p < 0.05$) improvement relative to pretherapy baseline values was observed for each of the primary efficacy parameters.

Gastrointestinal symptoms were the most frequently reported side effects (nine patients) in this study. These were generally mild to moderate in severity and improved spontaneously or in response to standard therapy. Three patients discontinued treatment because of side effects: one patient reported a rash after 35 days of active therapy, another reported an episode of tinnitus after 177 days of treatment, and a third patient reported a decrease in appetite after 356 days of treatment in the extension phase of the study. All symptoms resolved spontaneously when drug was discontinued.

REFERENCES

1. Renoux G, Renoux M. Levamisole inhibits and cures a solid malignant tumor and its pulmonmary metastasis in mice. Nature 1972; 240: 217.
2. Symoens J, Veys E, Mielants M, Pinals R. Adverse reactions to levamisole. Cancer Treat Rep 1978; 62:1721–30.
3. Gregory FJ. Thiazolobenzimidazole and thiazolobenzothiazole compounds as biological response modifiers. In: Fenichel R, Chirigos MA, eds. Immune modulation agents and their mechanisms. New York: Marcel Dekker, 1984:21–38.
4. Gilman SC, Carlson RP, Lewis AJ. Immunomodulatory activity of WY-18,251 (3-(*p*-chlorophenyl)thiazolo\[3,2-*a*] benzimidazole-2-acetic acid). J Immuno-pharmacol 1985; 7:79–98.
5. Colot M, Misksche M. Influence of thiabenzimidazole, WY-18,251, on cancer patients lymphocyte reactivity. J Immunopharmacol 1982–1983; 4:367–76.
6. Fenichel RL, Alburn HE, Schreck PA, Bloom R, Gregory FJ. Immunomodulating and antimetastatic activity of 3-(*p*-chlorophenyl)thiazolo[3,2-*a*] benzimidazole-2-acetic acid (WY-18,251, NSC 310633). J Immunopharmacol 1980; 2:491–508.
7. Fenichel RL, Dheer SK, Grant NH, Scott DP, Bloom R, Gregory FJ. Immunomodulating activity of 3-(*p*-chlorophenyl)thiazolo[3,2-*a*]benzimidazole-2-acetic acid (WY-18,251, NSC 310633) in mice implanted with Lewis lung tumor. Effect of WY-18,251 on lymphocyte proliferation and phagocytosis. J Immunopharmacol 1983; 5:333–40.
8. Smith KA. Interleukin 2. Immunol Rev 1980; 51:337–57.
9. Gilman SC, Carlson RP, Daniels JF, Datko L, Berner PB, Lewis AJ. Lymphoid abnormalities in rats with adjuvant-induced arthritis. II. Effect of antiarthritic therapy on immune function in relation to disease development. Int J Immunopharmacol 1987; 9:9–16.
10. Bardwick PA, Bleustein HG, Zvaifler NJ, Depper JM, Seegmiller JF. Altered regulation of Epstein–Barr virus induced lymphoblast proliferation in rheumatoid arthritis lymphoid cells. Arthritis Rheum 1980; 23:626–32.
11. Gilman SC, Bleustein HD. Effects of tilomisole, indomethacin and levamisole on regulation of Epstein–Barr virus induced B cell proliferation by peripheral blood mononuclear cells from normal individuals and patients with rheumatoid arthritis. Agents Actions 1987; 21:1–3.
12. Rogers CM, Rogers TJ, Gilman SC. Effects of WY-18,251 (3-(*p*-chlorophenyl)thiazolo[3,2-*a*]benzimidazole-2-acetic acid), levamisole and indomethacin on the generation of murine T suppressor cells in vitro. J Immunopharmacol 1985; 7:479–88.
13. Fenichel R, Dheer S. Inhibition of immunoglobulin synthesis by steroid sensitized human lymphocytes by a thiazolobenzimidazole compound (WY-18,251, NSC310633). Int J Immunopharmacol 1982; 4:332.
14. Herberman RB, ed. Natural cell-mediated immunity against tumors. New York: Academic Press, 1980: 1–1309.
15. Gilman SC, Carlson RP, Chang J, Lewis AJ. The antiinflammatory activity of the im-

munomodulator WY-18,251 (3-(*p*-chlorophenyl)thiazolo[3,2-*a*]benzimidazole-2-acetic acid). Agents Actions 1985; 17:53–9.

16. Lewis AJ, Parker J, DiLuigi J, Carlson RP. Immunomodulation delayed hypersensitivity to methylated bovine serum albumin (MBSA) in mice using subliminal and normal sensitization procedures. J Immunopharmacol 1981–1982; 3:289–307.
17. Calhoun W, Gilman SC, Datko LJ, Copenhaver TW, Carlson RP. Interaction studies of tilomisole, aspirin and naproxen in acute and chronic inflammation with assessment of gastrointestinal irritancy in the rat. Agents Actions 1991; 36:99–106.
18. Gilman SC, Carlson RP, Lewis AJ, Rogers TD, Scheffel J. Immunopharmacological modulation of antibody-forming cell responses. Agents Actions 1985; 16:611–12.
19. Billingham MEJ. Models of arthritis and the search for antiarthritic drugs. Pharmacol Ther 1983; 21:389–428.
20. Gilman SC, Daniels JF, Wilson RE, Carlson RP, Lewis AJ. Lymphoid abnormalities in rats with adjuvant-induced arthritis. I. Mitogen responsiveness and lymphokine synthesis. Ann Rheum Dis 1984; 43:847–55.
21. Kuehl FA Jr, Egan RW. Prostaglandins, arachidonic acid, and inflammation. Science 1980; 210:978–84.
22. Rola-Pleszcynski M. Immunoregulation by leukotrienes and other lipoxygenase metabolites. Immunol Today 1985; 6:302–7.
23. Wooley DE, Tetlo LC, Evanson JM. Collagenase immunolocalization studies of rheumatoid and malignant tissues. In: Wooley DE, Evanson JM, eds. Collagenases in normal and pathological connective tissue. Chichester: John Wiley 1980:105–25.
24. DiZio SM. WY-18,2512 Na: acute oral toxicity study in male mice. (Data on file at Wyeth–Ayerst Laboratories).
25. Burlingame PS, DiZio SM. WY-18,251 Na: acute oral toxocity study in rats. (Data on file at Wyeth–Ayerst Laboratories).
26. Tucker, CA, DiZio SM. WY-18,251 Na: acute oral toxicity study in dogs. (Data on file at Wyeth–Ayerst Laboratories).
27. Salamone R. WY-18,251 Na: three-month oral (capsule) drug safety evaluation in dogs. (Data on file at Wyeth–Ayerst Laboratories).
28. Janssen FW. Concentrations of WY-18,251 in the plasma of dogs given a single oral 6, 18 or 54 mg/kg dose of the sodium salt of the drug in a capsule. (Data on file at Wyeth–Ayerst Laboratories).
29. Janssen FW. Disposition of WY-18,251 in rhesus monkeys each given single 20 mg/kg intravenous and intragastric doses of ^{14}C-labeled WY-18,251. (Data on file at Wyeth–Ayerst Laboratories).
30. Janssen FW, Kirkman SK, Fenselau C, Sogniew M, Hoffman B, Young E, Ruelius H. Metabolic formation of N^{-} and *O*-glucuronides of 3-(*p*-chlorophenyl)thiazolo[3,2-*a*]benzimidazole-2-acetic acid. Drug Metab Dispos 1982; 10:599–604.
31. Knowles J, et al. Concentrations of WY-18,251 in human plasma and urine following a single 250 mg oral dose of the drug pilot study. (Data on file at Wyeth–Ayerst Laboratories).
32. Rooney TH, Horowitz P, Forster T, Koehnke R, Furst DE. Preliminary report of tilomisole: a new immunomodulator in active resistant rheumatoid arthritis (RA). Arthritis Rheum 1987; 30:560.

20

Leflunomide: A Novel Immunomodulating Drug

ROBERT R. BARTLETT, GILES CAMPION, PREDRAG MUSIKIC
and RUDOLPH SCHLEYERBACH
Hoechst AG Werk Kalle-Albert
Wiesbaden, Germany

THOMAS ZIELINSKI
J. Gutenberg University
Mainz, Germany

H.-ULRICH SCHORLEMMER
Behring Research Laboratories
Marburg, Germany

I. INTRODUCTION

The discovery of novel drugs, or any other thing in science, is very often pure serendipity.[*] Sometimes the finding may seem to have been serendipitous, but, in retrospect, was actually the luck of having the right people, who just happen to have had a "nose" for the right direction, coming together at the right time and place. This could very well apply to the story of leflunomide (HWA 486), an isoxazol derivative (Fig. 1).

The series of drugs from which leflunomide originated were synthesized as part of an agricultural herbicide project by G. Heubach, Hoechst AG. Another chemist from the same company, E. Wolf, thought the drugs could possess anti-inflammatory properties. Often chemists have such ideas, and just as often they are completely wrong, but this time the hunch was correct. Not the original series of compounds, butecessary variations, made by F. J. Kämmerer, led toward an antirheumatic drug with a truly different pharmacological profile.

Schleyerbach, using two animal models of human disorders (adjuvant arthritis and experimental allergic encephalomyelitis), first recognized leflunomide's anti-inflammatory and immunosuppressive characteristics. These early findings were then put on a sound scientific basis by Bartlett, who first separated this novel immunomodulating drug from classic anti-inflammatory and immunosuppressive agents and realized its clinical potential.

The first scientific paper, describing leflunomide's immunomodulating effects on the adjuvant arthritis model, was published in 1985 (1). Since that time, it has been found that this drug is not only very effective in combating an array of autoimmune diseases, but also in suppressing reactions leading to graft rejection. Leflunomide has been long in

---

* *serendipity*: making fortunate discoveries accidentally. This term was coined by Horace Walpole (ca. 1754) after the Persian fairy tale, "The Three Princes of Serendip," in which the princes make such discoveries.

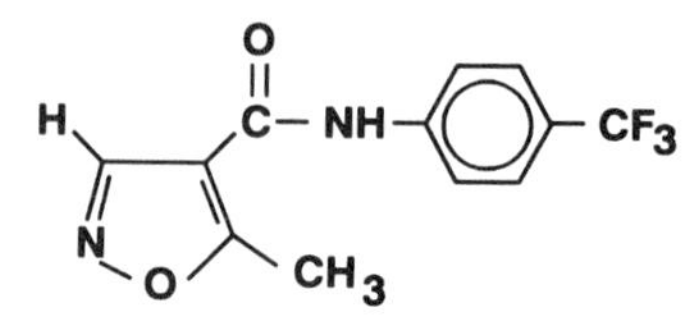

A77 1726

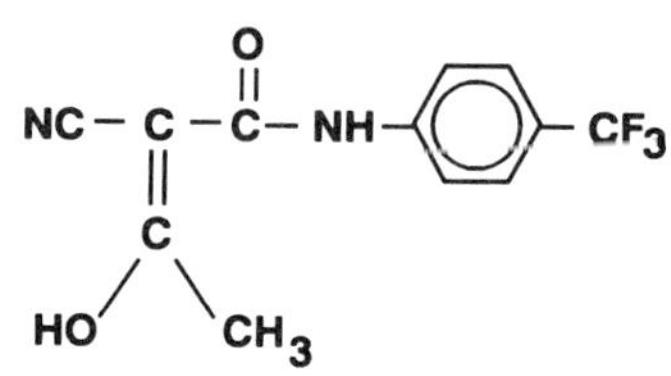

Figure 1 Leflunomide and its primary metabolite, A77 1726. Leflunomide, which has very good gastric tolerance, is a prodrug that is well absorbed in animals and humans, and rapidly converted to its active metabolite, A77 1726. This compound is eliminated by a combination of metabolism and fecal excretion, but is eliminated much more slowly in humans than in the other species. (Pidgen, Vose, et al., personal communication)

development and will still require several more years before it can be brought to the market as an antirheumatic agent.

In this chapter, we review the effects of leflunomide on inflammatory reactions, animal models of autoimmune disorders, and graft rejection, as well as our present knowledge of leflunomide's influence on the immune system. Additionally, our first clinical experience with this drug will be described.

II. ANTI-INFLAMMATORY, ANALGESIC, AND ANTIPYRETIC ACTIVITY OF LEFLUNOMIDE

The effects of leflunomide on inflammation are significant, but, when compared with most nonsteroidal anti-inflammatory drugs (NSAIDs) in classic inflammatory assays, could be judged as weak. For example, we have found that leflunomide is as active as phenylbutazone, yet not nearly as potent as indomethacin in the carrageenan paw edema assay. Furthermore, leflunomide demonstrated a protective effect, although distinctly weaker than phenylbutazone, on ultraviolet (UV) light-induced skin erythema (2).

Pertinent to the analgesic and antipyretic activity of leflunomide, this drug exhibited a weak, yet significant, and long-lasting antipyretic effect in rats that had yeast-induced fever (2). The analgesic activity of leflunomide was as strong as aminopyrine (aminophenazone) in the acetic acid writhing test in mice, much weaker than the same substance in the modified Randall–Selitto test, and completely ineffective in the rat tail-flick test (2). Thus, leflunomide has some, although relatively weak, effects on fever and pain.

III. EFFECTS OF LEFLUNOMIDE ON EXPERIMENTAL AUTOIMMUNE DISEASES OF ANIMALS

There is a great array of autoimmune diseases, ranging from organ-specific (attacking only one organ, e.g., uveitis) to non–organ-specific disorders (attacking several organs of the body, e.g., systemic lupus erythematosus). Leflunomide has been effective in the therapy of several autoimmune models in animals, and it may possess widespread application in human autoimmune diseases.

A. Adjuvant Arthritis

The adjuvant arthritic disorder of Lewis rats is perhaps the most often used animal model of chronic inflammation. With this model, we found that when leflunomide was applied in a therapeutic protocol designed to differentiate between NSAIDs and immunosuppressive agents, not only did leflunomide act like an immunosuppressive drug, but, unlike such agents, it could restore the diminished mitogen-induced lymphocyte response of the diseased animals (Figs. 2 and 3) (1). Although effective in this assay, leflunomide, surprisingly, did not seem to demonstrate immunosuppressive activity, at least in the ex vivo response of lymphocytes to mitogens in healthy rats (1). These results were independently confirmed by Hambleton and McMahon (3) and Pasternak et al. (4). Furthermore, Pasternak et al. (4) found that leflunomide significantly reduced edema, fibrinogen levels, and erythrocyte sedimentation rates. They also found that both leflunomide and cyclosporine reduced the delayed-type hypersensitivity (DTH) response to mycobacterial antigen on day 9, followed by a rebound to an enhanced DTH response on day 21. Hambleton and McMahon (3) confirmed the suppressive effects of leflunomide and cyclosporine on the early (day 10) DTH-reaction, yet, unlike Pasternak et al., found no effect on this reaction when tested on day 15. Similar results were observed when these animals were treated with prednisolone, whereas neither indomethacin nor tiaprofenic acid influenced the DTH reaction.

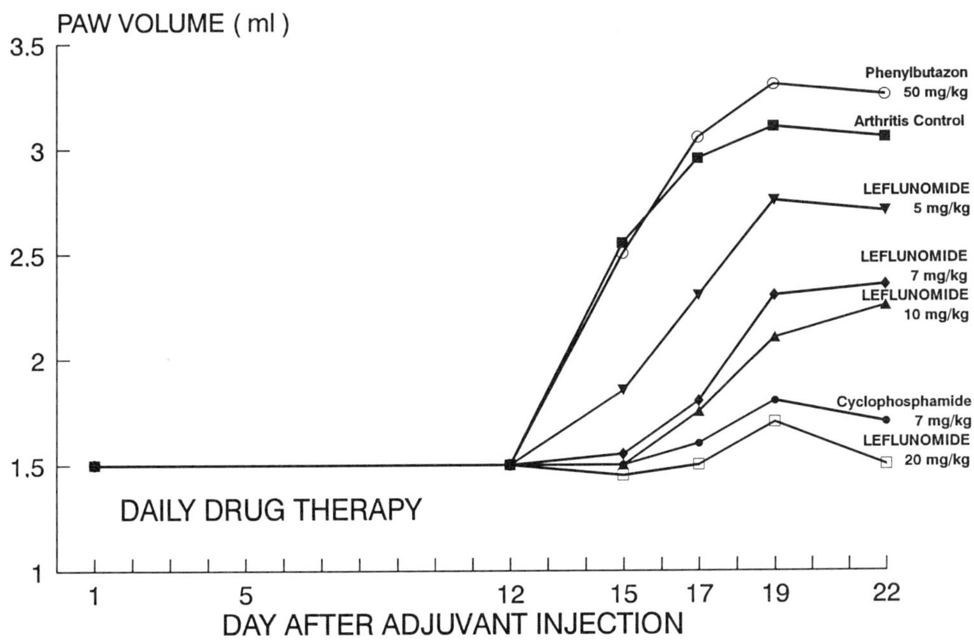

Figure 2 Effects of drugs on the development of adjuvant disease when the therapy is conducted from days 1–12 (assay for detecting immunosuppressive drugs). The disease was induced by injection of Freund's complete adjuvant into the left hind paw ($n = 10$). The severity of the disease was followed by measurement of the volume of the noninjected right hind paw (secondary lesion). Drugs were given daily, po, as indicated. The splenocytes from these animals were taken on day 22 and prepared for the lymphocyte proliferation assay (see Fig. 3). (Modified from Ref. 8)

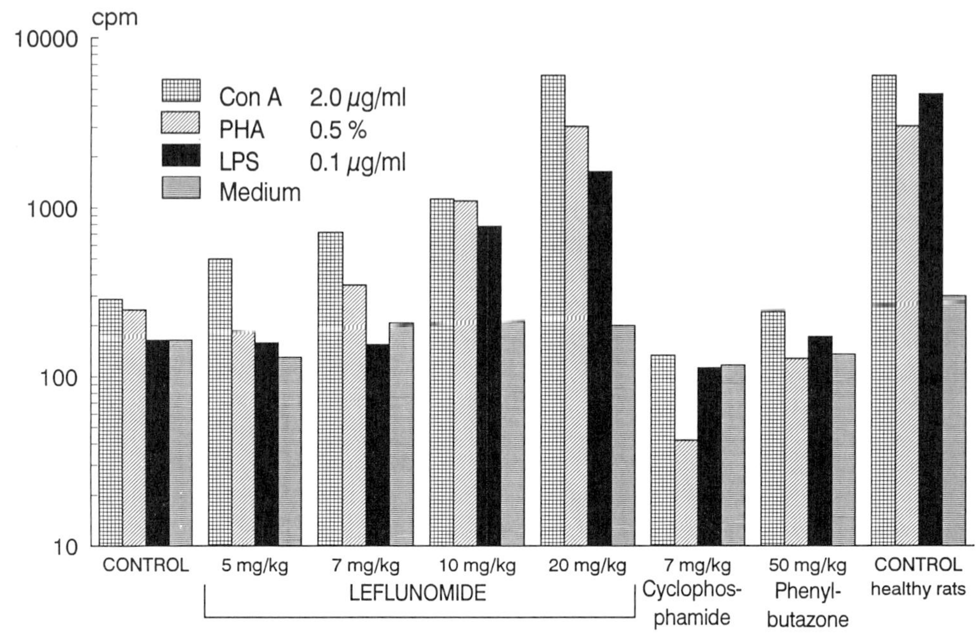

Figure 3 Adjuvant arthritis lymphocytic proliferation: from the animals depicted in Figure 2, the splenocytes were tested for their proliferative response to two T-cell mitogens, concanavalin A (Con A) and phytohemagglutinin (PHA), and a B-cell mitogen, lipopolysaccharide (LPS). Leflunomide, dose-dependently, restored the mitogenic response of adjuvant-diseased animals. (Modified from Ref. 8)

B. Murine Systemic Lupus Erythematosus

The most extreme example of a non–organ-specific autoimmune disease is systemic lupus erythematosus (SLE). The MRL Mpf lpr/lpr (MRL/lpr) mice spontaneously develop a severe disease with many symptoms very similar to human SLE; that is, hypergammaglobulinemia and glomerulonephritis, as well as symptoms of rheumatoid arthritis, such as paw swelling, pannus formation, proliferation of synovial tissue, degradation of articular cartilage, and the presence of circulating rheumatoid factor (RF) (5–8).

We have repeatedly found that treatment of MRL/lpr mice with leflunomide dose-dependently arrests disease progression and prevents the development of glomerulonephritis, both prophylactically (5,9) and, unlike cyclosporine or prednisolone, curatively (10). Leflunomide therapy resulted in the suppression of circulating immune complexes (11), which was a direct result of the greatly lowered autoantibody formation, such as those to double-stranded (ds)DNA (Fig. 4) or to immunoglobulins (i.e., RF) (5,9,10). Moreover, the large number of lymphocytes that accumulate in the lymph nodes and spleens of MRL/lpr mice were greatly suppressed, depressing the amount of the double-negative T cells [i.e., T lymphocytes possessing neither CD4 (T-helper cell phenotype) nor CD8 (T-suppressor cell phenotype) differential antigens (Fig. 5)] (11). At the same time, the ratio of CD4/CD8 T cells, which was greatly increased in untreated mice, was restored to normal values. These effects were also observed after treatment of these animals with cyclosporine (11). Furthermore, leflunomide therapy could restore not only the suppressed

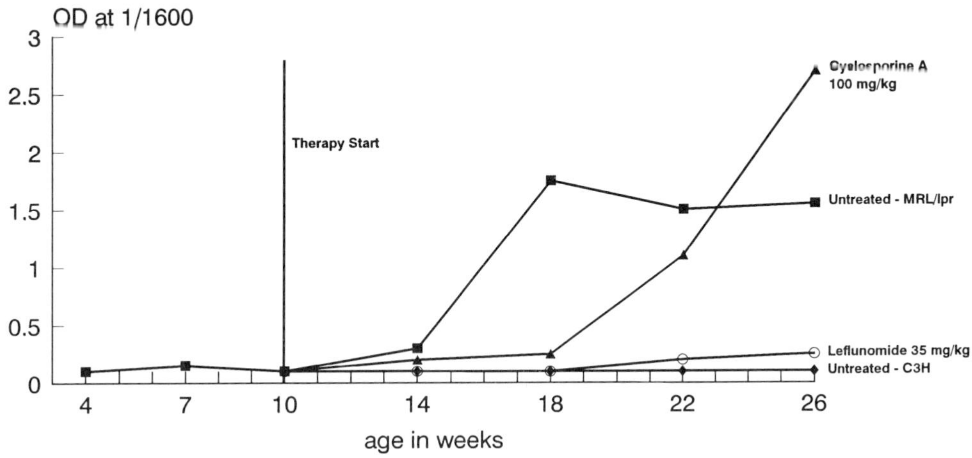

Figure 4 MRL/lpr female mice were treated with either 100 mg/kg of cyclosporine (CSA) or 36 mg/kg of leflunomide, starting when the animals were 10 weeks old. Every 2 weeks, serum levels of IgG class autoantibodies to double-stranded DNA (dsDNA) were determined. C3H mice served as healthy controls. Although CSA was effective in depressing the clinical symptoms of this murine disorder, the autoantibodies did develop, at a somewhat later time than in untreated MRL/lpr mice. Leflunomide prevented the development of these specific autoantibodies.

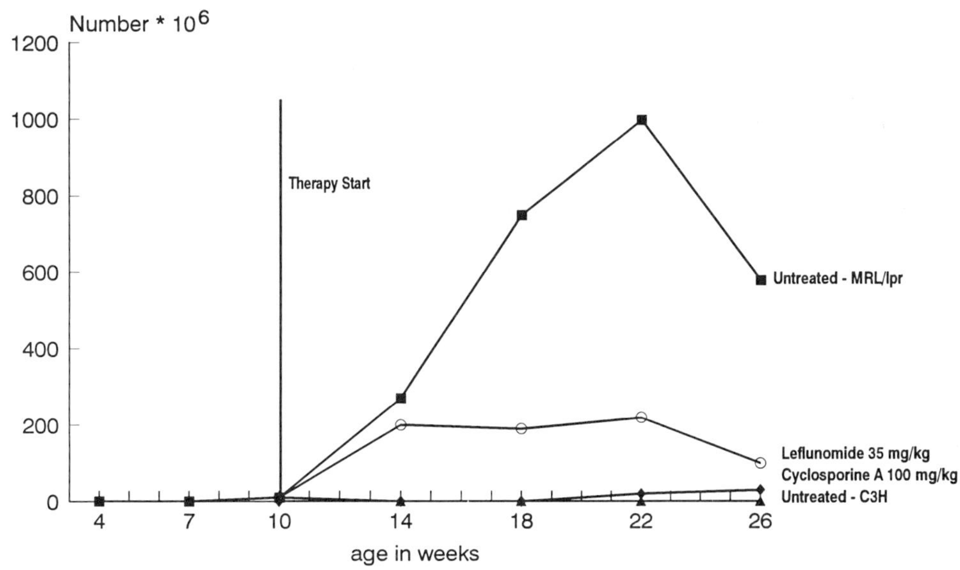

Figure 5 MRL/lpr mice were treated as described in Figure 4. The number of double-negative T cells (CD3 lymphocytes expressing neither CD4 nor CD8 phenotype) were determined by FACSCan analysis. Therapy with either leflunomide or cyclosporine resulted in a great reduction of these cells present in the lymph nodes of the autoimmune animals (Thy 1.2-positive cells per lymph node; preparactions were from three mesenteric lymph nodes per group).

proliferative response of lymphocytes to T-cell mitogens [phytohemagglutinin (PHA) and concanavalin A (Con A)], but also the depressed activity of macrophages to phorbol myristate acetate (PMA) (9).

Leflunomide's effects can be long-lasting. MRL/lpr mice that had undergone preventive therapy with this drug and become "healthy," did not show signs of the disease for several weeks after discontinuation of drug treatment (12). This is in contrast to the effects observed with cyclosporine therapy. The MRL/lpr mice treated preventively with cyclosporine develop symptoms of the disease almost immediately after discontinuation of therapy.

C. Proteoglycan-Induced Progressive Polyarthritis

Proteoglycan-induced arthritis in mice displays many similarities to human rheumatoid arthritis and ankylosing spondylitis (13). Initially, the disease begins as a polyarticular synovitis, usually in peripheral joints, and includes spondylitis, which becomes progressive, with extensive erosion of cartilage and bone within the joint. Proteoglycan-induced arthritis in BALB/c mice is dependent on the expression of both cell-mediated and humoral immunities to the mouse "self"-cartilage proteoglycan (14).

Leflunomide treatment of arthritic animals with an established disease resulted in suppression of acute inflammatory events and blocked the progression of chronic arthritis in previously involved joints (15). In addition, leflunomide treatment seemingly protected animals from development of further inflammation and prevented joints from developing new inflammatory episodes. Both the antibody response to the immunizing antigen (human proteoglycans) and the secondary autoantibody production declined significantly during the treatment. This suppressed response was still observed for the primary antibodies against human proteoglycans after 2 weeks and after 5–6 weeks for the autoantibodies after terminating drug therapy (15). Since the onset of arthritis and the appearance of autoreactive antibodies correlated in both primary and passively transferred arthritis, and the regression of inflammatory events and the decline of antibody levels showed a strong correlation during treatment with leflunomide, it appeared that the effect of this drug was primarily due to the suppression of autoreactive antibodies (15).

D. Experimental Allergic Encephalomyelitis as a Model for Multiple Sclerosis

Experimental allergic encephalomyelitis (EAE) is a T-cell-mediated, neurologic autoimmune disease that develops in susceptible animals following sensitization with either spinal cord homogenate or myelin basic protein (16). EAE is considered to be an appropriate model for multiple sclerosis (MS) in humans (17). Leflunomide demonstrated both preventive (12) and curative (2) effects on paralysis in an acute form of EAE in Lewis rats that was as effective as cyclosporine in this model.

E. Organ-Specific Nephritic Diseases

Leflunomide's effects on nephritic disorders have been reported from two independent laboratories using two different animal models. Thoenes et al. demonstrated that leflunomide was as effective as cyclosporine (18), but more efficacious than prednisolone, naproxen, or indomethacin in preventing disease development in experimental tubulointerstitial nephritis (TIN) in rats. Leflunomide was much more effective at inhibiting autoantibody formation to TIN than the other drugs tested.

Ogawa et al., who used an antibasement membrane antibody-induced glomerulonephritis in rats (19), showed that both preventive and curative therapy with leflunomide resulted in significant decreases in total urinary protein, plasma cholesterol, and fibrogen levels, as well as decreased incidences of fibrin, IgG, and C3 deposits.

F. Autoimmune Uveitis

Experimental autoimmune uveitis (EAU) is an autoimmune disease that becomes manifest after sensitization to retinal proteins, one of which is S-antigen (20). This disease, which is defined as an inflammation of the uveal tract and retina, can be induced in Lewis rats by injecting S-antigen into their footpad. The ensuing EAU, in these animals, is characterized by an initial cellular infiltration of the aqueous and vitreous humor between 9 and 11 days after antigen stimulation and culminates in the destruction and loss of function of photoreceptor cells between days 12 and 14. Serum and aqueous humor antibodies to S-antigen are detectable by day 8, and a cellular proliferative response is evident by day 14 (21). By using this animal model, Lang et al. found that daily topical administration of either leflunomide or cyclosporine suppressed the clinical symptoms of EAU in a dose-related manner (22). The minimum effective dose for both compounds, defined as a 90% or better inhibition of ocular disease, was about 4.5 mg/kg per day. Although only one eye was treated, both eyes improved, indicating that both drugs have a systemic therapeutic mechanism of action.

IV. LEFLUNOMIDE SUPPRESSES REACTIONS LEADING TO TRANSPLANTATION REJECTION

A. Graft-Versus-Host Diseases

Our first indication that leflunomide could be effective in suppressing transplantation rejection reactions was observed in mice undergoing chronic graft-versus-host (CG_vH) disease* (23). The animals suffering from this illness display symptoms very similar to SLE (see Sect. III.B). Leflunomide was just as effective as cyclophosphamide or prednisolone in inhibiting the clinical symptoms of the CGvH disorder. Furthermore, leflunomide therapy led to a restoration of the suppressed lymphocyte responses to T-cell mitogens (Con A and PHA), whereas prednisolone had no effect on this response. Depending on the dose, cyclophosphamide partly restored or inhibited these mitogen-induced responses of T cells (23,24).

B. Rejection of Transplanted Organs

Although we had results indicating that this agent was very effective in preventing the murine CGvH disease, it was necessary to examine the effects of this drug in preventing reactions leading to the rejection of transplanted organs. Chronic GvH disease is associated primarily with B cells and autoantibody formation, and we were not sure that leflunomide would necessarily prevent an acute organ rejection, which is primarily T-cell associated.

Thoenes et al. (25) removed kidneys from BN rats and transplanted one of them into each Lewis rat (RT 1l) in which both kidneys had been removed. In the untreated rats, these allografts were rejected within 8 days and the animals did not survive, whereas

*About 25% of patients transplanted with bone-marrow suffer from this disorder.

daily treatment with leflunomide for 30 days protected the graft, and all of these animals survived for the duration of the experiment (more than 60 days). The plasma creatinine levels, in these animals, were normal, indicating that the transplanted kidneys functioned normally, and the histological studies revealed virtually no signs of chronic rejection. The results obtained from cyclosporine therapy were very similar to those observed after leflunomide therapy, although neither azathioprine nor prednisolone offered any protection in this model.

After the success of the allokidney grafts, we decided to investigate the effects of leflunomide on alloskin grafts. By using two different strain combinations for our studies, DA into LEWIS (both MHC and non-MHC unidentical) and LEWIS into FISHER (only non-MHC unidentical), tail skin from the donor animals was grafted to the hosts. Therapy with leflunomide was started 1 day after transplantation and terminated on day 10. With use of this protocol, a dose-dependent inhibition of the rejection time could be observed in both transplant combinations (26).

With another protocol, whereby drug application was started 5 days after skin grafting, leflunomide was still very effective, whereas cyclosporine offered no protection (Fig. 6) (26). Interestingly, with the same protocol (from days 5 to 10), simultaneous use of both drugs resulted in substantially improved graft survival, over the use of either drug alone and without apparent increased toxicity (see Fig. 6) (26). These results suggested that the leflunomide and cyclosporine drug combination may have resulted in synergistic effects.

That the combination of leflunomide and cyclosporine is more effective than the sum of either alone, was also reported by Williams et al. (27), who used a rat cardiac allograft model. They found that even ineffective doses of either drug (1.25 mg/kg cyclosporine and 0.3 mg/kg leflunomide) were effective and synergistic when combined ($p = 0.003$ when assessed for synergy using the Cox stepwise proportional hazard model) (27).

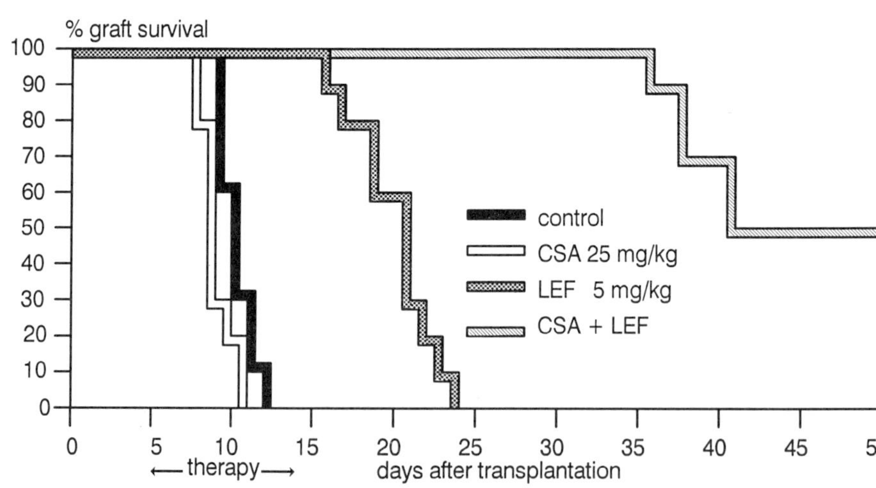

Figure 6 Comparison of leflunomide with cyclosporin in the tail skin transplantation model (DA → LEW) when therapy is delayed to day 5: Tail skins from DA rats (donor) were grafted to Lewis rats (receptor). Drug therapy was initiated on day 5, discontinued on day 10 (p.o. application), and graft rejection was monitored daily. Using this protocol, leflunomide (LEF), alone, was very effective, whereas monotherapy with cyclosporine (CSA) was not. The combination of both drugs offered substantially improved graft survival (50% long-term), suggesting synergistic effects.

C. Tolerance Induction

We often observed, in our various transplantation experiments, that leflunomide-treated animals displayed long-term graft survival, without any signs of rejection. We attempted to establish whether the drug had induced tolerance in these animals. This question was answered by Schorlemmer et al. (26) using the rat skin graft model. A second skin graft from the same donor was made to animals that had not rejected their primary grafts (>60 days). Additionally, a further skin graft from a third-party strain was made. All second-donor-specific grafts survived for the observation period (55 days after transplanting), regardless of leflunomide treatment regimen performed for the induction of long-term graft survival. All primary skin grafts survived for more than 120 days, and hair growth could be observed. In contrast, third-party control skin grafts were rejected rapidly, after about 8 days (Fig. 7). These results prove that leflunomide induces specific tolerance in rats.

Schorlemmer et al. investigated whether this tolerance could be transferred to naive animals (26). Splenocytes, from the aforementioned long-term skin graft survivor rats, were transferred into naive syngeneic animals. One day later, skin was grafted from the original donor animals, and graft rejection was monitored. As can be seen in Figure 8 (26), tolerance could be successfully transferred.

D. Allophile and Xenophile Antibody Production

Alloantibody formation is the cause of hyperacute graft rejection, which can take place within minutes, virtually during the transplantation operation, and is a problem for which there is no cure. Many patients with high titers of alloantibodies are excluded from transplantation; between 20 and 40% of patients are sensitized against 75% of donors, and most of these will never receive a transplant. Leflunomide is very effective in reducing

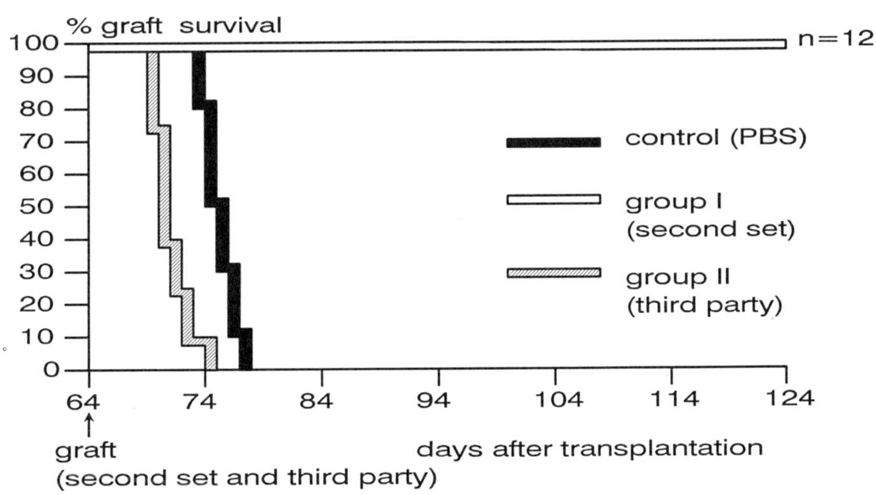

Figure 7 Tolerance induction by leflunomide in the (DA → LEW) tail skin transplant model: Rats that had not rejected their grafts (>60 days), owing to leflunomide therapy, were grafted a second time with second skin from the same donor and, additionally, skin from a third-party strain (BN rats). All primary skin grafts survived (>120 days) and had hair growth. In contrast, third-party control skin grafts were rejected rapidly.

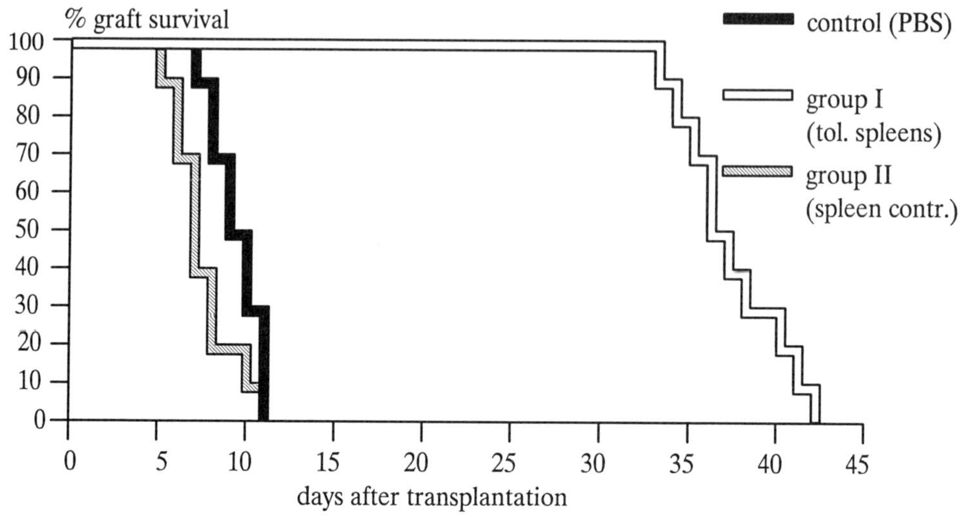

Figure 8 Transfer of specific tolerance induced by leflunomide in the DA → LEW tail skin transplant model (spleen cell transfer): Splenocytes, from long-term skin graft survivor rats depicted in Figure 7, were transferred into naive synergenic animals. One day later, skin was grafted from the original donor animals.

the titers of alloantibodies in rats (40) and, possibly, could offer a means to help such patients qualify for organ transplantation.

The unavailability of organs is perhaps one of the most limiting factors for transplantation. One potential way to alleviate this problem is to use organs from other animals, such as pigs or monkeys, at least until a human organ becomes available. Such xenotransplantations also offer their specific complications. For as yet unknown reasons, substantial amounts of naturally occurring xenophile antibodies can be detected in individuals and are a problem for the transplantation surgeon. Both natural and induced xenophilic antibodies are considered to be a major barrier to organ transplantation between phylogenetically discordant species and are held responsible for hyperacute and acute rejection of xenogeneic organs. As we had discovered in our studies with leflunomide's effects on alloantibodies, Ulrichs et al. (28) found that, in rats, both the naturally occurring and induced production of xenophilic antibodies could be effectively inhibited through therapy with leflunomide. This effect remained during the entire time of therapy (10 days), but antibodies returned to normal levels 20 days after termination of treatment. We are presently following this aspect in more detail. If leflunomide can suppress the titers of xenoantibodies in humans, this could offer a possibility for preventing xenorejection and, thus, a means of providing much-needed organs for patients.

V. STUDIES ON THE MODE OF ACTION OF LEFLUNOMIDE

A. Inhibition of the Passive Cutaneous Anaphylaxis Reaction

The passive cutaneous anaphylaxis (PCA) reaction in animals provides a means to study the immediate-type hypersensitivity. There are two classes of antibodies responsible for anaphylatic reactions, IgE and IgG1; IgE is the major class responsible for immediate hypersensitivity reactions in all mammalian species. By using an IgE antibody specific to dinitrophenyl (DNP) in a rat skin PCA model, a salt form of the primary metabolite of leflunomide, A77 1726A, was used to determine the antiallergic activity of this agent in the rat skin PCA assay. Leflunomide's metabolite dose-dependently inhibited the antigen-dependent PCA reaction (2). This indicates that leflunomide can inhibit mediator liberation from skin mast cells.

B. Effects on the Release of Histamine and Other Mediators from Mast Cells and Basophils

As demonstrated in animal models (DTH and PCA reactions), hypersensitivity reactions are modulated by leflunomide. The most important primary mediator of hypersensitivity is histamine, which binds to target cells (smooth-muscle cells, endothelial cells of blood vessels) by specific receptors. Leflunomide can inhibit the release of histamine from isolated human basophils and rat peritoneal mast cells (12). This is true for both calcium ionophore (A23 187)- and IgE-induced release. These in vitro results correlate with the in vivo PCA reaction observed in rat skin (2).

Not only histamine release, but also the formation and liberation of biologically active metabolites of arachidonic acid were, to varying degrees, inhibited by leflunomide's primary metabolite A77 1726. For example, the calcium ionophore-induced release of 5-hydroxyeicosatetraenoic acid (5-HETE) was strongly inhibited, although leukotriene B_4 (LTB_4) was much less suppressed, and prostaglandin E_2 (PGE_2) formation was not affected (12). Despite the limited ability to inhibit the generation of mediators from arachidonic acid, antagonism of contractive activity of one such mediator, $PGF_2\alpha$, has been reported (12). Moreover, we have observed that the generation of oxygen radicals during mediator liberation can be effectively prevented by treatment with leflunomide or its primary metabolite, A77 1726 (12).

Taken together, many of the antiphlogistic effects of leflunomide observed in animal models may result from the activity observed *in vitro* on various isolated inflammatory cells and their mediators.

C. Effects on Lymphocytes and Macrophages

It became obvious, very early on, that leflunomide asserts strong effects on B cells, either directly or by mediating T-cell products influencing B-cell activity. This was based on our findings that leflunomide seemed to be very effective in diseases in which primarily B cells and autoantibodies played a major role (i.e., SLE, TIN, EAE) and in the reduction of allo- and xenoantibodies. Lupus and other autoimmune diseases are T-cell-mediated; thus, it seemed reasonable that this agent must assert some effects on these lymphocytes. That T cells are affected by leflunomide has become clear from our results concerning transplantation rejection. Perhaps one of the primary, at the time misleading, results originated from the ex vivo experiments using healthy mice (29). Comparing the effects of leflunomide therapy on the immune response to those of cyclophosphamide, prednisolone, and cyclosporine, we found that, similar to the other three agents, leflunomide arrested the development of antibody-producing cells to the T-cell antigen sheep red blood cells (SRBC) and, thus, suppressed the production of their specific antibodies. Yet, unlike cyclophosphamide and prednisolone, neither cyclosporine nor leflunomide had inhibitory effects on the proliferative response of lymphocytes to the T–cell-independent B-cell mitogens, lipopolysaccharide (LPS) and dextransulfate (DXS). Contrary to the activities of the other drugs, leflunomide did not inhibit the response of lymphocytes to the T-cell mitogens Con A, PHA, nor, unexpectedly, to the preimmunized T-cell antigen SRBC. The reaction to SRBC was unanticipated, because leflunomide was able to reduce the antibody response to this specific antigen, yet the proliferative response was still detectable. Furthermore, not only was the oxidative burst of peritoneal macrophages not inhibited after PMA induction, as occurred after treatment with the three immunosuppressive substances, but this response was greatly enhanced after therapy with leflunomide (29).

These results suggested that leflunomide has suppressive activity on the development of T–lymphocyte-dependent antibody-producing cells and the formation of their specific antibody, but it does not interfere in the proliferative response of lymphocytes to this antigen. Because this agent did not inhibit T-cell responsiveness to mitogens, it seemed that leflunomide may influence the T–B-lymphocyte cooperation, without negatively influencing general T-cell or other leukocyte cooperation and function. That this interpretation was not fully correct became evident later when we obtained data indicating that T-cell activity is inhibited by leflunomide; for example, leflunomide suppressed T-cell-mediated DTH reaction to mycobacterial antigens of rats with adjuvant arthritis (3,4) and skin, kidney, and cardiac transplantation rejection (25–27). The reason for this misinterpretation from the *ex vivo* experimentation became apparent after examining the antiproliferative effects *in vitro*. Simply washing the cells was enough to allow the cells to resume proliferative activity. In vivo, these cells are, most likely, suppressed in their proliferative response, but as soon as they are washed free of substance and placed in culture, they can react normally to stimulation. That normal reactivity was found in autoimmune-diseased individuals after treatment with leflunomide is most likely a result of a reregulation of their immune response through this drug's activity.

We could demonstrate that T-dependent antibody production by healthy mice (29) and the formation of self-reactive antibodies (T-dependent) in autoimmune animals can be effectively suppressed, both preventively and curatively, by oral treatment with this drug (1,3,4,7,9–12,15,18,19). Also, disorders requiring T–T-cell cooperation, such as transplantation rejection, could be inhibited by leflunomide therapy. Thus, it was our feeling that leflunomide must somehow interfere in the interaction of lymphocytes, especially T and B cells, and that this interference is not limited to primary immune responses, but is effective on secondary immune reactions as well.

We first studied the effects of leflunomide's primary metabolite (A77 1726) on the in vitro PFC assay, to determine if we could observe the same effects we were seeing in vivo. A77 1726 could dose-dependently block the formation of PFC to SRBC, even when it was applied to the cultures as late as 4 days after their initiation and assayed on day 5 (12). This paralleled our experience in animal experiments (12).

D. Effects on Cytokines

The formation and release of cytokines (IL-1, IL-2, IL-3, IL-4, TRF-α, or INF-γ), formed by either Th_1 or Th_2 cells, are not inhibited by leflunomide (12). Thus, if this drug does have effects on cytokines, then it must somehow interfere with their activity.

The first evidence that leflunomide antagonizes T-cell products was obtained in an assay system for T-helper-cell-replacing factor (TRF) (12). Athymic lymphocytes from nu/nu mice are unable to generate antibody-producing plasma cells to SRBC because they lack T lymphocytes. It is possible to restore this humoral response by replacing helper cell function through the addition of T-cell products that act directly on B cells. When supernatant from Con A-stimulated T cells, containing TRF, is given into a culture of nu/nu splenocytes and SRBC on day 2, numerous PFC to this antigen can be detected on day 5. When A77 1726 was added to such cultures on day 0 or 2, a dose-dependent inhibition of specific plaque formation could be observed (12).

The activity of TRF has been attributed to interleukin-5 (IL-5), although it is difficult to ascribe these results with Con A supernatant to just one interleukin alone, because this activity most likely results from a combination of distinct factors interacting with each other.

With the availability of recombinant interleukins, it has become possible to study these factors individually. Leflunomide seems, to varying degrees, to interfere in the activities of several interleukins. We have found, for instance, that proliferative responses of IL-3 can be strongly suppressed by A77 1726, with a median inhibitory dose (ID_{50}) of about 3 μM (12). This inhibition could not be overcome by the addition of IL-3 to the cultures; therefore the effects were not likely due to antagonistic activity of leflunomide's primary metabolite. Interleukin-3 is a colony-stimulating factor, with varying effects on several hematopoietic cell lineages. Recently, it has been demonstrated that the sera of autoimmune MRL/lpr mice contain antibodies against the IL-3 receptor, inducing IL-3-like activity, which may play an important role in the pathology of these animals (30).

Not only the effects of IL-3, but also IL-4 were strongly suppressed by leflunomide (12). Interleukin-4 (BSF-1) also exerts multiple biological activities that affect various cells of hematopoietic lineages. Paul and Ohara proposed a principal role for IL-4 in the response of B cells to T-cell-dependent antigens (31). This interleukin promotes the formation of IgG_1 and IgE antibodies. Further, the activity of IL-2 is also suppressed ($ID_{50} \sim 50 \mu M$). Of the cytokines thus far tested, only IL-1 and interferon gamma (IFN-γ) are not affected in their activity by leflunomide. A77 1726, exhibited an antagonistic effect on IL-1-dependent IL-2 production observed at concentrations above 100 μM, although the IL-1-dependent proliferative response of thymocytes could be inhibited at relevant concentrations ($ID_{50} \approx 30$ μM). This effect was most likely due to inhibitory effects on IL-2, which is ultimately responsible for the proliferation of these cells.

We also have data showing that the cytokines: granulocyte colony-stimulating factor (G-CSF), granulocyte/macrophage-CSF (GM-CSF), and tissue necrosis factor-alpha (TNFα) are also depressed in their activity by A77 1726 (unpublished results). Thus, a principal portion of leflunomide's activity could be explained through its reduction of the activity of various cytokines.

E. Suppression of Interleukin-2 and Transferrin Receptor Expression

It is not possible to overcome the antiproliferative effects of leflunomide through the addition of cytokines such as IL-2. Because of this, we investigated the effects this drug has on the expression of cytokine receptors after cell activation. Zielinski et al. found that A77 1726 resulted in a dose-dependent suppression of both transferrin and IL-2 receptors after PHA or CD3 activation of human peripheral blood lymphocytes (39). Contrary to these findings, Chong et al., who used a similar experimental system, reported that leflunomide does not have effects on IL-2 receptor expression (32). A reason for this discrepancy may be the addition of PMA to the assay system used by Chong et al. that was not added in the test system of Zielinski et al. Addition of PMA to the cells overrides the effects of leflunomide, and the IL-2 receptor is expressed. It is known that PMA induces the activity of protein kinase C so that the inhibition of receptor expression by leflunomide is most likely upstream of protein kinase C activation. Interestingly, even though the cells express IL-2 receptor in the presence of PMA, the cells are still unable to proliferate in the presence of IL-2. This strongly indicates that leflunomide somehow interferes with signal transduction.

As yet, we have no data concerning the effects of this drug on other cytokine receptors, which may also be influenced.

F. Effects on Protein Kinases

From the data concerning leflunomide's inhibitory activity on various lymphokines, it appears that this agent does not specifically inhibit a discrete receptor for a certain lymphokine, but is more likely to influence a generalized mechanism common to these cytokines. Because we employed bioassays in which proliferation was determined for lymphokine dependency, we decided to investigate the antiproliferative activity of leflunomide's primary metabolite. We found that leflunomide's primary metabolite has a broad inhibitory activity on several cell types and is not species-specific nor limited to immune cells (11). There was, however, a wide range of sensitivity to this drug. Generally, the most sensitive of these cells were of B-cell origin (lymphocyte lines and hybridomas), which, with one exception, were about 10–40 times more sensitive than T-cell lines (11). The antiproliferative effects were not cytotoxic and were completely reversible (i.e., simple washing of the cells was enough to allow the cells to resume proliferative activity). Leflunomide is, thus, a cytostatic agent.

We have looked at tyrosine kinase inhibition as a hypothetical mechanism for the noncytotoxic and reversible antiproliferative activity of A77 1726. The data now assembled do offer support for the idea that tyrosine kinase inhibition, at least partially, may be responsible for leflunomide's antiproliferative action. We have found that the autophosphorylation of the epidermal growth factor (EGF) receptor could be inhibited by A77 1726 (11). However, newer data have been generated showing that this molecule was unable to directly inhibit a recombinant form of the enzyme (11). Thus, although our present working hypothesis states that tyrosine kinase is inhibited by leflunomide, there is still a great deal of work that must be pursued not only to verify this, but to determine where and how this enzyme is influenced.

Unlike tyrosine kinase, we found that after employing several assay systems (isolated enzyme, membrane, and intact cells), we could not observe any significant inhibitory effects on protein kinase C (unpublished data).

VI. CLINICAL EXPERIENCE IN PATIENTS WITH RHEUMATOID ARTHRITIS

As a result of leflunomide's promising effects on the various animal models of autoimmunity and due to advantageous tolerance studies in healthy human volunteers, it was decided to investigate the effects of leflunomide on patients suffering from rheumatic disorders. In a randomized, open clinical study, patients, fulfilling the criteria of the American Rheumatism Association for severe rheumatoid arthritis (RA), were divided into three groups ($n = 7$) and treated for 6 weeks with 5, 10, or 25 mg of leflunomide. Although the study was designed primarily to determine tolerability, clinical and immunological parameters before and after drug treatment were also evaluated (11).

The drug, even at the highest dose level, was very well tolerated. No clinically significant toxic signs could be detected in any of the patients. Along with clinical improvements (objective joint assessment and subjective assessment by the patients), the immunological parameters were largely improved. This included reduction in the erythrocyte sedimentation rate, amount of circulating immune complexes, and autoantibody titers (RF, type II collagen). Almost all of the patients in the 5- and 10-mg groups developed increased numbers of T and B cells, whereas those in the 25-mg group had significantly lowered numbers. The generally elevated CD4/CD8 (helper/suppressor) T-cell ratios of the patients, in all groups, were largely reduced, whereas the number of resting B cells (CD21) were increased, a sign of diminished immunological activity. Additionally, as we had seen in autoimmune-diseased animals, the depressed proliferative response of lymphocytes to mitogens (PHA, ConA, and PMA) was largely restored. The clinical and immunological improvements were dose-dependent, the 25-mg dose producing maximal effects (11).

These encouraging results motivated us to conduct further clinical studies (double-blind, placebo-controlled) that will be reported in the near future (Campion G, Musikic P, et al., manuscript in preparation). Leflunomide has now been administered to more than 500 patients, for more than 6 months, and the evolving conclusion is that this drug significantly reduces joint symptoms and serological markers in human RA, without producing serious toxicity (Campion G, Musikic P, et al., personal communication).

VII. CONCLUSIONS

Leflunomide is an antiphlogistic and immunomodulating if not an immunoregulating* agent that has been shown to be efficacious in preventing and treating autoimmune disorders and reactions leading to organ transplantation rejection. From our preliminary clinical data (11), we now have hope that these effects, observed in animals, may also be observed in the clinic.

Although we are far from understanding the mode of action of leflunomide, we are slowly gathering data that can offer us some insight. A good many of the immunosuppressive effects of leflunomide could be attributed to its inhibitory effects on the activity of many cytokines, most likely through receptor expression and signal transduction (possibly tyrosine kinase inhibition). Interference with the activity of IL-2 and IL-4 and consequent interference of cytotoxic T-cell formation may explain the inhibition of transplantation rejection. Increased IL-3-like activity has been reported in autoimmune MRL/lpr mice (30), which may contribute to the pathology of the disease (30), and it is speculated that leflunomide by interfering with this interleukin may, together with its interference with TRF activity (specifically, IL-4), explain some of its disease-modifying properties in animals with SLE-like and other autoimmune diseases. Also, it is possible that leflunomide modulates IL-6, which could be responsible for the suppression of acute-phase proteins observed in adjuvant-diseased rats (3) and patients with active rheumatoid arthritis (11).

Tyrosine kinase inhibition is a hypothetical mechanism for the noncytotoxic and reversible antiproliferative activity of A77 1726. Many known receptors for growth factors are associated with tyrosine kinase, including EGF (33); IL-2 (the intermediate binding, 75-kDa chain) (34); IL-3 (35): G-CSF; GM-CSF; and TNF-α (36). Leflunomide antagonizes the effects of all of these mediators. On the other hand, IL-1, which is not antagonized by leflunomide, is not associated with tyrosine kinase activation, but with threonine and serine kinase (37). More work is necessary before we can be sure that tyrosine kinase inhibition is important for leflunomide's mode of action. We know that

*Due to leflunomide's unique mode of action, a new classification for this class of drugs is evolving.

leflunomide does not inhibit protein kinase C directly, yet signal transduction is interrupted before this central enzyme system is activated. It is possible that additional enzyme systems upstream from protein kinase C could be responsible for leflunomide's activity.

The ability of leflunomide to inhibit the release of histamine from basophils and mast cells may also contribute to anti-inflammatory effects. Relating to our findings on leflunomide's activity on murine SLE-like disorders, it has been reported that SLE patients often exhibit abnormal production of antibodies to IgE, and that these autoantibodies may, by activating mast cells and basophils, play a consequential part in the release of vasoactive amines, thereby leading to generalized tissue injury (38).

That leflunomide was able to induce transferable tolerance to allogenic skin in rats is remarkable. Consequently, it is interesting that MRL/lpr mice, after discontinuation of leflunomide therapy (8 weeks), did not become ill during the entire observation period (8 weeks) (12). This might have been due to induction of tolerance. Further investigations concerning this possibility will have to be conducted before such questions can be answered.

We are confident that leflunomide will be an effective drug to combat transplantation rejection and human autoimmune disorders. Indeed, we already have preliminary clinical evidence for its beneficial effects in RA. Moreover, this drug will provide a tool in gaining new insight into the mechanisms leading to such ailments and their therapeutic control.

REFERENCES

1. Bartlett RR, Schleyerbach R. Immunopharmacological profile of a novel isoxazol derivative, HWA486, with potential antirheumatic activity—I. Disease modifying action on adjuvant arthritis of the rat. Int J Immunopharmacol 1985; 7:7–18.
2. Bartlett RR, Anagnosotpulos H, Zielinski T, Mattar T, Schleyerbach R. Effects of leflunomide on immune responses and models of inflammation. Springer Semin Immunopathol 1993; 14:381–94.
3. Hambleton P, McMahon S. Drug actions on delayed-type hypersensitivity in rats with developing and established adjuvant arthritis. Agents Actions 1990; 29:328–32.
4. Pasternak RD, Wadopian NS, Wright RN, Siminoff P, Gylys JA, Buyniski JP. Disease modifying activity of HWA 486 in rat adjuvant-induced arthritis. Agents Actions 1987; 21:241–3.
5. Bartlett RR, Raiss RX, Popovic S, Schleyerbach R. Immunologic, histologic and ultrastructural studies in autoimmune MRL/L mice. In: Kuettner KE, Schleyerbach R, Hascall VC, eds. Articular cartilage biochemistry. New York: Raven Press, 1986:391–412.
6. Fassbender HG. Joint destruction in various arthritic diseases. In: Kuettner KE, Schleyerbach R, Hascall VC, eds. Articular cartilage biochemistry. New York: Raven Press, 1986:371–89.
7. Hang M. Theofilopoulos AN, Dixon FJ. A spontaneous rheumatoid arthritis-like disease in MRL/L mice. J Exp Med 1982; 155:1690–701.
8. Theofilopoulos AN, Dixon FJ. Etiopathogenesis of murine SLE. Immunol Rev 1981; 55:179–216.
9. Popovic S, Bartlett RR. Disease modifying activity of HWA486 on the development of SLE in MRL/1-mice. Agents Actions 1986; 19:313–4.
10. Bartlett RR, Popovic S, Raiss RX. Development of autoimmunity in MRL/lpr mice and the effect of drugs on this murine disease. Scand J Rheumatol [Supp] 1988; 75:290–9.
11. Bartlett RR, Dimitrijevic M, Mattar T, Zielinski T, Germann T, Rüde E, Thoenes GH, Küchle CCA, Schorlemmer H-U, Bremmer E, Finnegan A, Schleyerbach R. Lariunomide (HWA 486), a novel immunomodulating compound for the treatment of autoimmune disorders and reactions leading to transplantation rejection. Agents Actions 1991; 32:10–21.
12. Bartlett RR, Mattar T, Weithmann U, Anagnostopulos H, Popovic S, Schleyerbach R.

Leflunomide (HWA 486): a novel immunorestoring drug. In: Lewis AJ, Doherty NS, Ackerman NR, eds. Therapeutic approaches to inflammatory diseases. New York: Elsevier Science Publishing, 1989:215–28.
13. Glant TT, Mikecz K, Arzornanian A, Poole A. Proteoglycan-induced arthritis in BALB/c mice: clinical features and histopathology. Arthritis Rheum 1987; 30:201–12.
14. Glant TT, Fülöp C, Mikecz K, Buzar G, Erhardt P. Proteoglycan-specific autoreactive antibodies and T-lymphocytes in experimental arthritis and human rheumatoid joint disease. Biochem Soc Trans 1990; 18:796–9.
15. Glant TT, Mikecz K, Bartlett RR, Deak F, Thonar EJ-MA, Williams JM, Mattar T, Kuettner KE, Schleyerbach R. Immunomodulation of proteoglycan-induced progressive polyarthritis by leflunomide. Int J Immunopharmacol 1992; 23:105–16.
16. McFarlin DF, Blank SE, Kibler RF, McKneally S, Shapira R. Experimental allergic encephalomyelitis in the rat: response to encephalitogenic proteins and peptides. Science 1973; 179:478–83.
17. Alvord EC. The challenge: how good a model of MS Is EAE today? In: Alvord EC, Kies MW, Suckling AJ, eds. Experimental allergic encephalomyelitis: a useful model for multiple sclerosis. New York: Alan R Liss, 1984:3–5.
18. Thoenes GH, Sitter T, Langer KH, Bartlett RR, Schleyerbach R. Leflunomide (HWA 486) inhibits experimental autoimmune tubulointerstitial nephritis in rats. Int J Immunopharmacol 1989; 11:921–9.
19. Ogawa T, Inazu M, Gotoh K, Hayashi S. Effects of leflunomide on glomerulonephritis induced by antibasement membrane antibody in rats. Agent Actions 1990; 31:321–8.
20. Wacker WB, Lipton MM. Experimental allergic uveitis: homologous retina as uvietigenic antigen. Nature 1965; 206:253–4.
21. de Kozak Y, Sakai J, Thillaye B, Faure JP. S antigen-induced experimental autoimmune uveo-retinitis in rats. Curr Eye Res 1982; 1:327–37.
22. Smith-Lang L, Glaser RL, Miller ST, Weimer LK, Robertson SM, Aoki KR, Yanni JM. Efficacy of novel immunomodulators leflunomide and rapamycin in autoimmune uveitis. 1992 FASEB J. 6(4):A1048, Part I.
23. Popovic S, Bartlett RR. The use of the murine chronic graft versus host (CGvH) disease, a model for systemic lupus erythematosus (SLE), for drug discovery. Agents Actions 1987; 21:284–6.
24. Bartlett RR, Cyclophosphamide. In: Bray MA, Morley J, eds. The pharmacology of lymphocytes. Berlin: Springer-Verlag, 1988;453–69.
25. Küchle CCA, Thoenes GH, Langer KH, Schorlemmer HU, Bartlett RR, Schleyerbach R. Prevention of kidney and skin graft rejection in rats by leflunomide, a new immunomodulating agent. Transpant Proc 1991; 23:1083–6.
26. Schorlemmer HU, Seiler FR, Bartlett RR. Prolongation of allogeneic transplanted skin grafts and induction of tolerance by leflunomide, a new immunosuppressive isoxazol derivative. Transplant Proc 1993; 2517:763–767.
27. Williams JW, Xiao F, Foster FF, Chong A, Sharma S, Bartlett RR, Sankary HN. Immunosuppressive effects of leflunomide in a cardiac allograft model. Transplant Proc 1993; 2517:745–746.
28. Ulrichs K, Kaitschick J, Bartlett RR, Müller-Ruchholtz W. Suppression of natural xenophile antibodies with the novel immunomodulating drug leflunomide. Transplant Proc 1992; 24:718–9.
29. Bartlett RR. Immunopharmacological profile of HWA486, a novel isoxazol derivative—II. In vivo immunomodulating effects differ from those of cyclophosphamide, prednisolone or cyclosporin A. Int J Immunopharmacol 1986; 8:199–204.
30. Ohta Y, Tamura S, Tezuka E, Sugawara M, Imai S, Tanaka H. Autoimmune MRL/lpr mice sera contain IgG with interleukin 3-like activity. J Immunol 1988; 140:520–5.
31. Paul WE, Ohara J. B cell stimulatory factor-1/interleukin 4. Annu Rev Immunol 1987; 5:429–59.

32. Chong AS-F, Gebel H, Finnegan A, Petraitis EE, Jiang XL, Sankary HN, Foster P, Williams JW. Leflunomide, a novel immunomodulatory agent. *In vitro* analyses of the mechanism of immunosuppression. Transplant Proc 1993; 25:747–749.
33. Waterfield MD. Epidermal growth factor and related molecules. Lancet 1989; 1:1243–6.
34. Mills GB, May C, McGill M, Fung M, Baker M, Sutherland R, Greene WC. Interleukin 2-induced tyrosine phosphorylation. Interleukin 2 receptor β is tyrosine phosphorylated. J Biol Chem 1990; 265:3561–7.
35. Pelech SL, Paddon HB, Charest DL, Federsppiel BS. IL-3-induced activation of protein kinases in the mast cell/megakaryocyte R6-X3 4 line. J Immunol 1990; 144:1759–66.
36. Evans JPM, Mire-Sluis AR, Hoffbrand AV, Wickremasinghe RG. Binding of G-CSF, GM-CSF, tumor necrosis factor-α and γ-interferon to cell surface receptors on human myeloid leukemia cells triggers rapid tyrosine and serine phosphorylation of a 75-kd protein. Blood 1990; 75:88–95.
37. Gasllis B, Pricket KS, Jackson J, Slack J, Schooley K, Sims JE, Dower SK. IL-1 induce rapid phosphorylation of the IL-1 receptor. J Immunol 1989; 143:3235–40.
38. Gruber BL, Kaufman LD, Marchese MJ, Roth W, Kaplan AP. Anti-IgE autoantibodies in systemic lupus erythematosus. Prevalence and biologic activity. Arthritis Rheum 1988; 31:1000–6.
39. Zielinski Th., Müller H-J, Bartlett RR. Effects of leflunomide (HWA486) on expression of lymphocyte activation markers. Agents and Actions. 1993:38 Spec Conf Issue.
40. Ulrichs K, Kaitschick J, Bartlett RR, Müller-Ruchholtz W. Suppression of natural xenophile antibodies with the novel immunormodulating drug leflunomide. Transplant Proc 1992:24/2:718–719.

21

Zileuton (A-64077)
A 5-Lipoxygenase Inhibitor

JUDITH COHN
Abbott Laboratories
Abbott Park, Illinois

I. INTRODUCTION

Zileuton (Abbott-64077; *N*-(1-benzo[*b*]thien-2-ylethyl)-*N*-hydroxyurea), is an orally active selective 5-lipoxygenase inhibitor. 5-Lipoxygenase (5-LO) is an enzyme that converts arachidonic acid (AA) to 5-hydroperoxyeicosa-6,8,11,14-tetraenoic acid (5-HPETE) in the pathway leading to the production of the leukotrienes (LTs). Leukotrienes have been implicated in the pathophysiology of numerous disease processes (1). Products of the lipoxygenase pathway have been identified in asthma (2–5) and other pulmonary diseases (6–10), ulcerative colitis, Crohn's disease (11–14), rheumatoid arthritis (15), atopic dermatitis (16), other allergic conditions (17), ischemic heart disease (18), and arteriosclerosis (19). Thus, inhibition of leukotriene synthesis may be postulated to have potential therapeutic benefits in these conditions. Both preclinical and clinical studies have confirmed that zileuton is a potent and specific 5-LO inhibitor that may be useful in the treatment of three of these conditions: ulcerative colitis, asthma, and rheumatoid arthritis.

Inflammation is a complicated response that involves recruitment of leukocytes, resulting in damage to local tissues. The vascular and cellular responses resulting from inflammatory injury are controlled by several different classes of chemical mediators. Because there is probably redundancy in the release and effects on target sites of various mediators, it would seem that neither inhibition of synthesis nor antagonism of the response to one group of mediators could provide significant benefit as a single therapy. However, there is persuasive evidence, some of which will be described in this chapter, that inhibition of leukotriene synthesis can produce important beneficial anti-inflammatory effects.

II. LEUKOTRIENES

A. Metabolic Pathway of Arachidonic Acid

The term *leukotrienes* was coined by Samuelsson et al. in 1979, because these mediators were originally demonstrated in soluble fractions of leukocyte cultures and because they contained a conjugated triene system in their structure (20). They are not stored in tissues, but rather, are synthesized from fatty acid precursors, such as arachidonic acid, on cell stimulation. One pathway of arachidonic acid metabolism involves the introduction of molecular oxygen to the fatty acid backbone, with the formation of an unstable hydroperoxy derivative (HPETE), which is controlled by lipoxygenase (Fig. 1). Unlike

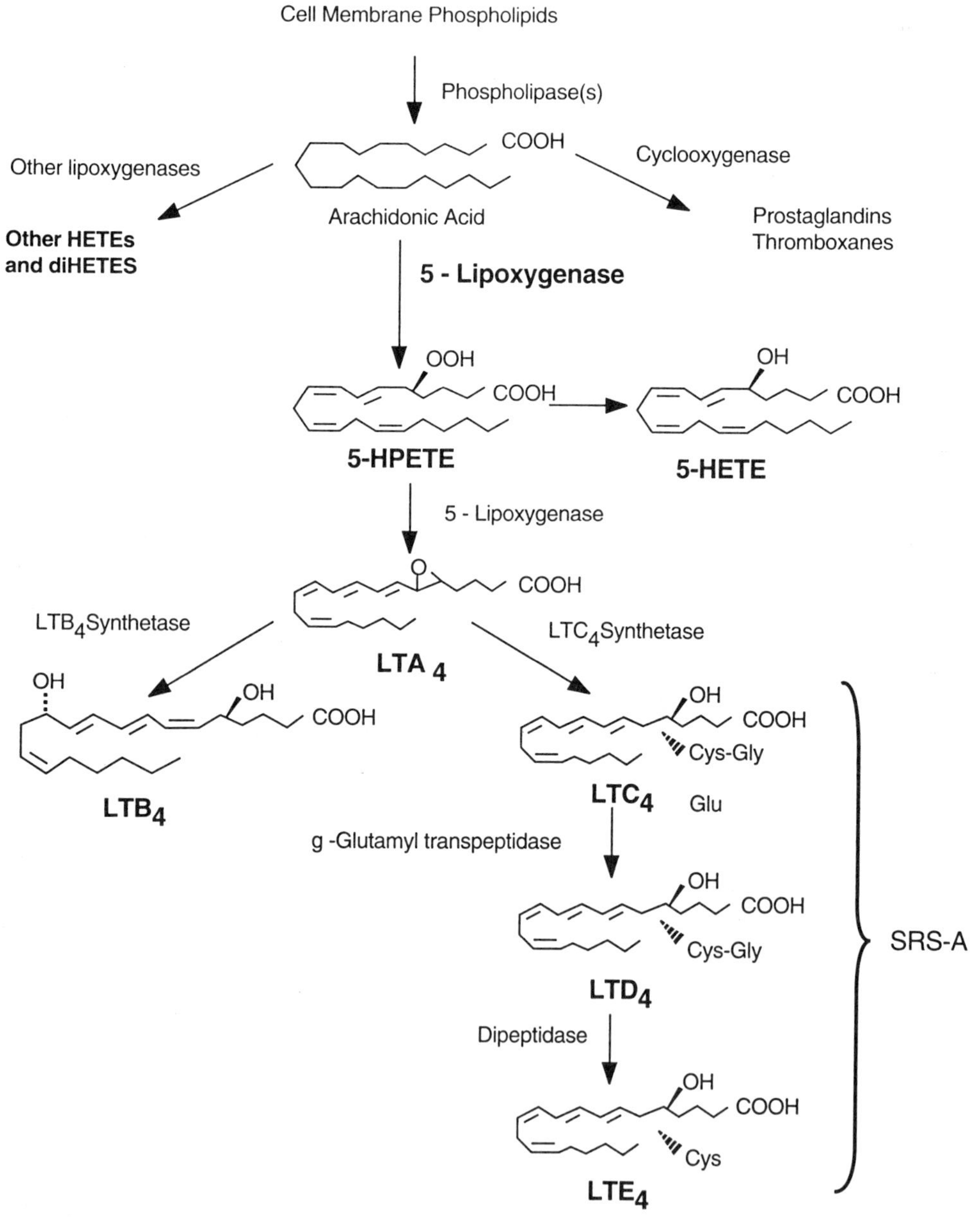

Figure 1 Metabolism of arachidonic acid.

cyclooxygenase (CO), which is widely distributed in mammalian cells, 5-LO is restricted mainly to neutrophils, eosinophils, monocytes, macrophages, and mast cells. In addition, 5-LO requires selective calcium-dependent activation, whereas CO does not. Third, it appears that on cell activation, 5-LO is translocated from cytosol to cell membrane. The translocation involves another protein with a relative molecular mass (M_r) of 18 kDa, which is called 5-LO-activating protein (FLAP) (21–24).

B. Biological Activities

The biological effects of leukotrienes are listed in Table 1. The most potent effects of LTB_4 include promoting the proinflammatory activity (chemotaxis, chemokinesis, adherence to endothelium, aggregation, degranulation, and superoxide generation by polymorphonuclear leukocytes; PMNs) (25–29). Eosinophil chemotaxis and release of peroxides also result directly from the effects of LTB_4 (30,31). Expression of complement receptors has been enhanced by LTB_4 (31). Although its significance is unclear, LTB_4 may influence lymphocyte responses, including B-cell production of immunoglobulins and T-cell regulation of this event (32).

The unstable hydroperoxy intermediate is rapidly further metabolized to an epoxide derivative (LTA_4; see Fig. 1). Another class of leukotrienes is formed from the further metabolism of LTA_4. This is a series of C-6 amino acid-substituted hydroxy fatty acids (LTC_4, D_4, E_4, and F_4) (33). The biological effects of the peptide LTs (LTC_4, D_4, and E_4) are mainly restricted to their ability to contract smooth muscle in a variety of tissues. This action has been studied primarily in models observing the microvasculature. Leukotriene C_4 and its cysteinylglycinyl product LTD_4 have a contractile activity at 1/1000, the molar dose of histamine (34). On the other hand, LTB_4 exhibits relatively weak smooth–muscle-contracting ability (35). Leukotrienes C_4, D_4, and E_4 are also responsible for an increase in blood vessel permeability, permitting the exudation of fluid from the plasma into the extravascular space (36). This contributes to the swelling of inflamed tissues and facilitates the transport of other inflammatory mediators to the site.

C. Interactions With Other Mediators of Inflammation

As with the prostaglandins, interactions between LTs and other substances have been observed. These interactions and mediator synergism are important phenomena in inflammation. Synergism occurs between the LTs and the vasodilatory PGs, causing plasma leakage and edema. Leukotriene C_4 stimulates release of PGE_2 and prostacyclin

Table 1 Biological Effects of the Leukotrienes

LTB_4	LTC_4, D_4, E_4
Activation of leukocytes	Smooth-muscle constriction
Chemokinesis	Leakage from venules
Chemotaxis	
Adherence	
Aggregation	
Degranulation	
Enhancement of C_{3b} receptors	
Suppression of lymphocytes	

(PGI_2) (37). This leads to a further increase in plasma exudate and an increase in the cyclic-adenosine monophosphate (cAMP) concentration.

Lipoxygenase products may also affect the production of other biologically active lipids, including platelet-activating factor (PAF) and thromboxane A_2 (TXA_2). In human neutrophils stimulated with the calcium ionophore, A23187, the production of PAF was greatly augmented by 5-HETE, 5-HPETE, and LTB_4 (38). It has been suggested that the 5-LO products may be acting by augmenting phospholipase A_2 activation. Evidence for this includes the demonstration in perfused lungs that leukotrienes augment thromboxane formation and in vitro experiments demonstrating PGE_2, PGI_2, and TXA_2 release from rat peritoneal macrophages after stimulation with LTC_4 and LTD_4 (37,39).

Pharmacological inhibition of LT production decreases interleukin-1 (IL-1) levels in vitro, suggesting that LTB_4 may enhance IL-1 production (40). Others have reported roles for exogenous LTB_4 and LTD_4 in stimulating synthesis of IL-1, IL-2, and interferon gamma (IFN-γ) from human monocyte and T-cell cultures (41,42). Leukotriene B_4 also promotes the differentiation of $CD8^+$ T lymphocytes (43). Human neutrophils and IL-3–primed basophils, stimulated with IL-8, have generated LTB_4 and LTC_4, respectively, through activation of the 5-LO enzyme (44,45).

Leukotrienes also stimulate superoxide anion production, the order of activity being $D_4 > C_4 > B_4$ (46). In turn, LTs can inactivate the hydroxyl ion (47).

III. ROLE OF LEUKOTRIENES IN INFLAMMATION

Both sulfidopeptide LTs and LTB_4 have been detected in a variety of secretions and tissues associated with experimental inflammatory lesions, or in human diseases with an inflammatory component (Table 2). For example, LTB_4 has been recovered from synovial fluid in arthritis (RA), colonic mucosa of inflammatory bowel disease patients, and psoriatic lesions (48–50). After disease-modifying therapy in patients with RA and spondylitis, there was a decrease in synovial fluid LTB_4 concentrations (51). Concentrations of LTB_4 rise quickly in experimental colitis and, importantly, agents that reduce LTB_4 concentrations also reduce inflammation. Sulfidopeptide LTs have been found in sputum from asthmatic patients, and elevated blood concentrations of sulfidopeptide LTs have been observed in children during an acute asthmatic attack (52,53). As noted in Table 2, increased concentrations of both sulfidopeptide LTs and LTB_4 have been detected in effusions from subjects with acute respiratory distress syndrome, allergic rhinitis, chronic inflammatory effusions from patients with cystic fibrosis, gout, urticaria, and allergic or irritant contact dermatitis (54–58). Leukotriene concentrations in experimental lesions or clinical diseases as well as the capacity for inflammatory cells to generate LTs are sufficient to induce many of the inflammation-related effects in the disease entities listed in the foregoing.

IV. CHEMISTRY OF ZILEUTON

Because of the potential importance of LTs as pathological mediators, considerable effort has been expended by the pharmaceutical industry in developing drugs to control either their release or action. The development of zileuton as a 5-LO inhibitor began with a search for a compound containing a hydroxamate moiety. This approach was based on the hypothesis that mammalian 5-LO, like soybean LO, contains a catalytically important iron (Fe) atom. Because hydroxamic acids are known to bind strongly to Fe^{+3} and have

Table 2 Leukotrienes and Human Disease

Condition/source	Stimulus	Products
Asthma		
Plasma	Asthmatic attack	"SRS-" C_4
Sputum		C_4, D_4
Lung tissue	Allergen challenge	C_4, D_4, E_4
Allergy		
Allergic rhinitis/nasal washout	Allergen	B_4, C_4, D_4, E_4
Allergic rhinoconjunctivitis/tear fluid	Allergen	C_4, D_4, E_4
Skin blister fluid	Allergen	C_4, D_4
Skin disease		
Psoriasis/skin blister fluid		C_4, D_4
Urticaria pigmentosa		B_4
Psoriasis/skin chamber		B_4, C_4, D_4
Inflammatory disease		
Inflammatory bowel disease/colonic mucosa		B_4
Spondylo, and rheumatoid arthritis/synovial fluid		B_4
Gout/synovial fluid		B_4
Chronic granulomatous disease/neutrophils	Ca I + AA	B_4
Hypereosinophilia/eosinophils	Ca I	B_4, C_4
Adult respiratory distress syndrome/lung edema fluid		B_4, C_4, D_4
Neonatal hypoxemia with pulmonary hypertension/lung lavage fluid	C_4, D_4	
Chronic bronchitis/sputum		B_4, C_4, D_4
Cystic fibrosis/sputum		B_4, D_4

been used to inhibit other metalloenzymes, it was postulated that a compound containing this moiety might exhibit potent binding to 5-LO (59–61). Although initially identified hydroxamates were potent in vitro inhibitors of 5-LO, their in vivo or ex vivo activity was unremarkable owing to their rapid metabolism to inactive carboxylic acids (62). After extensive analytical and metabolic studies, a compound with limited metabolism was identified (Fig. 2). The rest of this chapter will profile the in vivo and ex vivo 5-LO inhibitory properties and anti-inflammatory characteristics of this new compound, *N*-(1-benzo[*b*]thien-2-ylethyl-*N*-hydroxyurea), zileuton.

V. BIOCHEMICAL PHARMACOLOGY

The effects of zileuton and several commonly used reference inhibitors of eicosanoid synthesis on rat basophilic leukemia (RBL-1) cell lysates are presented in Table 3. Zileuton causes a concentration-dependent inhibition of 5-LO activity, with a median inhibitory concentration (IC_{50}) of 0.5 μM (63–65). Zileuton was approximately fourfold more potent than the reference agents BW755c and phenidone, and about half as active as nordihydroguaiaretic acid (NDGA). Inhibition of RBL-1 cell lysate 5-LO by zileuton was readily reversible and time-independent. In addition, the potency of zileuton was dependent on substrate concentration. Although the kinetics of 5-LO are not amenable to Michaelis–Menton analysis, the shift of IC_{50} for zileuton with substrate concentration would suggest this represents competitive inhibition of 5-LO.

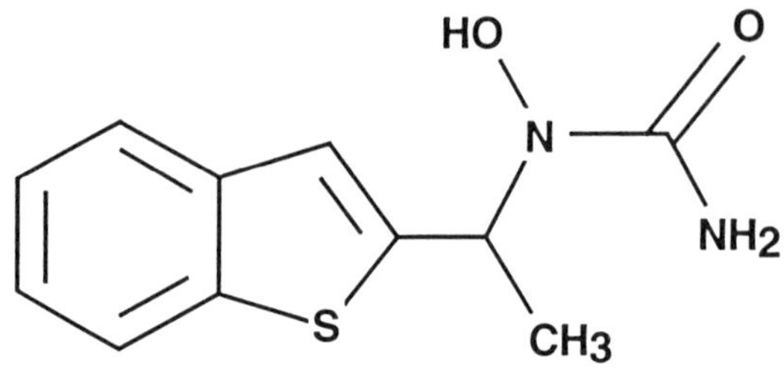

Figure 2 Chemical structure of Abbott-64077, zileuton.

Leukotriene B_4 release by intact RBL-1 cells passively sensitized with IgE antisera and subsequently challenged with antigen was inhibited by zileuton, with no effects on histamine release, although zileuton reversibly inhibited calcium ionophore A23187-stimulated synthesis of leukotrienes by intact rat polymorphonuclear leukocytes (PMNL) ($IC_{50} = 0.16$ μM) and human PMNL ($IC_{50} = 0.7$ μM) in vitro (63–64).

The selective inhibition of zileuton was evaluated by assessing its activity against several related enzymes (64). As shown in Table 4, the compound produces little or no inhibition of soybean lipoxygenase, human platelet 12-lipoxygenase, rabbit reticulocyte 15-lipoxygenase, or sheep seminal vesicle cyclooxygenase at concentrations up to and including 100 μM.

In rat PMNL, zileuton was more potent at inhibiting 5-LO ($IC_{50} = 0.16$ μM) than cyclooxygenase ($IC_{50} = 4.5$ μM) (63). This compared with an indomethacin IC_{50} for cyclooxygenase of 0.02 μM in the same cell population. Zileuton was more effective at inhibiting calcium ionophore A23187-stimulated LTB_4 production ($IC_{50} = 0.6$ μM) in human whole blood than thromboxane B_2 (TXB_2) generation ($IC_{50} = 20.0$ μM) (63). Unlike antioxidants, such as NDGA and phenidone, zileuton did not inhibit human PMNL myeloperoxidase. Zileuton was also ineffective as a receptor antagonist in inhibiting the binding of LTB_4 and C5a to human PMNL membranes and that of PAF to rabbit platelets.

The inhibitory activity of zileuton against ionophore A23187-stimulated LTB_4 biosynthesis in lung fragments from several species was examined. Zileuton inhibited LTB_4 synthesis in guinea pig ($IC_{50} = 3.6$ μM), rabbit ($IC_{50} = 0.7$ μM), cynomolgus and rhesus monkey ($IC_{50} = 0.51$ μM, 0.60 μM), sheep ($IC_{50} = 1.5$ μM), and human ($IC_{50} = 0.51$ μM) lung fragments. Leukotriene E_4 biosynthesis was also examined in some of these

Table 3 Inhibitory Effects of Zileuton and Reference Compounds on RBL-1 20,000 × *g* Supernatant 5-Lipoxygenase Activity

Compound	IC_{50} (μm)[a]
Zileuton	0.5 (0.4–0.6)
Phenidone	1.9 (1.5–2.8)
BW755c	2.0 (1.8–2.3)
NDGA	0.3 (0.2–0.3)
Indomethacin	12% at 100[b]

[a]IC_{50} values; 95% CL shown in parenthesis.
[b]Percentage of inhibition at highest tested concentration.

Table 4 Inhibitory Effects of Zileuton and Reference Compounds Against 12- and 15-Lipoxygenases and Cyclooxygenase Activity

	IC_{50}[a] (μm)		
Compound	Human platelet 12-lipoxygenase	Soybean 15-lipoxygenase	Sheep seminal vesicle cyclooxygenase
Zileuton	19% at 100[b]	NS at 100[c]	10% at 100[b]
Phenidone	0.1 (0.09–0.01)	0.4 (0.3–0.5)	94 (78–115)
BW755c	5% at 100[b]	213 (113–535)	97(85–111)
NDGA	0.2 (0.19–0.30)	2.0 1(1.7–2.3)	45% at 200[b]
Indomethacin	NS at 100[c]	NA at 100[c]	0.65 (0.57–0.74)

[a]IC_{50} values; 95% CL shown in parenthesis.
[b]Percentage of inhibition at highest tested concentration.
[c]No significant inhibition using one-way analysis of variance.

species and was inhibited at similar concentrations: human (IC_{50} = 0.73 μM), guinea pig (IC_{50} = 3.7 μM), and cynomolgus monkey (IC_{50} = 1.5 μM).

The actively sensitized guinea pig trachea has been used by several investigators as an in vitro model of antigen-induced airway smooth-muscle contraction (66). Zileuton inhibited the leukotriene component of this contraction in a dose-dependent manner, with an IC_{50} value of 7.1 μM.

The effect of zileuton on contraction of passively sensitized (with IgE) human bronchi in vitro was assessed (67). Zileuton inhibited the contraction caused by anti-IgE (Fig. 3).

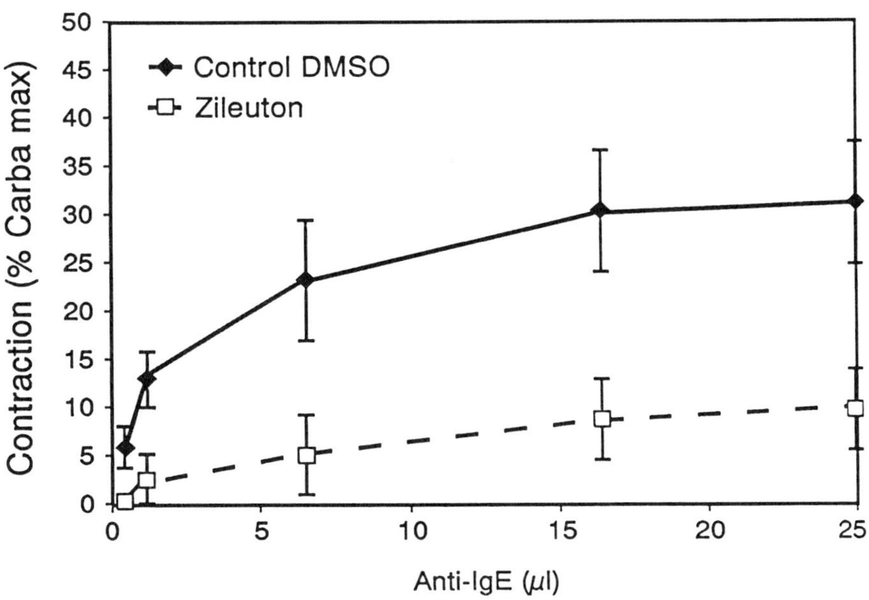

Figure 3 Human bronchi ring segments were passively sensitized by incubation with monoclonal IgE. Contraction was induced in the presence and absence of zileuton (10 μM) with monoclonal anti-IgE added to the bath (0.01–0.5 μg/ml).

This interference with an immunologically induced contraction would suggest a possible beneficial effect of zileuton in anaphylactic reactions in humans.

VI. ANIMAL PHARMACOLOGY

At oral doses from 0.5 to 5 mg/kg in the dog, zileuton produced a rapid and sustained inhibition of ex vivo blood LTB_4 biosynthesis that correlated with the pharmacokinetic behavior of the compound (64). At the lowest dose, peak inhibition (89%) of LTB_4 generation was observed 2 h after dosing and then declined gradually. In a similar ex vivo study in the rat, the compound displayed an oral ED_{50} of 2 mg/kg.

The ability of zileuton to inhibit biosynthesis of LTs in vivo after oral administration was demonstrated in the rat passive peritoneal anaphylaxis model. This is a modification of a method used to generate large quantities of slow-reacting substance of anaphylaxis (SRS-A) for study and characterization (67). After antigen challenge to passively sensitized rats, a rapid increase in 6-sulfidopeptide LT biosynthesis occurs, which peaks at 15 min. Oral administration of zileuton 1 h before antigen challenge resulted in a dose-dependent decrease in the formation of sulfidopeptide LTs. The calculated oral median effective dose (ED_{50}) was 3 mg/kg (Fig. 4).

The antiedema activity of zileuton was evaluated using the AA ear edema model. The acute edematous response resulting from the application of arachidonate to the mouse ear has been shown to involve the 6-sulfidopeptide LTs and be inhibited by 5-LO inhibitors and LTD_4 antagonists (69–71). Administration of zileuton at oral doses, ranging from 10 to 100 mg/kg, 15 min before AA challenge, produced a dose-related reduction of ear swelling (ED_{50} = 31 mg/kg).

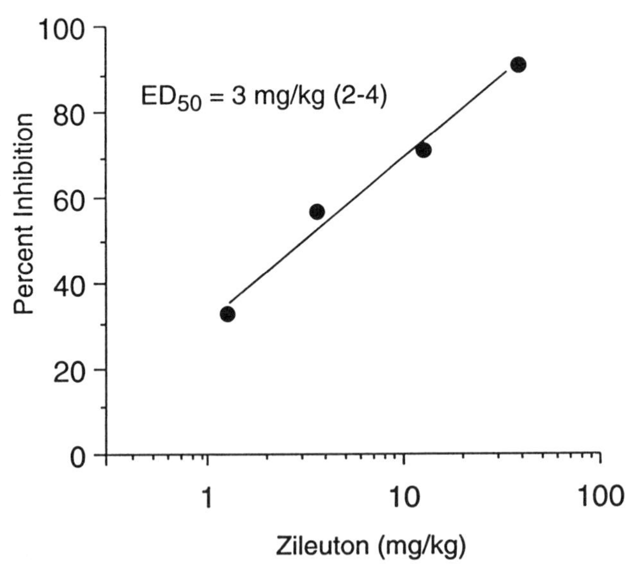

Figure 4 The effect of zileuton on sulfidopeptide LT biosynthesis in a rat peritoneal anaphylaxis assay. The compound was administered po to passively sensitized, fasted rats 1 h before challenge with bovine serum albumin (BSA). Results are expressed as mean inhibition of immunodetectable $LTC_4 \pm$ SEM (n = 14–16). Peritoneal fluids from control animals contained 344 ± 42 ng of LTC_4-like material per rat.

Plasma concentrations of zileuton were evaluated in several different species (dog, monkey, mouse, and rat) after oral administration of a 20-mg/kg dose (Fig. 5). The compound was absorbed rapidly in all species, and mean peak plasma levels were observed from 15 min to 1 h after dosing. Average peak concentrations ranged from a low of 5 μg/ml in the monkey, to a high of 20 μg/ml in the dog. Marked species differences were observed in the rate of plasma concentration decline after peak concentrations were noted. Studies in these same species after intravenous administration indicate that the elimination half-life of zileuton was 7.5, 0.3, 0.9, and 2.3 h in the dog, monkey, mouse, and rat, respectively.

An allergic sheep model was used to evaluate the effects of zileuton on antigen-induced early and late bronchial responses, airway inflammation, and airway hyperresponsiveness (72). Zileuton (10 mg/kg, oral) had no effect on the early response to antigen, but the drug inhibited the late response by 55% ($p < 0.05$). There was no significant increase in bronchoalveolar lavage eosinophils at 8 h postchallenge in zileuton-treated sheep. Furthermore, zileuton treatment blocked the airway hyperresponsiveness seen 24 h after challenge.

VII. HUMAN PHARMACOLOGY

A. Pharmacokinetics

Pharmacokinetics with zileuton were investigated during Phase I clinical trials in healthy male volunteers after oral administration of single 25- to 800-mg doses, after once-a-day

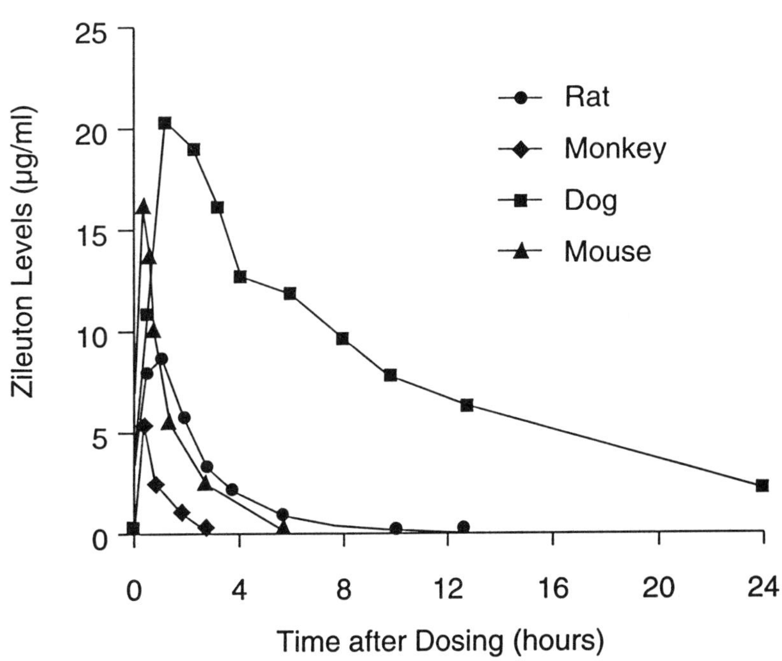

Figure 5 Plasma concentrations of zileuton in several laboratory animals after po administration. Zileuton was administered po to dogs, mice, monkeys, and rats, and blood samples were collected at selected times afterward. Plasma concentrations of zileuton were measured by high-performance liquid chromatography. Each point represents the mean concentration for at least two animals.

100- to 800-mg doses for 7 consecutive days, and after multiple doses for 14 consecutive days (200 mg qid, 400 mg tid, 800 mg bid, and 600 mg tid and qid; Fig. 6) (73). Mean peak plasma concentrations (C_{max}) ranged from 0.91 to 3.42 mg/L and were achieved in peak plasma times (t_{max}) ranging from 1.8 to 2.5 h after dosing (Table 1). The mean $t_{1/2}$ was 2.3 h, which was independent of zileuton dose. The mean apparent plasma clearance (*C/F*) was 737 ml/min and the mean apparent volume of distribution (*V/F*) was 167 L, both of which were dose-independent (the bioavailability factor F = fraction of drug absorbed × fraction surviving first-pass metabolism).

The areas under the plasma concentration–time curves (AUC) of zileuton increased proportionately with increasing dose size. With doses of 600 mg qid of zileuton, there begins to be nonlinearity of the curves. Generally, the pharmacokinetic constants for zileuton estimated after multiple dosing were similar to those after single-dose administration.

B. Organ Metabolism and Excretion

Zileuton is extensively metabolized by the liver through a first-pass effect, primarily by glucuronidation and, to a smaller extent, by dehydroxylation by intestinal flora. Zileuton is also highly protein-bound (93%) in human plasma, largely to albumin and to a minor degree to α_1-acid glycoprotein. Protein-bound zileuton is not displaced by other drugs, such as theophylline, salbutamol, prednisone, ibuprofen, sulfasalazine, and salicylate. These studies have found that zileuton is absorbed rapidly, with mean peak plasma levels at 1–3 h postdosing. Absorption is enhanced by a high-fat diet. The mean elimination half-life ranged from 1.0 to 2.3 h (Fig. 7) (73). Following a 600-mg qid dosage regimen, the mean peak concentrations of zileuton were 2.19 ± 0.66 μg/ml after the first dose and

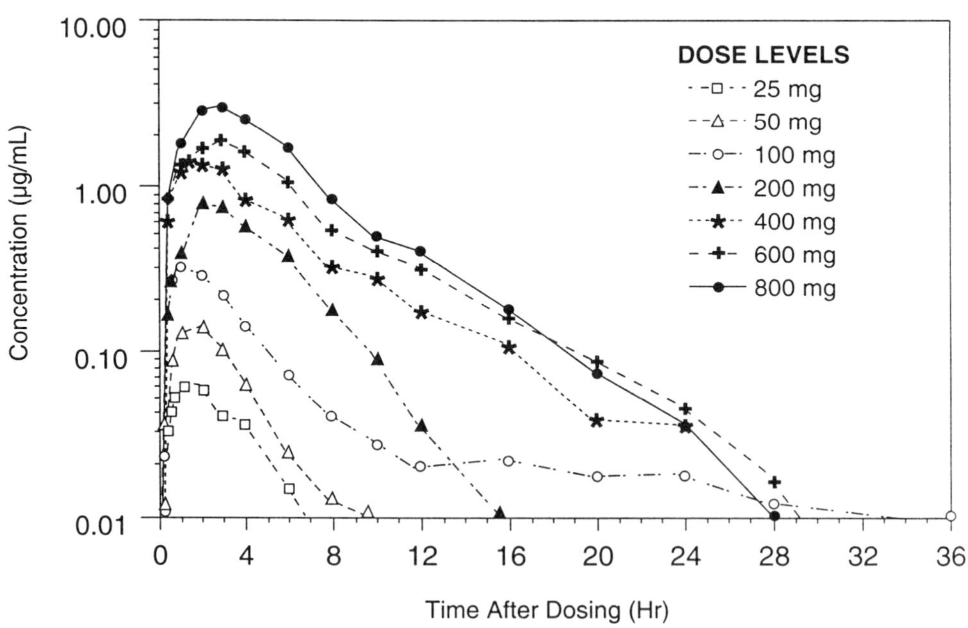

Figure 6 Mean plasma concentrations of Abbott-64077 in humans after simple oral administration.

4.16 ± 1.12 μg/ml at steady state. The corresponding mean trough levels were 0.90 ± 0.32 μg/ml after the first dose and 1.51 ± 0.52 μg/ml at steady state. The fluctuations of the plasma concentration, within each dosing interval (peaks to troughs), were smaller with more frequent dosing, and the qid regimen produced trough levels at steady state significantly higher than those after a single dose. The mean urinary recovery of total radioactivity after a single oral 400-mg [^{14}C] zileuton dose in four volunteers was 87.0 ± 4.2% after 24 h and 94.5 ± 6.4% after 7 days. Zileuton is excreted as a glucuronide, with about 2% appearing in the feces. Polar material and other unidentified metabolites represent most of the remainder. Unconjugated zileuton and the *N*-dehydroxylated metabolite are not found in urine, indicating that glucuronidation is the major metabolic pathway for zileuton in humans.

VIII. CLINICAL STUDIES: EVIDENCE OF ANTI-INFLAMMATORY RESPONSES

A. Single- and Multiple-Dose Clinical Studies

In a phase I clinical study, 25–800 mg of oral zileuton administered to 36 healthy male volunteers, was well tolerated, and produced a dose-related reduction in blood LTB_4 formation (74). In subjects receiving 400 mg tid for 14 consecutive days, the mean percentage inhibition of LTB_4 biosynthesis ranged from 46 to 79% between 2 and 6 h postdosing on 4 days. Subjects receiving 800 mg bid demonstrated a 69–90% inhibition during the same times (Fig. 8). This inhibition was higher than that observed with a single 400- or 800-mg dose. The duration of significant inhibition was longer for the 800-mg bid dosage. Individuals receiving 600 mg qid for 14-consecutive days demonstrated a

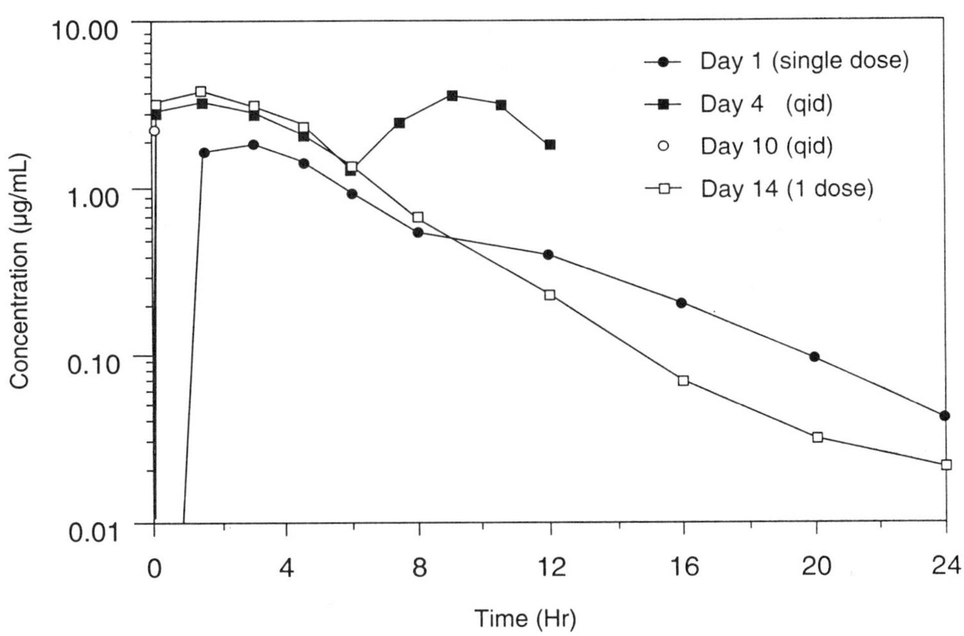

Figure 7 Mean plasma concentrations of Abbott-64077 in humans after multiple oral administration of 600 mg qid.

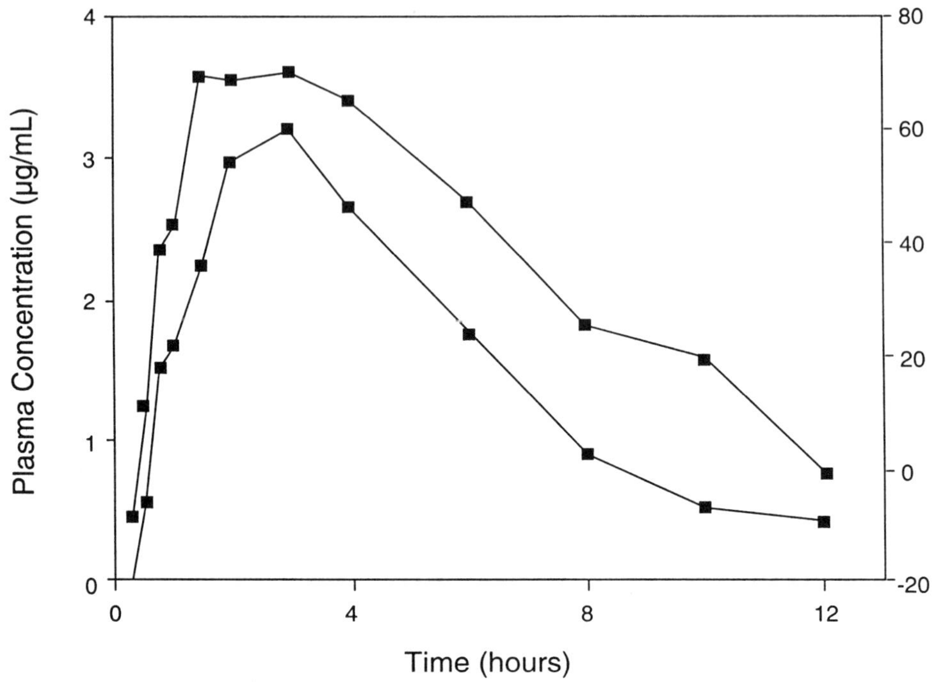

Figure 8 Six subjects were given 800 mg of zileuton. These curves represent the plasma concentration and ex vivo LTB4 inhibition after dosing.

mean maximum LTB_4 inhibition of 90% on day 4 of the study. After peak inhibition was reached, between 1.5 and 3 h postdose, it declined in parallel with the plasma levels of zileuton. There was complete reversal of inhibition 7 days postdosing. The extent and duration of inhibition is dose-related and correlates with the plasma concentration of the compound.

Reported adverse experiences included headache, gastrointestinal complaints, viral illnesses, fatigability, myalgia, and lightheadedness. Adverse events were reported in actively treated as well as placebo-treated subjects which were similar, were within the realm of individual variation, and were comparable in all Phase I studies. Table 5 is a compilation of the adverse events that were noted in Phase I and II trials for zileuton- and placebo-treated groups. The differences between these two groups were not statistically significant.

A battery of reproductive function variables, such as semen analysis, prostatic and testicular size, complete endocrine profiles, and sexual function questionnaires, were examined during these studies. No obvious clinically significant between-group differences or within-group trends were observed for any of these variables. Another trial measuring these variables is currently underway in 42 subjects for 18 weeks to confirm these results.

The influence of concomitant oral doses of zileuton and naproxen, and zileuton and sulfasalazine on the steady-state pharmacokinetics of both drugs was studied in healthy volunteers. It was concluded that the kinetics of zileuton were not changed by coadministration of naproxen or sulfasalazine. The steady-state plasma concentrations of

Table 5 Adverse Events from Phase I and Phase II Placebo-Controlled Studies that Occurred in 2% or More of Zileuton Patients

	Zileuton $N = 441$		Placebo $N = 323$	
Adverse	n	(%)	n	(%)
Any sign/symptom	268	(60.8)	170	(52.6)
Headache	112	(25.4)	70	(21.7)
Asthenia	49	(11.1)	27	(8.4)
Dizziness	29	(5.9)	14	(4.3)
Infection	24	(5.4)	23	(7.1)
Dyspepsia	23	(5.2)	12	(3.7)
Somnolence	20	(4.5)	11	(3.4)
Abdominal pain	18	(4.1)	6	(1.9)
Pharyngitis	17	(3.9)	13	(4.0)
Flu syndrome	17	(3.9)	6	(1.9)
Nausea	16	(3.6)	15	(4.6)
Insomnia	10	(2.3)	3	(0.9)
Pain	9	(2.0)	2	(0.6)
Back pain	9	(2.0)	3	(0.9)

naproxen were slightly elevated during the elimination phase by coadministration of zileuton, as compared with the levels measured after dosing with naproxen alone. The magnitude of the interaction was of negligible clinical significance. Indeed, the median normalized naproxen AUC increased by only 8%, compared with a coefficient of variation of 8–17% for the intersubject variability across the study.

The influence of multiple oral doses of zileuton on the steady-state pharmacokinetics of theophylline was studied in normal volunteers. The mean peak and trough concentrations of theophylline increased significantly from 12.14 ± 2.74 and 7.06 ± 2.09 μg/ml, respectively, after administration of theophylline alone, to 20.99 ± 3.46 and 15.92 ± 3.69 μg/ml after concurrent administration with zileuton. The significant decline of the theophylline clearance after zileuton coadministration (from 62.4 ± 15.4 to 31.8 ± 6.6 ml/min) was associated with an increase in the theophylline half-life, from 6.74 ± 1.30 to 8.36 ± 1.74 h. Because of the potential for developing theophylline toxicity, coadministration of zileuton and theophylline will most likely require a reduction in theophylline dose by approximately 50%.

B. Asthma

As described earlier, products of the 5-LO pathway have been detected in body fluids after experimentally induced bronchoconstriction and during spontaneous attacks of asthma (6,75–78). Until the development of zileuton, it remained to be shown that inhibition of the biosynthesis of these products was effective or safe in preventing asthmatic responses and improving lung function in asthmatic patients (79). Previous work examining the efficacy of several 5-LO inhibitors failed to demonstrate a positive effect on asthma (80–82). In those studies adequate blockade of 5-lipoxygenase could not be demonstrated.

In a double-blind, crossover trial evaluating the effects of a single 800-mg dose of zileuton on asthma provoked by inhalation of cold air, zileuton increased the respiratory heat loss required to cause a 10% ($p = 0.051$), 15% ($p = 0.004$), and 20% ($p = 0.008$) reduction in forced expiratory volume (FEV_1) by 47, 38, and 26%, respectively. [The amount of cold air response is measured by respiratory heat loss]. Zileuton also significantly increased the mean change from baseline in FEV_1 at 3 h after dosing (before the cold air challenge) (83).

Zileuton compared favorably with other drugs, such as inhaled terbutaline (43% increase in $PD_{10}FEV_1$) and theophylline (20% increase in $PD_{20}FEV_1$). Leukotriene B_4 production by calcium ionophore-stimulated whole blood ex vivo was also determined as a measure of 5-LO activity. Zileuton resulted in a 74% decrease in LTB_4 synthesis, compared with placebo. No effect on TXB_2 generation was observed, indicating selective 5-LO blockade, and also suggesting that shunting of AA to the cyclooxygenase pathway does not occur.

Eleven male asthmatics received a single oral dose (800 mg) of zileuton. The 5-LO inhibitor almost completely inhibited ex vivo LTB_4 production and reduced urinary excretion of LTE_4 by about half (84). The zileuton-induced reduction in maximum fall of FEV_1 in the early asthmatic response significantly correlated with the reduction in urinary LTE_4 excretion ($r = 0.8$), but not to the reduction in LTB_4 generation ex vivo.

In a study involving 145 mild-to-moderate asthmatic patients randomized to zileuton, 600 mg qid; zileuton, 800 mg bid; or placebo, there was significant improvement in airway function and symptomatology in patients receiving zileuton 600 mg qid. Acute effects included a 14.6% increase in FEV_1 60 min postinitial dosing (zileuton 600 mg qid ΔFEV_1 0.35 L, placebo $\Delta 0.07$ L; Fig. 9) (85). There was also a significant increase in both lung volumes (ΔFEV_1 of 0.32 L for zileuton, 600 mg qid, and $\Delta 0.05$ L for placebo) and morning

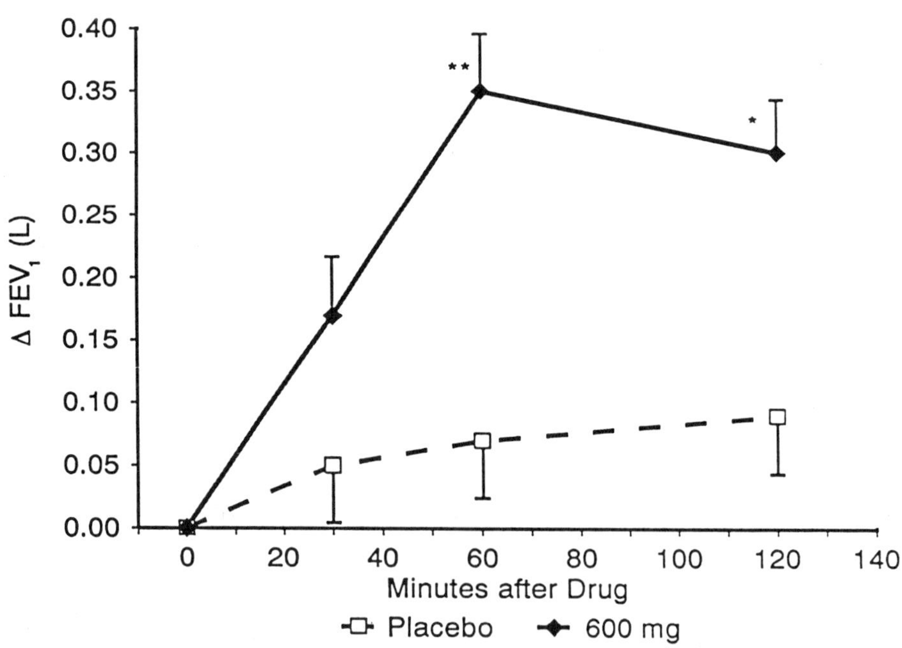

Figure 9 Change in FEV_1 over the 2 h after administration of zileuton (◆) or placebo (□). Zileuton (600 mg) produced a significant increase in FEV_1 at all time points ($p < 0.005$) over preadministration values (maximum improvement 0.35 ± 0.05 L). This change was significant, compared with placebo at 60 and 120 min (**$p < 0.001$, *$p = 0.01$). Values represent mean ± SEM.

peak expiratory flow rates (ΔPEF of 31 L/min for zileuton and Δ0.54 L/min for placebo) following 28 days of treatment (Figs. 10 and 11) (86). Daily symptom scores for patients given the 600-mg qid dose of zileuton showed a 37% ($p = 0.02$) improvement compared with placebo. There was a 24% decrease in occasions of β-agonist use in the zileuton-treated group after the 4 weeks of treatment, and no change in airway response to the β-agonist; that is, there was an additive bronchodilation with β-agonist (Fig. 12).

Because the long-term improvement in airflow obstruction was not associated with any change in β-agonist responsiveness, compared with placebo, it appears that the bronchodilation associated with 5-LO inhibition occurs by a mechanism that differs from that of the β-agonists. Zileuton, 2.4 g/day (600 mg qid), decreased urinary LTE_4 recovery by 39%, and this was significant compared with the placebo treatment group ($p<0.007$) (87). That the observed change in FEV_1 was due to zileuton's action on 5-LO is further substantiated by the observation that greater and more consistent inhibition of 5-LO, as measured by the reduction in urinary LTE_4 with 2.4 g/day was also associated with a greater improvement in airway function.

In a recently completed double-blind, placebo-controlled, crossover trial, 10 subjects who were allergic to ragweed received zileuton, 600 mg, qid, or placebo. Following 7 days of treatment, subjects underwent bronchoalveolar lavage (BAL) of a control lung segment, followed by segmental antigen challenge in the contralateral lung. The drug was continued, and BAL of the antigen-challenged segment was performed 24 h later. After a 3-week washout period, patients were crossed over to the alternative treatment. Antigen challenge led to a significant increase (nonparametric analysis) in total cells, neutrophils,

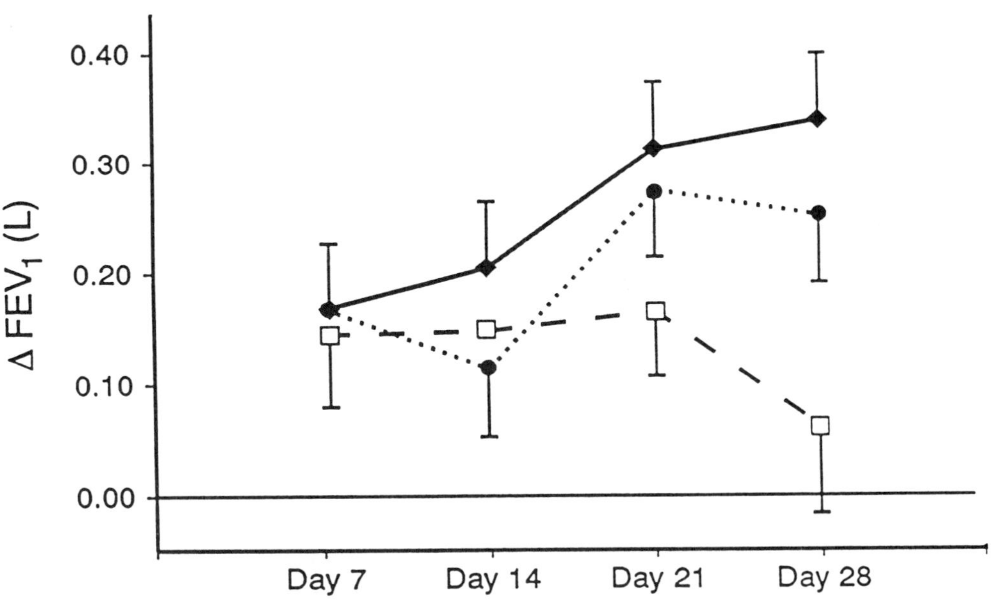

Figure 10 Change in FEV_1 after 4 weeks of administration of zileuton or placebo. Values represent the mean change in weekly FEV_1 (± SEM) compared with values at the end of the dummy lead-in. At 4 weeks the improvement in 2.4 g/day group was significant compared with placebo (*$p = 0.021$). At 4 weeks both zileuton groups were significantly improved compared with placebo lead-in (*$p < 0.001$, 2.4 g/day and $p < 0.003$, 1.6 g/day). The change in the placebo group was not significant ($p = 0.52$): (□) placebo; (●) 1.6 g/day; (◆) 2.4 g/day.

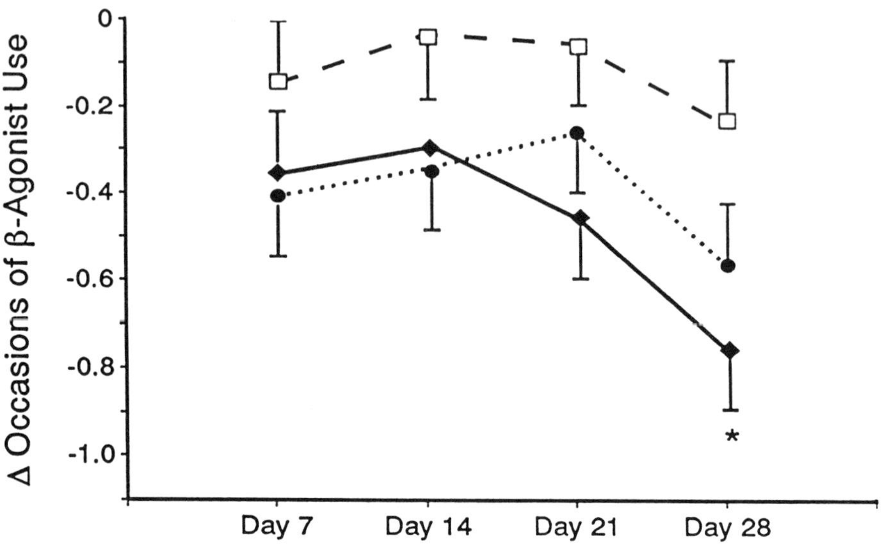

Figure 11 Change in occasions of daily β-agonist use during 4 weeks of treatment with zileuton (●, 1.6 g/d; ◆, 2.4 g/d) and placebo. Each point represents mean daily occasions of β-agonist use for the entire week ± SEM. At the end of 4 weeks of therapy the zileuton 2.4-g/day group had a 24% decrease (0.76 ± 0.21 occasions) compared with a 7% decrease (0.23 ± 0.20 occasions) in the placebo group (*$p = 0.031$): placebo (□); 1.6 g/day (●); 2.4 g/day (◆).

and eosinophils in subjects in both groups. Although seven of ten subjects had a smaller net cellular influx on the zileuton regimen, compared with control subjects, this difference did not reach statistical significance. The results suggest that zileuton may reduce cellular infiltration into the lung after antigen challenge.

C. Allergic Rhinitis

In a randomized, double-blind, single-dose, placebo-controlled, crossover study, zileuton, 800 mg (or placebo), was administered to nine patients with allergic rhinitis (88). Analysis revealed a statistically significant decrease in mean congestion scores (0 and 20 min postchallenge), when patients received zileuton, compared with placebo medication. Zileuton reduced the LTB_4 increase in nasal washings after allergen challenge from a mean increase of 22.3-fold to 2.4-fold. Ex vivo inhibition of LTB_4 in blood samples was about 90%; serum TXB_2 and 12-HETE levels were unaffected.

D. Ulcerative Colitis

The rationale for inhibition of 5-LO in ulcerative colitis is based on the increased generation of leukotrienes in the inflamed mucosa and their potent proinflammatory actions (49,89,90). A specific 5-LO inhibitor (L651,392, a phenothiazinone derivative) accelerated healing in a model of inflammatory bowel disease, and drugs with established efficacy in inflammatory bowel disease (corticosteroids, sulfasalazine, and its metabolite 5-aminosalicylic acid) seem to inhibit leukotriene synthesis (91–93).

The LTB_4 and PGE_2 concentrations were measured in rectal dialysis fluid from ten patients with active ulcerative colitis before and after oral administration of 800 mg of

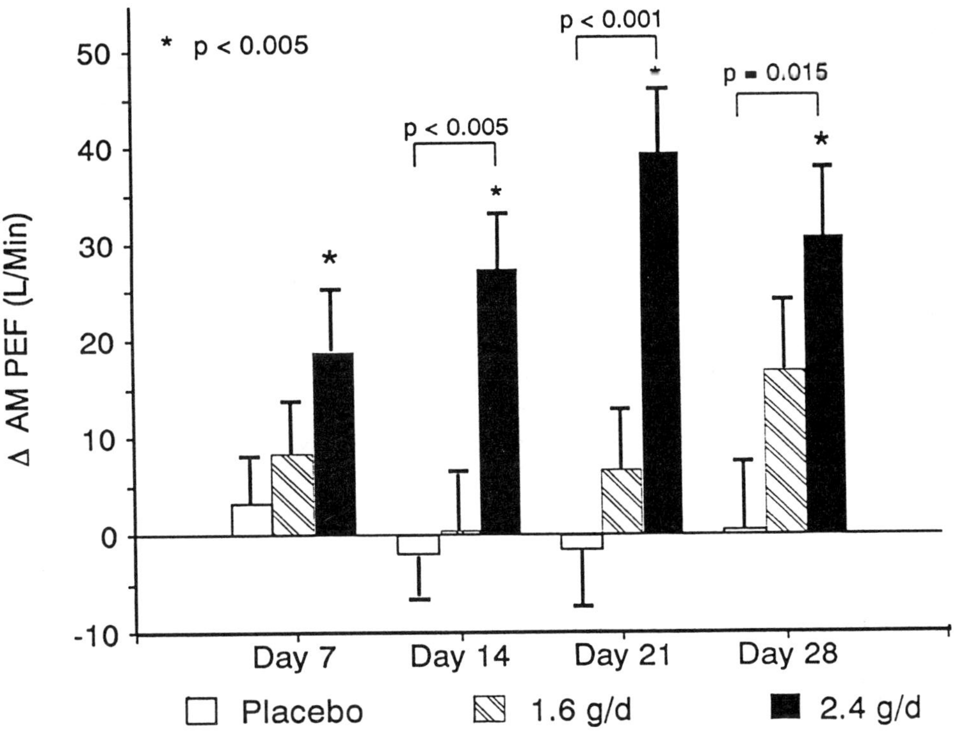

Figure 12 Change in AM (3a) peak expiratory flow during 4 weeks of treatment with zileuton. Bars represent mean of the peak flow for the entire week ± SEM (*$p = 0.015$, 2.4 g/day vs placebo). Zileuton produced a maximum increase of 39.5 ± 7.4 L/min in AM PEF, compared with the dummy lead-in ($p < 0.001$): placebo (□); 1.6 g/day ( ); 2.4 g/day (□).

zileuton (94). The median LTB_4 level fell significantly, from 4.9 ng/ml before treatment to 1.6 ng/ml after 4 h, and 0.7 ng/ml after 8 h; it had returned to pretreatment levels by 28 h. The concentration of PGE_2 did not change significantly.

The effects of zileuton in 11 patients with mild-to-moderately active ulcerative colitis were examined in an open label trial (95). The drug was administered in a daily oral dose of 800 mg for 28 days. Symptom assessment (scale 1–50) included stool character, rectal bleeding, abdominal and rectal pain, urgency, and general well being; at baseline, this index was 14.5 ± 6.3 and, after treatment, had declined to 7.5 ± 5.3 ($p < 0.01$). Sigmoidoscopic evaluation of disease severity (scale 1–15) included mucosal vascular pattern, erythema, granularity or ulcerations, friability, and exudate; at entry was 8.7 ± 2.5, and after treatment this had declined to 6.3 ± 2.5 ($p < 0.02$). Improvement in histologic appearance was seen in 4 patients, and no change in 7. Overall, 8 of 11 patients improved. No significant side effects occurred. This study further supports the potential use of 5-LO inhibitors in the treatment of ulcerative colitis.

In a larger clinical trial, involving 76 patients with ulcerative colitis for 4 weeks, a clinical response with combined improvement in both symptom and disease severity scores by sigmoidoscopy occurred more often in the zileuton group; this was significant ($p <$ 0.05) in the subset of patients without concurrent sulfasalazine. The individual symptoms assessed—urgency, rectal bleeding, abdominal or rectal pain, stool character—are each thought to be products of the inflammatory response. Total symptom score scale was 0–50; the zileuton-treated group, including patients with or without concurrent sulfasalazine, was 24.4 at baseline and fell to 18.2 at the end of the study, a 25% improvement. The baseline score for the placebo-treated patients was 21.04, with a statistically insignificant fall to 19.46 at the end of the study. Histologic features were rated on a scale of 0–3. In the group receiving zileuton, without concurrent sulfasalazine, there was a decrease from 2.17 to 1.78, whereas the placebo patients increased their score. The between-group comparison for the overall zileuton-treated group versus placebo was not significant for total sigmoidoscopic scores. No adverse events or toxicity indicating an unfavorable benefit/risk ratio were observed. Twenty-one patients being treated with zileuton (52.5%) and 11 patients treated with placebo medication (30.6%) reported adverse events during this study. Overall, the most prevalent adverse events were headache and nausea, with a distribution similar to that listed in Table 5. The LTB_4 concentrations in rectal dialysis fluid were significantly inhibited by zileuton, with a mean percentage inhibition of 65–70%. These data also demonstrate that, even though many different inflammatory mediators may be involved in the pathogenesis of ulcerative colitis, the selective inhibition of the synthesis of just one of these mediators can result in clinical improvement.

E. Rheumatoid Arthritis

One of the inflammatory diseases for which a leukotriene-modulating agent may be beneficial is rheumatoid arthritis (RA). Leukotriene B_4 is a potent chemotactic agent, and its ability to attract PMNLs may contribute to the observed accumulation of these cells in synovial fluid of persons with RA. A double-blind, placebo-controlled trial of 800 mg bid zileuton was conducted in 24 RA patients (96). Efficacy analysis revealed statistically significant mean decreases from baseline in the number of painful joints in both the treated and placebo groups. In addition, the zileuton-treated patients had significant decreases from baseline in the number of swollen joints and joint-swelling index (Fig. 13). Although trends favoring zileuton over placebo were evident in these studies, the improvement was marginal. This may be attributed to several factors, including strong placebo effects, small patient sample sizes, insufficient zileuton doses, and inadequate duration of therapy.

IX. ADVERSE EVENTS

The cumulative adverse event data from both Phase I and Phase II human clinical trials have been previously referred to (see Table 5). These data were collected from 754 patients who have been exposed to zileuton at doses up to 2400 mg/day and for treatment duration periods up to 6 months. A few patients have been treated with zileuton for more than 2 years. Most of the adverse events reported on zileuton treatment have been mild and self-limited and also occurred in placebo-treated subjects. Zileuton-treated patients have had no adverse effects involving cardiovascular or pulmonary function, electrocardiogram tracings, renal function, neurological examination, electroencephalogram, or ophthalmological examination. Mild, reversible hepatic transaminase elevations have occurred sporadically. There has been no evidence of increased infection, immunosuppression, or bone marrow suppression.

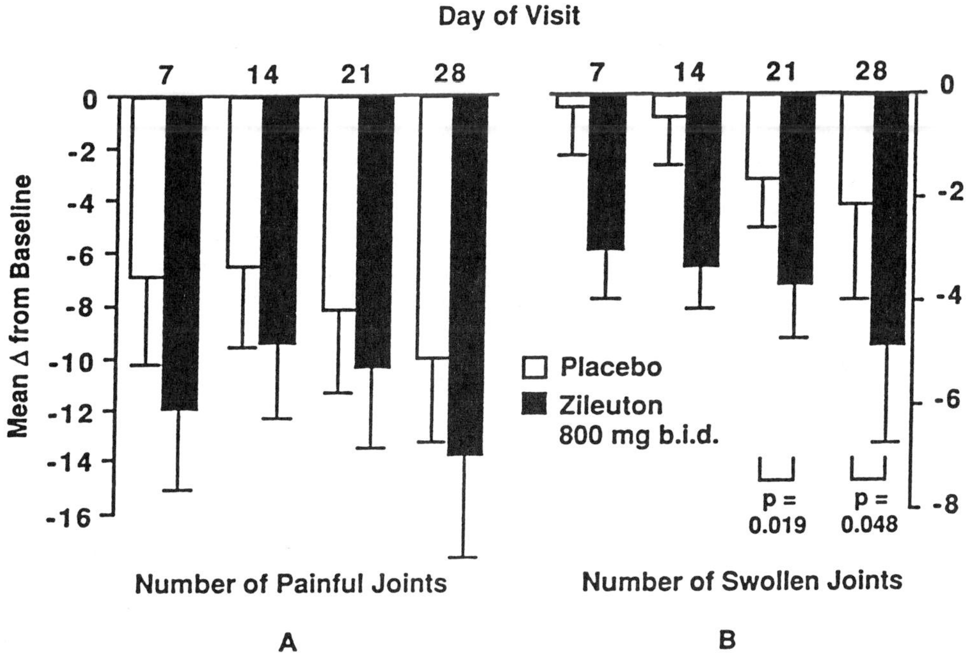

Figure 13 Effect of zileuton, 800 mg bid, compared with placebo in humans with rheumatoid arthritis over a 28-day course of treatment. (A) Changes in number of painful joints from baseline. (B) Changes in number of swollen joints from baseline. Results expressed as mean ± SE, with statistically significant differences indicated.

X. CONCLUSION

A potential role for 5–LO inhibitors in the treatment of human inflammatory diseases is suggested by previous studies showing elevation of leukotrienes in various disease states, coupled with evidence that administration of leukotrienes produces some of the key features of these diseases. The studies described with zileuton in this chapter have provided the first controlled evidence that leukotriene synthesis inhibition is a viable therapy for inflammatory disease states. The next few years should see a major increase in the number of clinical trials using leukotriene-modulating agents for the treatment of inflammatory diseases.

REFERENCES

1. Lewis RA, Austen KF, Soberman RJ. Leukotrienes and other products of the 5-lipoxygenase pathway. Biochemistry and relation to pathobiology in human disease. N Engl J Med 1990; 323:645–55.
2. Arm JP, Horton CE, House TJH, Clark TJH, Spur BW, Lee TH. Enhanced generation of leukotriene B_4 by neutrophils stimulated by unopsonized zymosan and by calcium ionophore after exercise-induced asthma. Am Rev Respir Dis 1988; 138:47–53.
3. Kohi F, Miyagawa H, Agrawal DK, Bewtra A, Townley RG. Generation of leukotriene B_4 and C_4 from granulocytes of normal controls, allergic rhinitis, and asthma subjects. Ann Allergy 1990; 65:228–32.
4. Takahasi K, Shimizu I, Namba K, Nakayama K, Okada C, Tsuzi M, Nakatoh K, Tada S,

Kimura I, Sudo M. Production of leukotrienes and superoxide from neutrophil-rich fraction of bronchial asthmatics. Jpn J Allergol 1988; 37:322–30.

5. Arm JP, O'Hickey SP, Spur BW, Lee TH. Airway responsiveness to histamine and leukotriene E_4 in subjects with aspirin induced asthma. Am Rev Respir Dis 1989; 140:148–53.
6. Wardlaw AJ, Hay H, Cromwell O, Collins JV, Kay AB. Leukotrienes, LTC_4 and LTB_4 in bronchoalveolar lavage in bronchial asthma and other respiratory diseases. J Allergy Clin Immunol 1989; 84:19–26.
7. Richards IM, Griffin RL, Oostveen JA, Morris J, Wishka DG, Dunn CJ. Effect of the selective leukotriene B_4 antagonist U-75302 on antigen-induced bronchopulmonary eosinophilia in sensitized guinea pigs. Am Rev Respir Dis 1989; 140:1712–18.
8. Stephenson AH, Lonigro AJ, Hyers TM, Webster RO, Fowler AA. Increased concentrations of leukotrienes in bronchoalveolar lavage fluid of patients with ARDS or at risk for ARDS. Am Rev Respir Dis 1988; 138:714–9.
9. Davis JM, Meyer JD, Barie PS, Yurt RW, Duhaney R, Dineen P, Shires GT. Elevated production of neutrophil leukotriene B_4 precedes pulmonary failure in critically ill surgical patients. Surg Gynecol Obstet 1990; 170:495–500.
10. David JM, Yurt RW, Barrie PS, Hudgins LC, Verma M, Dineen P, Shires GT. Leukotriene B_4 generation in patients with established pulmonary failure. Arch Surg 1989; 124:1451–55.
11. Goetzl EJ, Burrall BA, Baud L, Scriven KH, Levine JD, Koo CH. Generation and recognition of leukotriene mediators of hypersensitivity and inflammation. Dig Dis Sci 1988; 3(suppl): 36S–40S.
12. Vilaseca J, Salas A, Guarner F, Rodriguez R, Malagelada JR. Participation of thromboxane and other eicosanoid synthesis in the course of experimental inflammatory colitis. Gastroenterology 1990; 98:269–77.
13. Schumert R, Towner J, Zipser RD. Role of eicosanoids in human and experimental colitis. Dig Dis Sci 1988; 33(suppl):585–645.
14. Laursen LS, Naesdal J, Bukhave K, Lauritsen K, Rask-Madsen J. Selective 5-lipoxygenase inhibition in ulcerative colitis. Lancet 1990; 333:683–5.
15. Sperling RI, Coblyn JS, Larkin JK, Benincaso AI, Austen KF, Weinblatt ME. Inhibition of leukotriene B_4 synthesis in neutrophils from patients with rheumatoid arthritis by a single oral dose of methotrexate. Arthritis Rheum 1990; 33:1149–55.
16. Fogh K, Herlin T, Kragballe K. Eicosanoids in skin of patients with atopic dermatitis: prostaglandin E_2 and leukotriene B_4 are present in biologically active concentrations. J Allergy Clin Immunol 1989; 83:450–5.
17. Freeland HS, Pipkorn U, Schleimer RP, Bascom R, Lichtenstein LM, Naclerio RM, Petes SP. Leukotriene B_4 as a mediator of early and late reactions to antigen in humans: the effect of systemic glucocorticoid treatment in vivo. J Allergy Clin Immunol 1989; 83:634–42.
18. Mehta J, Dinerman J, Mehta P, Saldeen TGP, Lawson D, Donelly WH, Wallin R. Neutrophil function in ischemic heart disease. Circulation 1989; 79:549–56.
19. Lehr HA, Hubner C, Finckh B, Angermüller S, Nolte D, Beisiegel U, Kohnschutter A, Messmer K. Role of leukotrienes in leukocyte adhesion following systemic administration of oxidatively modified human low density lipoprotein in hamsters. J Clin Invest 1991; 88:9–14.
20. Samuelsson K, Borgeat P, Hammarstrom S, Murphy RC. Introduction of a nomenclature. Leukotrienes Prostaglandins, 1979; 17:785–7.
21. Rouzer CA, Kargman S. Translocation of 5-lipoxygenase to the membrane in human leukocytes challenged with ionophore A23187. J Biol Chem 1988; 263:10980–8.
22. Dixon RAF, Diehl RE, Opas E, Rands E, Vickers PJ, Evans JF, Gillard JW, Miller DK. Requirement of a 5-lipoxygenase-activating protein for leukotriene synthesis. Nature 1990; 343:282–4.
23. Miller DK, Gillard JW, Vickers PJ, Sadowski O, Leveille C, Mancini JA, Charleson P, Dixon RA, Ford-Hutchinson AW, Fortin R, et al. Identification and isolation of a membrane protein necessary for leukotriene production. Nature 1990; 343:278–81.

24. Rouzer CA, Ford-Hutchinson AW, Morton HE, Gillard JW. MK886, a potent and specific leukotriene biosynthesis inhibitor blocks and reverses the membrane association of 5-lipoxygenase in ionophore challenged leukocytes. J Biol Chem 1990; 265:1436–42.
25. Smith MJH. Biological activities of leukotriene B_4 (Isomer III). Adv Prostaglandin Thromboxane Leukotriene Res 1982; 9:283.
26. Showell HJ, Naccache PH, Borgeat P, Picard S, Vallerand P, Becker EL, Sha'afi RI. Characterization of the secretory activity of LTB_4 toward rabbit neutrophils. J Immunol 1982; 128:811–16.
27. Molski TFP, Naccache PH, Borgeat P, Sha'afi RI. Similarities in the mechanism by which formylmethionyl-leucyl-phenylalanine, arachidonic acid and leukotriene B_4 increase calcium and sodium influxes in rabbit neutrophils. Biochem Biophys Res Commun 1981; 103:227–32.
28. Bray MA, Cunningham RM, Ford-Hutchinson AW, Smith MJH. Leukotriene B_4: a mediator of vascular permeability. Br J Pharmacol 1981; 72:483–6.
29. Bray MA, Ford-Hutchinson AW, Smith MJH. Leukotriene B_4: an inflammatory mediator in vivo. Prostaglandins 1981; 22:213–22.
30. Palmer RMJ, Stepney RJ, Higgs GA, Eakins KE. Chemokinetic activity of arachidonic acid lipoxygenase products on leukocytes of different species. Prostaglandins 1980; 20:411–18.
31. Nagy L, Lee TH, Goetzl EJ, Pickett WC, Kay AB. Complement receptor enhancement and chemotaxis of human neutrophils and eosinophils by leukotrienes and other lipoxygenase products. Clin Exp Immunol 1982; 47:541–7.
32. Rogers TJ. The role of arachidonic acid metabolites in the function of murine suppressor cells. In: Goodwin JS, ed. Prostaglandins and immunity. Boston: Martinus Nyjhoff, 1985:80.
33. Charkin LW, Bailey D. The leukotrienes, chemistry and biology. Orlando: Academic Press, 1984.
34. Piper PJ. Pharmacology of leukotrienes. Br Med Bull 1983; 39:255–9.
35. Sirois P, Borgeat P, Jeanson A, Roy S, Girard G. The action of leukotriene B_4 (LTB_4) on the lung. Prostaglandins 1980; 5:429–44.
36. Samuelsson B. Leukotrienes: mediator of immediate hypersensitivity reactions and inflammation. Science 1983; 220:568–75.
37. Gimbrone MA, Brock AF, Schafer AI. Leukotriene B_4 stimulates polymorphonuclear adhesion to cultured vascular endothelial cells. J Clin Invest 1984; 74:1552–5.
38. Billah MM, Bryant RW, Siegel MI. Lipoxygenase products of arachidonic acid modulate biosynthesis of platelet-activating factor (1-*o*-alkyl-2-acetyl-SN-glycero-3-phosphocholine) by human neutrophils via phospholipase A_2. J Biol Chem 1985; 260:6899–906.
39. Feuerstein N, Foegh M, Ramwell PW. Leukotrienes C_4 and D_4 induce prostaglandin and thromboxane release from rat peritoneal macrophages. Br J Pharmacol 1981; 72:389–91.
40. Dinarello CA, Bisrai I, Rosenwasser LJ, Coceani F. The influence of lipoxygenase inhibitors in the in vitro production of human leukocyte pyrogen and lymphocyte activating factor (interleukin-1). Int J Immunopharmacol 1984; 6:43–50.
41. Rola-Pleszczynski M, Lemaire I. Leukotrienes augment interleukin 1 production by human monocytes. J Immunol 1985; 135:3958–66.
42. Rola-Pleszczynski M, Chabaillaz PA, Lemaire I. Stimulation of interleukin-2 and interferon gamma production by leukotriene B_4 in human lymphocyte cultures. Prostaglandins Leukotrienes Med 1986; 23:207–10.
43. Rola-Pleszczynski M, Borgeat P, Sirois P. Leukotriene B_4 induces human suppressor lymphocytes. Biochem Biophys Res Commun 1982; 108:1531–7.
44. Schroder JM. The monocyte-derived neutrophil activating peptide (NAP/interleukin 8) stimulates human arachidonate-5-lipoxygenase, but not the release of cellular arachidonate. J Exp Med 1989; 170:847–63.
45. Dahinden CA, Kurimoto Y, deWeck AL, Lindley I, Dewald B, Baggiolini M. The neutrophil-activating peptide NAF/NAP-1 induces histamine and leukotriene release by interleukin 3-primed basophils. J Exp Med 1989; 170:1787–1792.

46. Chopra M, Belch JJF, Smith WE. A comparison of the free radical scavenging activity of leukotrienes and prostaglandins. Free Radical Res Commun 1988; 5:95–9.
47. Belch JJF, Chopra M, Sturock RD, Smith WE. Leukotriene B_4 and its action with a free radical generating system. In: Higgs GA, Williams TJ, eds. Inflammatory mediators. London: Macmillan Press, 1986:240.
48. Klickstein LB, Shapleigh C, Goetzl EJ. Lipoxygenation of arachidonic acid as a source of polymorphonuclear leukocyte chemotactic factors in synovial fluid and tissue in rheumatoid arthritis and spondyloarthritis. J Clin Invest 1980; 66:1166–70.
49. Sharon P, Stenson WF. Enhanced synthesis of leukotriene B_4 by colonic mucosa in inflammatory bowel disease. Gastroenterology 1984; 86:453–60.
50. Brain SD, Camp RDR, Dowd PM, Kobza Black A, Greaves MW. The release of leukotriene B_4-like material in biologically active amounts from the lesional skin of patients with psoriasis. J Invest Dermatol 1984; 83:70–3.
51. Davidson EM, Rae SA, Smith MJH. Leukotriene B_4 a mediator of inflammation present in synovial fluid in rheumatoid arthritis. Ann Rheum Dis 1983; 42:677–9.
52. Zakrzewski JT, Barnes NC, Piper PJ. Quantitation of leukotrienes in asthmatic sputum. Br J Pharmacol 1985; 19:574.
53. Schwartzberg SB, Shelon SP, Van Praag D. Blood leukotriene levels during acute asthmatic attack in children. Prostaglandins Leukotrienes Med 1987; 26:143–55.
54. Matthay MA, Eschenbacher WL, Goetzl EJ. Elevated concentrations of leukotriene D_4 in pulmonary edema fluid of patients with the adult respiratory distress syndrome. J Clin Immunol 1984; 4:479–83.
55. Creticos PS, Peters SP, Adkinson NF, Naclero RM, Hayes EC, Norman PS, Lichtenstein LM. Peptide leukotriene release after antigen challenge in patients sensitive to ragweed. N Engl J Med 1984; 31:1626–30.
56. Shaw RJ, Fitzharris P, Cromwell O, Wardlaw AJ, Kay AB. Allergen-induced release of sulphidopeptide leukotrienes (SRSTA) and LTB_4 in allergic rhinitis. Allergy 1985; 40:1–6.
57. Cromwell O, Walport MJ, Morris HR, Taylor GW, Hodson ME, Batten J, Kay AB. Identification of leukotriene D_4 and B_4 in sputum from cystic fibrosis patients. Lancet 1981; 2:164–5.
58. Barr RM, Brain S, Camp RDR, Cilliers J, Greaves MW, Mallet AI, Misch K. Levels of arachidonic acid and its metabolites in the skin in human allergic and irritant contact dermatitis. Br J Dermatol 1984; 111:23–8.
59. Harris RB, Strong PDM, Wilson IB. Dipeptide hydroxamates are good inhibitors of angiotensin I-converting enzyme. Biochem Biophys Res Commun 1983; 116:394–9.
60. Corey EJ, Cashman JR, Kantner SS. Rationally designed, potent competitive inhibitors of leukotriene biosynthesis. J Am Chem Soc 1984; 106:1503–4.
61. Jackson WP, Islip PJ, Kneen G, Pugh A, Wates PJ. Acetohydroxamic acids as potent selective, orally active 5-lipoxygenase inhibitors. J Med Chem 1988; 31:499–500.
62. Summers JB, Grenn BP, Mazdizasni H, Gortze AM, Young PR, Bouska JB, Dyer RD, Brooks DW, Carter GW. In vivo characterization of hydroxamic acid inhibitors of 5-lipoxygenase. J Med Chem 1987; 30:2121–6.
63. Carter GW, Young PR, Albert DH, Bouska JB, Dyer RD, Bell RL, Summers JB, Brooks D, Gunn BP, Rubin P, Kesterson J. A-64077, a new orally active 5-lipoxygenase inhibitor. In: Zor Z, Naor Z, Dazon A, eds. Leukotrienes and prostanoids in health and disease. New trends in lipid mediators research. Basel: S Karger, 1989; 3:50.
64. Carter GW, Young PR, Albert DH, Bouska J, Dyer R, Bell RL, Summer JB, Brooks DW. 5-Lipoxygenase inhibitory activity of zileuton. J Pharm Exp Ther 1991; 256:929–37.
65. Bell RL, Young PR, Albert D, Lanni C, Summers JB, Brooks DW, Rubin P, Carter GW. The discovery and development of zileuton: an orally active 5-lipoxygenase inhibitor. Int J Immunopharmacol 1992; 14:505–9.
66. Burka JF, Paterson N. Evidence of lipoxygenase pathway involvement in allergic tracheal contraction. Prostaglandins 1980; 19:499–515.

67. Frossard N, LeGall G, Cohn J. Effect of a 5-lipoxygenase inhibitor, zileuton, on the immunologically induced contraction of human bronchi. Am Rev Respir Dis 1992; 145 (part 2):A289.
68. Orange RP, Valentine MD, Austen KF. Antigen-induced release of slow reacting substance of anaphylaxis (SRS-A rat) in rats prepared with homologous antibody. J Exp Med 1968; 127:767–82.
69. Carlson RP, O'Neill-Davis L, Chang J, Lewis AJ. Modulation of mouse ear edema by cyclooxygenase and lipoxygenase inhibitors and other pharmacologic agents. Agents Actions 1985; 17:197–204.
70. Opas EE, Bonnez RJ, Humes JL. Prostaglandin and leukotriene synthesis in mouse ears inflamed by arachidonic acid. J Invest Dermatol 1985; 84:253–6.
71. Young JM, Spires DA, Bedord CJ, Wagner B, Ballacon SJ, DeYoung LM. The mouse ear inflammatory response to topical arachidonic acid. J Invest Dermatol 1984; 82:367–71.
72. Abraham WM, Ahmed A, Cortes A, Sielczak MW, Hinz W, Bouska J, Lanni C, Bell RL. The 5-lipoxygenase inhibitor zileuton, blocks antigen-induced late airway responses, inflammation and airway hyperresponsiveness in allergic sheep. Eur J Pharmacol (in press).
73. Rubin P, Dube L, Braeckman R, Swanson L, Hansen R, Albert D, Carter G. Pharmacokinetics, safety and ability to diminish leukotriene synthesis by zileuton, an inhibitor of 5-lipoxygenase. Agents Actions (suppl)1991; 35:103–16.
74. Rubin P, Kesterson J, Swanson L, Lewkowski J, Albert D, Braeckman R, Carter GW. Safety, pharmacokinetics and leukotriene B_4 (LTB_4) inhibition of single doses of A64077 in normal male volunteers. J Clin Pharmacol Ther 1989; 45:187A.
75. Lam S, Chan H, LeRiche JC, Chan-Yeung M, Salari H. Release of leukotrienes in patients with bronchial asthma. J Allergy Clin Immunol 1988; 81:711–7.
76. Iikura Y, Nagakura T, Walsh GM, Akimoto K, Kisida M, Kondou T, Odajima Y, Okuma M, Akazawa A, Yukishita T. Role of chemical mediators after antigen and exercise challenge in children with asthma. J Allergy Clin Immunol 1988; 81:1050–5.
77. Taylor GW, Taylor I, Black P, Maltby NH, Turner N, Fuller RW, Dollery CT. Urinary leukotriene E_4 after antigen challenge and in acute asthma and allergic rhinitis. Lancet 1989; 1:584–8.
78. Pliss LB, Ingenito EP, Ingram RH Jr, Pichurko B. Assessment of bronchoalveolar cell and mediator response to isocapnic hyperpnea in asthma. Am Rev Respir Dis 1990; 142:73–8.
79. Lewis RA. A presumptive role for leukotrienes in obstructive airways diseases. Chest 1985; 88(suppl 2):98S–102S.
80. Fujmura M, Sasaki F, Nakatsumi Y, et al. Effects of a thromboxane synthetase inhibitor (OKY-046) and a lipoxygenase inhibitor (AA-861) on bronchial responsiveness to acetylcholine in asthmatic subjects. Thorax 1986; 41:955–9.
81. Fuller RW, Maltby N, Richmond R, et al. Oral nafazatrom in man: effect on inhaled antigen challenge. Br J Clin Pharmacol 1987; 23:677–81.
82. Mann JS, Robinson C, Sheridan AQ, Clement P, Back MK, Holgate ST. Effect of inhaled piripost (U60,257) a novel leukotriene inhibitor on allergen and exercise induced bronchoconstriction in asthma. Thorax 1986; 41:746–52.
83. Israel E, Dermarkarian R, Rosenberg M, Sperling R, Taylor G, Rubin P, Drazen JM. The effects of a 5-lipoxygenase inhibitor on asthma induced by cold, dry air. N Engl J Med 1990; 323:1740–4.
84. Hui KP, Taylor IK, Taylor GW, Rubin P, Kesterson J, Barnes NC, Barnes PJ. Effect of a 5-lipoxygenase inhibitor on leukotriene generation and airway responses after allergen challenge in asthmatic patients. Thorax 1991; 46:184–9.
85. Israel E, Rubin P, Pearlman H, Cohn J, Drazen J. 5-Lipoxygenase inhibition by zileuton causes acute bronchodilation in asthma. Am Rev Respir Dis 1992; 145(part 2):A16.
86. Israel E, Drazen J, Pearlman H, Cohn J, Rubin P. A double-blind multicenter study of zileuton, a potent 5-lipoxygenase (5-LO) inhibitor versus placebo in the treatment of spontaneous asthma in adults. J Allergy Clin Immunol 1992; 89(part 2):A236.

87. Israel E, Rubin P, Kemp JP, et al. The effect of inhibition of 5-lipoxygenase by zileuton in mild to moderate asthma. (submitted for publication).
88. Knapp HR. Reduced allergen-induced nasal congestion and leukotriene synthesis with an orally active 5-lipoxygenase inhibitor. N Engl J Med 1990; 323:1745–8.
89. Peskar BM, Drezling KW, Peskar BA, May B, Geobell H. Enhanced formation of sulfidopeptide-leukotrienes in ulcerative colitis and Crohn's disease: inhibition by sulfasalazine and 5-aminosalicylic acid. Agents Actions 1986; 18:381–3.
90. Lauritsen K, Laursen LS, Bukhave K, Rask-Madsen J. Effects of topical 5-aminosalicylic acid and prednisolone on prostaglandin E_2 and leukotriene B_4 levels determined by equilibrium in vivo dialysis of rectum in relapsing ulcerative colitis. Gastroenterology 1986; 91:837–44.
91. Wallace JL, MacNaughton WK, Morris GP, Beck PL. Inhibition of leukotriene synthesis markedly accelerates healing in a rat model of inflammatory bowel disease. Gastroenterology 1989; 96:29–36.
92. Stenson WF, Lobos E. Sulfasalazine inhibits the synthesis of chemotactic lipids by neutrophils. J Clin Invest 1982; 69:494–7.
93. Lauritsen K, Laursen LS, Bukhave K, Rask-Madsen J. In vivo effects of orally administered prednisolone on prostaglandin and leukotriene production in ulcerative colitis. Gut 1987; 28:1095–9.
94. Laursen LS, Naesdal J, Bukhave K, Lauritsen K, Rask-Madsen J. Selective 5-lipoxygenase inhibition in ulcerative colitis. Lancet 1990; 335:683.
95. Collawn C, Rubin P, Perez N, Bobadilla J, Cabrera G, Reyes E, Henson B, Kesterson J, Borovoy J, Kershenobich D. Phase II study of the safety and efficacy of a 5-lipoxygenase inhibitor in patients with ulcerative colitis. Am J Gastroenterol (in press).
96. Weinblatt ME, Kremer JM, Coblyn JS, Helfgott S, Maier AL, Petrillo G, Henson B, Rubin P, Sperling R. Zileuton, a 5-lipoxygenase inhibitor in rheumatoid arthritis. J Rheumatol (in press).

22

Pharmacological Properties of IX 207-887

ANDREW R. MACKENZIE
Sandoz Research Institute Berne Ltd.
Berne, Switzerland

I. INTRODUCTION

The prevention of chronic erosive joint disease has been a target of most pharmaceutical companies for many years. Until recently, attempts to control erosion were based on empirical screening in often less than satisfactory animal models of inflammatory arthritis. More recently, the molecular mechanisms involved have become clearer, and attempts have been made to identify agents designed to interfere with these mechanisms.

A key observation for the understanding of cartilage erosion was the discovery of a synovial cytokine originally named catabolin, which was able to induce cartilage proteoglycan loss from isolated live cartilage in culture (1). The subsequent discovery that catabolin was identical with the pleiotropic macrophage–monocyte cytokine, interleukin-1 (IL-1), led to the realization that the actions of this cytokine could, in principle, produce all of the features of erosive arthritis. Several extensive reviews have been written on the properties of the two forms of IL-1 (α and β) (2,3). The major properties relevant to erosive joint disease are (a) comitogenic action on lymphocytes, (b) induction of other cytokines from macrophages and fibroblasts [especially tumor necrosis factor (TNFα) and interleukin-6 (IL-6)], (c) induction of neutral proteinases synthesis and release from chondrocytes and synovial cells, (d) direct or indirect induction of acute-phase proteins, (e) induction of bone resorption, (f) induction of prostaglandin release from a wide variety of cell types, and (g) induction of pyrexia.

Subsequently, it has been found that in vivo, IL-1 can induce many of the features of erosive joint disease. A single dose of IL-1 given into rabbit knee joints produces a transient loss of proteoglycan, with recovery after a relatively short time (4). By contrast, continuous administration of low doses of IL-1 into rabbit knee joints by osmotic pump produces a complex pathological picture, strikingly reminiscent of antigen-induced arthritis, itself considered probably the best model of rheumatoid arthritis (RA) (5).

Some of the best recent evidence for the importance of IL-1 in the pathogenesis of erosive arthritis comes from experimental and clinical studies using monoclonal antibodies against IL-1α or IL-1β and the natural IL-1 receptor antagonist (IL-1ra). In antigen-induced arthritis in mice, both anti-IL-1 antibodies (6) and IL-1ra (7) inhibit the progress of the disease. In humans, a recent study (8) has shown that daily administration of IL-1ra, at the relatively high daily dose of 320 mg sc, reduces both clinical and laboratory parameters in RA. This study, although demonstrating the importance of IL-1 in RA, also shows that receptor antagonism may not be a very practical way to inhibit the effects of IL-1. This is probably because of the high affinity of the IL-1 receptor for IL-1 and the low receptor occupancy required for full biological activity, which means that very high IL-1ra levels must be maintained to bring about an effective blockade.

An alternative approach is to inhibit the production of IL-1. Several compounds have been reported that appear to have this activity. Most of these, however, appear to possess this property in addition to their more fundamental property of inhibiting either cyclooxygenase alone or cyclooxygenase and 5′-lipoxygenase. Examples are tenidap (9), SKF 86002 (10), SKF 105809 (11), and E-5110 (12). IX 207-887 appears to differ from all of these compounds in that it has inhibitory effects on IL-1 production at therapeutic concentrations, but is completely devoid of effects on prostaglandin cyclooxygenase and 5′-lipoxygenase.

II. CHEMISTRY

IX 207-887, *(Z)*-(10-methoxy-4*H*-benzo[4,5]cyclohepta[1,2-*b*]thiophene-4-yliden)acetic acid, is a low-molecular-weight heterocyclic compound (284.3) which has the structure shown in Figure 1. The synthesis of this compound has been described by Bollinger et al. (13).

IX 207-887 is a crystalline, pale yellow compound, with a melting point of 184–187°C. It is weakly acidic (pK_a = 6.82) and is stable in crystalline form and alkaline solution. In neutral and acidic solution it isomerizes to a mixture of the *Z*/*E* forms. In most studies reported in this review the free-acid form was used.

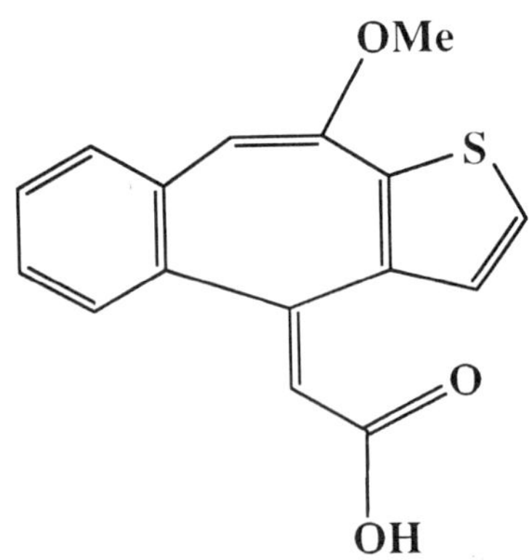

IX 207-887

Figure 1 Structure of IX 207-887.

III. PHARMACOKINETIC STUDIES

A. Human

In humans, the terminal plasma half-life following a single dose lay between 6 and 10 h. Up to an 800-mg dose proportionality was seen with low variability between subjects.

IX 207-887 is 99% protein-bound in plasma, this being mostly due to the diazepam site on albumin.

Following repeated administration of 800 mg/kg per day (bid), peak plasma levels of 220 μM and trough values of 30 μM were seen.

No tendency to accumulate was observed; in fact, a decrease in the area under the time–concentration curve (AUC) was observed over a 2-week period, possibly because of increased clearance through glucuronidation.

B. Rat

After oral administration, IX 207-887 was completely absorbed (100%). Enterohepatic circulation of 20% was also observed. The rate of absorption was high, with peak plasma levels occurring at 0.44 h. Bioavailability was good owing to a moderate first-pass effect. Distribution to the tissue was rapid, and maximal concentration in blood, kidney, liver, and lungs occurred at 2 h.

Metabolism occurred by three routes: oxidative ring hydroxylation at position 6 of the aromatic moiety; oxidation of the methoxy function to the 10-ketone; and conjugation through the carboxylic acid to form the 1-*O*-acyl glucuronide.

In urine, the major metabolite was the 10-ketone derivative; in the bile, it was the 1-*O*-acyl glucuronide; however, in plasma, the parent compound is the major component, of which 99% is bound to albumin. The elimination half-life (for radiolabeled compound) was 10 h, elimination occurring chiefly in the bile.

IV. IN VIVO ACTIVITIES OF IX 207-887

A. Antiarthritic Activity

1. *Adjuvant Arthritis*

When tested in the standard adjuvant arthritis test, using a therapeutic dosing schedule, IX 207-887 showed both a dose- and time-related effect (14). Figure 2 shows the effects of IX 207-887 on hind paw diameters in female Wistar rats treated orally for 10, 20, or 30 days, commencing 17 days after the injection of adjuvant, when the arthritis is fully developed. The results show that when treatment is extended to 20 or more days the potency appears to increase tenfold, compared with that seen after only 10 days therapy.

The effects of IX 207-887 are not limited to inhibition of soft-tissue swelling. The proteoglycan content of the femoral condyles of arthritic rats, with and without IX 207-887, has also been measured. The results in Figure 3 show a clear dose-related restoration of the proteoglycan content of the condyles by IX 207-887.

A similar protection against the bony changes was also seen when caudal vertebral mineralization was measured by a quantitative bone densitometric method (16). Table 1 shows that doses of 10 mg/kg po, or greater, markedly protect the bone from mineral loss and lead to a rate of bone density increase equivalent to a normal-growing rat. Histomorphometric analysis of nondecalcified bone sections further indicated that the

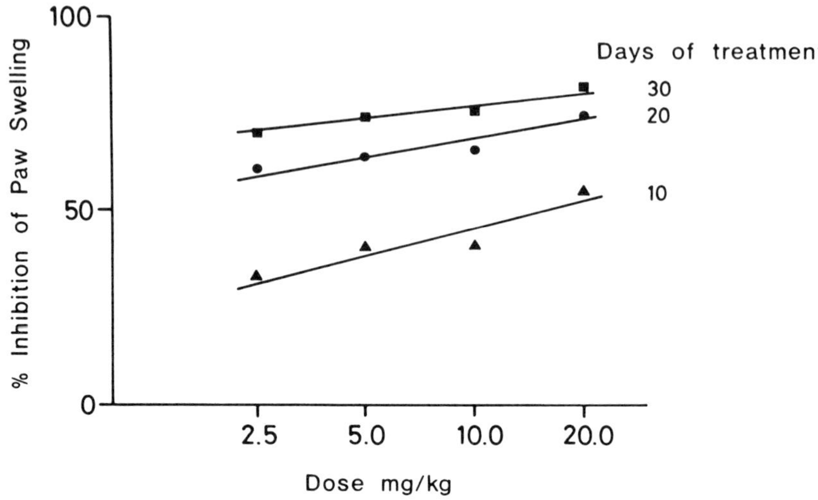

Figure 2 Effect of IX 207-887 on the paw swelling in adjuvant-induced arthritis. Compounds were dosed orally commencing 17 days after adjuvant had been injected at the base of the tail. Paw swelling was determined by measuring right and left hind paw diameter. Swelling was measured after 10, 20, and 30 days of treatment. (Only animals that had developed arthritis were included in the study.) (From Ref. 14)

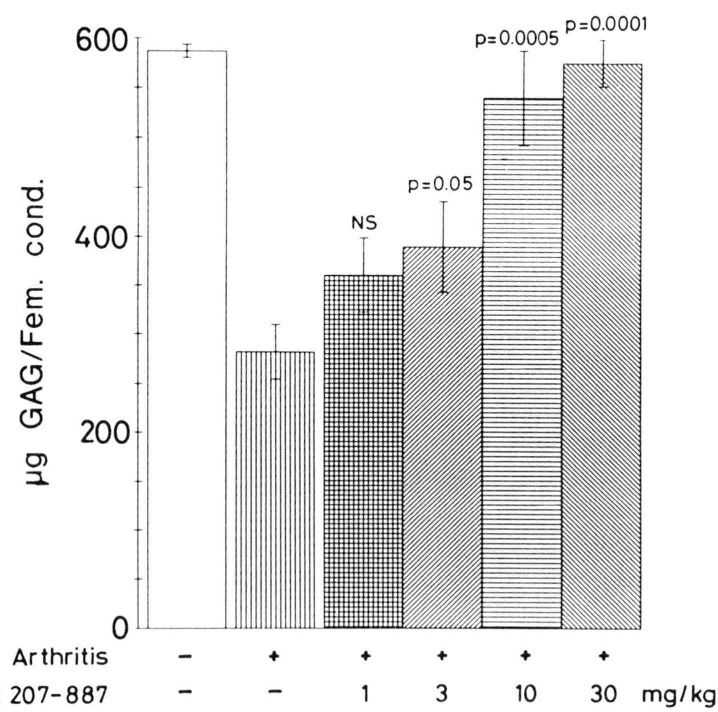

Figure 3 Protective effect of IX 207-887 against articular cartilage proteoglycan loss in adjuvant arthritic rats. Rats with established (17-day) adjuvant arthritis were treated orally for 21 days with IX 207-887. At the end of the dosing period the femoral condyles were dissected out and proteoglycan digested with papain. Solubilized glycosaminoglycans (GAGS) were detected spectrophotometrically following reaction with methylene blue (15). (From Ref. 14)

Table 1 Effect of IX 207-887 on the Bone Density of Caudal Vertebrae in Adjuvant Arthritis Rats

	Bone density[a] (relative optical density mU ± SEM)			
Treatment (po)	Day 0	Day 10	Day 20	Day 30
Normal control	555 ± 19	592 ± 10 (+37)	601 ± 27 (+46)	638 ± 15 (+83)
Arthritic control	598 ± 14	548 ± 12 (–50)	570 ± 29 (–28)	615 ± 16 (+17)
Arthritis + IX 207-887				
5 mg/kg	604 ± 13	562 ± 16 (–32)	605 ± 13 (+1)	617 ± 13 (+13)
10	578 ± 15	594 ± 9 (+16)	616 ± 14 (+38)	652 ± 17 (+74)
20	578 ± 9	585 ± 25 (+7)	590 ± 12 (+12)	668 ± 9 (+90)

[a]Numbers in parenthesis; milliunits change from day 0 (pretreatment) value.
X-ray films were taken of the caudal vertebrae, together with a standard stepped-wedge on each radiograph to allow proper standardization. Density analysis was made on the radiograph of the second and third vertebrae by an image analysis program (Imaging Research Inc., Ontario, Canada) adapted for use "in-house." The density is expressed in arbitrary optical density units.

normalization of bone parameters under the influence of IX 207-887 occurs (16). Trabecular volume and area of osteoclastic resorption are normal following therapeutic administration of 10 mg/kg per day po of IX 207-887 for 40 days. Plasma osteocalcin, which is considered a marker of new bone formation, was also normalized. Interestingly, the percentage of unmineralized osteoid remained slightly elevated, possibly indicating that the repair process is still continuing slowly at this time.

Consistent with the view that IX 207-887 acts by the inhibition of IL-1 production is the effect seen on the rat acute-phase protein, α_2-macroglobulin (Table 2). Caution,

Table 2 Effect of IX 207-887 on Plasma α_2-Macroglobulin Levels in Adjuvant Arthritic Rats

	α_2-Macroglobulin (% of pretreatment level, mean ± SEM)		
Treatment (po)	Day 8	Day 15	Day 22
Arthritic control	85.7 ± 30.6	58.6 ± 40.8	64.4 ± 36.1
Normal control		< limits of detection	
IX 207-887			
1 mg/kg	71.5 ± 23.6	62.3 ± 34.2	81.5 ± 66.5
3	63.6 ± 34.8	53.0 ± 45.2	69.7 ± 68.4
10	36.0 ± 7.8	6.2 ± 1.1	1.1 ± 0.1
30	24.8 ± 7.2	6.3 ± 1.9	0.7 ± 0.1

Plasma samples taken on the indicated days were assayed for α_2-macroglobulin by rocket electrophoresis using a high-titre rabbit antiserum to purified α_2-macroglobulin.

however, is required in this interpretation, since the acute phase in adjuvant arthritis, unlike human RA, may be reduced by some classic nonsteroidal anti-inflammatory drugs (NSAIDs).

2. Collagen Arthritis

IX 207-887 has been evaluated in both the developing and established models of rat collagen-induced arthritis. It can be seen in Table 3 that the incidence of disease is substantially reduced over the oral dose range 5–15 mg/kg per day. In the established disease, a short 7-day course produced a 65% inhibition of paw swelling at 10 mg/kg. By comparison, 3 mg/kg indomethacin was required to produce a similar effect. Over this period, IX 207-887 was substantially better than cyclosporin A (Sandimmune), which has relatively weak effects on paw swelling in this model, but appears to have a greater effect on the bony changes (17).

B. Acute Anti-Inflammatory Activity

1. Carrageenan Edema

IX 207-887 possesses acute anti-inflammatory properties in the carrageenan paw edema test. Interestingly, the median effective dose (ED_{50}) of 11.3 mg/kg po, is similar to the dose required in a standard adjuvant arthritis test over a 7-day therapeutic treatment period. This contrasts strongly with NSAIDs, such as indomethacin, for which the dose required in an acute test is severalfold higher than that required in adjuvant arthritis.

Additional experiments carried out in adrenalectomized rats showed a similar ED_{50}, indicating that the anti-inflammatory effect is not due to the release of endogenous corticosterone.

2. Lipopolysaccharide Pouch

To investigate whether IX 207-887 has effects on prostaglandin production in vivo, studies were conducted in which an inflammatory exudate was induced in a subcutaneous air pouch on the dorsum of a rat. The cells in the exudate were subsequently stimulated with lipopolysaccharide (LPS) to induce prostaglandin (PG) secretion.

The results in Figure 4 show that IX 207-887 has only very modest effects on PGE_2

Table 3 Effect of IX 207-887 and Reference Compounds on the Developing Collagen Arthritis

Compound	Dose (mg/kg, po)	Incidence of disease	ED_{50} (mg/kg, po)
Control		8/10	
IX 207-887	5	6/10	ca 10
	15	2/10	
Indomethacin	1	4/10	ca 1
	3	3/10	
Cyclosporine (Sandimmun)	3	3/10	ca 10
	10	3/10	

Wistar rats were immunized with native type II rat collagen by intradermal route in Freund's incomplete adjuvant (3 mg/0.1 ml). Symptoms are usually seen after approximately 2 weeks. Disease was assessed by determining the incidence of arthritis in groups of ten mice. The ED_{50} = the dose required to reduce the disease incidence by 50% (i.e., to 4/10).

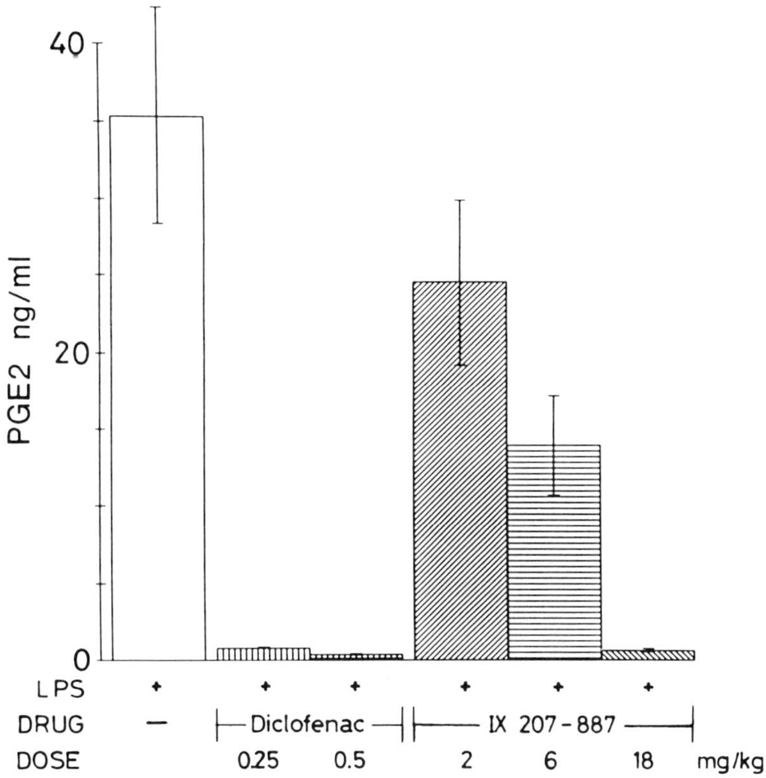

Figure 4 In vivo inhibition of PGE_2 production at sites of inflammation by IX 207-887. Air pouches were created on the backs of rats, and an inflammatory exudate was induced 24 h later by the injection of 5 ml of 2% carboxylmethylcellulose (CMC). After a further 24 h period, 50 μg of LPS was injected into the pouch. Exudates were collected 5 h later. Drug administration: 1 h before and 6 h after CMC and 1 h before LPS; route: po; assessment: measurement of PGE_2 by radioimmunoassay (RIA). (From Ref. 14)

production over the therapeutic range effective in adjuvant arthritis (3–15 mg/kg per day). By contrast, the cyclooxygenase inhibitor, diclofenac showed complete suppression of prostaglandin synthesis at doses substantially below the arthritis ED_{50} (Table 4). These and other data shown in Section IV.D indicate that IX 207-887 is not acting as a general cyclooxygenase inhibitor.

Table 4 Comparison of the ED_{50} Values of IX 207-887 and Diclofenac Against 7-Day Therapeutic Adjuvant Arthritis and PGE_2 Secretion in the LPS Pouch

	ED_{50}		ED_{50} ratio
Compound	Arthritis	Pouch	Arth/Pouch
IX 207-887	10 mg/kg	4 mg/kg	2.5
Diclofenac	3 mg/kg	<<0.25 mg/kg	>>12

3. *Effects on Leukocyte Migration*

To investigate the effect on leukocyte migration, polystyrol sponges, soaked in carrageenan solution were implanted subcutaneously in rats for 24 h. When dosed over the entire 24-h period, IX 207-887 had no effects on leukocyte migration at 10 mg/kg. By contrast, dexamethasone profoundly inhibited cell accumulation, whereas indomethacin caused a moderate enhancement. The latter effect is commonly interpreted as being due to the increased availability of arachidonic acid as substrate for the 5′-lipoxygenase pathway and the resulting increase in the chemokinetic mediator, leukotriene B_4 (LTB_4). This may be taken as further evidence that IX 207-887 differs from classic NSAIDs in that it does not inhibit cyclooxygenase. It can also be concluded that IX 207-887 is acting differently from glucocorticoids.

4. *Effects on the Acute-Phase Response (α2-Macroglobulin)*

As shown in Table 2, IX 207-887 suppresses the acute-phase response in adjuvant arthritis. An acute-phase response that is more difficult to inhibit can also be induced in rats by the administration of a single dose of bacterial lipopolysaccharide (LPS). It can be seen from Table 5 that very few agents used in the therapy of RA reduce the acute-phase response in this situation. Indeed, several NSAIDs increase the acute-phase response, possibly because of subclinical gastrointestinal irritation, which itself will provoke an acute-phase response. IX 207-887 appears unusual in its ability to inhibit this reaction and is consistent with a mechanism of action that involves the inhibition of IL-1 production; IL-1 being one of the cytokines induced by LPS, which can directly or indirectly induce the synthesis of acute-phase proteins in the liver. The only other compound that has some effect on this model is indomethacin, but only at doses that are fourfold higher than the arthritis therapeutic dose.

Table 5 Effect of IX 207-887 and a Range of NSAIDs and Other Antirheumatic Agents on the LPS-Induced Increase in the Acute-Phase Plasma Protein α_2-Macroglobulin

Drug	Dose (mg/kg, po)	% of LPS-control[a] (mean ± SD)	
IX 207-887	6	75 ± 24*	(10)
	20	60 ± 26**	(24)
Indomethacin	2	78 ± 20$^+$	(10)
Etodolic acid	10	90 ± 13	(5)
Naproxen	4	98 ± 28	(5)
Piroxicam	3	98 ± 14	(5)
Diclofenac	4	158 ± 35$^+$	(5)
Cyclosporin A (Sandimmun)	20	127 ± 37	(4)
d-Penicillamine	20	149 ± 33$^+$	(4)
Levamisole	20	84 ± 17	(4)
Cyclophosphamide	10	102 ± 12	(4)

[a]Numbers in parentheses = number of rats
Significance vs control: ^+p = <0.05; $^*p$ = <0.01; $^{**}p$ = <0.001.
The acute-phase response was induced by the subcutaneous injection of 100 μg/kg LPS from *Salmonella abortus equi*. The drug was given three times before LPS and twice afterward. Plasma samples for determination of α_2-macroglobulin were collected 24 h after LPS administration.

C. Antipyretic Activity

IX 207-887 inhibits both yeast- and LPS-induced pyrexia in rats. The ED_{50} in both models is about 20 mg/kg po (results not shown), which is approximately twice the antiarthritic dose over 7 days. [No effects on normothermic rats have been seen.] Because IX 207-887 does not produce the dramatic reductions in prostaglandin levels in vivo seen with NSAIDs, the antipyretic effect is presumably due to some other mechanism. Inhibition of IL-1 production would be consistent with these results.

D. Ex Vivo Effects on Prostanoid Production

To determine whether IX 207-887 has effects on generalized prostanoid production, ex vivo experiments were performed, in which rabbits were treated orally with 12, 60, or 300 mg/kg po of IX 207-887, given as the arginine salt. Three hours later platelet-rich plasma (PRP) was prepared and mesenteric arteries and gastric mucosa were excised. The spontaneous generation of PGE_2 by the gastric mucosa was measured, as was the generation of PGI_2-like activity from the mechanically stimulated arterial slices.

Prostanoid generation in PRP was evaluated by measuring ADP-induced aggregation of platelets. The readout in this test is the threshold amount of exogenous arachidonic acid necessary to produce aggregation.

The results in Table 6 show that, at doses up to 300 mg/kg po, IX 207-887 has no effect on platelet aggregation, nor on spontaneous PGE_2 production from the gastric mucosa. A weak inhibitory effect, however, was seen on PGI_2 production from arterial slices, which was subsequently shown not to be due to inhibition of prostacyclin synthetase. Naproxen, at a high dose, substantially inhibited all parameters.

The lack of effects on platelet aggregation were confirmed in guinea pigs, at doses up to 100 mg/kg po (results not shown). Taken together, these results show that IX 207-887 has no generalized effects on prostanoid production in vivo.

Table 6 Ex Vivo Effects of IX 207-887 Arginine Salt (ARG) and IX 207-887 Acid (S) on Prostanoid Production in the Rabbit

Compound	Dose (mg/kg po IX 207-887 base)	*n*	Generation of PGE_2 by gastric mucosa (spontaneous) (ng/g ± SD)	Generation of PGI_2 by arterial slices (mech. stimulation) (ng/mg ± SD)	AA-threshold in platelet-rich plasma (PRP) (μM ± SD)
Control		6	88 ± 20	1.41 ± 0.28	67 ± 24
IX 207-887	12	7	70 ± 27	1.32 ± 0.36	55 ± 17
(ARG)[a]	60	7	220 ± 78	0.67 ± 0.14[c,d]	50 ± 19[d]
	300	4	77 ± 27	0.27 ± 0.16[c]	63 ± 12
Control		6	96 ± 19[b]	1.78 ± 0.38	85 ± 32
IX 207-887 (S)	62.5	7	226 ± 51[b,c]	0.39 ± 0.12[c]	86 ± 15[d]
Naproxen	100	7	40 ± 15[c,d]	0.20 ± 0.13[c]	168 ± 25[c,d]

[a]Given as arginine salt; dose given as base equivalent.
[b]$n = 5$.
[c]$p < 0.001$.
[d]$n = 6$.

E. Antinociceptive Properties

In view of the lack of generalized effects on prostanoid production, it was not surprising to find that IX 207-887 has no antinociceptive effects in pain models in which prostaglandin-mediated hyperalgesia plays a prominent role (e.g., Randall–Selitto inflamed paw pressure test and phenylbenzoquinone writhing model).

Interestingly, after single-dose administration of IX 207-887 to rats with established, untreated adjuvant arthritis, antinociception was seen as early as 2 h after dosing (Table 7). The mechanism of this effect is unknown.

F. Immunosuppressive Properties

In a range of immune function tests, IX 207-887 appears to be devoid of activity. A summary of the results is shown in Table 8.

The systems used were (a) 4-day primary antibody response in mice to sheep erythrocytes, assessed by counting splenic plaque-forming cells (PFC); (b) local (footpad) graft-versus-host (GvH) reaction induced by the injection of Wistar/Furth (WF) spleen cells into female (F344 WF) F_1 recipients; (c) 5-day contact sensitization in mice by

Table 7 Antinociceptive Activity of IX 207-887

Test	IX 207-887	Paracetamol (acetaminophen)	Acetylsalicyclic acid (aspirin)
Rat (OFA)			
Arthritis	7 (2–18)	142 (92–206)	90 (1–131)
Randall–Selitto paw edema	>320 (n = 10)	203 (32–292)	ca 509 (–)
Mouse (OF1)			
Writhing: phenylbenzoquinone-induced	48 (28–83) (n = 20)	50 (27–92)	240 (160–360)

Results are expressed as ED_{50} values (mg/kg po), with 95% confidence limits.
Arthritis pain test: Adjuvant arthritic rats were used 18 days after injection of adjuvant. Hind paw flexion pressure, necessary to produce vocalization was used to measure nociception. Assessment was made 2 h after a single dose of drug.

Table 8 Immunosuppressive Effects of IX 207-887 In Vitro

	ED_{50} (mg/kg po)	
Test[a]	IX 207-887	Cyclosporin A (Sandimmun)
LHG	>50	55
Local graft-vs-host reaction	>50	36
Contact sensitivity (oxazolone)	>50	70
DTH *(P. acnes)*	>30	15
PCA	>100	>100

[a]LHG, local hemolysis in gel, used to evaluate the 4-day primary antibody response to sheep erythrocytes in mice; DTH, delayed-type hypersensitivity; PCA, passive cutaneous anaphylaxis.

oxazolone; (d) delayed-type hypersensitivity (DTH) to *Propionibacterium acnes* in rats; (e) rat passive cutaneous anaphylaxis (PCA).

On the basis of these results, it is unlikely that IX 207-887 will induce immunosuppression in patients being treated for RA.

G. Gastrointestinal Effects

1. Castor Oil-Induced Diarrhea

Oral administration of castor oil to fasted rats induces a diarrhea that is readily reversed by the administration of cyclooxygenase inhibitors (NSAIDs) and, thus, is considered to be prostaglandin-dependent (18). It can be seen in Table 9 that even a very high dose of IX 207-887, of 30 mg/kg, produced no significant control of the diarrhea. Diclofenac, by contrast, showed good protection even at 3 mg/kg po.

This finding further reinforces the conclusion that IX 207-887 does not cause an inhibition of mucosal PGE_2 production.

2. Ulcerogenicity

In view of the weak effects on prostaglandin production in vivo (see Sect. IV.D), it was predicted that IX 207-887 would have a low ulcerogenic potential. This was substantiated in subacute ulcerogenicity studies in which doses up to 500 mg/kg were applied orally on 5 consecutive days to rats. Inspection of the stomach for ulcers was made 6 h after the last dose.

The results in Table 10 show that, even at doses more than 50-fold higher than the arthritis therapeutic dose, no ulceration was seen. By contrast, a dose of indomethacin that is only 18-fold the arthritis therapeutic dose produced death through peritonitis resulting from perforated ulcers. Under these condition, the threshold dose for gastric ulceration with indomethacin is only 2–3 mg/kg.

V. IN VITRO ACTIVITIES OF IX 207-887

A. Plasma Concentrations

To ensure that only relevant concentrations of IX 207-887 were used in vitro the plasma levels achieved in vivo were taken into account. As shown in Section III, multiple dosing of 800 mg po to humans gave peak plasma levels of 220 μM and trough levels of 30 μM.

Table 9 Effect of IX 207-887 and Diclofenac on Castor Oil-Induced Diarrhea in the Rat[a]

Drug	Dose (mg/kg, po)	Inhibition of diarrhea (%)
Control		
IX207-887	30	19
Diclofenac	3	51
	10	77

[a]Mean values from three experiments; $n = 5$. Following castor oil, rats were kept individually in small cages on grids for 4 h. After this time the feces were collected and weighed. The results are expressed as percentage inhibition relative to the stool weight of the control.

Table 10 Ulcerogenic Activity of IX 207-887 in the Normally Fed Rat

Drug	Dose (mg/kg, po)	Rats with ulcers/ total number tested
Control		0/10
IX 207-887	100	0/10
	500	0/10
Indomethacin	9	8/10[a]

[a]Three of ten rats died on the fifth day.
Animals were dosed orally for 5 days by gavage, and the stomachs were examined 6 h after the last dose.

B. Inhibition of Cytokine Release

1. *Human Monocytes*

Human monocytes, stimulated with LPS, release IL-1β, which may be detected in the culture medium. Interleukin-1β is also found in the cell lysates, in which it probably exists mainly or entirely in the inactive 33-kDa pro-form.

IX 207-887 inhibits the release of IL-1β to the outside, but appears to have a negligible effect on the cellular compartment, as shown in Figure 5 (19,20). IX 207-887, therefore, appears to act at a posttranslational level. This was supported by the finding that mRNA for IL-1β, detected by Northern blotting, was not reduced by IX 207-887.

Because of the low levels of IL-1α secreted by human monocytes, it is not known if IX 207-887 has the potential to inhibit IL-1α in humans.

Further studies on the release of TNFα and IL-6 from LPS-stimulated monocytes showed that the effects are relatively selective. No significant effects were seen on TNFα except at 100 μM. However, a weak, but consistent, inhibitory effect was seen on IL-6 secretion (20–30% inhibition at 30–100 μM) (20). Because of this selectivity, it seems unlikely that IX 207-887 is acting as a general protein synthesis inhibitor, a conclusion that is further confirmed by the observation that IX 207-887 has no effects on the constitutive macrophage–monocyte product, lysozyme.

Moreover, at concentrations of compound that inhibit IL-1, no cytotoxicity occurs, as judged by the lack of any increase in lactate dehydrogenase (LDH) leakage.

2. *Mouse Macrophages*

Mouse macrophages, unlike human monocytes, produce preponderantly IL-1α. The results in Figure 6 show that IX 207-887 reduces, but does not completely inhibit, IL-1 production from mouse macrophages. These results suggest that the release of both species of IL-1 are inhibited, although experiments on cells secreting significant quantities of both have not been performed.

C. Effects on Neutrophil Functions

1. *Effects on Granule Exocytosis*

When freshly isolated human neutrophils, primed with cytochalasin B, are stimulated with the peptide *N*-formyl-methionyl-leucyl-phenylalanine (FMLP), exocytosis of both azurophil and specific granules occur. Several marker enzymes can be measured to monitor the extent of granule release.

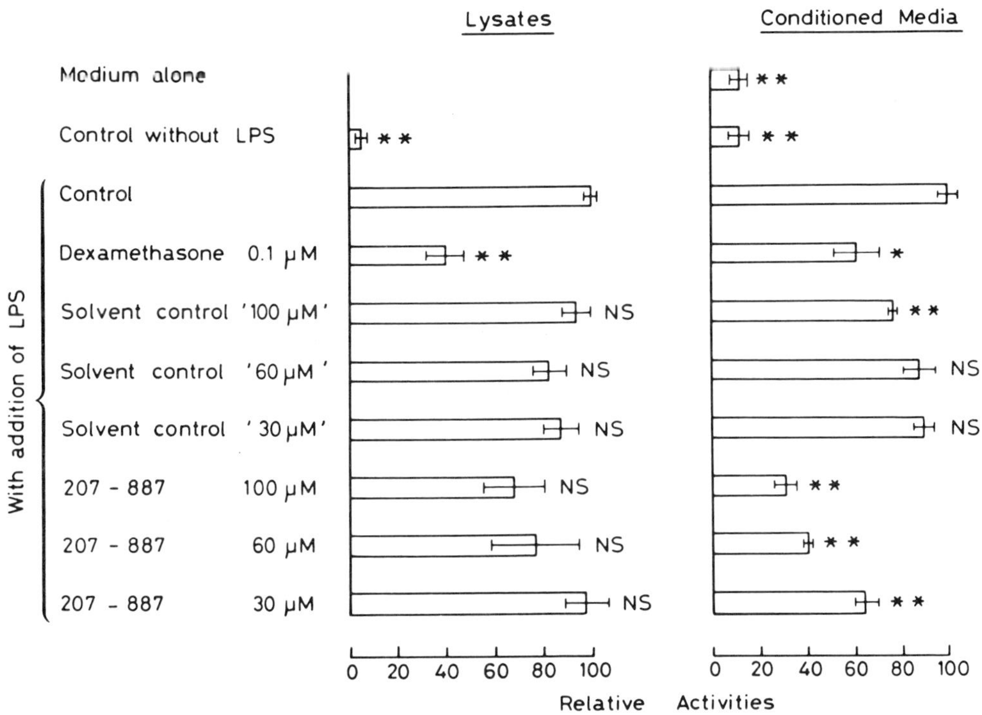

Figure 5 Effect of IX 207-887, dimethyl sulfoxide (DMSO; solvent), and dexamethasone on the synthesis and release of IL-1. Conditioned media and lysates from human monocytes were prepared and the IL-1 content was monitored by the RIA test. The data are expressed as percentage of the LPS controls. The absolute values (ng/ml; means ± SEM; *N*) of the IL-1 content in the LPS controls of lysates and conditioned media were:

	Lysates	Conditioned media
LPS control 1	12.6 ± 5.41 (3)	3.8 ± 0.76 (3)
LPS control 2	11.3 ± 4.35 (3)	4.0 ± 1.15 (3)

(From Ref. 20)

Under optimal conditions for granule exocytosis (i.e., with preincubation with cytochalasin B), IX 207-887 produced a dose-dependent inhibition of both azurophil granules (vitamin B_{12}-binding protein) and specific granules (peroxidase and β-glucuronidase), with a median inhibitory concentration (IC_{50}) of between 30 and 100 μM (21). At the same time, LDH leakage did not significantly increase, showing that the effect was not due to cytotoxicity. The inhibition of exocytosis in neutrophils is in contrast with mouse peritoneal macrophages, in which the release of β-glucuronidase is not inhibited. Inhibition of release was not seen when the physiological ligands IL-8 or aggregated IgG were used. The physiological relevance of the effect with FMLP is, therefore, uncertain.

2. *Effect on Superoxide Production from Neutrophils*

In an attempt to identify the site of action of IX 207-887 in the neutrophil, further studies were carried out in which superoxide release was measured. As with the granule-release

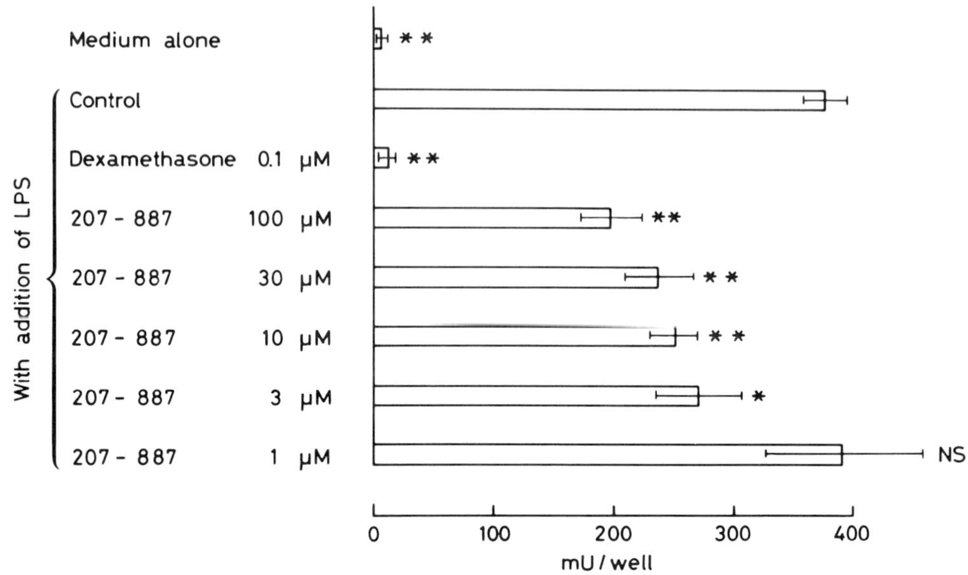

Figure 6 Effect of IX 207-887 and dexamethasone on IL-1 release from mouse peritoneal macrophages. Adherent and freshly explanted cells were preincubated 3 h with the test drugs, the medium was changed, and the cells were stimulated with LPS. After 1 day, the conditioned media were diluted 1:1 with fresh medium and added to confluent chondrocytes to monitor the metalloproteinase-inducing activity as a measure of IL-1. The data from two to five experiments with triplicate cultures as expressed in milliunits per well (means ± SEM). (From Ref. 20)

experiments, IX 207-887 inhibited O_2^- production induced by FMLP in the presence of cytochalasin B (EC_{50} 30–100 μM).

The signal transduction cascade for FMLP is thought to proceed as follows: Following ligand binding to the receptor which is G–protein-coupled, phospholipase C is activated. This leads to the generation of both inositol triphosphate, which induces calcium mobilization and diacylglycerol. Both these ligands activate protein kinase C (PK-C); by a poorly understood series of phosphorylation events, this leads to activation of NADP oxidase through which O_2^- is generated.

In an attempt to locate the site of action of IX 207-887, studies were carried out with agents that bypass one or more of these reactions. A summary is shown in Table 11.

The results show that sodium fluoride stimulation, which directly activates G-proteins (22), is also inhibited by IX 207-887, suggesting that IX 207-887 acts on an event after receptor ligand interaction. By contrast, phorbol myristate acetate (PMA) activation, which directly activates PK-C was unaffected by IX 207-887, showing that the inhibited step is earlier in the cascade.

Studies with concanavalin A (Con A), which directly activates PL-C, and the calcium ionophore A23187 are somewhat contradictory. Con A-induced O_2^- production is unaffected, whereas that induced by calcium ionophore is inhibited, although relatively weakly (37% inhibition at 100 μM). Because calcium mobilization occurs as a consequence of PL-C activation this result is difficult to rationalize.

Nevertheless, it seems probable in this system that IX 207-887 operates during early activation, certainly before PK-C and, possibly, through an interaction with G-protein.

Table 11 IC_{50} Values[a] of the Effect of IX 207-887 on Stimulus-Induced Superoxide Release From Human Neutrophils

Stimulus[b]	Control value (nmol/10^6 cells)	Inc. time (min)	IC_{50} (μM)	n
FMLP 10^{-7}M	12.4 ± 0.8	10	45 ± 5	8
NaF 20 mM	6.5 ± 0.4	30	66 ± 14	3
Con A 100 μg/ml	5.9 ± 1.8	30	>200	3
PMA 20 ng/ml	12.4 ± 0.6	10	>100	3
A23187 10^{-6}M	3.5 ± 0.3	10	>100	3
C5a 1 μg/ml	6.2	30	>200	1

[a]IC_{50} values are given as mean ± SEM, calculated from curves consisting of at least four points in duplicate. When the IC_{50} is greater than the highest concentration tested, the percentage of control at that concentration of substance is given; n number of separate experiments performed.
[b]NaF, sodium floride; Inc. time, incubation time; FMLP, Con A, PMA, see text.

D. Effects on Arachidonic Acid Metabolism

1. *Cyclooxygenase*

IX 207-887 has no inhibitory effects on prostaglandin synthase or cyclooxygenase derived from bovine seminal vesicles at concentrations up to 5 mM.

It is unlikely that IX 207-887 is converted to a cyclooxygenase inhibitor in vivo, since most of the compound circulates as the parent drug. The 10-keto metabolite is formed in vivo, but a synthetic version of this compound was devoid of cyclooxygenase inhibitory activity.

2. *Phospholipase A2*

Although IX 207-887 does not inhibit cyclooxygenase, it might indirectly reduce prostaglandin production by inhibition of substrate (arachidonic acid) generation. Studies at concentrations, up to 100 μM, had no effect on porcine pancreatic PLA_2.

3. *Cellular Secretion of Prostaglandins*

a. Resident Mouse Peritoneal Macrophages. Somewhat surprisingly in view of the results in the foregoing Sections D.1 and D.2, it was observed that when IX 207-887 was tested on zymosan-stimulated peritoneal macrophages, PGE_2 release was inhibited with an IC_{50} of near 50 μM. By contrast, the 5-lipoxygenase product, LTC_4 was stimulated at concentrations up to 60 μM (Table 12). Additional studies in human neutrophils (results not shown) indicate that IX 207-887 has no effects on 5′-, 12′, or 15′-lipoxygenase.

Further studies were carried out to explain the discrepancy between the foregoing observations and the previously described lack of cyclooxygenase inhibition. It was found that when cells are stimulated with exogenous arachidonic acid (which also induces PGE_2), IX 207-887 is ineffective (results not shown). To eliminate a possible effect on arachidonic acid release, macrophages were prelabeled with [^{3}H]arachidonic acid and stimulated with zymosan in the presence of cyclooxygenase and 5′-lipoxygenase inhibitors to prevent further metabolism of released arachidonic acid. Under these conditions, IX 207-887 also failed to have an effect.

The effects on prostaglandin production from macrophages cannot yet be adequately

Table 12 Effect of IX 207-887 on Zymosan-Induced Acid Metabolism in Murine Macrophages

Drugs/ concentrations	ZYM-induced PGE$_2$ production[a]		LTC$_4$ production[a]	
Control	0.5 ± 0.13	(5)	0.34 ± 0.12	(2)
Zymosan	11.7 ± 1.19	(5)	24.1 ± 8.8	(2)
IX 207-887				
200 μM	3.6 ± 0.61	(4)	34.3 ± 14.4	(2)
30	6.4 ± 0.08	(3)	32.4 ± 14.1	(2)
10	8.6 ± 0.28	(3)	31.9 ± 12.8	(2)
3	10.0 ± 0.73	(3)	29.3 ± 11.2	(2)
Control	3.8 ± 0.42	(2)	0.34 ± 0.14	(2)
Zymosan	33.2 ± 6.13	(2)	41.7 ± 0.55	(2)
Indomethacin				
1 μM	4.2 ± 0.5	(2)	58.2 ± 3.8	(2)

[a]Mean ± SEM (ng/well) from *(N)* experiments with three parallel determinations.
The cells were preincubated with drug for 24 h before the addition of zymosan. After a further 1 h, the supernatants were harvested for determination of the concentration of each mediator. PGE$_2$ was determined by immunoassay and LTC$_4$ by thin-layer chromatography.

explained, but these experiments suggest that IX 207-887 may be interfering with membrane transport of PGE$_2$.

b. Human Monocytes. In contrast with the rapid burst in mouse macrophages, monocyte PGE$_2$ release occurs much more slowly and to a smaller extent in human monocytes. In this model, IX 207-887 was more potent, having an IC$_{50}$ of about 3 μM.

Findings were similar with the human promonocyte line, THP-1 (23). When these cells interact with IFN-γ they differentiate into a monocytelike state in which LPS will induce PGE$_2$ secretion. Under these conditions, IX 207-887 shows almost complete inhibition at 10 μM (21).

c. Bone and Cartilage Cells. One of the most potent effects yet seen with IX 207-887 is the inhibition of PGE$_2$ release from mouse bone cells stimulated with IL-1. Inhibition occurred with an IC$_{50}$ near 1 μM. It is unclear why these cells should be so sensitive, but it may be pertinent that the total PGE$_2$ released is much smaller and occurs more slowly than from macrophages.

Similar effects were seen with human trabecular bone cells (24) for which the IC$_{50}$ is approximately 10 μM.

By contrast, PGE$_2$ release from human articular chondrocytes was only weakly inhibited by 100 μM IX 207-887 (ca 20%) (Russell RGG, personal communication).

4. *Further Effects on Bone and Cartilage Cells*

a. Interleukin-6 Production. Interleukin-6 is produced by both chondrocytes (24) and bone cells (25), and it is thought that this cytokine may play an important role in both bone and cartilage erosion (26).

Studies in human bone cells, stimulated with IL-1, showed that IL-6 secretion is weakly inhibited (30% at 100 μM). By contrast, in human chondrocytes, the same concentration induced a 70% inhibition of IL-6 (Russell RGG, personal communication).

IX 207-887, therefore, appears to have highly selective effects that differ depending on the cell type. In bone cells, PGE_2, but not IL-6, is inhibited, whereas the opposite pattern is seen with chondrocytes.

5. In Vitro Immunosuppression

IX 207-887 has no overt immunosuppressive effects in vivo. In general in vitro studies support these findings.

IX 207-887 had no effect on either IL-1- or IL-2-driven thymocyte proliferation at concentrations up to 100 μM (19).

Other studies showed that the mixed lymphocyte reaction is unaffected at 50 μM, whereas the primary antibody response (Mischell–Dutton test) was inhibited with an IC_{50} of 50 μM (this contrasts with the lack of effect on primary antibody responses in vivo).

Somewhat surprisingly, Con A- and LPS-induced proliferation of mouse splenic mononuclear cells was inhibited at 2 and 0.5 μM, respectively. These latter models probably involve a major IL-1-driven component (from accessory cells) that amplifies the lymphocyte proliferative response.

In spite of the effects IX 207-887 had on macrophage secretory function, it has no significant effect on immune (opsonized sheep erythrocytes) or nonimmune phagocytosis (tanned sheep erythrocytes) at concentrations up to 200 μM.

VI. CLINICAL EXPERIENCE

Two clinical studies of IX 207-887 in rheumatoid arthritis have been reported.

In a preliminary open dose-finding study (27), 12 patients were treated (9 rheumatoid arthritis and 3 nonrheumatoid arthropathies). The median dose given was 800 mg/day.

Of ten patients who completed the course, four showed clinical improvement, according to Ritchie index and pain score and also showed falls in the erythrocyte sedimentation rate (ESR) and in C-reactive protein (CRP). A 16-week double-blind, placebo-controlled study was reported by Dougados et al. (28). In this trial, 20 patients at each of two doses (800 mg and 1200 mg/day) were compared with 20 placebo-treated patients.

Treatment with corticosteroids, NSAIDs, analgesics, or combinations thereof, was maintained during the trial. Patients, however, all underwent a 3-month washout of all slow-acting disease-modifying drugs. (Most patients had previously received gold salts and at least one other second SAARD.) Both IX 207-887-treated groups showed significant falls in pain, Ritchie index, morning stiffness, and Lee functional index. Significant changes were also seen in several biological parameters (α_1-glycoprotein, CRP, latex and Rose–Waaler tests for rheumatoid factor), suggesting that the drug has disease-modifying properties.

Tolerability was considered acceptable with two patients withdrawing from the placebo group (two through lack of efficacy) and nine from the treatment groups, through side effects: skin rash, five; intestinal disturbance, two; hepatitis, one; and meningitis, one.

Overall, the authors concluded that IX 207-887 had acceptable tolerability in RA patients, and that it is an efficient slow-acting drug in rheumatoid arthritis.

VII. SUMMARY AND CONCLUSIONS

From the summary of properties shown in Tables 13 and 14, it can be seen that IX 207-887 has a profile of activity that appears distinct from existing anti-inflammatory or

Table 13 Summary of Main In Vivo Properties

Acute anti-inflammatory activity
Antiarthritic activity in adjuvant and collagen arthritis models
Antiarthritic effects time-dependent
Prevents cartilage proteoglycan loss and osteopenia in arthritic rats
Antipyretic
Reduces the acute-phase response to LPS
No generalized inhibition of prostanoid synthesis in vivo
Weak inhibition of PGE_2 in inflammatory exudates
No ulcerogenic effects at >50 times the therapeutic dose
Not immunosuppressive

Table 14 Summary of Main In Vitro Properties

Inhibits IL-1 and, to smaller extent, IL-6 at therapeutic concentrations
Does not antagonize IL-1
Inhibits IL-6 release from chondrocytes
Inhibits neutrophil O_2^- release and granule exocytosis in response to FMLP, but not other stimulants
Inhibits PGE_2 from bone cells and monocytes–macrophages
Does not inhibit seminal vesicle cyclooxygenase at 5 mM
Does not inhibit PLA_2 nor 5'-lipoxygenase
Not cytotoxic at 100 μM

antirheumatic agents. Importantly, IX 207-887 is devoid of any inhibitory action on bovine seminal vesicle cyclooxygenase and does not cause a general inhibition of prostaglandin production in vivo. Two consequences of this profile are that (a) IX 207-887 is extremely well tolerated by the gastrointestinal tract, and (b) the compound does not possess acute antinociceptive activity in standard models. Therefore, it was anticipated (and confirmed by clinical experience) that the use of IX 207-887 in RA patients would require concomitant therapy with an NSAID.

In isolated macrophages and bone cells and at sites of inflammation in vivo, IX 207-887 does produce an inhibition of prostaglandin production by a mechanism that is unknown. This inhibition in vivo at sites of inflammation is, however, very weak, compared with classic NSAIDs and is probably a secondary *result* of the anti-inflammatory effect of the compound on other mechanisms, rather than the direct effect on prostanoids.

The mechanism of action of IX 207-887 is not fully understood, but appears to involve the highly selective inhibition of the release of several inflammatory mediators from monocytes–macrophages, neutrophils, and bone and cartilage cells. Of particular importance is the effect of IX 207-887 on IL-1 secretion and, to a smaller extent, IL-6 secretion from monocytes–macrophages.

The molecular mechanism is not understood, but at least for IL-1, it is clear that transcription is unaffected, and the cellular content of the IL-1 protein appears relatively unchanged.

Since cell activation by LPS is not generally impaired by IX 207-887 (e.g., TNFα production is normal), it seems likely that the effect is on the secretory process or membrane transport. Because it is not known how IL-1α and β are released from the cell, it is difficult to further investigate this process.

This conclusion is, however, somewhat contradicted by the observed effects of IX 207-887 on neutrophils. The inhibitory effects are highly selective for the particular stimulating ligand, even when the terminal event (O_2 release or degranulation) remains constant in these experiments. Here, the early events in membrane receptor–effect coupling seem to be the target.

The findings may be reconcilable, because membrane transport systems operate both during cell stimulation and mediator release. The principal interest of IX 207-887 is that what ever the exact molecular mechanism, the result is a compound with a very selective effect, both in terms of which cell types and which particular secreted products are affected.

The early clinical experience with IX 207-887 has been encouraging, but further trials will be necessary to confirm these results and to establish the place of the compound in the therapy of rheumatoid arthritis.

ACKNOWLEDGMENTS

The author wishes to thank Dr. J. Schnyder and Dr. P. Cooper for their critical review of the manuscript and helpful suggestions. Thanks are also due to Mrs. C. Weber for her painstaking secretarial assistance in the preparation of the manuscript.

REFERENCES

1. Saklatvala J, Dingle JT. Identification of catabolin: a protein from synovium which induces degradation of cartilage. Biochem Biophys Res Commun 1980; 96:1225–31.
2. Dinarello CA. Interleukin-1 and its biologically related cytokines. Adv Immunol 1989; 44:153–205.
3. di Giovine FS, Duff GW. Interleukin 1: the first cytokine. Immunol Today 1990; 11:13–20.
4. Pettifer ER, Higgs GA, Henderson B. Interleukin-1 induces leukocyte infiltration and cartilage proteoglycan degradation in the synovial joint. Proc Natl Acad Sci USA 1986; 83:8749–53.
5. Feige U, Karbowski A, Pataki A. Histopathology of arthritis induced by continuous infusion of hr-interleukin-1-α into the rabbit knee joint. Calcified Tiss Int 1990; 46(suppl 2):A52.
6. van den Berg WB, van de Loo F, Otterness I, Arntz O, Joosten LA. In vivo evidence for a key role of IL-1 cartilage destruction in experimental arthritis. Agents Actions [Suppl] 1991; 32:159–63.
7. Wooley PH, Whalen JD, Chapman DL, Berger AE, Aspar DG, Richard KA, Staite ND. The effect of an interleukin-1 receptor antagonist protein on type II collagen and antigen induced arthritis in mice. Arthritis Rheum 1990; 33:520.
8. Lebsack ME, Paul CC, Bloedow DC, Burch FX, Sack MA, Chase W, Catalano MA. Subcutaneous IL-1 receptor antagonist in patients with rheumatoid arthritis. Arthritis Rheum 1991; 34(suppl 9):S45.
9. Otterness IG, Bliven ML, Downs JT, Natoli EJ, Hanson DC. Inhibition of interleukin 1 synthesis by tenidap: a new drug for arthritis. Cytokine 1991; 3:277–83.
10. Lee JC, Griswold DE, Votta B, Hanna N. Inhibition of monocyte IL-1 production by the anti-inflammatory compound, SK&F 86002. Int J Immunopharmacol 1988; 10:837–43.
11. Marshall PJ, Griswold DE, Breton J, Webb EF, Hillegass LM, Sarau HM, Newton J Jr, Lee JC, Bender PE, Hanna N. Pharmacology of the pyrroloimidazole, SK&F 105809—I. Inhibition of inflammatory cytokine production and of 5-lipoxygenase- and cyclooxygenase-mediated metabolism of arachidonic acid. Biochem Pharmacol 1991; 42:813–24.
12. Shirota H, Goto H, Hashida R, Yamatsu I, Katayama K. Inhibitory effects of E-5110 on interleukin-1 generation from human monocytes. Agents Actions 1989; 27:322–4.

13. Bollinger P, Cooper PH, Gubler HU, Leutwiler A, Payne TG. (Benzo[4,5]cyclohepta[1,2-*b*]thiophene-4-ylidene)acetic acids; novel non-ulcerogenic antiinflammatory agents. Helv Chim Acta 1990; 73:1197–204.
14. Mackenzie AR, Bollinger P, Cooper PH, del Pozo E, Elford P, Graeber M, Gubler H-U, Leutwiler A, Payne TG, Ruch W, Schnyder J, Wuethrich H-J. Pharmacological effects of a new antiarthritic agent, IX 207-887. Br J Rheumatol 1991; 30(suppl 2):75–8.
15. Farndale RW, Buttle DJ, Barrett AJ. Improved quantitation and discrimination of sulphate glycosaminoglycans by use of dimethylmethylene blue. Biochim Biophys Acta 1986; 883:173–7.
16. del Pozo E. Manuscript in preparation.
17. Borel JF, Gubler H-U, Hiestand PC, Wenger RM. Immunopharmacological properties of cyclosporine (Sandimmune) and val^2-dihydrocyclosporine and their prospect in chronic inflammation. Adv Inflamm Res 1986; 11:277–91.
18. Niemeggeers CJE, Lenaerts FM, Janssen PAJ. Loperamide (R 18553), a novel type of antidiarrheal agent. Part 1: in vivo oral pharmacology and acute toxicity. comparison with morphine, codeine, diphenoxylate and difenoxine. Arzneimitteltforschung 1974; 24:1633–6.
19. Schnyder J, Bollinger P, Payne TG. Inhibition of monokine release by IX 207-887. Agents Actions 1990; 29:108–10.
20. Schnyder J, Bollinger P, Payne T. Inhibition of interleukin-1 release by IX 207-887. Agents Actions 1990; 30:350–62.
21. Schnyder J, Cooper PH, MacKenzie A. Modulation of secretory processes of phagocytosis by IX 207-887. Springer Semin Immunopathol 1993; 14:345–52.
22. Gabler WL, Creamer HR, Bullock WW. Fluoride activation of neutrophils: similarities to formylmethionylleucyl-phenylalanine. Inflammation 1989; 13:47–58.
23. Tsuchiya S, Yamabe M, Yamaguchi Y, Kobayashi Y, Konno T, Tada K. Establishment and characterization of a human acute monocytic leukemia cell line (THP-1). Int J Cancer 1980; 26:171–6.
24. Bunning RAD, Russell RGG, Van Damme J. Production of interleukin-6 by human articular chondrocytes and its role in the induction of prostaglandin E_2. Calcified Tiss Int 1990; 46(suppl 2):A31.
25. Ishimi Y, Miyaura C, Jin CH, Akatsu T, Abe E, Nakamura Y, Yamaguchi A, Yoshiki S, Matsuda T, Hirano T, Kishimoto T, Suda T. IL-6 is produced by osteoblasts and induces bone resorption. J Immunol 1990; 145:3297–303.
26. Kurihara N, Bertolini D, Suda T, Akiyama Y, Roodman GD. IL-6 stimulates osteoclast-like multinucleated cell formation in long term human marrow cultures by inducing IL-1 release. J Immunol 1990; 144:4226–30.
27. Seibel MJ, Brückle W, Respondek M, Beveridge T, Schnyder J, Müller W. Erste klinische Erfahrungen in der Behandlung chronischer Polyarthritiden mit einem neuen Monokin-Release-Inhibitor. Z Rheumatol 1989; 48:147–51.
28. Dougados M, Combe B, Beveridge T, Bondeix I, Lallemand A, Amor B, Sany J. IX 207-887 in rheumatoid arthritis: double blind placebo controlled dose-ranging study. Arthritis Rheum 1992; 35:999–1006.

23

Pharmacological Properties of E5090

An Orally Active Inhibitor of Interleukin-1 Generation

HIROSHI SHIROTA, KEN-ICHI CHIBA, MASAKI GOTO, and KOUICHI KATAYAMA
Eisai Co., Ltd.
Tsukuba-shi, Japan

ISAO YAMATSU
Eisai Co., Ltd.
Tokyo, Japan

I. INTRODUCTION

Interleukin-1 (IL-1), which is a cytokine produced and released mainly by stimulated monocytes–macrophages, has been recognized as an essential mediator in inflammatory as well as immune responses (1–3). Therefore, it is expected that inhibitors of IL-1 generation or IL-1 receptor antagonists (4,5) will be useful tools for the control of inflammatory responses. The anti-inflammatory steroids are well known as potent inhibitors of IL-1 generation (6–9). However, the main mechanism of steroidal anti-inflammatory effects remains unclear because the steroids widely inhibit the generation of many inflammatory mediators, including the products of the arachidonate cascade and some cytokines. Recently, several nonsteroidal anti-inflammatory drugs (NSAIDs) that inhibit the generation or release of IL-1 in in vitro systems have been reported (10–14). However, there are few reports about the in vivo inhibitory effects of these compounds on IL-1 generation in inflammatory foci.

E5090, (*z*)-3-[4-(acetyloxy)-5-ethyl-3-methoxy-1-naphthalenyl]-2-methyl-2-propenoic acid (Fig. 1), is a newly synthesized orally active inhibitor of IL-1 generation that was found by using both in vitro and in vivo screening systems (15). When orally administered, E5090 is rapidly absorbed and transformed to the pharmacologically active form, DA-E5090, by deacetylation in rats, and is mainly distributed as this active form in the body (16). E5090 is clearly different from the classic NSAIDs, such as indomethacin (IND), because neither E5090 nor DA-E5090 has any direct inhibitory action on arachidonate cyclooxygenase.

In this chapter, we describe the inhibitory effects of this compound on both in vitro and in vivo IL-1 generation and its anti-inflammatory properties in some inflammatory animal models.

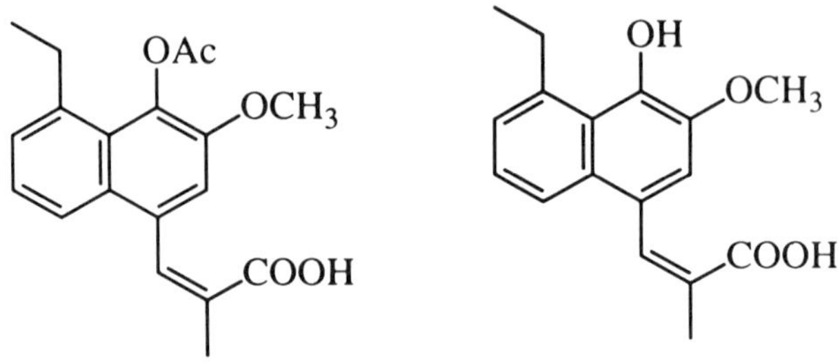

E5090 DA-E5090

Figure 1 Chemical structures of E5090 and DA-E5090.

II. IN VITRO INHIBITORY EFFECTS ON INTERLEUKIN-1 GENERATION

The inhibitory effects of DA-E5090, which is the pharmacologically active form of E5090, on in vitro IL-1 generation were investigated in human monocytes (17). The monocytes were prepared by the reported method (18), and cultured with 1 μg/ml of lipopolysaccharide (LPS) for 18 h in the presence or absence of DA-E5090. Interleukin-1 contents in the cultured medium and cell lysate of the monocytes were determined by using the thymocyte costimulator (LAF) assay with C3H/HeJ mouse cells (18) and by enzyme-linked immunosorbent assay (ELISA) for both IL-1α and IL-1β. As shown in Table 1, 1–10 μM DA-E5090 dose-dependently reduced the amount of both intra- and extracellular IL-1 activity enhanced by LPS, as determined by the LAF assay. The results from the ELISA showed that IL-1α was detected mainly intracellularly and IL-1β extracellularly. DA-E5090 inhibited the generation of both IL-1α and β. The inhibitory effect of DA-E5090 on IL-1 generation was not due to a nonspecific inhibition of protein biosynthesis, because DA-E5090 had no effect on [^{35}S]methionine incorporation into the cultured monocytes, even at a concentration of 10 μM.

The effect of DA-E5090 on the expression of IL-1α and β mRNAs induced by LPS in cultured human monocytes was examined. Human monocytes were cultured for 4 h with 1 μg/ml of LPS in the presence or absence of DA-E5090. After the cultivation, RNA isolation and Northern blotting analysis were performed, as described previously (19), by using DNA probes of human IL-1α, IL-1β, and β-actin. DA-E5090 suppressed

Table 1 Inhibitory Effect of DA-E5090 on IL-1 Generation by Human Monocytes Stimulated With LPS

	LAF (units/ml)		ELISA (pg/ml) IL-1α		ELISA (pg/ml) IL-1β	
	Supernatant	Cell	Supernatant	Cell	Supernatant	Cell
Medium	4.4	4.2	0	0	0	0
LPS (1 μg/ml)	46.2	44.0	106	1286	1114	241
+ DA-E5090 1 μM	49.0	27.4	72	792	929	147
3 μM	27.4	29.9	61	620	748	49
10 μM	13.0	7.1	52	175	377	33

Each value is the mean of triplicate samples.

the expression of both IL-1α and β mRNAs at concentrations of 3 and 10 μM, but did not affect the level of β-actin mRNA. These results in human monocytes show that DA-E5090 inhibits IL-1 generation through the suppression of IL-1 mRNA expression, and this inhibitory effect was not due to a nonspecific suppression of mRNA biosynthesis.

Furthermore, the inhibitory effects of DA-E5090 on IL-1 generation are commonly observed in several in vitro systems, using resident or exudate macrophages of rats or mice stimulated with LPS (1 ng/ml), opsonized zymosan (1 mg/ml), or immune complexes, and are similar to those of an anti-inflammatory steroid, prednisolone (PRED).

III. IN VIVO INHIBITORY EFFECTS ON INTERLEUKIN-1 GENERATION

A well-established inflammatory animal model that is suitable for quantitative measurements of IL-1 in inflammatory foci is not yet available, especially for evaluation of a drug effect. We used air pouch models in rats (20,21) to quantitatively measure the IL-1 activity produced in the inflammatory focus. Various experimental conditions in the air pouch models, such as the kinds and amount of stimuli, timing of treatment with stimuli, the time course of the production of several inflammatory mediators, and indexes of inflammatory responses, were investigated before evaluation of the drug effects. We were able to establish suitable experimental conditions for both nonallergic and allergic air pouch models, that are useful as in vivo IL-1-generating systems (Fig. 2).

In the carboxymethylcellulose (CMC)–LPS air-pouch model, LPS was used as a nonallergic stimulus of inflammation. The inflammation was provoked by injection of 5 ng of LPS into a previously prepared CMC air pouch. The IL-1 activity, which was measured by LAF assay, was detected mainly in the exudate cells of the pouch fluid only during the acute phase, within 24 h, and peaked at 4 h after the LPS injection. As other inflammatory mediators, prostaglandin E_2 (PGE_2), tumor necrosis factor (TNF), and IL-6 were determined by radioimmunoassay, L-P3 cytotoxicity assay (22), and MH60.BSF2 growth assay (23), respectively. These mediators were also detected during the acute phase of inflammation, but unlike IL-1, they were found mainly in the supernatant of the

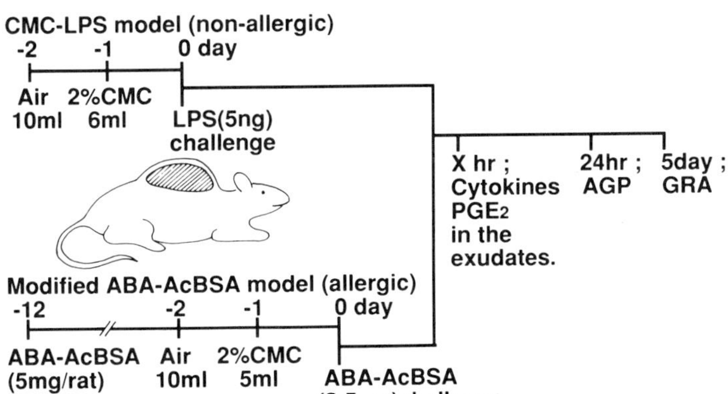

Figure 2 Experimental procedures for the nonallergic and allergic air-pouch models in rats: CMC, carboxymethylcellulose; ABA–AcBSA, azobenzenearsonate-conjugated acetyl bovine serum albumin. Low-endotoxin ABA–AcBSA was used for the challenge injection. AGP, serum α1-acid glycoprotein; GRA, granuloma wet weight.

pouch fluid. As inflammatory symptoms, enhancement of serum α_1-acid glycoprotein (AGP) was observed 24 h after the LPS injection, and granuloma was formed 5 days after.

In the allergic air-pouch model, azobenzenearsonate-conjugated acetyl bovine serum albumin (ABA–AcBSA) was injected into a previously prepared CMC air pouch of rats preimmunized with ABA–AcBSA. Low-endotoxin ABA-AcBSA was used as the antigen for the challenge injection into the pouch. In this allergic air pouch model, IL-1 and other inflammatory mediators in the pouch fluid were detected in the acute phase within 24 h, and peaked at 6 h after the challenge injection. The amounts of these mediators in this model were almost the same as in the CMC–LPS model, although that of TNF was less than in the CMC–LPS model. As the main inflammatory symptom, granuloma formation was observed 5 days after the challenge injection.

By using these air pouch models, the inhibitory effects of orally administered E5090 on the generation of IL-1 and the anti-inflammatory effects of the drug were investigated, and were compared with those of PRED and IND (24).

Figure 3 shows the effects of E5090 and reference drugs on the generation of IL-1 and PGE_2 in the CMC–LPS model. Both E5090 and PRED dose-dependently inhibited the generation of IL-1 and PGE_2, in dose ranges of 25–200 mg/kg and 5–20 mg/kg, respectively; 3 mg/kg of IND completely inhibited the generation of PGE_2, but had no effect on IL-1 generation. Figure 4 shows the effects of these tested drugs on the enhancement of AGP and granulmoa formation, which reflect the severity of inflammation

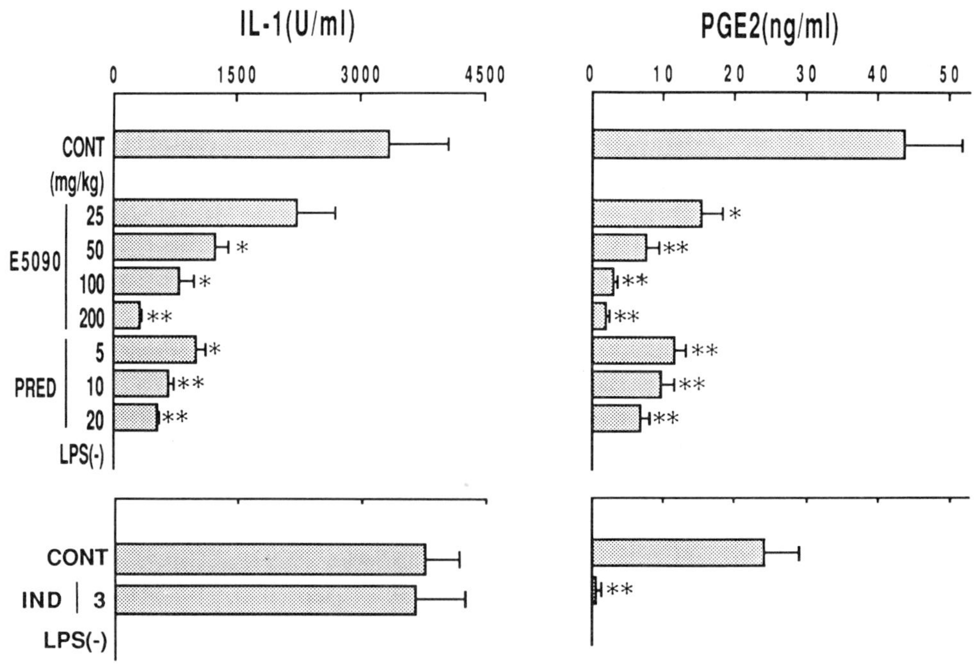

Figure 3 Effects of E5090 and reference drugs on IL-1 and PGE_2 generation in the CMC–LPS air-pouch model of rats. The test drugs were administered orally 2 h before the LPS injection. IL-1 activity and PGE_2 content in the exudate were measured at 4 h after the LPS injection. Each column shows the mean with SE of four to six animals: $^*p < 0.05$, $^{**}p < 0.01$, significant difference from control.

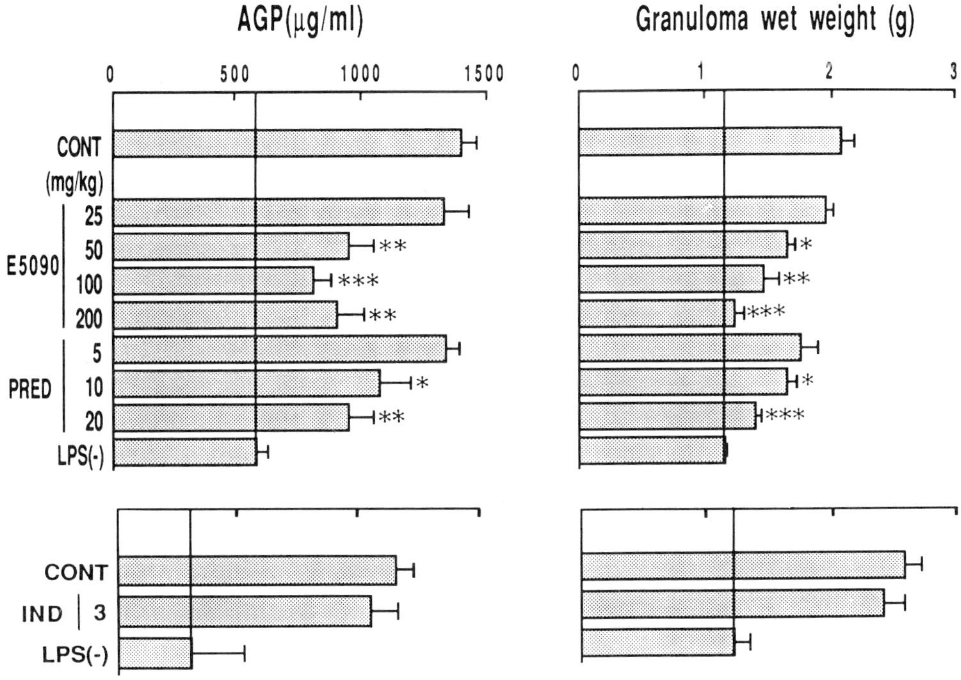

Figure 4 Effects of E5090 and reference drugs on the enhancement of AGP and granuloma formation in the CMC–LPS air-pouch model of rats. The test drugs were administered singly 2 h before the LPS injection. The AGP level and granuloma wet weight were measured at 24 h and 5 days after the LPS injection, respectively. Each column shows the mean with SE of four to six animals: $*p < 0.05$, $**p < 0.01$, $***p < 0.001$, significant difference from control.

in the CMC–LPS model. E5090 suppressed both enhancement of AGP and granuloma formation in the same way as PRED by single administration at 2 h before the LPS injection. However, IND had no suppressive effect on either of the inflammatory indexes.

Figure 5 shows the effects of E5090 and reference drugs on the generation of IL-1 and PGE_2, and on granuloma formation in the ABA–AcBSA model. In this allergic inflammatory model, E5090 again inhibited the generation of IL-1 and PGE_2 in the acute phase, and suppressed chronic granuloma formation on daily repeated administration in the same way as PRED. However, IND did not inhibit either IL-1 generation or granuloma formation, in spite of complete inhibition of PGE_2 generation, similarly to the results in the CMC–LPS model.

The inhibitory mechanism of E5090 on PGE_2 generation in both models is not yet clear, although it may be due to the inhibition of IL-1 generation by E5090 in the inflammatory focus. Nevertheless, because of the ineffectiveness of IND, it was clarified that PGE_2 was not an essential mediator of chronic granuloma formation in these air pouch models.

We also investigated the effects of E5090 and reference drugs on the generation of TNF and IL-6, which are inflammatory cytokines similar to IL-1, in both models. It was clarified that IND had no inhibitory effect, and PRED had nonspecific inhibitory effects on the generation of all of these inflammatory cytokines. On the other hand, E5090

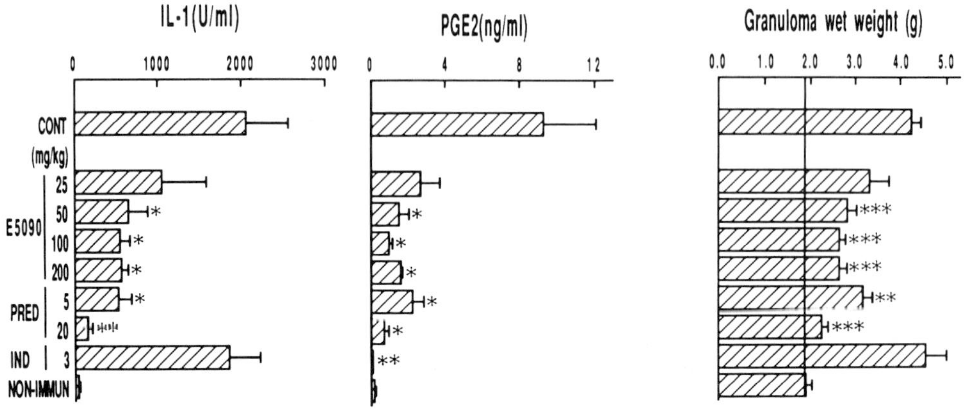

Figure 5 Effects of E5090 and reference drugs on IL-1 and PGE_2 generation and on granuloma formation in the allergic air-pouch model of rats. The rats were immunized with ABA–AcBSA 12 days before the induction of allergic response. The antigen was injected into the air pouch 2 h after the oral administration of test drugs. IL-1 activity and PGE_2 content in the exudate were measured at 6 h after the challenge injection. The drug administration was continued once daily, and the granuloma wet weight was measured at 5 days after the challenge injection. Each column shows the mean with SE of three to eight animals: $^{*}p < 0.05$, $^{**}p < 0.01$, $^{***}p < 0.001$, significant difference from control.

inhibited IL-6 generation only in the CMC–LPS model, and tended to inhibit TNF generation only in the ABA–AcBSA model. However, these inhibitory effects of E5090 on TNF or IL-6 generation were less potent than that on IL-1 generation. These results indicate that E5090 more specifically inhibits the generation of IL-1 in vivo. Furthermore, the suppressive effect of E5090 on the granuloma formation was reasonably well correlated with the inhibition of IL-1 among the cytokines determined in both models. An important role for IL-1 generated at the acute phase in the chronic granuloma formation is indicated.

IV. INHIBITORY EFFECTS ON ARTHRITIC MODELS

Effects of E5090 on both adjuvant-induced and type-II collagen-induced arthritis of rats were investigated and were compared with those of PRED and IND (25).

In adjuvant arthritis, daily oral administration of E5090 suppressed the swelling of both adjuvant-treated and untreated paws at a dose of more than 25 mg/kg (Fig. 6). The anti-inflammatory potency of E5090 was estimated to be about one-tenth of that of PRED.

As systemic inflammatory symptoms, enhancements of erythrocyte sedimentation rate (ESR) and of peripheral blood leukocyte (PBL) number were observed in this arthritic model. As shown in Figure 7, E5090 suppressed both symptoms as effectively as PRED. On the other hand, 1 mg/kg of IND showed no effect on these systemic inflammatory symptoms, although it markedly suppressed the paw inflammation. The effect of E5090 on adjuvant arthritis is similar to that of PRED in these respects, but different from that of IND.

In this arthritis model, marked changes in the weights of immunologically significant organs, such as spleen and thymus, were observed. As shown in Figure 8, both E5090 and PRED improved the splenomegaly, whereas IND had no effect. E5090 also tended to improve the thymus atrophy at higher doses, although the effect of E5090 was less marked than that of IND. Conversely, PRED further aggravated the atrophy, even at the lowest dose used, indicating the immunological toxicity of the steroid.

These findings in adjuvant arthritis suggest that the efficacies of E5090 are similar to those of PRED, but not IND, whereas E5090 does not show steroidlike immunological toxicities. The roles of cytokines in adjuvant arthritis remain to be fully established (26–28), but the suppressive effects of an inhibitor of IL-1 generation, E5090, especially on these systemic symptoms, may suggest the participation of IL-1 in this arthritis.

In type-II collagen-induced arthritis (29), daily oral administration of E5090 dose-dependently suppressed both paw swelling and joint destruction, as determined by x-ray radiography, from the dose of 25 mg/kg; however, the maximum potency of E5090 was weaker than that of PRED or IND. It was indicated that prostaglandins may play a dominant role in this arthritic model in rats because 3 mg/kg of IND completely suppressed the development of both swelling and joint destruction of the paws. However, it is of great importance that as an inhibitor of IL-1 generation, without direct cyclooxygenase-inhibiting activity, E5090 causes the suppression of joint destruction as well as swelling in this arthritis.

V. INHIBITORY EFFECTS ON ACUTE INFLAMMATION, INFLAMMATORY PAIN, AND PYREXIA

Table 2 shows the anti-inflammatory, analgesic, and antipyretic effects of orally administered E5090 and reference drugs on several inflammatory models in rats (25).

In the acute inflammatory models, E5090 suppressed carrageenan-induced paw swelling (30) at doses of more than 100 mg/kg, and also suppressed adjuvant-induced local hyperthermia (31) at doses of 10–30 mg/kg. The inhibitory potency of E5090 on these acute inflammatory models was estimated to be 1/10–1/30 that of PRED.

E5090 showed analgesic effects against inflammatory pain, tested by using both flection pain in chronic adjuvant arthritis (32) and lame-walking reaction of rats with adjuvant-induced primary paw inflammation (33), at doses of 25 and 50 mg/kg, respectively. The analgesic potency of E5090 in these models was estimated to be 1/5–1/10 of that of PRED.

E5090 also showed antipyretic effects on the pyrexia induced by both intravenous injection of LPS (10 μg/kg) and subcutaneous injection of yeast suspension (34) at doses of 50 mg/kg and 10–30 mg/kg, respectively. The potency of E5090 on these pyrexia models in rats was estimated to be 1/5–1/10 of that of PRED.

As shown in the results for IND, these inflammatory animal models are very sensitive to classic NSAIDs, so prostaglandins may play a dominant role in these models. However, as an inhibitor of IL-1 generation, without direct inhibitory activity on cyclooxygenase, E5090 was also effective on the major inflammatory symptoms, such as swelling, pain, and fever. These findings suggest that inhibitors of IL-1 generation, other than cyclooxygenase inhibitors such as NSAIDs, may be useful tools for the control of these major inflammatory symptoms.

VI. CONCLUSION

In addition to several in vitro systems of IL-1 generation, we investigated the air-pouch models in rats as in vivo systems of IL-1 generation. We have established in detail experimental conditions for both nonallergic (CMC–LPS) and allergic (ABA–AcBSA) air-pouch models that are suitable for the quantitative measurement of IL-1 in the

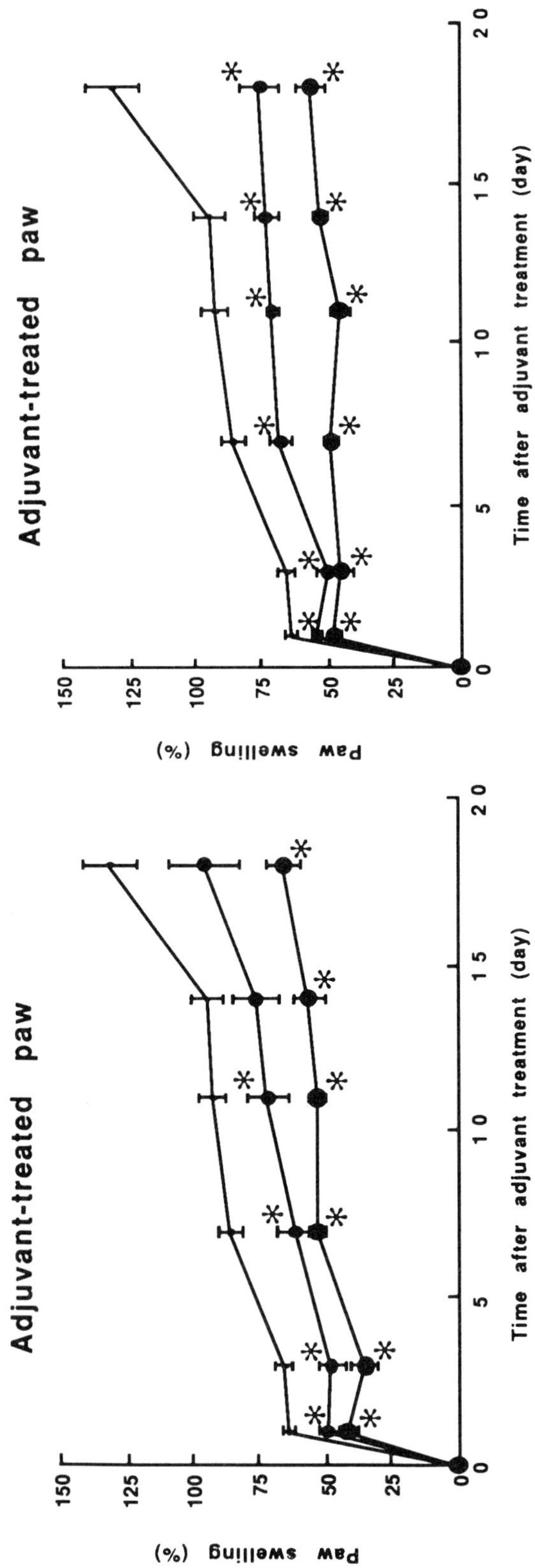
Prednisolone
Adjuvant-treated paw
Paw swelling (%)
150
125
100
75
50
25
0
0
5
10
15
20
Time after adjuvant treatment (day)
E5090
Adjuvant-treated paw
Paw swelling (%)
150
125
100
75
50
25
0
0
5
10
15
20
Time after adjuvant treatment (day)

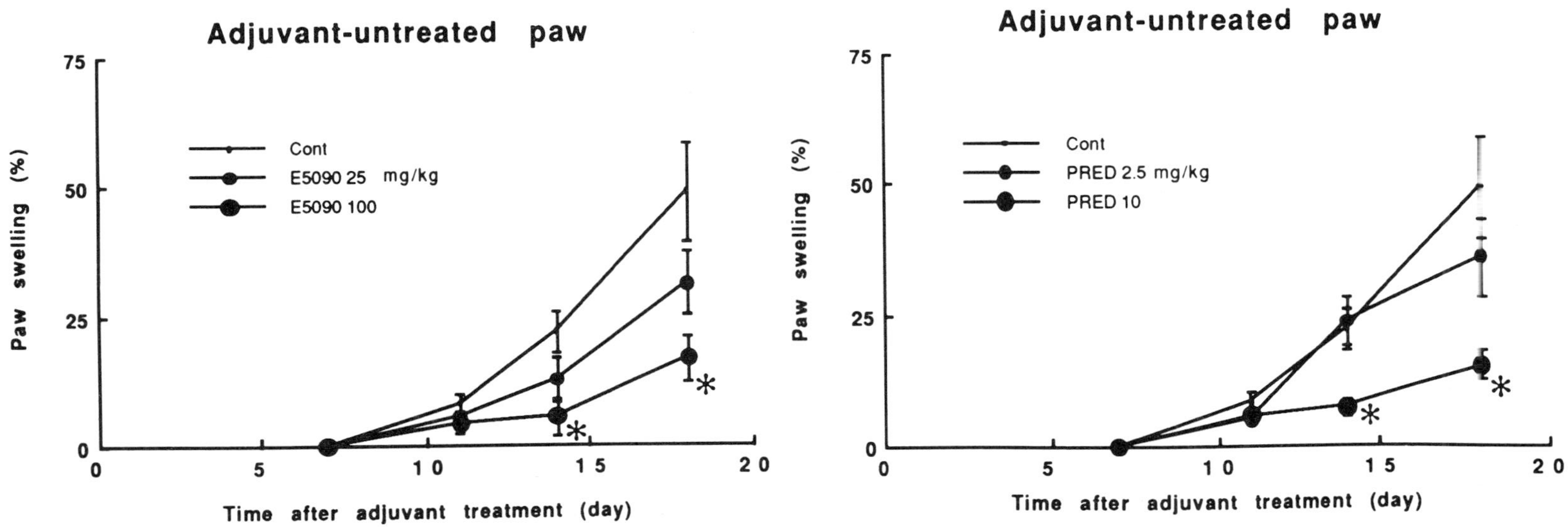

Figure 6 Effects of E5090 and PRED on the paw inflammation in adjuvant arthritis of rats. The test drugs were orally administered once daily from the first day of the adjuvant treatment. Each point shows the mean with SE of six to nine animals: *p <0.05, significant difference from control.

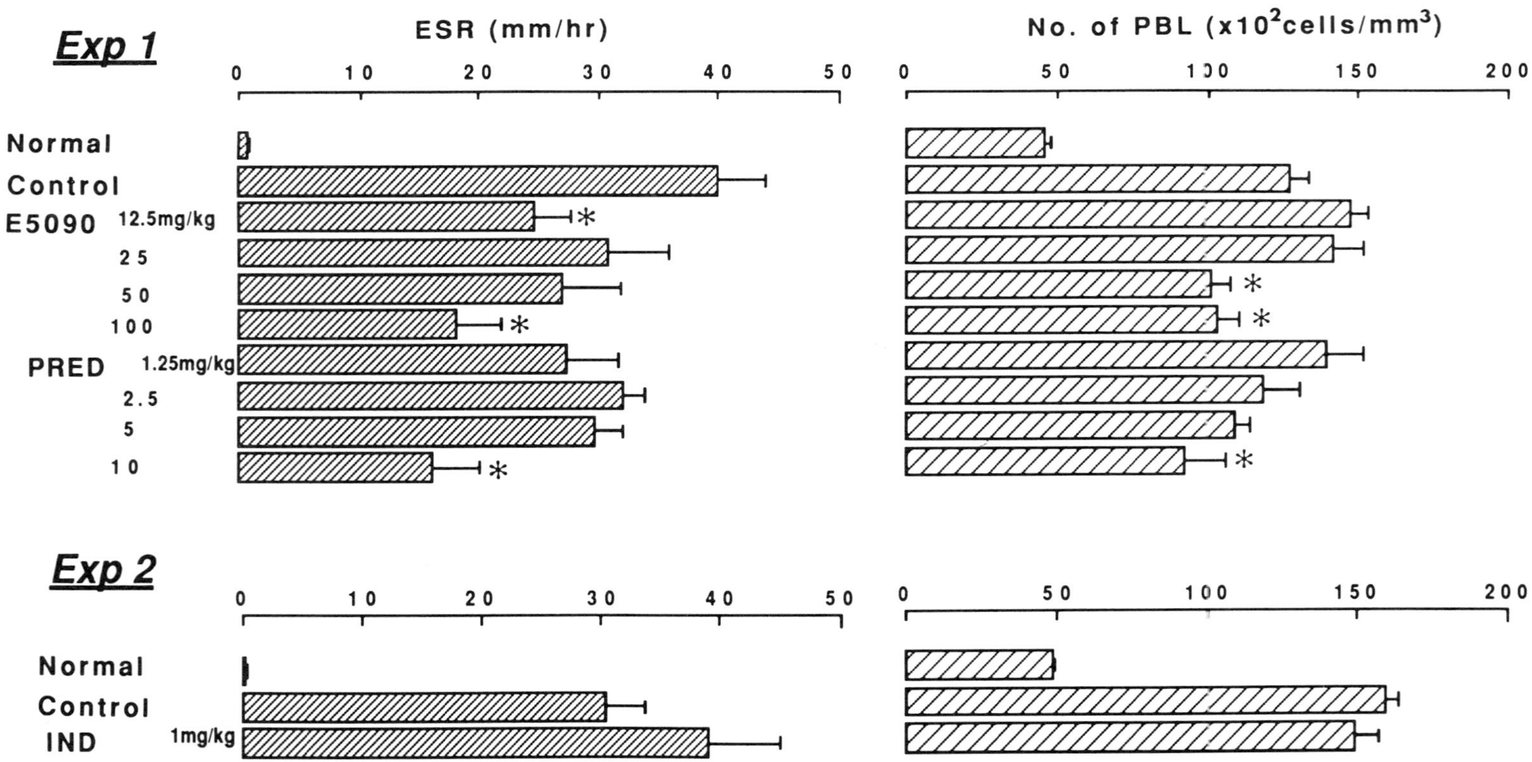

Figure 7 Effects of E5090 and reference drugs on the enhancements of ESR and number of PBL in adjuvant arthritis of rats. Each column shows the mean with SE of six to nine animals determined at the 18th day (Exp 1) or the 19th day (Exp 2) after the adjuvant treatment: $*p < 0.05$, significant difference from control.

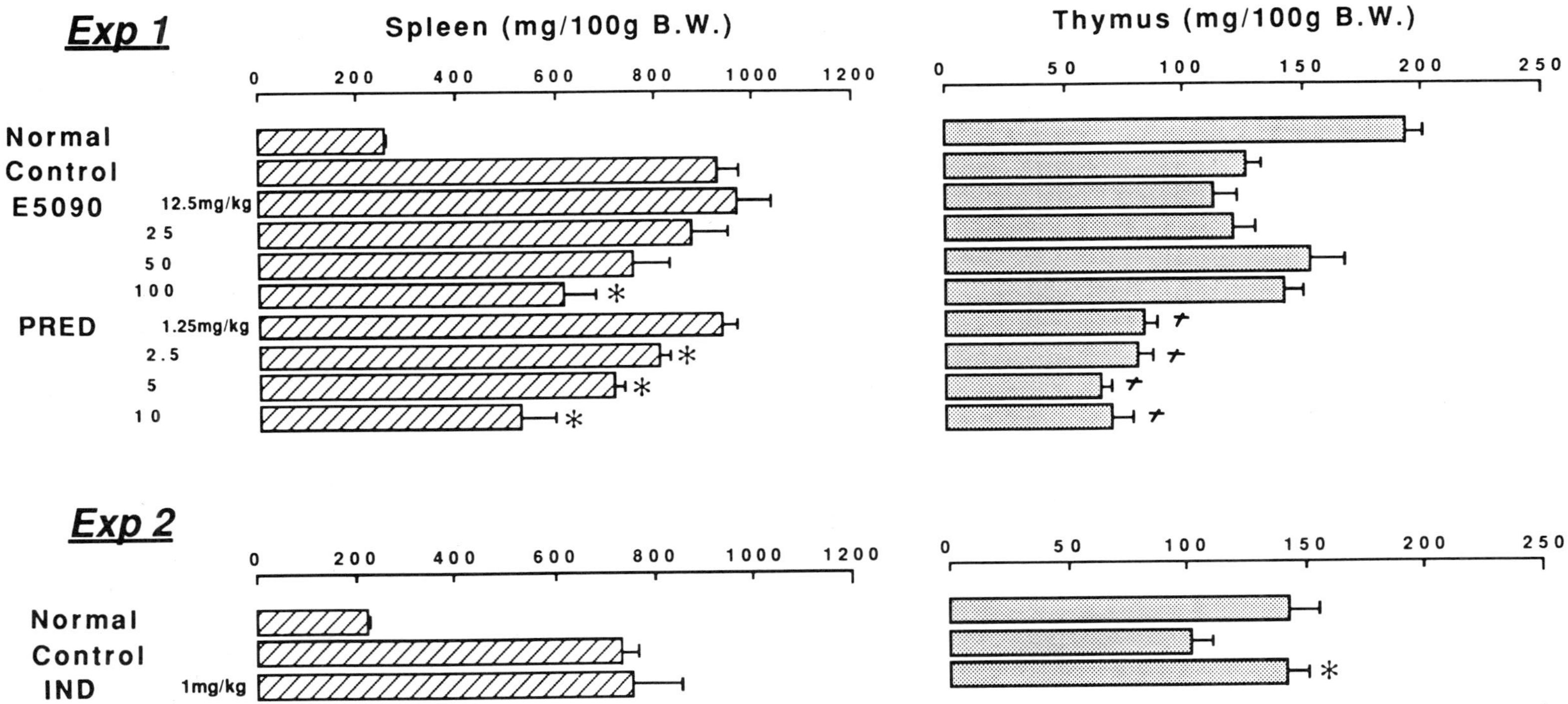

Figure 8 Effects of E5090 and reference drugs on the weight changes in immunologically significant organs in adjuvant arthritis of rats. Each column shows the mean with SE of six to nine animals determined at the 18th day (Exp 1) or the 19th day (Exp 2) after the adjuvant treatment: $^{*}p < 0.05$, improvement vs control; $^{\dagger}p < 0.05$, aggravation vs control.

Table 2 Inhibitory Effects of E5090 and Reference Drugs on Acute Inflammation, Inflammatory Pain, and Pyrexia in Rats

Inflammatory model	E5090	PRED	IND
Acute inflammation			
carageenan-induced paw edema	100	5	1
Adjuvant-induced local hyperthermia	10–30	1	0.3
Inflammatory pain			
Arthritic flection pain	25	5	1
Lame-walking reaction	50	5	<3
Pyrexia			
LPS-induced pyrexia	50	10	2.5–10
Yeast-induced pyrexia	10–30	1–3	<3

Each value shows the minimum effective does (mg/kg, po).

inflammatory foci. By using not only in vitro systems, but also these newly characterized animal models, E5090 was found to be an orally active inhibitor of IL-1 generation. The in vitro studies with human monocytes have clarified that DA-E5090, the pharmacologically active form of E5090, inhibited both IL-1α and β generation by the inhibition of IL-1 mRNA expression. The studies with the air-pouch models strongly indicated that orally administered E5090 showed steroidlike anti-inflammatory effects, such as the suppression of chronic granuloma formation, probably by the inhibition of IL-1 generation at the acute phase in the inflammatory foci. In adjuvant arthritis, E5090 also showed steroidlike anti-inflammatory effects, such as suppression of the enhancements of ESR and of PBL number, and of splenomegaly. On the other hand, thymus atrophy, which is potently induced by steroids, was not observed in the treatment with E5090. These findings suggest that this inhibitor of IL-1 generation, E5090, shows steroidlike anti-inflammatory efficacies, but does not show a representative steroidlike immunological toxicity.

VII. SUMMARY

E5090 is a newly synthesized, orally active inhibitor of IL-1 generation, without cyclooxygenase inhibiting activity. When orally administered, E5090 is rapidly absorbed and transformed to the pharmacologically active form, DA-E5090, by deacetylation. In in vitro systems using human monocytes stimulated with LPS, DA-E5090 dose-dependently inhibited IL-1 generation by the inhibition of IL-1 mRNA expression. The in vitro inhibitory effects of DA-E5090 on IL-1 generation were also confirmed in several systems using peritoneal exudate or resident macrophages of rats and mice. In in vivo systems of IL-1 generation, which were newly established rat air-pouch models induced by nonallergic or allergic stimuli, orally administered E5090 dose-dependently inhibited the generation of IL-1 activity and the chronic granuloma formation, its action being similar to that of a steroidal anti-inflammatory drug, prednisolone. On the other hand, a nonsteroidal anti-inflammatory drug, indomethacin, had no effect on IL-1 generation or granuloma formation, in spite of its complete inhibition of prostaglandin E_2 generation. Quantitative studies concerning other inflammatory cytokines such as TNF and IL-6 suggest that IL-1 is a main mediator for the granuloma formation in both air-pouch models. In adjuvant arthritis of rats, E5090 suppressed not only paw inflammation, but also the enhancement of ESR and peripheral blood leukocyte number, similar to prednisolone, but different from indomethacin. These results indicate that inhibitors of IL-1 generation may show steroidlike anti-inflammatory effects.

REFERENCES

1. Oppenheim JJ, Kovacs EJ, Matsushima K, Durum SK. There is no more than one interleukin 1. Immunol Today 1986; 7:45–56.
2. Dinarello CA. Biology of interleukin 1. FASEB J 1988; 2:108–15.
3. di Giovine FS, Duff GW. Interleukin 1: the first interleukin. Immunol Today 1990; 11:13–20.
4. Carter DB, Deibel MR, Dunn CJ, Tomich CSC, Laborde AL, Slightom JL, Berger AE, Biehlowski MJ, Sun FF, McEwan RN, Harris PKW, Yem AW, Waszak GA,, Chosay JG, Hardee MM, Zurcherneely HA, Reardon IM, Heinrikson RL, Truesdell SE, Shelly JA, Eessalu TE, Taylor BM, Tracey DE. Purification, cloning, expression and biological characterization of an interleukin-1 receptor antagonist protein. Nature 1990; 343:633–8.
5. Hannum CH, Wilcox CJ, Arend WP, Joslin FG, Dripps DJ, Heimdal PL, Armes LG, Sommer A, Eisenberg SP, Thompson, RC. Interleukin-1 receptor antagonist activity of a human interleukin-1 inhibitor. Nature 1990; 343:336–40.
6. Snyder DS, Uannue ER. Corticosteroids inhibit murine macrophage la expression and interleukin 1 production. J Immunol 1982; 129:1803–5.
7. Stosic-Grujicic S, Simic MM. Modulation of interleukin 1 production by activated macrophages: in vitro action of hydrocortisone, colchicine, and cytochalasin B. Cell Immunol 1982; 69:235–47.
8. Simon WL, Ann-Ping T, Hardy C, Jan T, Karen P, Elsie ME, Anthony CA. Glucocorticoids selectively inhibit the transcription of the interleukin 1β gene and decrease the stability of interleukin 1β mRNA. Proc Natl Acad Sci USA 1988; 85:1204–8.
9. Lew W, Oppenheim JJ, Matsushima K. Analysis of the suppression of IL-1α and IL-1β production in human peripheral blood mononuclear adherent cells by a glucocorticoid hormone. J Immunol. 1988; 140:1895–1902.
10. McDonald B, Loose L, Rosenwasser LJ. The influence of a novel arachidonate inhibitor, CP66, 248, on the production and activity of human monocyte IL-1 [abstract]. Arthritis Rheum 1988; 31 (suppl 4):5–17.
11. Otterness IG, Bliven ML, Downs JT, Hanson DC. Effects of CP66,248 on IL-1 synthesis by murine peritoneal macrophages [abstract]. Arthritis Rheum 1988; 31:5–90.
12. Lee JC, Griswold DE, Votta B, Hanna N. Inhibition of monocyte IL-1 production by the anti-inflammatory compound, SK&F86002. Int J Immunopharmacol 1988; 10:835–43.
13. Shirota H, Goto M, Hashida R, Yamatsu I, Katayama K. Inhibitory effects of E5110 on interleukin-1 generation from human monocytes. Agents Actions 1989; 27:322–4.
14. Schnyder J, Bollinger P, Payne T. Inhibition of interleukin-1 release by IX 2077-887. Agents Actions 1990; 30:350–62.
15. Okita M, Tanaka M, Kaneko T, Tagami K, Hibi S, Okamoto Y, Chiba K, Goto M, Sakurai H, Shirota H. Structure activity relationship of 3-(1-naphthalenyl)-2-propenoic acids; orally active inhibitor on IL-1 generation [abstract]. IAIS symp Drugs Inflamm, The Netherlands. 1990:1.
16. Sakurai H, Chiba K, Yokohama H, Yamatsu I, Horie T. The correlation between pharmacokinetics and pharmacodynamics of E5090 in rat air-pouch models [abstract]. IAIS Symp Drugs Inflamm, The Netherlands, 1990:2.
17. Goto M, Chiba K, Hashida R, Shirota H. In vitro inhibitory effects on the generation of IL-1 by human monocytes. Agents Actions [Suppl]. 1991; 32:255–9.
18. Oppenheim JJ, Shneyour A, Kook AI. Enhancement of DNA synthesis and cAMP content of mouse thymocytes by mediator(s) derived from adherent cells. J Immunol 1976; 116:1466–72.
19. Sambrook J, Fritsch EF, Maniatis T. Extraction, purification, and analysis of messenger

RNA from eukaryotic cells. In: Molecular cloning. vol 1, 2nd ed. New York: Cold Spring Harbor Laboratory Press. 1989:Chap. 7.
20. Fukuhara M, Tsurufuji S. The effect of locally injected anti-inflammatory drugs on the carrageenin granuloma in rats. Biochem Pharmacol 1969; 18:475–84.
21. Tsurufuji S, Yoshino S, Ohuchi K. Induction of an allergic air-pouch inflammation in rats. Arch Allergy Appl Immunol 1982; 69:189–98.
22. Hishinuma I, Nagakawa J, Hirota K, Miyamoto K, Tsukidate K, Yamanaka T, Katayama K. Involvement of tumor necrosis factor-α in development of hepatic injury in galactosamine-sensitized mice. Hepatology 1990; 12:1187–91.
23. Matsuda T, Hirano T, Kishimoto T. Establishment of an interleukin 6 (IL6)/B cell stimulatory factor 2-dependent cell line and preparation of anti-IL6 monoclonal antibodies. Eur J Immunol 1988; 18:951–6.
24. Chiba K, Goto M, Shirota H. A novel inhibitor of IL-1 generation. E5090: in vivo inhibitory effect on the generation of IL-1-like factor and on granuloma formation in an air pouch model. Agents Actions [Suppl] 1991; 32:231–5.
25. Shirota H, Chiba K, Goto M, Hashida R, Ono, H. Antiinflammatory properties of E5090, a novel orally active inhibitor of IL-1 generation. Agents Actions [Suppl] 1991; 32:219–23.
26. Phadke K, Carlson DJ, Gitter BD, Butler LD. Role of interleukin 1 and interleukin 2 in rat and mouse arthritis models. J Immunol 1986; 136:4085–91.
27. Johnson WJ, DiMartino MJ, Hanna N. Macrophage activation in rat models of inflammation and arthritis: determination of markers of stage activation. Cell Immunol 1986; 103:54–64.
28. Lee JC, DiMartino MJ, Votta BJ, Hanna N. Effect of auranofin treatment on aberrant splenic interleukin production in adjuvant arthritic rats. J Immunol 1987; 139:3268–74.
29. Terato K, Hashida R, Miyamoto K, Morimoto T, Katoh Y, Kobayashi S, Tajima T, Otake S, Hori H, Nagal Y. Histological, immunological and biochemical studies on type II collagen-induced arthritis in rats. Biomed Res 1982; 3:495–505.
30. Winter CA, Risley EA, Nuss GW. Carrageenin-induced edema in hind paw of the rat as an assay for anti-inflammatory drugs. Proc Soc Exp Biol Med 1962; 111:544–7.
31. Shirota H, Goto M, Katayama K. Application of adjuvant-induced local hyperthermia for evaluation of anti-inflammatory drugs. J Pharmacol Exp Ther 1988; 247:1158–63.
32. Kuzuna S, Kawai K. Evaluation of analgesic agents in rats with adjuvant arthritis. Chem Pharm Bull 1975; 23:1184–91.
33. Higuchi S, Osada Y, Shioiri Y, Tanaka N, Ootomo S, Aihara H. Effects of anti-inflammatory drugs on the lame walking reaction in adjuvant-induced edematous rats. Folia Pharmacol Jpn 1984; 84:243–9.
34. Kaneko T, Ozaki S, Okawa I, Yamatsu K. Pharmacological studies on *dl*-2-[3-(2′-chlorophenoxy)phenyl] propionic acid: analgesic and antipyretic effects. Folia Pharmacol, Jpn 1983; 81:481–92.

IV
Future Developments

24

Future Therapy for Arthritis

IVAN G. OTTERNESS and E. ROY PETTIPHER
Pfizer Inc.
Groton, Connecticut

I. INTRODUCTION

There are several drugs that have been used with some success for the treatment of rheumatoid arthritis and osteoarthritis. Unfortunately, there are no cures for either disease; the mainstay of treatment remains anti-inflammatory therapy. For rheumatoid arthritis patients who cannot be maintained on anti-inflammatory therapy alone, second-line drugs, such as gold, *d*-penicillamine, chloroquine, sulfasalazine, methotrexate, and azathioprine, are available. Large-scale cooperating clinical trials have enabled the physician to better understand comparative therapeutic and side effect profiles of these second-line agents. Meta-analysis, by providing statistical methodology for pooling results from many smaller studies, has the potential to further deepen our understanding of the relative therapeutic profiles of these agents (1). However, none of these second-line drugs, even the antimetabolites methotrexate and azathioprine, act on an identified pathological mechanism. Thus, one can seek a folic acid antagonist with improved safety, as in the trials of 10-deazaaminopterin (2), but one cannot seek to increase safety by improving drug targeting to a validated therapeutic mechanism. This limits rational approaches for improving the effectiveness of these drugs.

Current approaches to the discovery of new drugs to treat arthritis are largely mechanism-based. Mechanism-based approaches to drug discovery have two important advantages: First, demonstration of clinical efficacy expands our understanding of arthritic disease by confirming the importance of a mechanism in the disease pathology. Second, demonstration of clinical efficacy defines a mechanism that can be optimized rationally to achieve improved therapeutic effectiveness and tolerance. Over the past decade, many discrete immunological and biochemical mechanisms have been defined which may contribute to the pathology of rheumatoid arthritis or osteoarthritis. These mechanisms are largely based on in vitro studies with human tissue and by use of animal models that are believed to mimic key aspects of arthritic disease. However, the importance of any particular mechanism in the disease process will have to be defined by drugs that (a) are selective for that mechanism and (b) attain blood and tissue concentrations in humans sufficient to block the mechanism under clinical investigation. Because of these considerations, this review of future therapeutic developments is focused on attempts to inhibit specific mechanisms of arthritic disease.

There are major mechanistic differences between rheumatoid arthritis (RA) and osteoarthritis (OA). Rheumatoid arthritis has an immunological basis, demonstrated by T- and B-cell infiltration of the synovial lining and an ongoing influx of inflammatory cells [i.e., polymorphonuclear neutrophils (PMNs) and monocytes] into the synovial fluid and the synovial lining. Although there can be some inflammation associated with OA, this is not a major characteristic of the disease.

The sites and mechanisms of cartilage loss appear substantially different between OA and RA. Cartilage loss in RA is most severe at the cartilage–pannus junction, and there is extensive bony erosion at the margins of the cartilage. This contrasts with OA in which there is surface fibrillation and ulceration of the cartilage and eventual eburnation. Pannus is absent and, instead of marginal bony erosions, there is often marginal osteophyte formation and subchondral sclerosis.

Cartilage metabolism responds differently to the two diseases. The RA cartilage is characterized by a suppression of proteoglycan synthesis and decreased proteoglycan content in diseased areas. The OA cartilage, at least in the early stages, is characterized by enhanced proteoglycan synthesis and proteoglycan content. These pathological differences presumably reflect different disease mechanisms. Thus, most approaches to therapy are specific for either RA or OA, and only a few therapies (e.g., the use of analgesics and intra-articular glucocorticoids) are of use for the treatment of both forms of arthritis.

II. RHEUMATOID ARTHRITIS

A. Inhibitors of Cytokines, Their Synthesis and Actions

1. Interleukin-1

Several studies have shown that interleukin-1 (IL-1) is potentially an important mediator of arthritis. It induces the synthesis of the metalloproteinases, which may have a role in cartilage loss (3); induces the expression of adhesion molecules important for the migration of cells into inflamed tissue (4); induces the synthesis of chemotactic cytokines, such as IL-8 (5); and induces the synthesis of other cytokines, such as colony-stimulating factor (6), that prime cells for enhanced synthesis of inflammatory mediators. Moreover, direct injection of IL-1 into animal knee joints will induce an arthritis (7). Administration of IL-1 will induce a flare of a quiescent, preexisting arthritis (e.g., streptococcal arthritis; 8) and will increase the incidence and severity of arthritis in animals primed for arthritis (e.g., collagen arthritis; 9). These studies in animals provide strong support for the view that therapies that inhibit IL-1 synthesis or actions may show efficacy in RA.

Recent therapeutic studies in animal models strengthen the case that IL-1 may play a significant role in arthritis. Schwab et al. (10) showed that administration of the IL-1 receptor antagonist inhibited the flareup of streptococcal arthritis induced by streptococcal cell walls. van de Loo et al. (11), studying monoarticular antigen arthritis, showed that antimurine IL-1 antibody protects against inhibition of proteoglycan synthesis and loss of cartilage.

a. Interleukin-1 Receptor Antagonist

A natural IL-1 receptor antagonist (IL-1RA) has been isolated and characterized. It is a 22-kDa protein (17 kDa when it is not glycosylated) that has extensive structural homology with IL-1β. A single amino acid change of aspartic acid to lysine converts IL-1RA into an agonist (12). It binds to both IL-1 receptors (13), has been effective in the streptococcal cell wall model of arthritis (10) and in models of shock (14,15), and is currently in clinical trials for both shock and RA.

Because IL-1RA is a protein, it cannot be administered orally. To treat a chronic disease, such as arthritis, a subcutaneous dosage form has been developed that appears to compensate for the short in vivo half-life of IL-1RA. It provides, in effect, a continuous-release depot. Similar to IL-1, IL-1RA seems to be reasonably resistant to proteinases in blood; hence, its fast clearance rate seems to be the limiting factor in maintaining therapeutic levels of antagonist. Initial studies in RA have been reported (16). In four patients treated with 6 mg/kg IL-1RA sc, a mean reduction in the number of tender joints from 24 to 10 was reported within 2 weeks, and that reduction was maintained for 2 weeks after discontinuation of receptor antagonist. The concentration of C-reactive protein (CRP), an acute-phase reactant the synthesis of which is considered IL-1–dependent, was also reduced by greater than 50%. Additional patients will have to be studied to validate these early results.

b. Soluble Interleukin-1 Receptor

An alternative method to inhibit the actions of IL-1 is to bind it with a soluble circulating IL-1 receptor (sIL-1R) or with an anti-IL-1 antibody. The sIL-1R or the anti-IL-1 antibody, by binding tightly to IL-1, keeps IL-1 from binding to its receptor and eliciting a biological response. Both an anti-IL-1 antibody and sIL-1R should have advantages over the receptor antagonist. Because sIL-1R only need bind and neutralize IL-1, it need not be present in much more than stoichiometric amounts compared with IL-1. By contrast, IL-1RA requires nearly a 1000 times higher concentration than IL-1 to prevent significant receptor occupancy, giving an advantage in amount of protein that must be administered. Initial studies with the sIL-1R have been reported in rodents (17) and in experimental autoimmune encephalomyelitis (18). These appear to strengthen the premise that inhibition of IL-1 is a useful therapeutic target.

The clinical use of sIL-1R has many of the same problems as IL-1RA. It is a protein and, therefore, it cannot be administered orally. Because of its higher molecular weight, sIL-1R has a modestly longer in vivo half-life. Since both IL-1RA and sIL-1R are proteins, questions about allergic sensitization after repeated administration must be closely monitored during Phase II and III chronic studies.

c. Antisense Inhibition of Interleukin-I Receptor Expression

An alternative mode of inhibiting IL-1 activity is to inhibit expression of the IL-1 receptor by using antisense synthetic oligonucleotides. An antisense oligonucleotide forms a duplex with its complementary sense mRNA and prevents transcription (19,20). Although the method has been demonstrated in tissue culture and a few in vivo settings, difficulties in transport, uptake, and targeting of the oligonucleotides (21) have so far prevented the successful application of the method to human disease. Although IL-1R is as yet the only published target for antisense therapy in RA, it is clear that the approach, if in vivo effects can be achieved, could have general applicability to any protein that is a rational therapeutic target.

d. *Inhibitors of Interleukin-1 Synthesis and Actions*

There are now multiple drugs reported to have an effect on IL-1 synthesis or actions in vitro [e.g., glucocorticoids (22), E-5090 (see Chap. 23), tenidap (23,24), IX 207-887 (see Chap. 22), SKF-86,002 (25), and chloroquine (26)]. The selectivity and effectiveness of these compounds on IL-1 in vivo are insufficiently understood to draw definitive statements about IL-1 actions as part of their in vivo activity in animal models of arthritic disease. None of these drugs show complete selectivity for inhibition of IL-1. Thus, most of the drugs have additional activities that affect other metabolic pathways (e.g., prostaglandins, leukotrienes, or other cytokines).

IX-207-887 and tenidap have advanced into clinical trials. Clinical improvement has been reported for patients treated with IX-207-887 (27) and with tenidap (28,29). Elevated levels of the acute-phase reactant CRP have been associated with increased disease activity and x-ray progression of disease (30); its concentration is not influenced by nonsteroidal anti-inflammatory drugs (NSAIDs; 31). Glucocorticoids (32), IL-1RA (16), tenidap (33,34), and IX-207-887 (27) reduce CRP levels in clinical studies. These results suggest that these drugs may be more effective than conventional NSAIDs in RA patients.

e. *Inhibitors of Interleukin 1β Processing*

Considerable ongoing preclinical effort has been made to synthesize inhibitors of the specific IL-1β convertase that cleaves biologically inactive pro-IL-1β to an active 17-kDa molecule (35). Interleukin-1β has been shown to be important for several systemic effects of IL-1 [i.e., fever, IL-6 production, acute-phase reactant production (36), and leukocyte infiltration (37)]. However, in the single study that has examined separately the effects of IL-1α and IL-1β in the arthritic joint, therapeutic effects could be obtained only by blocking both forms of IL-1 with antibody (11). If our animal studies can be extrapolated to human clinical effects, inhibition of systemic IL-1 effects may be accomplished with an IL-1β convertase inhibitor. Such inhibition would improve the patients' sense of well-being and their general activity level. However, inhibition of both IL-1α and IL-1β together would be required to affect the pathology occurring locally in the arthritic joint.

2. *Tumor Necrosis Factor*

Tumor necrosis factor (TNF) and IL-1 possess many of the same activities in inflammation and the immune response. Although that might lead one to conclude that they are redundant cytokines, this clearly is not so. Production of TNF is regulated differently at both the level of synthesis and secretion. Thus, in rheumatoid arthritis, there is ample evidence for cellular activation and TNF production (38). Moreover, TNF receptors are localized in the synovial tissue and cartilage–pannus junction in patients with RA, whereas in OA, both TNF and TNF receptors appear to be present only at a very low level (39). Consequently, it is unlikely that TNF is a major cytokine in OA. Anti-TNF antibodies have been effective in several animal models of inflammation and autoimmune disease. Transgenic mice with excessive TNF production have developed arthritis (40), and TNF, administered into knee joints of animals can give rise to an acute arthritis (41,42). Thus there is ample data justifying clinical trials of agents that would block TNF activity.

a. *Soluble Tumor Necrosis Factor Receptors*

Seckinger et al. (43) and Cope et al. (44) showed that soluble TNF receptors (sTNF-R) are shed during many types of inflammatory and immune responses. These shed receptors can bind circulating TNF and block its activity. Unlike the anti-TNF antibodies that bind only TNFα, the sTNF-R inactivates both TNFα and TNFβ. When TNF production is in excess of the blocking activity of circulating shed receptors, additional shed receptors could be of therapeutic use. Piguet et al. (45) have shown that recombinant soluble TNF receptor administered at 1 and 3 weeks after immunization to type II collagen prevented the development of collagen arthritis. By preparing a chimeric molecule (fusion of IgG and sTNF-R to form a bivalent sTNF-R) cTNF-R, a molecule with six- to eightfold higher affinity for TNF than sTNF-R or cell surface TNF-R has been formed (46). In addition, the formation of the chimera extends the half-life compared with the sTNF-R. Lesslauer et al. (47) have also prepared a cTNF-R and demonstrated that it could protect against lipopolysaccharide (LPS)-induced lethality. The possibility that some form of the TNF-R will be of therapeutic usefulness in humans remains to be tested.

b. Anti-Tumor Necrosis Factor Antibody

Antimurine TNF antibody inhibits the paw swelling and histological appearance of murine collagen arthritis when administered before disease onset (48,49). It does not affect the incidence of arthritis or the level of circulating anticollagen antibody. When administered after the onset of arthritis, it reduces the clinical score, paw swelling, and histology of the disease, suggesting it would be of therapeutic value for treatment of established disease. Anti-TNF antibody also protects against experimental allergic encephalomyelitis (50). The use of chimeric human–murine anti-TNF–blocking antibodies is being tested in the clinic as a mode of therapy for RA, and preliminary results in nine patients suggest it may be of value (51).

B. Immunosuppressive Approaches to Treatment of Rheumatoid Arthritis

1. Rationale

The pathological characteristics of rheumatoid arthritis resemble a misdirected immune response; hence, the classification of RA as an autoimmune disease. Most animal models of RA can be inhibited by prophylactic treatment with immunosuppressive drugs, such as cyclosporine, cyclophosphamide, or azathioprine. In some models, therapeutic treatment (i.e., treatment after the disease is established) is also effective. In human RA, treatments that suppress the immune response, such as the cyclophosphamide (52), azathioprine (53), cyclosporine (54), thoracic duct drainage (55), total lymphoid irradiation (56), and leukopheresis (57), are effective, although not well tolerated. Newer agents or their analogues are in testing [e.g., FK 506, rapamycin, and leflunomide; see Chap. 20). In addition, there is an ongoing search for more selective and safe methods of immunosuppression for treatment of severe RA.

2. Nonspecific T-Cell Approaches

a. Antibodies to T-Cell Antigens

One of the problems in developing specific therapy for RA is defining key immune mechanisms that will allow more specific targeting. A number of observations suggest that the T cell is critical for maintaining a chronic synovitis (58). One approach that has been taken is to ablate T cells by using monoclonal antibodies.

CD4. CD3 is a pan–T-cell marker. Elimination of $CD3^+$ T cells should give results equivalent to thoracic duct drainage in the treatment of RA. However, poor tolerance to the first injection of anti-CD3 antibodies has been a major problem; it is associated with the release of a wide variety of cytokines into the circulation (59). Although this effect can be ameliorated by glucocorticoid administration in most patients (6), it can be life-threatening in a small proportion of patients. Thus, for RA, selectivity has been sought by targeting T-cell subsets.

CD4, CD5, CD7. CD4 is a T-cell surface antigen that is found in association with class II major histocompatibility complex (MHC) antigens and is generally associated with T–helper-cell activity. In RA, the perivascular lymphoid aggregates are preponderantly CD4 T cells (61). Anti-CD4 antibodies can be used to suppress levels of CD4 T cells and, correspondingly, their activities. Treatment of RA patients with anti-CD4 monoclonal antibodies results in a depletion of CD4 T cells and a subsequent amelioration of the symptoms of arthritis, beginning within 7 days in most patients and lasting for up to 6 months in some patients (62,63). Fever and flulike symptoms were the major side effect. Most patients treated with mouse monoclonal antibodies developed antimouse antibody, sometimes specific for the idiotypic determinants (64).

Favorable results have also been reported with anti-CD5 antibody (65) and with anti-CD7a antibody (66). An anti-CD5 monoclonal antibody conjugated with the toxin ricin has also given favorable results in early clinical trials, and Verwilghen et al. (48) suggest that these antibodies, but not anti-CD3 or CD28 antibodies, are selective for inhibition of proliferation of T cells in synovial fluid. All three antibodies inhibit proliferation of peripheral blood T cells.

b. Humanized Antibodies

After repeated administration of murine monoclonal antibodies, patients can develop an immune response to the murine antibodies. This can result in neutralization of the monoclonal antibody so that it becomes ineffective as a therapeutant, or it can result in an allergic response. One potential solution is to convert the murine antibody to a more humanlike molecule. A chimeric antibody can be generated—a human Fc region joined to a murine Fab region—or a humanized antibody can be constructed (67). The latter is carried out by reconstructing the antibody, maintaining the variable region contact residues of the murine antibody and substituting a human framework and constant regions residues for the murine ones. This results in an essentially human antibody. An anti-CD4 chimeric antibody is currently under study (68,69). Results suggest that improvement (greater than 50% reduction in swollen joints count) was noted in 43% of patients at 5 weeks and 33% at 6 months. They found a very prolonged depression of CD4 cells. Only two patients developed very low levels of antivariable region antibodies. The alternative approach of humanizing the murine monoclonal antibody has been taken with the Campath 1 antibody.

Campath 1 is a murine antibody against CDw52, an antigen on most lymphocytes and monocytes, which has been tested primarily in patients undergoing bone marrow transplantation and, after humanization, was named Campath 1H. It is being tested in a limited number of patients with severe RA. In one RA patient treated with Campath 1H (70), there was a rapid onset of clinical improvement, within 24 h of administration of the antibody, that lasted 12–14 weeks. No immune response was found to Campath 1H. Rheumatoid factor was suppressed, but not CRP or the erythrocyte sedimentation rate (ESR). Lymphocyte counts remained suppressed for 7 months after treatment. In a separate study of eight patients, seven showed therapeutic benefit lasting up to 7 months (71). Improvement in the Ritchie index and joint score was found across the group for 4 months.

c. Anti-Interleukin-2 Receptor Antibody

Animal experiments strongly suggest that T cells are required for establishing chronic disease. Exposure to antigen in the absence of an effective T-cell limb of the immune response (nude rats, for example) results in an acute inflammation that does not become chronic. Antigen or mitogen stimulation of T cells leads to expression of IL-2R. Thus, it could be reasoned that removal of activated IL-2R–expressing T cells, particularly during bouts of active disease, could provide a selective way to remove those T cells involved in the disease. A single limited trial of anti-IL-2R has been reported (72).

d. Interleukin-2 Fusion Proteins

The possibility that high-affinity IL-2 receptors are a specific marker of activated T cells has been exploited to specifically ablate those T-cell clones proliferating during the disease process. Diphtheria toxin–IL-2 (a chimeric toxin–IL-2 fusion protein) was used to block insulin-dependent diabetes in the nonobese diabetic (NOD) mouse (73). Pseudomonas exotoxin chimeric IL-2 (IL-2–PE40) was tested in adjuvant arthritic rats (74). Administration of IL-2–PE40 before the establishment of overt clinical disease proved an effective modifier of adjuvant arthritis. Continuous infusion, rather than twice-a-day administration, improves effectiveness (75). However, it was not as complete an inhibitor of disease as cyclophosphamide pretreatment, suggesting that not all clones are removed by this therapy. Indeed, it would be expected that there might be quiescent clones present at most stages of the disease. These would not be activated during a 10-day therapeutic course and would be a much larger problem in established disease. Toleration was good, although specific antibodies to the IL-2–PE40 molecule were detected after 10 days of therapy, suggesting there would be a limitation to its long-term use.

3. Selective T-Cell Approaches

The foregoing approaches suffer from the problem that all cells with certain cell surface molecules are blocked and no advantage is taken of the antigen specificity of the immune response. Rheumatoid arthritis is, in all likelihood, a disease driven by specific sets of antigen-responsive cells. Thus, inhibition of the antigen-specific T cells could provide a therapy that does not suppress general immune function and would not be life-threatening despite complete ablation of the antigen-specific response.

a. Oral Tolerance. It has been known for years that oral exposure to antigen can result in a long-lasting tolerance to that antigen. Thus, oral exposure to antigen can prevent the subsequent induction of autoimmune disease (76–78). Although it is possible that induction of hyporesponsiveness to type II collagen could be of benefit for RA, as it is for adjuvant arthritis (79) and collagen arthritis (76), it is equally likely that type II collagen is not the antigen critical for the onset and perpetuation of RA. Consequently, there is an ongoing search for a disease-inducing antigen. In addition, few studies have been carried out to determine how to induce tolerance or hyporesponsiveness after an autoimmune disease has been established. An appropriate antigen needs to be defined before this approach can be translated from animals to humans.

b. Major Histocompatibility Complex Peptides. The HLA class II molecules function by presenting peptide antigens to CD4 T cells. They are heterodimeric molecules encoded within the human major histocompatibility complex (MHC). The association of RA with the HLA-DR4 haplotype was identified first (80). As the DR genes were sequenced, it became apparent that the linkage with RA was localized to a specific amino acid sequence in the third variable region of the DR β-chain (81). This sequence provides a target for development of specific therapy.

Synthetic peptides can passively block MHC class II-restricted activation of T cells

(82). The therapeutic validity of this approach has been demonstrated in the murine model of experimental allergic encephalomyelitis (EAE; 83), in which the encephalogenic peptide is identified. For RA, an arthrogenic peptide is not known. Thus, other methods are being used to approach the problem. Empirical selection of agents that block peptide presentation by appropriate DR haplotypes, (i.e., DR4 haplotypes Dw4 and Dw14, and DR1), but not by disease-unrelated haplotypes, (i.e., DR4 Dw10), may provide a method to circumvent the need to identify an RA-specific antigen.

c. T-Cell Vaccination. During disease transfer of EAE by T-cell lines specific for myelin basic protein, it was noted that some T-cell lines would transfer disease, whereas others would protect against the disease. Administration of specific T-cell lines that protect against disease has been called T-cell vaccination. T-cell vaccination protects against adjuvant arthritis (84) and type II collagen arthritis (85) as well as other diseases in animal models. T-cell vaccination has also been used to treat established adjuvant arthritis (86).

Vaccination is believed to amplify a natural immunoregulatory network that depends on idiotypic determinants on the T-cell receptor (i.e., in murine EAE there is evidence for preferential use of the Vβ 8 gene by encephalogenic T cells), and CD8 T cells appear to be required for the clonal unresponsiveness (87). Methods of expanding T-cell clones from arthritic patients are being explored to identify the appropriate T-cell clones and, eventually, T-cell receptor peptides for vaccination. In the absence of an antigen, Kingsley et al. (88) have immunized three patients with autologous synovial mononuclear cells and three patients with saline. In one patient, there was clear improvement accompanied by a steadily increasing antivaccine response. No other patients had an antivaccine response.

4. *Summary*

Enough data has been accumulated to strongly suggest that significant therapeutic effects could be obtained with antigen-specific therapeutics targeted to T cells. However, results to date are all in animal models for which the inciting antigen is defined. Until an inciting antigen is identified for RA, nonspecific immunosuppression by drugs or antibodies will continue to be the approach from which new therapeutic agents will arise.

C. Inhibitors of Leukocyte Migration Into Inflammatory Lesions

1. *Introduction*

The synovial joints of RA patients contain large numbers of leukocytes. The chronically inflamed synovial lining is infiltrated with monocyte–macrophages, T cells, B cells, and plasma cells. Although relatively few neutrophils are present in the synovial lining, RA synovial fluid contains a neutrophil-rich exudate, and this effusion increases dramatically during a flare. The relative contribution of each type of leukocyte to the pathology of RA is still unclear, but it is widely believed that disease activity is orchestrated by activated T lymphocytes that elaborate lymphokines to, in turn, activate resident and infiltrating macrophages. Thus, T-cell depletion by thoracic duct drainage (55) or by more recent monoclonal antibody-based approaches has a major effect on disease activity in RA. Although there are no clinical studies that have examined the effects of monocyte depletion in RA, monocytes–macrophages are major sources of cytokines, such as IL-1 and TNFα, and the presence of cells with the macrophage phenotype correlates with the degree of synovial lining hypertrophy and the progression of radiographic joint destruction (89,90). Neutrophil infiltration contributes to the swelling of acutely inflamed joints (91). However, based on histological examination of RA joints (89,90,92) and the effects of neutrophil depletion in animal models of arthritis (91), it appears that these cells are not responsible for the destruction of cartilage and bone that leads to loss of joint function and deformity. Despite this, inhibition of neutrophil accumulation is likely to have a major effect on the symptoms of disease, many of which are not controlled adequately by NSAID-therapy.

Although inhibition of neutrophil or mononuclear cell migration to inflamed joints has long been recognized as a rational strategy for developing novel RA therapies, it is only recently that significant insights have been gained into the molecular mechanisms of leukocyte adhesion and emigration.

2. *Mechanisms of Leukocyte Adhesion and Emigration*

Neutrophil emigration into inflamed tissues is preceded by interactions of the leukocytes with the microvascular endothelium that, first, involves rolling and, then, firm adhesion before transendothelial migration or diapedesis. These interactions occur almost exclusively in postcapillary venules and occur rapidly on application of an inflammatory stimulus. Each of these processes involves discrete ligand–receptor interactions. The rolling is mediated by the expression of lectins on the surface of neutrophils and endothelial cells. One such lectin is termed L-selectin, since it is found on lymphocytes and is postulated to be involved in the homing of lymphocytes to peripheral lymph nodes. L-selectin is expressed constitutively on neutrophils and, since neutrophils do not roll to any great extent under normal conditions, it is suggested that this molecule undergoes an affinity change upon chemotactic receptor occupation (93). Although antibodies directed against L-selectin block neutrophil rolling in vivo (94), it is unclear what the ligand or counterreceptor for L-selectin is on the endothelial cell. Indirect evidence, using blocking antibodies, suggests that L-selectin can bind to E-selectin expressed on endothelial cells. Certainly, artificial preparations of E-selectin can support leukocyte rolling. However, this molecule is not constitutively expressed and has to be synthesized in response to cytokines, such as IL-1 and TNF; therefore, it is unlikely to be responsible for the rapid induction of leukocyte rolling. At sites of ongoing inflammation, E-selectin is continously expressed (95) and may contribute to leukocyte rolling under these circumstances. Induction of rolling may occur within minutes as a result of activation of endothelial cells by stimuli, such as thrombin or histamine. These mediators cause rapid surface expression of a preformed molecule stored in Weibel–Palade bodies, termed P-selectin (96). Neutrophils can bind to P-selectin with high affinity, an interaction shown to mediate rolling in vitro.

Rolling allows intimate contact of neutrophils with the endothelium on which endothelial-derived and other chemotactic factors can engage their receptors on the neutrophil and initiate the process of firm adhesion and subsequent transendothelial migration. This involves an increase in the affinity or avidity of the β2 integrins (CD11b/CD18) on the neutrophil surface for intercellular adhesion molecule (ICAM)-1, its receptor on the endothelium. The importance of this interaction is demonstrated by the ability of neutralizing antibodies directed against CD18 or ICAM-1 to block neutrophil adhesion to and migration through cytokine-activated endothelium in vitro. In vivo, antibodies against both CD18 or ICAM-1 block neutrophil infiltration in response to a variety of stimuli. Mononuclear cell adhesion and emigration in inflamed tissues may occur in a manner similar to those described for neutrophils, although both lymphocytes and monocytes express a different adhesion molecule, VLA-4. VLA-4 is not found on neutrophils and mediates adhesion by interaction with VCAM-1 expressed on cytokine-activated endothelium (97).

The molecular mechanisms involved in leukocyte infiltration offer a variety of potential points to reduce inflammation in diseases such as rheumatoid arthritis. Some of those being attempted are discussed in the following.

3. *Drugs Interfering With the Production or Action of Chemotactic Factors*

a. *Leukotriene B4 Antagonists and 5-Lipoxygenase Inhibitors*

Leukotriene B_4 (LTB_4) is an arachidonic acid metabolite of the lipoxygenase pathway that possesses potent chemotactic activity for neutrophils and monocytes (98). Infiltrating neutrophils, rather than resident connective tissue cells, are believed to be the chief source of LTB_4 at sites of inflammation (99). Therefore, LTB_4 can be thought of as a mediator that amplifies an ongoing inflammation, rather than one that initiates leukocyte emigration. Leukotriene B_4 has been detected in the synovial effusions of patients afflicted with RA and gout (100); consequently, inhibition of the synthesis or action of LTB_4 is a rational approach to reduce the degree of neutrophil accumulation and accompanying symptoms of disease.

SC-41930 is an orally bioavailable LTB_4 antagonist, with submicromolar potency, that has demonstrated efficacy in animal models of dermal inflammation, reperfusion injury, colitis, and encephalitis (101). Its activity in arthritis models is at present unknown. More potent LTB_4 antagonists are in development, and it is hoped that one of these compounds will be evaluated in RA in the future. The 5-lipoxygenase inhibitor zileuton, which blocks the formation of LTB_4, is in early RA trials (102). At a dose of 800 mg, twice a day, LTB_4 production in peripheral blood ex vivo was inhibited by about 70%, although clinical changes were not differentiated from those of the placebo. More extensive trials are expected and, in particular, it will be revealing to determine the effect of combining a 5-lipoxygenase inhibitor with an NSAID, as there is preliminary evidence of a synergistic interaction between these classes of compounds in experimental arthritis. Perhaps the most promising compound in development in this area is the non-redox–inhibitor of 5-lipoxygenase, ICI D2138, which is approximately ten times more potent than zileuton and has a longer duration of action after oral administration in animals (103).

b. *C5a*

The complement split product, C5a, is a potent chemotactic factor derived from plasma activated by immune complexes, endotoxin, and other stimuli. It plays a central role in leukocyte recruitment in a range of acute inflammatory reactions. Investigators have used a recombinant soluble form of the complement type 1 receptor (sCR1) to probe the role of C5a in acute inflammation, as this molecule inactivates C3 and C5 convertases (104). Recombinant sCR1 has suppressed myocardial reperfusion injury (105), edema associated with the Arthus reaction (106), and pulmonary edema associated with systemic administration of endotoxin or platelet-activating factor (PAF; 107). There are as yet no reports of the activity of sCR1 in models of arthritis or in RA clinical trials; however, as C5a is present in RA effusions (108) and collagen arthritis is C5-dependent (109), sCR1 looks like a promising treatment for RA. Phase 1 clinical studies are in progress.

The G-protein-linked C5a chemotactic receptor has been cloned and is a member of the rhodopsin superfamily of compounds that have seven hydrophobic domains spanning the cell membrane (110). As antagonists of this receptor family have already been discovered (e.g., the PAF receptor), this may facilitate the design of C5a receptor antagonists. A series of diaminoquinolines with C5a antagonist activity may serve as a starting point for the design of more potent and specific compounds (111).

c. *Interleukin-8*

Interleukin-8 is a chemotactic cytokine (molecular weight 7500), produced by tissue macrophages, fibroblasts (including synovial cells), and endothelial cells in response to endotoxin, IL-1, or TNFα. This mediator may serve as a sentinel cytokine to initiate and maintain leukocyte recruitment to sites of inflammation. Neutralizing antibodies directed against IL-8 can inhibit transendothelial migration of neutrophils through endothelium in vitro (112), illustrating the importance of endothelial cell-derived IL-8 in leukocyte emigration. Several groups have detected high levels of IL-8 in RA synovial fluid (113–115). Intra-articular injection of IL-8 leads to neutrophilic and monocytic synovitis in rabbits (114,116), suggesting that IL-8 may be an important mediator in inflammatory arthritis. Two high-affinity IL-8 receptors have been cloned and belong to the G–protein-linked superfamily of receptors with seven transmembrane domains (117). There are now no reports of biological or synthetic IL-8 antagonists, although a quinolylmethoxy-phenylamine (ETH 615) which inhibits IL-8 biosynthesis has been reported (118).

2. *Inhibition of Leukocyte Adhesion*

a. *Inhibition of Integrin Interactions With Endothelial Cells*

Monoclonal antibodies that prevent the interaction of integrins with ICAM-1 are effective inhibitors of neutrophil emigration and resultant tissue damage in a wide range of animal models.

The murine monoclonal antibody 60.3 recognizes CD18, the β2 chain of leukocyte integrins and has been shown to block human neutrophil adhesion in vitro. In vivo, it displays dramatic anti-inflammatory activity. It prevents neutrophil emigration into rabbit skin sites injected with chemotactic factors or cytokines (119,120), increases survival in hemorrhagic shock in rabbits and primates (121,122), and reduces synovitis in rabbits with antigen-induced arthritis (123). Interestingly, 60.3 does not increase the mortality rates in rabbits with abdominal sepsis (124), which suggests that short-term inhibition of integrin function does not compromise host defense to a dangerous extent. The monoclonal antibody IB4 also recognizes CD18 and reduces neutrophil infiltration, but not monocyte infiltration, in rabbits after injection of IL-8 (116). This antibody has recently been humanized.

Monoclonal antibodies directed against adhesion molecules expressed on endothelial cells have also been tested in animal models of inflammation. Blocking anti-ICAM-1 antibodies inhibit neutrophil adhesion in the rabbit mesentery in response to C5a (125) and reduce eosinophil infiltration and airway hyperreactivity in a model of allergic asthma (126). In RA patients, rapid clinical improvement was obtained in 9 of 13 patients and, in some patients, improvements were sustained for more than 2 months after anti-ICAM therapy (127).

b. *Selectins*

Antibodies against L-selectin, E-selectin, and P-selectin, all suppress neutrophil emigration in a variety of in vivo systems, presumably by inhibiting the early obligatory rolling stage before neutrophil emigration. An L-selectin chimera also inhibits neutrophil accumulation (128). However, as the ligand for E-selectin is thought to be related to the carbohydrate blood group Lewis antigen (i.e., sialyl Lewis^{x}), investigators are focusing on understanding these lectin–carbohydrate interactions to discover low molecular weight inhibitors with oral bioavailability. Sialyl Lewis^{a} is also a good ligand for E-selectin, and as Lewis[x] and Lewis[a] bind with much less affinity, the epitopes recognized by E-selectin probably involve sialic acid and fucose residues (129).

D. Inhibition of Angiogenesis

Neovascularization is important physiologically in would healing and in the development of the corpus luteum. Growth of rheumatoid pannus, too, is dependent on neovascularization, particularly in the early stages, and selective inhibition of angiogenesis in RA may limit disease progression. Fumagillin is a naturally occurring fungal antibiotic, derived from *Aspergillus fumigatus fresenius*, which was serendipitously discovered to inhibit endothelial cell growth in infected cultures (130). A synthetic analogue of fumagillin has been described, AGM 1470 (130), and this compound suppresses collagen arthritis when administered prophylactically and therapeutically (131).

III. OSTEOARTHRITIS

A. Intervention With Biological Products

1. Hyaluronan

Hyaluronan (hyaluronic acid) is a natural component of synovial fluid and of the proteoglycan molecules of articular cartilage. Its synthesis by synovial lining cells is stimulated by IL-1, perhaps as a protective response. As hyaluronan is a lubricant of articular cartilage and an inhibitor of several in vitro pathological processes, it has been suggested that administration of excess hyaluronan could provide protection to the articular cartilage during times of inflammatory stress (132). Clinical trials that suggest a beneficial effect in OA have been carried out on the effects of intraarticular hyaluronan (133,134). However, more extensive studies need to be carried out to fully evaluate the potential of this therapy. Hylan, a lightly cross-linked hyaluronan, has a higher molecular weight, a longer resident time in biological applications (135), and appears to have the same protective action on cartilage in vitro (136). It is currently undergoing clinical trials.

2. Glycosaminoglycan Polysulfate Esters

Glycosaminoglycan polysulfate esters (GAGPS) inhibit cartilage degrading enzymes both in vitro and in vivo (137–139) and may stimulate the metabolism of chondrocytes and synovial cells. Therapeutic studies in dogs (137,139–141) show improvement in the joint status determined by macroscopic and histological examination of GAGPS-treated anterior cruciate ligament transected (ACLT) dogs, compared with placebo-treated ACLT dogs. Similar results were obtained in rabbit ACLT and menisectomy models (142,143). These results suggest that intra-articular injection of GAGPS should be of value for treatment of OA. In spite of the favorable results obtained in animal models, few controlled human clinical trials have been published. Raatikainen et al. carried out a 1-year placebo-controlled (intra-articular physiological saline) study and reported favorable responses (144). Kannus et al. completed a detailed study of the patellofemoral pain syndrome in which injections of physiological saline or GAGPS were compared with uninjected patients (145). In all three cases, conservative treatment (i.e., strengthening the quadriceps muscle) was also instituted. There was no advantage for GAGPS injections compared with saline, and both injection protocols were better than no injections at 6 weeks, but not at 6 months, suggesting a placebo effect. The therapeutic effect at 6 months could be attributed to the strengthening of the quadriceps and not to the GAGPS therapy.

The demonstration of therapeutic effects in animal models of OA, but not in humans, is problematic. It could be a result of the animals' more rapid turnover of articular cartilage and their relatively young age (repair is more likely). An alternative explanation is that experimentally induced OA evolves rapidly so the effects of treatment can be readily observed. Whatever the cause, a clear demonstration of therapeutic benefit for intra-articular GAGPS treatment in humans is still lacking.

In response to reports that GAGPS could be active when given orally, Baici et al. (146) examined whether oral GAGPS would lead to its significant GAGPS concentration in synovial fluid. They found no evidence for sufficient absorption of intact GAGPS to elevate synovial levels of GAGPS. They concluded that the only possible effect of oral GAGPS was an interaction with orally administered NSAID to make them more tolerated in the gastrointestinal tract and give a better analgesic effect. A simple placebo effect is an alternative explanation.

B. Intervention With Drugs

The use of drugs to treat OA is a controversial area. Anti-inflammatory drugs have been the mainstay of therapy, because they minimize pain and thereby help maintain movement. It has been suggested that because there is little inflammation in many cases of OA, simple analgesics should be sufficient therapy (147,148). To the extent that analgesia encourages overuse of a damaged joint, the recovery from joint injury could be impaired by too effective analgesia (76). On the other hand, effective anti-inflammatory therapy can also promote moderate exercise, which stimulates cartilage proteoglycan synthesis, and is known to diminish pain perception. There is now insufficient data to resolve this controversy. However, new types of analgesic drugs are on the horizon. Substance P (149,150) and kinin (151) antagonists have been tested in animal models and are in clinical trials in humans. It is likely that they would find use in inflammatory OA and in RA.

1. *Cytokine Inhibitors*

The therapeutic usefulness of the cytokine inhibitors may be different in OA than in RA. Synovial explants from human OA knees (152) and dog knees (153) after anterior cruciate ligament transection produce both IL-1α and IL-β in tissue culture, with IL-1β being the preponderant form. Additional stimulation with LPS further elevated the levels of IL-β. Tumor necrosis factor was not detected in either the stimulated or the unstimulated synovial explants. Interleukin-1 receptors in OA are up-regulated (154), whereas TNF receptors occur at only low levels (39). Whether these results suggest a greater role for IL-1 in OA will have to be determined with cytokine-specific therapy in the clinic.

Cytokine therapy for OA will have to await development of small-molecule drugs, as most of the cartilage degradation is believed to be driven by the chondrocyte. Neither antibodies or chimeric receptor–immunoglobulin molecules will penetrate cartilage. Moreover, long-term administration of proteins therapeutics would be expected to lead to an immune response against the protein.

2. *Proteinase Inhibitors*

Although we have classified the proteinase inhibitors under the heading of therapeutics for OA, it should be clear that they could be equally effective in RA. In fact, if chronic tolerance is a problem with proteinase inhibitors, they could end up being used exclusively in RA, for which their application could be limited to periods of disease exacerbation.

a. Metalloproteinases. The metalloproteinases, so-called because of the involvement of zinc in their active site, are considered important in cartilage remodeling.

Compelling evidence has been presented for their elevation in OA (80) and for an imbalance between the tissue inhibitors of the metalloproteinases (TIMPs) and the metalloproteinases, leaving an excess of enzyme activity in OA (155). It seems probable that inhibition of metalloproteinase activity could reduce the rate of cartilage degeneration in OA. Reduction of the rate of cartilage loss could both slow the disease progression and give opportunity for new synthesis to compensate for loss of cartilage.

Inhibitors of Metalloproteinases. Collagenase, gelatinase, and stromelysin, all are potentially involved in cartilage breakdown; accordingly, general inhibitors of metalloproteinases have been therapeutic targets for prevention of cartilage loss. Although little testing has been reported in vivo, general metalloproteinase inhibitors have been reported to prevent IL-1-induced cartilage degradation in vitro (156–158), and at least one (157) shows some evidence of cartilage-protective activity in an animal model of arthritis. Inhibitors with better bioavailability are under development.

Tetracyclines. Tetracycline was shown to inhibit human synovial collagenase activity (159). Yu et al. (160) also examined doxycycline and found it inhibited type XI collagenolytic activity (gelatinase activity) in extracts of human osteoarthritic cartilage. It may work by chelating Zn^{2+}. This implies that doxycycline should be a general inhibitor of all the metalloproteinases, including stromelysin. In subsequent in vivo studies, Yu et al. found a significant reduction in the severity of canine ACLT-induced OA (161). They measured gelatinase and collagenase levels in the articular cartilage and found a decrease in amount and activity of the enzymes in the OA cartilage of the treated dogs compared with control dogs. These results, coupled with those of Greenwald et al. (162), who showed that the tetracyclines inhibit the expression of metalloproteinase activity in adjuvant arthritis, suggest that prophylactic treatment using metalloproteinase inhibitors can have a beneficial effect in animal models of arthritis. Whether they will be beneficial in animal models of established OA or in human OA remains an open question.

b. Inhibitors of Thiol Proteinases. The cathepsins B and L are lysosomal thiol endopeptidases. Buttle et al. showed that an inhibitor of cysteinyl proteinases inhibits IL-1-mediated cartilage breakdown (163,164). This suggests that these enzymes either directly cause cartilage damage or may act secondarily by activating the metalloproteinases to carry out cartilage degradation. van Noorden et al. first showed a thiol proteinase inhibitor to inhibit the methylated BSA model of arthritis (165). Ahmed et al. showed a structurally related compound to inhibit the severity of inflammation and the extent of cartilage and bone damage in adjuvant-induced arthritis (166). Cathepsin B activity in liver also was reduced after treatment. The inhibitors had no effect on the incidence or onset of disease, suggesting the compound's effects were limited to proteinase-mediated damage. Inhibition of this lysosomal proteinase leads to engorgement of the phagocytic cells with undigested debris (167). Whether this will be a problem in the long run needs to be determined.

c. Plasminogen Activator and Plasmin. Plasmin may play an important role in cartilage destruction by activating latent collagenase (168), and plasmin has been detected in experimental OA cartilage (169). The degradation of collagen by IL-1-stimulated chondrocytes is facilitated by the addition of plasminogen, indicating that these cells can express plasminogen activator activity (168,170). However, proteoglycan degradation in cartilage cultured with IL-1 occurs maximally without addition of plasminogen or plasmin (171).

Tranexamic Acid. Tranexamic acid is a potent inhibitor of plasminogen activator and thus might be expected to inhibit collagen loss from cartilage. Telhag first studied oral administration of tranexamic acid in the Hulth model of osteoarthritis (i.e., both meniscectomy and cruciate ligament section; 172). After treatment, he found reduced hexosamine loss and normalization of the elevated chondroitin sulfate synthesis that occurs after disease induction. Butler et al. examined the effect of tranexamic acid in rabbits with partial meniscectomy and sesamoid and collateral ligament section (173). Tranexamic acid was administered by intra-articular injections 7 and 14 days after surgery. Improvement in most measures of cartilage degeneration (i.e., clone formation, chondrocyte loss, proteoglycan loss, cartilage ulceration, and erosions) was found. Vignon et al. studied the effect of tranexamic acid after anterior cruciate ligament transection in the rabbit (174). After 3 times per week intra-muscular administration, the number of cartilage erosions, as well as the amount of bone exposure, were significantly decreased. These three studies suggest that articular cartilage can be protected after ligament transection by brief treatment with tranexamic acid during the period following surgery.

Tranexamic acid has been used in humans as an antifibrinolytic and in C1s deficiency. However, inhibition of plasminogen activator could predispose to thrombosis and intravascular coagulation. Thus, until a plasminogen activator inhibitor can be selectively targeted to the cartilage, this approach is unlikely to result in a successful drug.

d. Tissue Inhibitor of Metalloproteinases. The natural tissue inhibitor of metalloproteinases (TIMP) was present in amounts insufficient to inhibit the metalloproteinase present in OA (155). One possible remedy is to stimulate the production of TIMP. Interleukin-6 is known to induce TIMP (81), but although IL-6 does not induce the metalloproteinases by itself, it does enhance the synthesis of collagenase and stromelysin in combination with IL-1 (175). In the absence of known selective inducers of the TIMPs, their intra-articular administration might be a practical approach to therapy. The TIMPs do not block IL-1-induced cartilage proteoglycan loss (156). This finding has reduced confidence that they will be effective in OA when administered exogenously.

IV. PROSPECTS AND FUTURE POSSIBILITIES

During the past decade, basic biomedical research has uncovered many potential targets for the development of therapeutic agents to treat RA and, to a smaller degree, OA. Numerous approaches have been described in this chapter, but the list was not exhaustive. Of the approaches discussed, in many cases, clinical trials are ongoing and, for some cases, early clinical data is available.

An almost bewildering number of mediators have been postulated to be involved in the pathogenesis of inflammatory conditions such as RA. This leads one to wonder whether inhibition of a single mediator is likely to bestow significant clinical efficacy. However, it is reassuring to observe that mediators often act synergistically and that inhibition of one mediator alone is sufficient to inhibit disease pathology. This is exemplified in shock where inhibition of IL-1 or TNFα is beneficial; it is not necessary to inhibit both mediators. In arthritis, too, it is clear that IL-1 and TNFα act synergistically (41) and that inhibition of either IL-1 or TNFα is efficacious in animal models (10,11,49). Moreover, inhibitors of both metallo- and cysteine proteinases are effective in preventing IL-1-induced cartilage degradation in vitro, suggesting a cascade of activation processes in which both classes of enzymes are intimately involved. Thus, fortunately, it seems that redundancy is rare in biological systems.

In RA, many of these approaches are currently being tested in the clinic so that there can be some optimism for better therapy in the next decade. For OA, the short-term outlook is not so optimistic. Surgical intervention to correct unstable or deformed joints, muscle-strengthening exercises, and joint replacement are likely to remain the most effective therapies in the near term. Until good, accepted surrogate biochemical markers or more accurate, sensitive-imaging techniques are developed, OA clinical trials for chondroprotective drugs will remain long and expensive. Promising work in both biochemical markers and imaging is emerging, but without a breakthrough, improvement in analgesic treatment will be the only probable advance in OA treatment in this decade.

REFERENCES

1. Felson DT, Anderson JJ, Meenan RF. Use of short-term efficacy/toxicity tradeoffs to select second-line drugs in rheumatoid arthritis. A metaanalysis of published clinical trials. Arthritis Rheum 1992; 35:1117–25.
2. Alarcón GS, Castaneda O, Ferrándiz M, Krumdieck CL, Koopman WJ. Efficacy and safety of 10-deazaaminopterin in the treatment of rheumatoid arthritis. A one-year continuation, double-blind study. Arthritis Rheum 1992; 35:1318–21.
3. Woessner JF Jr. Matrix metalloproteinases and their inhibitors in connective tissue remodeling. FASEB J 1991; 5:2145–54.
4. Dustin ML, Rothlein R, Bhan AK, Dinarello CA, and Springer TA. Induction by IL-1 and interferon-γ: tissue distribution, biochemistry, and function of a natural adherence molecule (ICAM-1). J Immunol 1986; 137:245–54.
5. DeMarco D, Kunkel SL. IL-1-induced gene expression of neutrophil activating peptide (IL-8) and monocyte chemotactic peptide in human synovial cells. Biochem Biophys Res Comm 1991; 174:411–6.
6. Fibbe WE, Van Damme JBA, Voogt PJ, Duinkerken N, Kluck PMC, Falkenburg JHF. Interleukin-1 (22-K factor) induces release of granulocyte–macrophage colony-stimulating activity from human mononuclear phagocytes. Blood 1986; 68:1316–21.
7. Pettipher ER, Higgs GA, Henderson B. Interleukin 1 induces leukocyte infiltration and cartilage proteoglycan degradation in the synovial joint. Proc Natl Acad Sci USA 1986; 83:8749–53.
8. Stimpson SA, Dalldorf FG, Otterness IG, Schwab JH. Exacerbation of arthritis by IL-1 in rat joints previously injured by peptidoglycan-polysaccharide. J Immunol 1988; 140:2964–9.
9. Hom JT, Bendele AM, Carson DG. In vivo administration with IL-1 accelerates the development of collagen-induced arthritis in mice. J Immunol 1988; 141:834–41.
10. Schwab JH, Anderle SK, Brown RR, Dalldorf FG, Thompson RC. Pro- and anti-inflammatory roles of interleukin-1 in recurrence of bacterial cell wall-induced arthritis. Infect Immun 1991; 59:4436–42.
11. van de Loo FAJ, Arntz OJ, Otterness IG, van den Berg WB. Protection against cartilage proteoglycan synthesis inhibition by antiinterleukin 1 antibodies in experimental arthritis. J Rheumatol 1992; 19:348–56.
12. Ju G, Labriola-Tomkins E, Campen CA, Benjamin WR, Karas J, Plocinski J, Biondi D, Kaffka KL, Kilian PL, Eisenberg SP, Evans RJ. Conversion of the interleukin 1 receptor antagonist into an agonist by site-specific mutagenesis. Proc Natl Acad s (TNF),ci USA 1991; 88:2658–62.
13. Dripps DJ, Verderber E, Ng RK, Thompson RC, Eisenberg SP. Interleukin-1 receptor antagonist binds to the type II interleukin-1 receptor in B cells and neutrophils. J Biol Chem 1991; 266:20311–5.

14. Ohlson KO, Björk P, Bergenfeldt M, Hageman R, Thompson RC. Interleukin-1 receptor antagonist reduces mortality from endotoxin shock. Nature 1990; 348:550–2.
15. Alexander HR, Doherty GM, Buresh CM, Venzon DJ, Norton JA. A recombinant human receptor antagonist to interleukin 1 improves survival after lethal endotoxemia in mice. J Exp Med 1991; 173:1029–32.
16. Lebsack ME, Paul CC, Bloedow DC, Burch FX, Sack A, Chase W, Catalano MA. Subcutaneous IL-1 receptor antagonist in patients with rheumatoid arthritis. Arthritis Rheum 1991; 34:S45.
17. Fanslow WC, Sims JE, Sassenfeld H, Morrissey PJ, Gillis S, Dower KD, Widmer MB. Regulation of alloreactivity in vivo by a soluble form of the interleukin-1 receptor. Science 1990; 248:739–42.
18. Jacobs CA, Baker PE, Roux ER, Picha KS, Toivola B, Waugh S, Kennedy MK. Experimental autoimmune encephalomyelitis is exacerbated by IL-1α and suppressed by soluble IL-1 receptor. J Immunol 1991; 146:2983–9.
19. Wickstrom D, ed. Prospects for antisense nucleic acid therapy of cancer and AIDS. New York: Wiley-Liss. 1991.
20. Lattuada D, Mazzei M, Meazza R, Nicolin A. Therapeutic implications of antisense oligonucleotides. Int J Clin Lab Res 1992; 21:296–9.
21. Budker VG, Knorre DG, Vlassov VV. Cell membranes as barriers for antisense constructions. Antisense Res Dev 1992; 2:177–84.
22. Lee SW, Tsou A-P, Chan H, Thomas J, Petrie K, Euglui EM, Allison AC. Glucocorticoids selectively inhibit the transcription of the interleukin 1β gene and decrease the stability of interleukin 1β mRNA, Proc Natl Acad Sci USA 1988; 85:1204–8.
23. Otterness IG, Bliven ML, Downs JT, Natoli EJ, Hanson DC. Inhibition of interleukin 1 synthesis by tenidap: a new drug for arthritis. Cytokine 1991; 3:277–83.
24. Sipe JD, Bartle LM, Loose LD. Modification of proinflammatory cytokine production by the antirheumatic agents tenidap and naproxen. J Immunol 1992; 148:480–4.
25. Lee JC, Griswold DE, Votta B, Hanna N. Inhibition of monocyte IL-1 production by the antiinflammatory compound SKF 86002. Int J Immunopharmacol 1988; 10:835–43.
26. Rainsford KD. Effects of antimalarial drugs on interleukin 1-induced cartilage proteoglycan degradation in vitro. J Pharm Pharmacol 1986; 38:829–33.
27. Dougados M, Combe B, Beveridge T, Bourdeix I, Lallemand A, Amor B, Sany J. IX 207-887 in rheumatoid arthritis. A double-blind placebo-controlled study. Arthritis Rheum 1992; 35:999–1006.
28. Davis, JS, Loose LD, Borger AP. Clinical efficacy of CP-66,248 [5-chloro-2,3-dihydro-2-oxo-3-(2-theinylcarbonyl)-indole-1-carboxaminde] in osteoarthritis (OA). Arthritis Rheum 1988; 31:S72.
29. Katz P, Borger AP, Loose LD. Evaluation of CP-66,248 [5-chloro-2,3-dihydro-2-oxo-3-(2-theinylcarbonyl)-indole-1-carboxaminde] in rheumatoid arthritis (RA). Arthritis Rheum 1988; 31:S52.
30. Larsen A. The relation of radiographic changes to serum acute-phase proteins and rheumatoid factor in 200 patients with rheumatoid arthritis. Scand J Rheumatol 1988; 17:123–9.
31. McConkey B, Crockson RA, Crockson AP, Wilkinson AR. The effects of some antiinflammatory drugs on the acute phase proteins in rheumatoid arthritis. Q J Med 1973; 42:785–91.
32. McConkey B, Davies P, Crockson RA. Effects of gold, dapsone, and prednisone on serum C-reactive protein and haptoglobin and the erythrocyte sedimentation rate in rheumatoid arthritis. Ann Rheum Dis 1979; 38:141–4.
33. Loose LD, Sipe JD, Kirby DS, Kraska AR, Weiner ES, Shanahan WR, Leeming MRG, Farrow P, Stack CB, Ting N. Reduction of acute-phase proteins with tenidap sodium, a cytokine-modulating antirheumatic drug. Br J Rheumatol 1993; 32:19–25.
34. Loose LD, Littman BH, Sipe JD. Modulation of acute phase proteins by tenidap, a new antiinflammatory, antirheumatic drug. Arthritis Rheum 1990; 38:579A.
35. Cerretti DP, Kozlosky CJ, Mosley B, Nelson N, van Ness K, Greenstreet TA, March CJ,

Kronheim SR, Druck T, Cannizzaro LA, Huebner K, Black RA. Molecular cloning of the interleukin-1β converting enzyme. Science 1992; 256:97–100.
36. Otterness IG, Bliven JL, Carreras I, Sipe JD. In vivo roles of IL-1α and IL-1β. Cytokine 1991; 3:513.
37. Perretti M, Solito E, Parente L. Evidence that endogenous interleukin-1 is involved in leukocyte migration in acute experimental inflammation in rats and mice. Agents Actions 1992; 35:71–8.
38. Chu C-Q, Field M, Feldmann M, Maini RN. Localization of tumor necrosis factor α in synovial tissues and at the cartilage–pannus junction in patients with rheumatoid arthritis. Arthritis Rheum 1991; 34:1125–32.
39. Deleuran BW, Chu C-Q, Field M, Brennan FM, Mitchell T, Feldmann M, Maini RN. Localization of tumor necrosis factor receptors in the synovial tissue and cartilage–pannus junction in patients with rheumatoid arthritis. Implications for local actions of tumor necrosis factor α. Arthritis Rheum 1992; 35:1170-8.
40. Keffer J, Probert L, Cazlaris H, Georgopoulos S, Kaslaris E, Kiossis D, Kollias G. Transgenic mice expressing human tumour necrosis factor: a predictive genetic model of arthritis. EMBO J 1991; 10:4025–31.
41. Henderson B, Pettipher ER. Arthritogenic actions of recombinant IL-1 and tumour necrosis factor α in the rabbit: evidence for synergistic interactions between cytokines in vivo. Clin Exp Immunol 1989; 75:306–10.
42. O'Byrne EM, Blancuzzi V, Wilson DE, Wong M, Jeng AY. Elevated substance P and accelerated cartilage degradation in rabbit knees injected with interleukin-1 and tumor necrosis factor. Arthritis Rheum 1990; 33:1023–8.
43. Seckinger P, Zhang JH, Hauptmann B, Dayer JM. Characterization of a TNFα inhibitor. Evidence of immunological cross-reactivity with the TNF receptor. Proc Natl Acad Sci USA 1990; 87:5188–92.
44. Cope AP, Aderka D, Doherty M, Engelmann H, Gibbons D, Jones AC, Brennan FM, Maini RN, Wallach D, Feldmann M. Increased levels of soluble tumor necrosis factor receptors in the sera and synovial fluid of patients with rheumatic diseases. Arthritis Rheum 1992; 35:1160–9.
45. Piguet PF, Grau GE, Vesin C, Loetscher H, Gentz R, Lesslauer W. Evolution of collagen arthritis in mice is arrested by treatment with antitumor necrosis factor (TNF) antibody or a recombinant soluble TNF receptor. Immunology 1992; 77:510–4.
46. Askenazi A, Marsters SA, Capon DJ, Chamow SM, Figari IS, Pennica D, Goeddel DV, Palladino MA, Smith DH. Protection against endotoxic shock by a tumor necrosis factor receptor immunoadhesin. Proc Natl Acad Sci USA 1991; 88:10535–9.
47. Lesslauer W, Tabuchi H, Gentz R, Brockhaus M, Schlaeger EJ, Grau G, Piguet PF, Pointaire P, Vassalli P, Loetscher H. Recombinant soluble tumor necrosis factor receptor proteins protect mice from lipopolysaccharide-induced lethality. Eur J Immunol 1991; 21:2883–6.
48. Verwilghen J, Kingsley GH, Ceuppens JL, Panayi G. Inhibition of synovial fluid T cell proliferation by anti-CD5 monoclonal antibodies. A potential mechanism for their immunotherapeutic action in vivo. Arthritis Rheum 1993; 35:1445–51.
49. Williams RO, Feldmann M, Maini RN. Anti-tumour necrosis factor ameliorates joint disease in murine collagen-induced arthritis. Proc Natl Acad Sci USA 1991; 89:9784–8.
50. Selmaj K, Raine CS, Cross AH. Anti-tumor necrosis factor therapy abrogates autoimmune demyelination. J Neurol 1991; 30:694–700.
51. Elliot MJ, Maini RN, Feldmann M, Williams RO, Brennan FM, Chu CQ. Treatment of rheumatoid arthritis with chimeric monoclonal antibodies to TNFα: safety, clinical efficacy and control of the acute-phase response. J Cell Biochem 1993; 17B:145.
52. Co-operating Clinics Committee of the American Rheumatoid Association. A controlled trial of cyclophosphamide in rheumatoid arthritis. N Engl J Med 1970; 283:883–9.
53. Urowitz MB, Gordan DA, Smythe HA, Pruzanski W, Ogryzlo MA. Azathioprine in rheumatoid arthritis. A double-blind crossover study. Arthritis Rheum 1973; 16:411–8.

54. Dougados M, Awada H, Amor B. Cyclosporin A in Rheumatoid arthritis: a double blind placebo controlled study in 52 patients. Ann Rheum Dis 1988; 47:127–33.
55. Paulus HE, Machleder HI, Levine S, Yu DTY, MacDonald NS. Lymphocyte involvement in rheumatoid arthritis: studies during thoracic duct drainage. Arthritis Rheum 1977; 20:1249–62.
56. Trentham D, Belli JA, Anderson RJ, Buckley JA, Goetzl EJ, David JR, Austen KF. Clinical and immunological effects of fractioned total lymphoid irradiation in refractory rheumatoid arthritis. N Engl J Med 1981; 305:976–82.
57. Karsh J, Klippel JH, Plotz PH, Decker JL, Wright DG, Flye MW. Lymphophoresis in rheumatoid arthritis. Arthritis Rheum 1981; 24:867–73.
58. Panayi G, Lanchbury JS, Kingsley GH. The importance of the T cell in initiating and maintaining the chronic synovitis of rheumatoid arthritis. Arthritis Rheum 1992; 35:729–35.
59. Chatenoud L, Ferran C, Reuter A, Legendre C, Gevaert Y, Kreis H, Franchimont P, Bach JF. Systemic reaction to the monoclonal antibody OKT3 in relation to serum levels of tumor necrosis factor and interferon γ. N Engl J Med 1989; 320:1420.
60. Chatenoud L, Legendre C, Ferran C, Bach JF, Kreis H. Corticosteroid inhibition of the OKT3 induced cytokine-related syndrome—dosage and kinetics prerequisites. Transplantation 1991; 51:334–8.
61. Duke O, Panayi GS, Janossy G, Poulter LW. An immunohistological analysis of lymphocyte subpopulations and their microenvironment in the synovial membranes of patients with rheumatoid arthritis using monoclonal antibodies. Clin Exp Immunol 1982; 49:22–30.
62. Horneff G, Burmeister GR, Emmrich F, Kalden JR. Treatment of rheumatoid arthritis with an anti-CD4 monoclonal antibody. Arthritis Rheum 1982; 34:129–40.
63. Wendling D, Wijdenes J, Racadot E, Morel-Fourrier B. Therapeutic use of monoclonal anti-CD4 antibody in rheumatoid arthritis. J Rheumatol 1991; 18:325–7.
64. Horneff G, Winkler T, Kalden J, Emmrich F, Burmeister G. Human anti-mouse antibody response induced by anti-CD4 monoclonal antibody therapy in patients with rheumatoid arthritis. Clin Immunol Immunopathol 1991; 59:89–103.
65. Strand V, Fishwild D. Rheumatoid arthritis investigators group. Treatment of rheumatoid arthritis with anti-CD5 immunoconjugate: clinical and immunologic findings and preliminary results of re-treatment. Arthritis Rheum 1990; 33:S25.
66. Kirkham B, Chikanza I, Pitzalis C, Kingsley GH, Grahame R, Gibson T, Panayi GS. Response to monoclonal CD7 antibody in rheumatoid arthritis. Lancet 1988; 2:589.
67. Reichmann L, Clark M, Waldmann H, Winter G. Reshaping human antibodies for therapy. Nature 1988; 332:323–7.
68. Reiter C, van der Lubbe PA, Breedveld F. Chimeric monoclonal CD4 antibody cM-T412 induces a long lasting CD4 cell depletion in rheumatoid arthritis (RA) patients. Arthritis Rheum 1991; 34:91.
69. Moreland LW, Bucy RP, Tilden A, Pratt PW, LoBuglio AF, Khazaeli M, Everson MP, Daddona P, Ghrayeb J, Kilgarriff C, Sanders ME, Koopman WJ. Use of a chimeric anti-CD4 antibody in patients with refractory rheumatoid arthritis. Arthritis Rheum 1993; 36:307–18.
70. Kyle V, Roddy J, Hale G, Hazleman BL, Waldmann H. Humanized monoclonal antibody treatment in rheumatoid arthritis. J Rheumatol 1991; 18:1737–8.
71. Issacs JD, Watts RA, Hazleman BL, Hale G, Waldmann H. Humanized monoclonal antibody therapy in rheumatoid arthritis. Arthritis Rheum 1992; 35:S43.
72. Kyle V, Coughlan RJ, Tighe H, Waldmann H, Hazleman BL. Beneficial effect of monoclonal antibody to interleukin 2 receptors on activated T cells on rheumatoid arthritis. Ann Rheum Dis 1989; 48:428–9.
73. Pacheco-Silva A, Bastos MG, Muggia RA, Pankewycz O, Nichols J, Murphy ZR, Strom TB, Rubin-Kelley VE. Interleukin 2 receptor targeted fusion toxin (DAB486-IL-2) treatment blocks diabetogenic autoimmunity in non-obese diabetic mice. Eur J Immunol 1992; 22:697–702.
74. Case J, Lorberboum-Galski H, Lafyatis R, FitzGerald D, Wilder R, Pastan I. Chimeric

cytotoxin IL-2–PE40 delays and mitigates adjuvant-induced arthritis in rats. Proc Natl Acad Sci USA 1991; 86:287–91.

75. Lorberboum-Galski H, Lafyatis R, Case JP, FitzGerald D, Wilder RL, Pastan I. Administration of IL-2–PE40 via osmotic pumps prevents adjuvant induced arthritis in rats. Improved therapeutic index of IL-2–PE40 administrated by continuous infusion. Int J Immunopharmacol 1991; 13:305–15.
76. Nagler-Anderson C, Bober LA, Robinson ME, Siskind GW, Thorbecke GJ. Suppression of type II collagen-induced arthritis by intragastric administration of soluble type II collagen. Proc Natl Acad Sci USA 1986; 83:7443–6.
77. Higgins PJ, Weiner HL. Suppression of experimental autoimmune encephalomyelitis by oral administration of myelin basic protein and its fragments. J Immunol 1988; 140:440–5.
78. Zhang ZJ, Davidson L, Eisenbarth G, Weiner HL. Suppression of diabetes in nonobese diabetic mice by oral administration of porcine insulin. Proc Natl Acad Sci USA 1991; 88:10252–6.
79. Zhang J, Lee C, Lider O, Weiner HL. Suppression of adjuvant arthritis in Lewis rats by oral administration of type II collagen. J Immunol 1990; 145:2489–93.
80. Martel-Pelletier J, Pelletier J-P, Cloutier J-M, Howell DS, Ghandur-Mnaymneh L, Woessner JF Jr. Neutral proteases capable of proteoglycan digesting activity in osteoarthritic and normal human articular cartilage. Arthritis Rheum 1984; 24:305–12.
81. Lotz M, Guerne P-A. Interleukin-6 induces the synthesis of tissue inhibitor of metalloproteinases-1/erythroid potentiating activity (TIMP1/EPA). J Biol Chem 1991; 266:2017–20.
82. Adorini L. The molecular basis of antigen presentation to T lymphocytes: novel possibilities for immunointervention. Int Rev Immunol 1990; 6:1–88.
83. Lamont AG, Sette A, Fujinami R, Colon SM, Miles C, Grey HM. Inhibition of experimental autoimmune encephalomyelitis induction in SJL/J mice by using a peptide with high affinity for I-A molecules. J Immunol 1990; 145:1687–93.
84. Cohen IR, Holoshitz J, Van Eden W, Frenkel A. T lymphocyte clones illuminate pathogenesis and effect therapy of experimental arthritis. Arthritis Rheum 1985; 28:841–5.
85. Kakimoto K, Katsuki M, Hirofuji T, Iwata H, Koga T. Isolation of a T cell line capable of protecting mice against collagen-induced arthritis. J Immunol 1988; 140:78–83.
86. Lider O, Karin N, Shinitzky M, Cohen IR. Therapeutic vaccination against adjuvant arthritis using autoimmune T lymphocytes treated with hydrostatic pressure. Proc Natl Acad Sci USA 1987; 84:4577–80.
87. Gaur A, Haspel R, Mayer JP, Gathman CG. Requirement for $CD8^+$ cells in T cell receptor peptide-induced clonal unresponsiveness. Science 1992; 259:91–4.
88. Kingsley G, Verwilghen JI, Panayi GS. T cell vaccination (TCV) in rheumatoid arthritis (RA): a controlled double-blind pilot study. Arthritis Rheum 1992; 35:S59.
89. Bromley M, Woolley DE. Histopathology of the rheumatoid lesion. Identification of cell types at sites of cartilage erosion. Arthritis Rheum 1984; 27:857–63.
90. Muirden KD. Lysosomal enzymes in synovial membrane in rheumatoid arthritis. Relationship to joint damage. Ann Rheum Dis 1972; 31:265–71.
91. Pettipher ER, Henderson B, Moncada S, Higgs GA. Leucocyte infiltration and cartilage proteoglycan loss in immune arthritis in the rabbit. Br J Pharmacol 1988; 95:169–76.
92. Fassbender HG, Seibel M, Hebert T. Pathways of destruction in metacarpal and metatarsal joints of patients with rheumatoid arthritis. Scand J Rheumatol 1992; 21:10–6.
93. Spertini O, Kansas GS, Munro JM, Griffin JD, Tedder TF. Regulation of leukocyte migration by activation of the leukocyte adhesion molecule-1 (LAM-1) selectin. Nature 1991; 349:691–4.
94. Von Andrian UH, Hansell P, Chambers JD, Berger EM, Filho IT, Butcher EC, Arfors K-E. L-selectin function is required for β2-integrin-mediated neutrophil adhesion at physiological shear rates in vivo. Am J Physiol 1992; 263:H1034–44.
95. Koch AE, Burrows JC, Haines GK, Carlos TM, Harlan JM, Leibovich SJ. Immunolocaliza-

tion of endothelial and leukocyte adhesion molecules in human rheumatoid and osteoarthritic synovial tissues. Lab Invest 1991; 64:313–20.

96. McEver RP. Selectins: novel receptors that mediate leukocyte adhesion during inflammation. Thromb Haemost 1991; 65:223–8.
97. Osborn L, Hession C, Tizard R, Vassallo C, Luhowskyj S, Chi-Rosso G, Lobb R. Direct expression cloning of vascular cell adhesion molecule 1, a cytokine-induced endothelial protein that binds to lymphocytes. Cell 1989; 59:1203–11.
98. Bray MA. The pharmacology and pathophysiology of leukotriene B_4. Br Med Bull 1983; 39:249–54.
99. Simmons PM, Salmon JA, Moncada S. The release of leukotriene B_4 during experimental inflammation. Biochem Pharmacol 1983; 32:1353–9.
100. Rae SA, Davidson EM, Smith MJH. Leukotriene B_4, an inflammatory mediator in gout. Lancet 1982; 2:1122–4.
101. Djuric SW, Fretland DJ, Penning TD. The leukotriene B_4 receptor antagonists—a most discriminating class of antiinflammatory agent? Drug Future 1992; 17:819–30.
102. Weinblatt ME, Kremer JM, Coblyn JS, Helfgott S, Maier AL, Petrillo G, Henson B, Rubin P, Sperling R. Zileuton, a 5-lipoxygenase inhibitor in rheumatoid arthritis. J Rheumatol 1992; 19:1537–41.
103. McMillan RM, Spruce KE, Crawley GC, Walker ERH, Foster SJ. Pre-clinical pharmacology of ICI D2138, a potent orally-active nonredox inhibitor of 5-lipoxygenase. Br J Pharmacol 1992; 107:1042–7.
104. Iida K, Nussenzweig V. Complement receptor is an inhibitor of the complement cascade. J Exp Med 1981; 153:1138–50.
105. Weisman HF, Bartow T, Leppo MK, Marsh HC, Carson GR, Concino MF, Boyle MP, Roux KH, Weisfeldt ML, Fearon DT. Soluble human complement receptor type 1: in vivo inhibitor of complement suppressing post-ischemic myocardial inflammation and necrosis. Science 1990; 249:146–51.
106. Yeh CG, Marsh HC, Carson GR, Berman L, Concino MF, Scesney SM, Kuestner RE, Skibbens R, Donahue KA, Ip SH. Recombinant soluble human receptor type 1 inhibits inflammation in the reversed passive Arthus reaction in rats. J Immunol 1991; 146:250–6.
107. Rabinovici R, Yeh CG, Hillegass LM, Griswold DE, DiMartino MJ, Vernick J, Fong K-LL, Feuerstein G. Role of complement in endotoxin/platelet-activating factor-induced lung injury. J Immunol 1992; 149:1744–50.
108. Jose PJ, Moss IK, Maini RN, Williams TJ. Measurement of the chemotactic complement fragment C5a in rheumatoid synovial fluids by radioimmunoassay: role of C5a in the acute inflammatory phase. Ann Rheum Dis 1990; 49:747–52.
109. Watson WC, Townes AS. Genetic susceptibility to murine collagen II autoimmune arthritis. Proposed relationship to the IgG autoantibody subclass response, complement C5, major histocompatibility complex (MHC) and non-MHC loci. J Exp Med 1985; 162:1878–91.
110. Gerard NP, Gerard C. The chemotactic receptor for human C5a anaphylotoxin. Nature 1991; 349:614–7.
111. Lanza TJ, Durette PL, Rollins T, Siciliano S, Cianciarulo DN, Kobayashi SV, Caldwell CG, Springer MS, Hagmann WK. Substituted 4,6-diaminoquinolines as inhibitors of C5a receptor binding. J Med Chem 1992; 35:252–8.
112. Huber AR, Kunkel SL, Todd RF, Weiss SJ. Regulation of transendothelial neutrophil migration by endogenous interleukin-8. Science 1991; 254:99–102.
113. Brennan FM, Zachariae CO, Chantry D, Larsen CG, Turner M, Maini RN, Matsushima K, Feldmann M. Detection of interleukin 8 biological activity in synovial fluids from patients with rheumatoid arthritis and production of interleukin 8 mRNA by isolated synovial cells. Eur J Immunol 1990; 20:2141–4.
114. Endo H, Akahoshi T, Takagishi K, Kashiwazaki S, Matsushima K. Elevation of interleukin 8 (IL-8) levels in joint fluids of patients with rheumatoid arthritis and the induction by IL-8

of leukocyte infiltration and synovitis in rabbit joints. Lymphokine Cytokine Res 1991; 10:245–52.
115. Rampart M, Herman AG, Grillet B, Opdenakker G, Van Damme J. Development and application of a radioimmunoassay for interleukin 8: detection of interleukin 8 in synovial fluids from patients with inflammatory joint disease. Lab Invest 1992; 66:512–8.
116. Forrest MJ, Eiermann GJ, Meurer R, Walakovits LA, MacIntyre DE. The role of CD 18 in IL-8 induced dermal and synovial inflammation. Br J Pharmacol 1992; 106:287–94.
117. Lee J, Horuk R, Rice GC, Bennett GL, Camerato T, Wood WI. Characterization of two high affinity human interleukin-8 receptors. Biol Chem 1992; 267:16283–7.
118. Larsen CG, Paludan K, Kristensen M, Deleuran B, Thomsen MK, Pedersen FS, Matsushima K, Thestrup-Pedersen K. ETH 615, a novel inhibitor of interleukin-8 (IL-8) production. J Invest Dermatol 1990; 95:478.
119. Arfors K-E, Lundberg C, Lindbom L, Lundberg K, Beatty PG, Harlan JM. A monoclonal antibody to the membrane glycoprotein complex CD18 inhibits polymorphonuclear leukocyte accumulation and plasma protein leakage in vivo. Blood 1987; 69:338–40.
120. Nourshargh S, Rampart M, Hellewell PG, Jose PJ, Harlan JM, Edwards AJ, Williams TJ. Accumulation of ^{111}In-neutrophils in rabbit skin in allergic and non-allergic inflammatory reactions in vivo. Inhibition by neutrophil pretreatment in vitro with a monoclonal antibody recognizing the CD18 antigen. J Immunol 1989; 142:3193–8.
121. Vedder NB, Winn RK, Rice CL, Chi E, Arfors K, Harlan JM. A monoclonal antibody to the adherence promoting leukocyte glycoprotein CD 18 reduces organ injury and improves survival from hemorrhagic shock and resuscitation in rabbits. J Clin Invest 1988; 81:939–44.
122. Mileski WJ, Winn RK, Vedder NB, Pohlman TH, Harlan JM, Rice CL. Inhibition of CD 18-dependent neutrophil adherence reduces organ injury after hemorrhagic shock in primates. Surgery 1990; 108:206–12.
123. Jasin HE, Lightfoot E, Davis LS, Rothlein R, Faanes RB, Lipsky PE. Amelioration of antigen-induced arthritis in rabbits treated with monoclonal antibodies to leukocyte adhesion molecules. Arthritis Rheum 1992; 35:541–9.
124. Mileski WJ, Winn RK, Harlan JM, Rice CL. Transient inhibition of neutrophil adherence with the anti-CD 18 monoclonal antibody 60.3 does not increase mortality rates in abdominal sepsis. Surgery 1991, 109:497–501.
125. Argenbright LW, Letts LG, Rothlein R. Monoclonal antibodies to the leukocyte membrane CD 18 glycoprotein complex and to intercellular adhesion molecule-1 inhibit leukocyte–endothelial adhesion in rabbits. J Leukocyte Biol 1991; 49:253–7.
126. Wegner CD, Gundel RH, Reilly P, Haynes N, Letts LG, Rothlein R. Intercellular adhesion molecule-1 (ICAM-1) in the pathogenesis of asthma. Science 1990; 247:456–9.
127. Kavanaugh AF, Nichols LA, Lipsky PE. Treatment of refractory rheumatoid arthritis with an anti-CD54 (intracellular adhesion molecule-1, ICAM-1) monoclonal antibody. Arthritis Rheum 1992; 35:S43.
128. Watson SR, Fennie C, Lasky LA. Neutrophil influx into an inflammatory site inhibited by a soluble homing receptor-IgG chimera. Nature 1991; 349:164–7.
129. Berg EL, Robinson MK, Mansson O, Butcher EC, Magnani JL. A carbohydrate domain common to both sialyl Lewis^a and sialyl Lewis^x is recognized by the endothelial cell leukocyte adhesion molecule ELAM-1. J Biol Chem 1991; 266:14869–72.
130. Ingber D, Fujita T, Kishimoto S, Sudo K, Kanamaru T, Brem H, Folkman J. Synthetic analogues of fumagillin that inhibit angiogenesis and suppress tumour growth. Nature 1990; 348:555–7.
131. Peacock DJ, Banquerigo ML, Brahn E. Angiogenesis inhibition suppresses collagen arthritis. J Exp Med 1992; 175:1135–8.
132. Strachan RK, Smith P, Gardner DL. Hyaluronate in rheumatology and orthopaedics: is there a role? Ann Rheum Dis 1990; 49:949–52.
133. Grecomoro G, Martorana U, Di Marco C. Intra-articular treatment with sodium hyaluronate in gonarthritis controlled clinical trial versus placebo. Pharmatherapeutics 1987; 5:137–41.

134. Punzi L, Schiavon F, Ramonda R, Malatesta V, Gambari, Todesco S. Intra-articular hyaluronic acid in the treatment of inflammatory and non-inflammatory knee effusions. Curr Ther Res 1988; 43:643–7.
135. Balazs EA, Bland PA, Denlinger JL, Goldman AI, Larsen NE, Leshchiner EA, Leshchiner A, Morales B. Matrix engineering. Blood Coagulation Fibrinolysis 1991; 2:173–8.
136. Larsen NE, Lombard KM, Parent E, Balazs EA. Effect of hylan on cartilage and chondrocyte cultures. J Orthop Res 1992; 10:23–32.
137. Howell DS, Carreno MR, Pelletier J-P, Muniz OE. Articular cartilage breakdown in a lapine model of osteoarthritis: action of glycosaminoglycan polysulfate ester (GAGPS) on proteoglycan degrading enzyme activity, hexuronate, and cell counts. Clin Orthop 1986; 213:69–76.
138. Burkhard D, Ghosh P. Laboratory evaluation of glycosaminoglycan polysulphate ester for chondroprotective activity: a review. Curr Ther Res 1986; 40:1034–53.
139. Altman RD, Howell DS, Muniz OE, Dean DD. The effect of glycosaminoglycan polysulfuric acid ester on articular cartilage in experimental arthritis: effects on collagenolytic enzyme activity and cartilage swelling properties. J Rheumatol 1987; 14:127–9.
140. Carreno MR, Muniz OE, Howell DS. The effect of glycosaminoglycan polysulfuric acid ester on articular cartilage in experimental osteoarthritis: effects on morphological parameters of disease severity. J Rheumatol 1986; 12:490–7.
141. Altman RD, Dean DD, Muniz OE, Howell DS. Prophylactic treatment of canine osteoarthritis with glycosaminoglycan polysulfuric acid ester (GAGPS). Arthritis Rheum 1989; 32:759–62.
142. Dean DD, Muniz OE, Rodriguez I, Carreno MR, Morales S, Agundez A, Madan ME, Altman RD, Annefeld M, Howell DS. Amelioration of lapine osteoarthritis by treatment with glycosaminoglycan–peptide association complex (Rumalon). Arthritis Rheum 1991; 34:304–13.
143. Moskowitz RW, Reese JH, Young RG, Fein-Krantz D, Malemud DM, Caplan AI. The effects of Rumalon, a glycosaminoglycan peptide complex, in a partial meniscectomy model of osteoarthritis in rabbits. J Rheumatol 1991; 18:205–9.
144. Raatikainen T, Väänänen K, Tamelander G. Effect of glycosaminoglycan polysulphate on chondromalacia patellae: a placebo controlled 1-year study. Acta Orthop Scand 1990; 61:443–8.
145. Kannus P, Natri A, Niittymäki S, Järvinen M. Effect of intraarticular glycosaminoglycan polysulfate treatment on patellofemoral pain syndrome. Arthritis Rheum 1992; 35:1053–61.
146. Baici A, Hörler D, Moser B, Hofer HO, Fehr K, Wagenhäuser FJ. Analysis of glycosaminoglycans in human serum after oral administration of chondroitin sulfate. Rheumatol Int 1992; 12:81–8.
147. Bradley JD, Brandt KD, Katz BP, Kalasinski LA, Ryan SI. Comparison of an antiinflammatory dose of ibuprofen, and analgesic dose of ibuprofen, and acetaminophen in the treatment of patients with osteoarthritis of the knee. N Engl J Med 1991; 325:87–91.
148. Sanders PA, Grennan DM. Non-steroidal anti-inflammatory drugs versus simple analgesics in the treatment of arthritis. Baillieres Clin Rheumatol 1990; 4:371–85.
149. Snider RM, Constantine JW, Lowe JA, Longo KP, Lebel WS, Woody HA, Drozda SE, Desai MC, Vinick FJ, Spencer RW, Hess H-J. A potent nonpeptide antagonist of the substance P (NK1) receptor. Science 1991; 251:435–7.
150. Lowe JAI. Substance P antagonists. Drugs Future 1992; 17:1115–21.
151. Bhoola KD, Elson CJ, Dieppe PA. Kinins—key mediators in inflammatory arthritis? Br J Rheumatol 1992; 31:509–18.
152. Pelletier J-P, Roughley PJ, DiBattista JA, McCollum R, Martel-Pelletier J. Are cytokines involved in osteoarthritic pathophysiology? J Rheumatol 1991; 20:12–25.
153. Pelletier J-P, Faure M-P, DiBattista JA, Wilhelm S, Visco D, Martel-Pelletier J. Coordinate synthesis of stromelysin, interleukin-1, and oncogene proteins in experimental osteoarthritis. An immunohistochemical study. Am J Pathol 1993; 142:95–105.
154. Martell-Pelletier J, McCollum R, DiBattista J, Faure M-P, Chin JA, Fournier S, Sarfati M,

Pelletier J-P. The interleukin-1 receptor in normal and osteoarthritic human articular chondrocytes. Identification as the type I receptor and analysis of binding kinetics and biological function. Arthritis Rheum 1992; 35:530–40.

155. Dean DD, Martel-Pelletier J, Pelletier J-P, Howell DS, Woessner JF Jr. Evidence for metalloproteinase and metalloproteinase inhibitor imbalance in human osteoarthritic cartilage. J Clin Invest 1989; 84:678–85.
156. Andrews HJ, Plumpton TA, Harper GP, Cawston TE. A synthetic peptide metalloproteinase inhibitor, but not TIMP, prevents the breakdown of proteoglycan within articular cartilage in vitro. Agents Actions 1992; 37:147–53.
157. DiMartino MJ, Wolff CE. Anti-inflammatory and chondroprotective activities of a potent metalloproteinase inhibitor. J Cell Biochem Suppl 1991; 15E:179.
158. Nixon JS, Bottomley KMK, Broadhurst MJ, Brown PA, Johnson WH, Lawton G, Marley J, Sedgwick AD, Wilkinson SE. Potent collagenase inhibitors prevent interleukin-1-induced cartilage degradation in vitro. Int J Tissue React 1991; 13:237–43.
159. Greenwald RA, Golub LM, Lavietes B, Ramamurthy NS, Gruber B, Laskin RS, McNamara TF. Tetracyclines inhibit human synovial collagenase in vivo and in vitro. J Rheumatol 1987; 14:28–32.
160. Yu LPJ, Smith GN, Hasty KA, Brandt KD. Doxycycline inhibits type XI collagenolytic activity of extracts from human osteoarthritic cartilage and of gelatinase. J Rheumatol 1991; 18:1450–2.
161. Yu LPJ, Smith GNJ, Brandt KD, Myers SL, O'Connor BL, Brandt DA. Reduction of the severity of canine osteoarthritis by prophylactic treatment with oral doxycycline. Arthritis Rheum 1992; 35:1150–9.
162. Greenwald RA, Moak SA, Ramamurthy NS, Golub LM. Tetracyclines suppress matrix metalloproteinase activity in adjuvant arthritis and in combination with flurbiprofen, ameliorate bone damage. J Rheumatol 1992; 19:927–38.
163. Buttle DJ, Saklatvala J, Tamai M, Barrett AJ. Inhibition of interleukin 1-stimulated cartilage proteoglycan degradation by a lipophilic inactivator of cysteine endopeptidases. Biochem J 1992; 282:175–7.
164. Buttle DJ, Saklatvala J. Lysosomal cysteine endopeptidases mediate interleukin 1-stimulated cartilage proteoglycan degradation. Biochem J 1992; 287:657–61.
165. van Noorden CJF, Smith RE, Rasnick D. Cysteine proteinase activity in arthritic rat knee joints and the effects of a selective systemic inhibitor, Z-Phe-AlaCH_2F. J Rheumatol 1988; 15:1526–35.
166. Ahmed NK, Martin LA, Watts LM, Palmer J, Thornberg L, Prior J, Esser RE. Peptidyl fluoromethyl ketones as inhibitors of cathepsin B. Implication for treatment of rheumatoid arthritis. Biochem Pharmacol 1992; 44:1201–7.
167. van Noorden CJF, Everts V. Selective inhibition of cysteine proteinases by Z-phe-alaCH_2F suppresses digestion of collagen by fibroblasts and osteoclasts. Biochem Biophys Res Commun 1991; 178:179–84.
168. Eeckhout Y, Vaes G. Further studies on the activation of procollagenase. Effect of lysosomal cathepsin B, plasmin and kallikrein and spontaneous activation. Biochem J 1977; 166:21–31.
169. Pelletier J-P, Mineau F, Fauve M-P, Martel-Pelletier J. Imbalance between the mechanisms of activation and inhibition of metalloproteases in the early lesions of experimental osteoarthritis. Arthritis Rheum 1990; 33:1466–76.
170. Cruwys, SC, Davies DE, Pettipher ER. Co-operation between interleukin 1 and the fibrinolytic system in the degradation of collagen by articular chondrocytes. Br J Pharmacol 1990; 100:631–5.
171. Saklatvala J, Sarsfield SJ. How do interleukin 1 and tumor necrosis factor induce degradation of proteoglycan in cartilage? In: Glauert A, ed. The control of tissue damage. Amsterdam: Elsevier, 1988.
172. Telhag H. (1973). Effect of tranexamic acid (Cyklokapron) on the synthesis of chondroitin

sulphate and the content of hexosamine in the same fraction on normal and degenerated joint cartilage in the rabbit. Acta Orthop Scand 1988; 44:249–55.
173. Butler M, Colombo C, Hickman L, O'Byrne E, Steele R, Steinetz B, Quintavalla J, Yokoyama N. A new model of osteoarthritis in rabbits III. Evaluation of anti-osteoarthritis effects of selected drugs administered intraarticularly. Arthritis Rheum 1983; 26:1380–86.
174. Vignon E, Mathieu P, Bejui J, Descotes J, Hartmann D, Patricot LM, Richard M. Study of an inhibitor of plasminogen activator (tranexamic acid) in the treatment of experimental osteoarthritis. J Rheumatol 1991; 18:131–3.
175. Ito A, Itoh Y, Sasaguri Y, Morimatsu M, More Y. Effects of interleukin-6 on the metabolism of connective tissue components in rheumatoid synovial fibroblasts. Arthritis Rheum 1992; 35:1197–201.

Index

A-78773, 89
α_1-acid glycoprotein, 414
α_2-macroglobulin, 395
Abdominal hysterectomy, 257
Absorption, 273
ACE Inhibitors, 225
Acetaminophen, 34, 97, 103, 107, 108, 109, 172, 173, 186, 201, 218, 221, 278, 281, 291, 299, 300, 305, 308, 312
  acetaminophen plus codeine, 255, 312, 313
Acetanilide, 97
Acetic acid derivatives, 102
Acetylsalicyclic acid (aspirin), 400
Acne, 77
Acute cerebral ischemia, 59
Acute ischemic injury, 56
Acute pulmonary edema, 228
Acute renal failure, 230
Acute tendonitis, 84
Acute traumatic injuries, 81
Acute tubular nephrotoxicity, 311
Acute-phase proteins, 318, 323, 325, 395
Acute-phase response, 398
Adenylate cyclase, 299
Adjuvant arthritis, 318, 416
Adult respiratory distress syndrome (ARDS), 43
Adverse, 378
Adverse drug reactions (*see also* Adverse events), 217
Adverse effects, 343
Adverse events, 260, 284, 313, 326, 378, 379, 384
Adverse reactions, 87
Aglycones, 275
AGM 1470, 438
Agranulocytosis, 228
AHR 10240, 275
AHR 10282 (*see also* Bromfenac), 275
AHR 11665, 275
AIDS, 230
Airway hyperresponsiveness, 375
Airway inflammation, 375
Alclofenac, 223, 226
Alkaline phosphatase, 175
Allergic interstitial nephritis, 199
Allergic rhinitis, 382
Alloantibody formation, 357
Allografts, 355
Allophile, 357
Aminoalkylindole, 297
Aminoglycosides, 225
Aminotransferase, 175
Aminotransferase level, 178
Amiopyrine (aminophenazone), 350
Amphenac, 173
Analgesic, 269, 297, 311, 350, 417
  analgesic effects, 286

Anaphylaxis, 260, 358
Angiogenesis, 438
Angiotensin-converting enzyme (ACE) inhibitors, 197, 221
Ankle sprain, 82
Ankylosing spondylitis, 354
Anthralin, 72
Anti-CD3 antibodies, 431
Anti-CD5 antibody, 432
Anti-CD7a antibody, 432
Anti-DNA autoantibody, 321
Anti-inflammatory, 250, 269, 288, 333, 350, 377, 396, 417
Anti-tumor necrosis factor antibody, 431
Antiarthritic, 318, 393
Antibody production, 357
Antibody-dependent cellular cytotoxicity (ADCC), 337
Anticollagen antibody, 319
Antihypertensive drugs, 221
Antinociceptive, 269, 297, 302, 400
Antiplatelet agents, 63
Antiproliferative, 362
Antiproliferative effects, 360
Antipyretic, 250, 271, 289, 339, 350, 399, 417
Antipyretic analgesics, 100, 104, 105
Antisense, 429
Aplastic anemia, 228
Arachidonate metabolism, 322
Arachidonate metabolites, 46
Arachidonic acid, 55, 74, 207, 342, 359, 367, 401
Arterial hypoxemia, 51
Arthritis, 283, 416
Articular cartilage, 6
2-Arylpropionates, 133
Aseptic meningitis, 230
Aspirin, 1, 28, 34, 60, 97, 102, 107, 108, 109, 172, 184, 196, 211, 214, 218, 219, 221, 261, 268, 278, 279, 283, 286, 287, 288, 305, 308, 339, 340, 341, 343, 345
  aspirin hypersensitivity, 220
Asthma, 379
Atopic dermatitis, 71
Aurum the Gold, 87
Autoimmune diseases, 350
Autoimmune hemolytic anemia, 229
Autoimmune uveitis, 355
Autologous mixed leukocyte reactions (auto-MLR), 334
Autophosphorylation, 362
Azapropazone, 103, 136, 173, 184
Azathioprine, 321, 356
Azurophil granules, 403

β-agonist, 381
B-cell mitogen, 352
B cells, 359
β2 integrins, 435
BALB/c mice, 354
Bendazac, 727, 786
BenGay, 87
Benorilate, 173, 186
Benoxaprofen, 12, 17, 21, 73, 178, 179, 201, 210
Benzoic acid, 72, 108
Benzoic acid derivatives, 102
Benzydamine, 71, 72, 86
Betamethazone valerate, 80
Bioavailability, 272, 273, 343
Biodisposition, 306
Bleeding, 148
Blood dyscrasias (phenylbutazone sulindac), 212
Blood-brain barrier, 254
BMY 30094, 89
Bone density, 395
Bone erosion, 340
Bradykinin, 207, 291, 304, 322
BRL 20459, 89
Bromfenac, 267
Bronchoalveolar lavage, 381
Bufexamac, 72, 77, 83, 86
Buprenorphine, 260
Bursitis, 83
BW755c, 371, 372, 373

C-reactive protein (CRP), 330, 429
C5a, 436
Caffeine, 109, 201
Calcium ionophore, 359, 372
Campath 1H, 432
Cannabidol, 301
Cannabinoid receptor agonist, 298
Carboxylic acids, 209
Cardiovascular side effects, 221
Carprofen, 130, 132, 173, 181, 308
Cartilage (*see also* Articular cartilage), 5, 428
Cartilage erosion, 391
Cartilage-pannus junction, 343
Catabolin, 391

Cathepsin B, 7, 440
Cathepsins L, 440
CD3, 431
CD4, 432
CD5, 432
CD7, 432
Cellular Immunity, 333
Central nervous system, 230
Cerebral vasospasm, 58, 60
Cerebral vessels, 56
Cerebrovascular diseases, 56
Ceruloplasmin, 324
Chiral, 127
Chiral inversion, 134
Chirality, 289
Cholecystectomy, 257
Cholestatic jaundice (diflunisal), 212
Choline magnesium trisalcylate, 223
Chondrocytes, 13
Chondroprotective, 11
Chronic active hepatitis, 176
Chronic hepatitis, 175, 176
Cimetidine, 163, 277
Cinchophen, 171, 173
Cinnamic aldehyde, 72
cis-retinoic acid, 77
Clidanac, 128
Clobenoside, 86
Clobetasol, 74
Clobuzarit, 317, 323, 324, 325
  clozic, 317
Clofibrate, 327
Clometacin, 173, 176
CNS effects (indomethacin, naproxen), 212, 230
CoA thioester intermediates, 133
Cognitive function, 231
Collagen, 6
Collagen arthritis (*see also* Collagen-induced arthritis), 318
Collagen-induced arthritis, 342
Collagenase, 343, 440
Committee of Safety of Medicines, 180
Concanavalin A (Con A), 333
Corticosteroids, 11, 15, 43, 187, 200, 226
Cox stepwise proportional hazard model, 356
CP-55940, 301
Crohn's disease, 152
Cutaneous toxicity, 207, 213
Cyclooxygenase, 369
Cyclooxygenase inhibitor, 247, 297
Cyclophosphamide, 351, 352, 355, 359, 398
Cyclosporine (Sandimmune), 352, 355, 356, 359, 396, 398
Cyclosporine A (*see also* Cyclosporine), 353
Cytochalasin B, 402
Cytokines, 8, 45, 360, 402, 411, 413, 428
  cytokine inhibitors, 438, 439

d-Penicillamine, 338, 398
DA-E5090, 412
Dangerous drug interactions, 110
Delayed-type hypersensitivity, 338, 351
Dermatitis, 77
Dermatological effects, 226
Dermatology, 207
Dexamethasone, 398, 403, 404
Diaphragm disease, 149
Diarrhea, 151, 212, 262, 401
Diazepam, 393
Diclofenac (*see also* Diclofenac sodium), 1, 3, 72, 101, 102, 107, 172, 173, 174, 196, 223, 250, 251, 267, 397, 398, 401
Diclofenac sodium, 31, 213
Diflunisal, 102, 107, 173, 196, 213, 214
Digoxin, 224
Dimethyl sulfoxide (DMSO), 403
Dinitrophenyl, 359
Dipyridamole, 63, 211
Dipyrone, 103, 107, 108
Disease-modifying antirheumatic drugs (DMARDs), 317
Distribution, 273
Dithanol, 75
Diuretics, 197, 225
Diverticulitis, 151
Double-negative T cells, 352
Drug Exanthem, 214
Drug interactions, 223
Duodenal ulcers, 159
Dyskinesia, 231
Dyspepsia, 262

E-selectin, 435
E5090, 411
E6080, 89
Eczema, 71, 77
Eczematous dermatitis, 210
Elderly patients, 199, 220, 222, 228, 230, 231, 277, 353
Eliminated by the urine, 276
Elimination, 275

Enantiomers, 127
Encephalopathy, 231
Endothelium, 56
Enolic acids, 209
Enoxolone, 80, 86
Epicondylitis, 82
Epidermolysis bullosa simplex, 77
Epilepsy, 231
Erythema, 211
Erythema multiforme, 213, 226
Erythrocyte sedimentation rate, 416
ETH615, 437
Ethanesulfonate, 311
Etodolac, 130, 136, 196, 286, 287, 288
Etodolic acid, 398
Etofenamate, 72, 86, 258
Etofenamic acid O, 173
Excretion, 376
Experimental allergic encephalomyelitis, 354
Extrapyramidal symptoms, 231

FDA, 145, 171, 220
Fecal excretion, 343, 350
Felbinac, 71, 72, 86
Fenamates, 100, 102, 174
Fenbufen, 102, 173, 179, 226
Fenclofenac (Flenac), 178, 220
Fenclofenamic acid, 173
Fenclozic, 173
Fenclozic Acid (Myalex), 178
Fenoprofen (*see also* Fenoprofen calcium; Nafon), 101, 103, 107, 130, 173, 179, 200, 229
Fenoprofen calcium, 37, 196
Fentiazac (Flogene), 72, 173, 178
Feprazone, 173
First-pass effect, 376, 393
Fixed drug eruption, 214
FLAP, 76
Flex-All 87, 454
Floctafenine, 173, 174
Flufenamic acid, 102, 173, 174
Flunoxaprofen, 72, 86, 89, 128, 130
Fluocinolone acetonide, 77
Flurbiprofen, 72, 103, 107, 129, 130, 173, 181, 196, 226
FMLP, 402
FPL 62064, 89
Fumagillin, 438
Fungal infections, 77
Furosemide, 254

G-proteins, 404
Gastric
  irritancy, 339
  toxicity, 271
  ulcers, 159
Gastroduodenal side effects, 145
Gastrointestinal
  adverse reactions, 220
  bleeding, 60, 261
  effects, 401
  irritancy, 250, 308
Gelatinase, 440
Glafenine (Glifan), 173, 175, 258
Glomerulonephritis, 352
Glucocorticoid receptors, 16
Glucuronidation, 343, 376, 393
Glucuronide conjugates, 275
Glusuria, 313
Glutathione, 186, 201
Glycosaminoglycans, 6, 394
Glycosaminoglycan Polysulfate Esters (GAGPS), 438
GM 7050, 89
Gold, 338, 345
Gold compounds, 187
Graft-versus-host diseases, 355
Granule exocytosis, 402
Granulocyte colony-stimulating factor (G-CSF), 361
Gualenic acid, 80, 86

Haptoglobin, 323
Headache (diflunisal, indomethacin), 212
Hematological adverse reactions, 228
Heparin, 59
Hepatic
  cholestasis, 180
  disease, 171
  dysfunction, 253
  effects, 323
  injury, 182
  peroxisomal proliferation, 323
  transaminase elevations, 384
Hepatitis, 182
Hepatomas, 323
Hepatotoxicity, 218
5-HETE, 291, 342
15-HETE, 342
Heterocyclic, 392
Histamine, 359
Histamine antagonists, 163
HIV, 230
Hoffmann, 97

Human pharmacodynamics, 277
Human pharmacokinetics, 274
Humanized antibodies, 432
Humoral and cell-mediated immunity, 321
Humoral immunity, 338
Hyaluronan, 438
5-Hydroxyelcosatetraenoic acid (5-HETE), 359
Hydroxyperoxyacids, 74
Hyperacute graft rejection, 357
Hypergamma-globulinemia, 352
Hyperkalemia, 196, 202, 223
Hypertension, 221

Ibufenac (Motrin), 172, 173, 178
Ibuprofen, 1, 2, 9, 47, 60, 71, 72, 86, 100, 101, 103, 107, 108, 127, 129, 130, 151, 173, 178, 196, 199, 200, 210, 223, 226, 230, 231, 250, 251, 278, 279, 286, 287, 288, 299, 300, 305, 308, 376
Ibuproxam, 86
ICAM-1, 435
Icy Hot, 87
Idiosyncrasy, 175, 180
IgE antibody, 358
IgG1 antibody, 358
Interleukin
  IL-1, 6, 322
  IL-1α, 322
  IL-1β, 46
  IL-1β convertase, 430
  IL-1RA, 429
  IL-2-PE40, 433
  IL-6, 46
  IL-8, 403
  Interleukin-2 (IL-2), 334
  Interleukin-1, 322, 411, 428
  Interleukin-1 receptor antagonist, 429
  Interleukin-1α, 402
  Interleukin-1β, 402
  Interleukin-2, 361, 432
  Interleukin-2 fusion proteins, 433
  Interleukin-3, 361
  Interleukin-4, 361
  Interleukin-5, 361
  Interleukin-6, 406
  Interleukin-8, 437
  soluble Interleukin-1 Receptor, 429
Ileal dysfunction, 148
Ileitis, 146
Immediate-type hypersensitivity, 358
Immunomodulating, 333, 349
Immunosuppression, 407
Immunosuppressive, 351, 400, 431
Indoleacetic acid, 27
Indomethacin (Indocin), 12, 13, 33, 49, 59, 60, 72, 102, 173, 176, 196, 197, 211, 221, 226, 228, 229, 230, 250, 251, 268, 287, 288, 299, 300, 305, 308, 322, 335, 336, 339, 340, 341, 343, 354, 372, 373, 396, 398, 401, 402, 406, 414, 415, 422
Indoprofen, 131, 173, 223
Inflammatory bowel disease, 147
Inflammatory dermatoses, 71
Insulin-like growth factor-1 (IGF-1), 6
Integrin, 437
Interferon gamma (INF-γ), 334
Interstitial nephritis, 195, 222, 292
Intraventricular hemorrhage, 58
Ischemic stroke, 61
Ischemic tubular necrosis, 222
Isoxepac, 173
Isoxicam, 173, 184
IX 207-887, 392, 430

Jaundice, 172, 175

Kebuzone, 173, 184
Ketobemidone, 258
Ketoenolic acids, 103, 104
6-Keto-PGF$_{1\alpha}$, 291
Ketoprofen, 12, 13, 38, 72, 101, 103, 107, 108, 131, 132, 173, 181, 196, 223, 250, 251, 267, 287, 327
Ketorolac, 33, 73, 247, 250, 251, 269
Kidney dysfunction, 110
Killer cell activity, 337

L 651,392, 89, 382
L-651,896, 89
L-selectin, 435
Lee functional index, 407
Leflunomide, 349
Leukocyte
  adhesion, 435, 437
  emigration, 435
  migration, 398, 434
Leukotriene B4, 291, 332, 359, 372
Leukotriene B4 antagonists, 436
Leukotrienes, 47, 74, 200, 207, 367
Levamisole, 333, 335, 336, 337, 338, 339, 340, 342, 343, 398

Levonantradol, 301, 303, 306
Lichenoid eruptions, 220
Lipid mediators, 45
5-Lipoxygenase, pathway inhibitors, 7, 63, 67, 367, 405, 436
15-Lipoxygenase, 342
Lithium, 224
  toxicity, 223
Liver cirrhosis, 252
Lonapalene (RS43179), 75, 89, 210
Lupus, 342
Lymphocytes, 45

Macrophages, 45
Major histocompatibility complex peptides, 433
Masoprocol, 89
Meclofenamate, 12, 50, 60, 75, 76, 174, 214
Meclofenamate sodium, 196
Meclofenamic acid, 102, 173
Medicone Derma, 87
Mefenamic acid, 31, 37, 102, 173, 196, 200, 223, 229
Menstrual migraine, 38
Meperidine, 256, 269
Metabolism, 252, 274, 376
Metalloproteinases, 7, 439
Metamizole, 105
Methotrexate, 187, 224
Methyl nicotinate, 72
Methylprednisolone, 338
Metoprolol, 34
Migraine, 27
Mischell-Dutton test, 407
Misoprostol, 17, 160, 162
Mitogen-induced lymphocyte response, 351
MK-886, 76, 89
Models of skin inflammation, 72
Monoarticular antigen arthritis, 428
Monocytes, 45
Morniflumate, 86
Morphine, 257, 286, 302, 305
MRL/1 mice, 342
MRL/lpr mice, 320, 354
Multiple sclerosis, 354
Muramyl peptide, 342
Muscular pain, 81
Musculoskeletal adverse reactions, 229

N-acetyl-benzoquinoneimine, 201
Nabilone, 306
Naloxone, 269, 287, 292
Naproxen, 14, 29, 35, 60, 72, 101, 103, 107, 108, 128, 151, 173, 178, 196, 221, 223, 226, 230, 231, 287, 288, 299, 300, 305, 340, 354, 378, 398, 399
Naproxen (Naprosen), 179
Natural killer (NK) cells, 337
NDGA, 372, 373
Neonatal intraventricular hemorrhage, 60
Nephritic diseases, 354
Nephritis (diflunisal fenoprofen fenamic acid), 212
Nephrotic syndrome, 195, 198, 199, 222
Neutrophils, 44
Nifenazone, 86
Niflumic acid, 72, 86, 173, 174, 230
Nonopiate analgesic, 293
Nonspecific T-cell approaches, 431
Nordihydroguaiaretic acid, 342, 371
Noxema Medicated Skin Cream, 87
NPC-15199, 89
NPC567, 292
NSAID-induced asthma, 221
NSAID-induced renal toxicity, 195
nu/nu mice, 350

Ocular inflammation, 251
Omeprazole, 165
Opthalmic application, 255
Opthalmic pharmacology, 252
Oral surgery, 277, 278
Oral tolerance, 433
Orthopedic pain, 281
Orthopedic surgery, 278
Osteoarthritis, 5, 6, 81, 82, 146, 229, 283
Osteocalcin, 395
OTC, 98, 195
Oxaceprol, 80, 86
Oxaprozin (Oxapro), 173, 181
Oxicams, 184
Oxygen free radicals, 57
Oxygen radicals, 359
Oxyphenbutazone (Tanderil), 136, 173, 184, 220, 226, 228,
Oxyphenbutazone, 184
OZP, 89

P-8892, 89
P-8977, 89
Pain intensity difference (PID), 279
Pannus formation, 352

Papillary necrosis, 200, 202, 292
Paracetamol (*see also* Acetaminophen), 29, 400
Parenteral analgesic, 247
Patent ductus arteriosus, 60
Pemedolac, 269, 285, 287, 288
(+)-pemedolac, 289
(–)-pemedolac, 290
Penicillamine, 187, 345
Pentazocine, 258
Peptic ulcers, 261
Peripheral analgesic, 285
Peripheral neuropathy, 231
Peroxisomal proliferation, 323
PGE_2, 291
PGI_2, 55
Phagocytosis, 337
Pharmacodynamics, 199
Pharmacokinetic(s), 71, 100, 224, 252, 271, 326, 344, 375, 393
Phenacetin, 109, 201, 222
Phenazone (antipyrine), 97, 100, 103, 107, 108, 173
  derivatives, 103
Phenidone, 371, 373
Phenylbutazone (Butazolidine), 12, 13, 72, 103, 172, 173, 182, 196, 200, 201, 212, 214, 220, 222, 223, 226, 228, 229, 288, 350, 351, 352
Phospholipase A2, 322, 405
Photosensitivity, 88, 214, 227
Phytohemagglutinin (PHA), 333
Piketoprofen, 86
Piroxicam (Feldene), 13, 14, 15, 60, 71, 72, 86, 103, 151, 173, 184, 196, 214, 269, 286, 287, 288, 398
Pirprofen (Rengasil), 13, 33, 173
Pizotifen, 37
Plasma clearance, 326
Plasma transaminases, 218
Plasmin, 440
Plasminogen activator, 7, 440
Platelet-activating factor, 46
Pneumonitis, 228
Postmarketing surveillance, 218
Postoperative wound hematomas, 261
Potassium-sparing, 225
Pranosal, 86
Pravadoline, 297, 300, 301, 305, 306, 308
Prednisolone, 351, 352, 354, 355, 356, 359, 414, 415, 418, 422
Prednisone, 345, 376
Pregnancy and the fetus, 231
Probenecid, 225, 254
Proctocolitis, 220
Propoxyphene, 258
Propranolol, 37
Propyphenazone, 103, 107, 108
Proquazone, 173
Prostacyclin, 55
Prostaglandin E_2 (PGE_2), 291, 298, 322, 342, 359
Prostaglandins, 8, 74, 162, 165, 405
Prostanoid, 399
Protein kinase, 12, 362
Protein kinase C, 404
Protein loss, 148
Protein-binding, 273
Proteinase inhibitors, 439
Proteinuria, 200, 313
Proteoglycanase, 7
Proteoglycans, 6, 354, 393
Psoriasis, 71, 74
Pulmonary adverse reactions, 227
Pulmonary hypertension, 51
Purazinobutazone, 86
Pure red cell anemia, 229
Pyranocarboxylic acid, 290

R68151, 80, 89
R70795, 89
(R)-etodolac, 132
(R)-flurbiprofen, 129
Ranitidine, 160
Reactive oxygen, 44
Rectal administration, 151
Rectal suppository, 254
Regulatory authorities, 98
Renal and biliary excretion, 271
Renal
  clearance, 252, 326
  colic, 257
  dialysis, 253
  effects, 311
  failure, 197
  impairment, 252, 253
  insufficiency, 223
  lithotripsy, 261
  papillary necrosis, 223
  prostaglandins, 197
  toxicity, 195
Reversible glucuronidation, 327
Reversible hyponatremia, 196
Reye's syndrome, 177, 186, 219
Rheumatoid arthritis, 5, 146, 283, 320, 333, 345, 354, 362, 384, 407, 428

Rhuligel, 87
Ritchie Articular Index (RI), 330, 407
Ro 31-3948/000, 325
Romazarit, 317
Rose-Waaler test, 407

(S)-etodolac, 132
(S)-ibuprofen, 129
S-antigen, 355
Safety profile, 284
Salbutamol, 376
Salicylate therapy, 222
Salicylates, 12, 100, 102, 107, 108, 173, 184, 201, 218, 231, 376
Salicylic acid, 72, 87, 102, 107
SC-41930, 436
SC-45662, 89
Scald burns, 72
Seizures (fenamic acids), 212
Selectins, 437
Sepsis, 198
Seromucoid, 324
Serotonin, 27, 207
Serum amyloid, 323
Serum creatinine, 60
Serum transaminase, 219
Sialadenitis, 220
Sjogren's syndrome, 220
SK&F 87002, 14
Slow-reacting substance of anaphylaxis (SRS-A), 374
Small-intestinal damage, 146, 150
Small-intestinal strictures, 149
Sodium retention, 202
Soft-tissue injuries, 81, 258
Soluble TNF receptors (sTNF-R), 430
Sprains, 81, 84
Staphylococcal enterotoxin B (SEB), 336
Stereoselective metabolism, 132
Stereoselective pharmacodynamics, 128
Stereoselective pharmacokinetics, 129
Stereoselective protein binding, 132
Stevens-Johnson syndrome, 180, 213, 226
Stomatitis, 220
Stroke, 55
Stromelysin, 7, 440
Sucralfate, 161, 165
Sudoxicam, 60, 173
Sulfasalazine, 376, 378
Sulindac (Clinoril), 136, 172, 173, 177, 196, 214, 223, 230
  sulfate, 12
Sunburn, 77
Superoxide, 403
Superoxide dismutase, 80, 89
Suppositories, 151
Suppressor T cells, 336
Suprofen (Suprol), 131, 181, 201, 269
Synergistic effects, 356
Systemic anaphylactoid reactions, 223
Systemic lupus erythematosus, 185, 342, 350, 352

T-cell mitogens, 352
T-cell vaccination, 434
T-helper cell-replacing factor, 360
Tendonitis, 83, 84
Tenidap, 14, 89, 430
Tenoxicam, 103
Teratogenicity, 231
Terbutaline, 380
Tetracycline, 210, 440
Δ9-Tetrahydrocannabinol, (THC), 298, 301, 303, 306
Δ9-THC (*see* Δ9-Tetrahydrocannabinol)
Theophylline, 376, 380
Thrombocytopenia, 229
Thromboembolic events, 59
Thromboxane, 55
Thromboxane A_2 (TXA_2), 268
Thromboxane B_2, 291, 372
Tiaprofen, 103
Tiaprofenic acid, 12, 13, 15, 33, 131, 351
Ticlopidine, 63
Tilomisole, 333
Timegadine, 305
TIMP, 441
TIMP-1, 7
Tinnitus, 346
Tissue inhibitor of metalloproteinases (*see also* TIMP), 441
Tissue necrosis factor-alpha, 361
TMK 688, 89
TN873R, 89
TNFα (*see also* tumor necrosis factor-alpha), 6, 45
Tolfenamic acid, 33, 173, 174
Tolmetin (Tolectin), 12, 102, 173, 177, 196, 223, 230
Tooth extraction, 279
Topic, 255
Topical, 208
  application, 71
  gel, 258
  nonsteroidal anti-inflammatory drugs, 71

Toxic epidermal necrolysis, 213
  Lyall's syndrome, 226
Toxic hepatitis (sulindac, phenylbutazone), 212
Tranexamic acid, 441
Transaminase elevations, 384
Transferrin, 361
Transforming growth factor-b (TFG-b), 6
Transplantation rejection, 355
Triamcinolone acetanide, 80
Triamterene, 225
Trimethoprim-sulfamethoxazole, 230
Tubular nephrosis, 292
Tubulo-interstitial nephritis, 354–55
Tumor necrosis factor, 430
Type-II collagen-induced arthritis, 416
Tyrosine kinase, 362

Ufenamate, 80, 86
Ulcerative colitis, 151, 152, 382
Ulcerogenic, 288
Ulcerogenic potency, 251
Ulcerogenicity, 401
Unwanted drug effects, 106
UR 10324, 89
Uric acid crystal, 202
Uricosuria (diflunisal, meclofenamate sodium), 212
Urticaria, 214
UV-induced erythema, 72
UVB, 77

Vasodilators, 225
VCAM-1, 435
Vitamin B_{12}-binding protein, 403
VLA-4, 435

Water retention, 195
Weber effect, 217
WIN 31041, 298, 306, 308
WIN 48098, 297
WIN 55212-2, 298, 301, 303, 306
WIN 56098, 298, 299, 302
WY-50295, 89

Xenoantibodies, 359
Xenotransplantations, 358

Zenophile, 357
Zileuton (A-64077), 367, 372, 373, 436
Zomepirac, 223, 269, 286, 299, 300, 302, 305, 309
Zomepirac (Na), 308
Zomepirac (Zomax), 177

About the Editors

ALAN J. LEWIS is Vice President of Research at Wyeth-Ayerst Research, Princeton, New Jersey. The author or coauthor of over 100 scientific journal articles and book chapters and the editor of five books related to inflammation research, Dr. Lewis is President of the International Association of Inflammation Societies (IAIS) and a past President of the Inflammation Research Association. He is also a member of the British Pharmacological Society, the Mid-Atlantic Pharmacology Society, the American Society for Clinical Pharmacology and Therapeutics, and the American Rheumatism Association, among others. Dr. Lewis' major research interests are in the areas of allergy, respiratory pharmacology, inflammation, and immunomodulation. He received the B.Sc. degree (1967) in physiology and biochemistry from the University of Southampton, Hampshire, England, and the Ph.D. degree (1970) in pharmacology from the University of Wales Institute of Science and Technology (now University of Wales College of Cardiff), Cardiff.

DANIEL E. FURST is Clinical Director of the Virginia Mason Research Center, Seattle, Washington, and Director of the Clinical Research Programs at the same institution. He is also Clinical Professor of Medicine and Rheumatology at the University of Washington, Seattle. The author, coauthor, editor, or coeditor of more than 160 publications, including (with Jonathan S. Dixon) *Second-Line Agents in the Treatment of Rheumatic Diseases* and (with Michael E. Weinblatt) *Immunomodulators in the Rheumatic Diseases* (both titles Marcel Dekker, Inc.), Dr. Furst is a Fellow of the American College of Physicians and a member of the American College of Rheumatology, the American Society for Clinical Pharmacology and Therapeutics, the New York Academy of Sciences, and the American Federation for Clinical Research. He received the B.A. degree (1964) and the M.D. degree (1968) from The Johns Hopkins University, Baltimore, Maryland, and completed Fellowships in rheumatology (1975) at the University of California, Los Angeles, and in clinical pharmacology (1977) at the University of California, San Francisco.